# Chemosensitivity

# METHODS IN MOLECULAR MEDICINE™

## *John M. Walker,* SERIES EDITOR

118. **Antifungal Agents:** *Methods and Protocols,* edited by *Erika J. Ernst and P. David Rogers,* 2005

117. **Fibrosis Research:** *Methods and Protocols,* edited by *John Varga, David A. Brenner, and Sem H. Phan,* 2005

116. **Inteferon Methods and Protocols,** edited by *Daniel J. J. Carr,* 2005

115. **Lymphoma:** *Methods and Protocols,* edited by *Timothy Illidge and Peter W. M. Johnson,* 2005

114. **Microarrays in Clinical Diagnostics,** edited by *Thomas Joos and Paolo Fortina,* 2005

113. **Multiple Myeloma:** *Methods and Protocols,* edited by *Ross D. Brown and P. Joy Ho,* 2005

112. **Molecular Cardiology:** *Methods and Protocols,* edited by *Zhongjie Sun,* 2005

111. **Chemosensitivity:** *Volume 2, In Vivo Models, Imaging, and Molecular Regulators,* edited by *Rosalyn D. Blumethal,* 2005

110. **Chemosensitivity:** *Volume 1, In Vitro Assays,* edited by *Rosalyn D. Blumethal,* 2005

109. **Adoptive Immunotherapy:** *Methods and Protocols,* edited by *Burkhard Ludewig and Matthias W. Hoffman,* 2005

108. **Hypertension:** *Methods and Protocols,* edited by *Jérôme P. Fennell and Andrew H. Baker,* 2005

107. **Human Cell Culture Protocols,** *Second Edition,* edited by *Joanna Picot,* 2005

106. **Antisense Therapeutics,** *Second Edition,* edited by *M. Ian Phillips,* 2005

105. **Developmental Hematopoiesis:** *Methods and Protocols,* edited by *Margaret H. Baron,* 2005

104. **Stroke Genomics:** *Methods and Reviews,* edited by *Simon J. Read and David Virley,* 2004

103. **Pancreatic Cancer:** *Methods and Protocols,* edited by *Gloria H. Su,* 2004

102. **Autoimmunity:** *Methods and Protocols,* edited by *Andras Perl,* 2004

101. **Cartilage and Osteoarthritis:** *Volume 2, Structure and In Vivo Analysis,* edited by *Frédéric De Ceuninck, Massimo Sabatini, and Philippe Pastoureau,* 2004

100. **Cartilage and Osteoarthritis:** *Volume 1, Cellular and Molecular Tools,* edited by *Massimo Sabatini, Philippe Pastoureau, and Frédéric De Ceuninck,* 2004

99. **Pain Research:** *Methods and Protocols,* edited by *David Z. Luo,* 2004

98. **Tumor Necrosis Factor:** *Methods and Protocols,* edited by *Angelo Corti and Pietro Ghezzi,* 2004

97. **Molecular Diagnosis of Cancer:** *Methods and Protocols, Second Edition,* edited by *Joseph E. Roulston and John M. S. Bartlett,* 2004

96. **Hepatitis B and D Protocols:** *Volume 2, Immunology, Model Systems, and Clinical Studies,* edited by *Robert K. Hamatake and Johnson Y. N. Lau,* 2004

95. **Hepatitis B and D Protocols:** *Volume 1, Detection, Genotypes, and Characterization,* edited by *Robert K. Hamatake and Johnson Y. N. Lau,* 2004

94. **Molecular Diagnosis of Infectious Diseases,** *Second Edition,* edited by *Jochen Decker and Udo Reischl,* 2004

93. **Anticoagulants, Antiplatelets, and Thrombolytics,** edited by *Shaker A. Mousa,* 2004

92. **Molecular Diagnosis of Genetic Diseases,** *Second Edition,* edited by *Rob Elles and Roger Mountford,* 2004

91. **Pediatric Hematology:** *Methods and Protocols,* edited by *Nicholas J. Goulden and Colin G. Steward,* 2003

90. **Suicide Gene Therapy:** *Methods and Reviews,* edited by *Caroline J. Springer,* 2004

89. **The Blood–Brain Barrier:** *Biology and Research Protocols,* edited by *Sukriti Nag,* 2003

88. **Cancer Cell Culture:** *Methods and Protocols,* edited by *Simon P. Langdon,* 2003

87. **Vaccine Protocols,** *Second Edition,* edited by *Andrew Robinson, Michael J. Hudson, and Martin P. Cranage,* 2003

86. **Renal Disease:** *Techniques and Protocols,* edited by *Michael S. Goligorsky,* 2003

85. **Novel Anticancer Drug Protocols,** edited by *John K. Buolamwini and Alex A. Adjei,* 2003

84. **Opioid Research:** *Methods and Protocols,* edited by *Zhizhong Z. Pan,* 2003

83. **Diabetes Mellitus:** *Methods and Protocols,* edited by *Sabire Özcan,* 2003

82. **Hemoglobin Disorders:** *Molecular Methods and Protocols,* edited by *Ronald L. Nagel,* 2003

**METHODS IN MOLECULAR MEDICINE™**

# Chemosensitivity

*Volume 2*

*In Vivo Models, Imaging,
and Molecular Regulators*

Edited by

## Rosalyn D. Blumenthal

*Garden State Cancer Center, Belleville, NJ*

HUMANA PRESS ✱ TOTOWA, NEW JERSEY

© 2005 Humana Press Inc.
999 Riverview Drive, Suite 208
Totowa, New Jersey 07512

www.humanapress.com

All rights reserved. No part of this book may be reproduced, stored in a retrieval system, or transmitted in any form or by any means, electronic, mechanical, photocopying, microfilming, recording, or otherwise without written permission from the Publisher. Methods in Molecular Medicine™ is a trademark of The Humana Press Inc.

The content and opinions expressed in this book are the sole work of the authors and editors, who have warranted due diligence in the creation and issuance of their work. The publisher, editors, and authors are not responsible for errors or omissions or for any consequences arising from the information or opinions presented in this book and make no warranty, express or implied, with respect to its contents.

This publication is printed on acid-free paper. ∞
ANSI Z39.48-1984 (American Standards Institute)

Permanence of Paper for Printed Library Materials.

Cover illustrations: *Foreground illustration*: Figure 4, from Chapter 24, "$^{99m}$Tc-Annexin A5 Uptake and Imaging to Monitor Chemosensitivity," by Tarik Z. Belhocine and Francis G. Blankenberg. *Background illustration*: Figure 4, from Chapter 22 (Volume 2), "Assessing Growth and Response to Therapy in Murine Tumor Models," by C. P. Reynolds et al.

Cover design by Patricia F. Cleary.

For additional copies, pricing for bulk purchases, and/or information about other Humana titles, contact Humana at the above address or at any of the following numbers: Tel.: 973-256-1699; Fax: 973-256-8341; E-mail: humana@humanapr.com; or visit our Website: www.humanapress.com

**Photocopy Authorization Policy:**
Authorization to photocopy items for internal or personal use, or the internal or personal use of specific clients, is granted by Humana Press Inc., provided that the base fee of US $30.00 per copy is paid directly to the Copyright Clearance Center at 222 Rosewood Drive, Danvers, MA 01923. For those organizations that have been granted a photocopy license from the CCC, a separate system of payment has been arranged and is acceptable to Humana Press Inc. The fee code for users of the Transactional Reporting Service is: [1-58829-586-9/05 $30.00].

Printed in the United States of America. 10 9 8 7 6 5 4 3 2 1

E-ISBN 1-59259-889-7
Library of Congress Cataloging in Publication Data
Chemosensitivity / edited by Rosalyn D. Blumenthal.
              v. ; cm. — (Methods in molecular medicine ; 110-111)
    Includes bibliographical references and index.
    Contents: v. 1. In vitro assays — v. 2 In vivo models, imaging, and molecular regulators.
    ISBN 1-58829-586-9 (hardcover : alk. paper)
    1. Cancer—Chemotherapy—Laboratory manuals. 2. Antineoplastic agents—Effectiveness—Laboratory manuals. 3. Cancer cells—Laboratory manuals. 4. Cancer--Molecular aspects—Laboratory manuals.
    [DNLM: 1. Antineoplastic Agents—pharmacology. 2. Drug Screening Assays, Antitumor—methods. 3. Drug Resistance, Neoplasm. 4. Models, Animal. 5. Neoplasms—drug therapy. QV 269 C5177 2005] I. Blumenthal, Rosalyn D. II. Series.

RC271.C5C396 2005

616.99'4061—dc22
                                              2004012494

# Preface

Chemotherapy is used to treat many types of cancer. A large number of drug classes are in use, including the vinca alkaloids, taxanes, antibiotics, anthracyclines, DNA alkylators, other DNA damaging agents, hormones, and interferons. More potent analogs of existing drugs and novel agents directed at new targets are continuously being developed. Over the last few years, agents that affect COX-2, PPARγ, and various signal transduction pathways have received much attention. To identify which agents are effective for which types of tumors, it is important to develop accurate in vitro and preclinical in vivo screening systems that can identify the cytotoxic and/or cytostatic potential of an agent on established tumor cell lines or cells isolated from individual fresh cancer biopsy specimens removed from cancer patients. Chemosensitivity testing allows the selection of drugs that appear sensitive in the laboratory, thus offering patients a better chance of response.

One of the main problems associated with chemotherapy has been that patient tumors with the same histology do not necessarily respond identically to the same agent or dose schedule of multiple agents. Identifying the presence of resistance mechanisms and other determinants for drug sensitivity in order to classify tumors into response categories has been an ongoing research effort. Advances in our understanding of the genetic and protein fingerprints of primary tumors and their metastases has opened a door to the possibility of customizing therapy to individuals. There is accumulating evidence suggesting that laboratory screening of samples from a patient's tumor may help select the appropriate treatment(s) to administer, thereby avoiding ineffective drugs, and sparing patients the side effects normally associated with these agents.

The aim of these two volumes on *Chemosensitivity* of the *Methods in Molecular Medicine* series, is to comprehensively present protocols that can be used to (a) assess chemosensitivity in vitro and in vivo, and (b) assess parameters that modulate chemosensitivity in individual tumors. Volume I presents an overview in Chapter 1 and then covers *In Vitro Measures of Chemosensitivity*, includes clonogenic, colorimetric, fluorometric, and histochemical approaches. Volume II, Part I, *Measurements of DNA Damage, Cell Death, and Regulators of Cytotoxicity*, includes methods to detect chromosome loss and breakage, changes in cell cycle, expression of members of the bcl-2 family of proteins, expression of caspases and PARP cleavage, metabolic factors influencing sensitivity, measurements of drug retention, expression of drug resistance proteins, and measurements of ceramide and sphingolipids associated with drug sensitivity. Volume

II, Part II, *Genomics, Proteomics, and Chemosensitivity,* addresses DNA microarrays for gene profiling, genetic manipulation to identify genes regulating chemosensitivity, proteomics using 2D-PAGE and mass spectrometry, and bioinformatics approaches. The last part, *In Vivo Animal Modeling of Chemosensitivity,* covers protocols to establish clinically meaningful metastatic and orthotropic models of solid and liquid tumors, statistical approaches to analyze preclinical data, and animal imaging approaches that can be used to assess chemosensitivity such as GFP-tagged genes, SPECT using $^{99m}$Tc-annexin, PET imaging with $^{18}$FDG, and magnetic resonance imaging.

Each chapter is written by someone experienced with the methodology and contains a detailed introductory section with references of how the technique has been used in the past, a list of materials and equipment needed to perform the assay, and a step-by-step set of instructions for each method. At the end of each chapter a "Notes" section is included with useful information, helpful hints, and problems and pitfalls to be aware of, in order to make the assay run smoothly and allow for easy interpretation of data.

*Rosalyn D. Blumenthal*

# Contents

Preface .................................................................................................. v
Color Plate ............................................................................................ xi
Contributors ........................................................................................ xiii
Contents of Volume 1 ......................................................................... xvii

**PART I. MEASUREMENTS OF DNA DAMAGE, CELL DEATH,
AND REGULATORS OF CYTOTOXICITY**

1 In Vitro Micronucleus Technique to Predict Chemosensitivity
  *Michael Fenech* ............................................................................ 3
2 Cell Cycle and Drug Sensitivity
  *Aslamuzzaman Kazi and Q. Ping Dou* ....................................... 33
3 TUNEL Assay as a Measure of Chemotherapy-Induced Apoptosis
  *Robert Wieder* ............................................................................ 43
4 Apoptosis Assessment by the DNA Diffusion Assay
  *Narendra P. Singh* ...................................................................... 55
5 PARP Cleavage and Caspase Activity to Assess Chemosensitivity
  *Alok C. Bharti, Yasunari Takada, and Bharat B. Aggarwal* ....... 69
6 Diphenylamine Assay of DNA Fragmentation
  for Chemosensitivity Testing
  *Cicek Gercel-Taylor* ................................................................... 79
7 Immunodetecting Members of the Bcl-2 Family of Proteins
  *Richard B. Lock and Kathleen M. Murphy* ................................ 83
8 Correlation of Telomerase Activity
  and Telomere Length to Chemosensitivity
  *Yasuhiko Kiyozuka* ..................................................................... 97
9 Application of Silicon Sensor Technologies to Tumor Tissue In Vitro:
  *Detection of Metabolic Correlates of Chemosensitivity*
  *Pedro Mestres-Ventura, Andrea Morguet, Anette Schofer,
  Michael Laue, and Werner Schmidt* ........................................ 109
10 Overview of Tumor Cell Chemoresistance Mechanisms
   *Laura Gatti and Franco Zunino* ............................................... 127
11 Flow Cytometric Monitoring of Fluorescent Drug
   Retention and Efflux
   *Awtar Krishan and Ronald M. Hamelik* ................................... 149

12  Flow Cytometric Measurement of Functional
    and Phenotypic P-Glycoprotein
    *Monica Pallis and Emma Das-Gupta* .................................................. 167

13  Measurement of Ceramide and Sphingolipid Metabolism in Tumors:
    *Potential Modulation of Chemosensitivity*
    *David E. Modrak* ..................................................................... 183

## PART II. GENOMICS, PROTEOMICS, AND CHEMOSENSITIVITY

14  Gene Expression Profiling to Characterize
    Anticancer Drug Sensitivity
    *James K. Breaux and Gerrit Los* ....................................... 197

15  Identifying Genes Related to Chemosensitivity
    Using Support Vector Machine
    *Lei Bao* ................................................................................ 233

16  Genetic Manipulation of Yeast to Identify Genes
    Involved in Regulation of Chemosensitivity
    *Giovanni L. Beretta and Paola Perego* ............................................... 241

17  Real-Time RT-PCR (Taqman®) of Tumor mRNA
    to Predict Sensitivity of Specimens to 5-Fluorouracil
    *Tetsuro Kubota* ..................................................................... 257

18  Use of Proteomics to Study Chemosensitivity
    *Julia Poland, Silke Wandschneider, Andrea Urbani,
    Sergio Bernardini, Giorgio Federici, and Pranav Sinha* ............... 267

## PART III. IN VIVO ANIMAL MODELING OF CHEMOSENSITIVITY

19  Clinically Relevant Metastatic Breast Cancer
    Models to Study Chemosensitivity
    *Lee Su Kim and Janet E. Price* ............................................. 285

20  Orthotopic Metastatic (MetaMouse®) Models
    for Discovery and Development of Novel Chemotherapy
    *Robert M. Hoffman* ........................................................ 297

21  Preclinical Testing of Antileukemic Drugs
    Using an In Vivo Model of Systemic Disease
    *Richard B. Lock, Natalia L. Liem, and Rachael A. Papa* ................... 323

22  Assessing Growth and Response
    to Therapy in Murine Tumor Models
    *C. Patrick Reynolds, Bee-Chun Sun, Yves A. DeClerck,
    and Rex A. Moats* ..................................................................... 335

## Contents

23  Evaluation of Chemosensitivity of Micrometastatses
    with Green Fluorescent Protein
    Gene-Tagged Tumor Models in Mice
    **Hayao Nakanishi, Seiji Ito, Yoshinari Mochizuki,
    and Masae Tatematsu** .................................................................. *351*

24  $^{99m}$Tc-Annexin A5 Uptake and Imaging to Monitor Chemosensitivity
    **Tarik Z. Belhocine and Francis G. Blankenberg** ........................... *363*

25  Magnetic Resonance Imaging
    of Tumor Response to Chemotherapy
    **Richard Mazurchuk and Joseph A. Spernyak** ................................ *381*

26  Metabolic Monitoring of Chemosensitivity with $^{18}$FDG PET
    **Guy Jerusalem and Tarik Z. Belhocine** ......................................... *417*

Index .................................................................................................. *441*

# Color Plate

The following illustrations appear in the color plate that follows page 238.

**Chapter 24:**

Figure 1, p. 364, Molecular basis for Annexin A5 imaging.

Figure 2, p. 365, Molecular structure of human Annexin A5.

Figure 5, p. 373, $^{99m}$Tc-Annexin A5 uptake as seen by SPECT and autoradiography.

Figure 6, p. 374, Evaluation of tumor regression post-doxorubicin treatment.

**Chapter 26:**

Figure 1A, p. 418, Glucose uptake into tumor cells.

Figure 1B, p. 419, $^{18}$FDG uptake into tumor cells.

Figure 3B, p. 427, Semiquantitative assessment of $^{18}$FDG uptake with the primary cervical tumor.

# Contributors

BHARAT AGGARWAL • *Department of Experimental Therapeutics, University of Texas M.D. Anderson Cancer Center, Houston, TX, USA*
LEI BAO • *Department of Molecular Sciences, The University of Tennessee Health Science Center, Memphis, TN, USA*
TARIK Z. BELHOCINE • *Department of Nuclear Medicine, Jules Bordet Cancer Institute, Brussels, Belgium*
GIOVANNI L. BERETTA • *Istituto Nazionale Tumori, Milan, Italy*
SERGIO BERNARDINI • *Laboratorio di Biochimica Clinica, Universita di Roma "Tor Vergata," Roma, Italy*
ALOK C. BHARTI • *Department of Experimental Therapeutics, University of Texas M.D. Anderson Cancer Center, Houston, TX, USA*
FRANCIS G. BLANKENBERG • *Division Pediatric Radiology, Stanford University School of Medicine, Palo Alto, CA, USA*
ROSALYN D. BLUMENTHAL • *Garden State Cancer Center, Belleville, NJ, USA*
JAMES K. BREAUX • *Rebecca and John Moores UCSD Cancer Center, University of California–San Diego, La Jolla, CA, USA*
EMMA DAS-GUPTA • *Academic Haematology, Nottingham City Hospital, Nottingham, UK*
YVES A. DECLERCK • *Division of Hematology-Oncology, Keck School Medicine, University Southern California, Los Angeles, CA, USA*
Q. PING DOU • *Wayne State University School of Medicine, Detroit, MI, USA*
GIORGIO FEDERICI • *Laboratorio di Biochimica Clinica, Universita di Roma "Tor Vergata," Roma, Italy*
MICHAEL FENECH • *CSIRO Health Science and Nutrition, South Australia, Australia*
LAURA GATTI • *Istituto Nazionale Tumori, Milan, Italy*
CICEK GERCEL-TAYLOR • *Department of Obstetrics and Gynecology and Women's Health, University of Louisville, Louisville, KY, USA*
RONALD M. HAMELIK • *Division of Experimental Therapeutics, University of Miami, Miami, FL, USA*
ROBERT M. HOFFMAN • *Department Surgery, University of California–San Diego, and AntiCancer Inc., San Diego, CA, USA*
SEIJI ITO • *Department of Gastroenterological Surgery, Aichi Cancer Center Research Institute, Chikusa-ku, Nagoya, Japan*

GUY JERUSALEM • *Department of Hemtology/Oncology, University Hospital of Liège, Liège, Belgium*
ASLAMUZZAMAN KAZI • *Moffitt Cancer Center & Research Institute, University of South Florida, Tampa, FL, USA*
LEE SU KIM • *Department of Cancer Biology, University of Texas M.D. Anderson Cancer Center, Houston, TX, USA*
YASUHIKO KIYOZUKA • *Department Pathology II, Kansai Medical University, Osaka, Japan*
AWTAR KRISHAN • *Division of Experimental Therapeutics, University of Miami, Miami, FL, USA*
TETSURO KUBOTA • *Department of Surgery, Keio University, Tokyo, Japan*
MICHAEL LAUE • *Institute Anatomy & Cell Biology, University of Saarland, Germany*
NATALIA L. LIEM • *Children's Cancer Institute Australia for Medical Research, South Australia, Sydney, Australia*
RICHARD B. LOCK • *Children's Cancer Institute Australia for Medical Research, South Australia, Sydney, Australia*
GERRIT LOS • *Rebecca and John Moores UCSD Cancer Center, University of California– San Diego, La Jolla, CA, USA*
RICHARD MAZURCHUK • *Roswell Park Cancer Institute, Buffalo, NY, USA*
PEDRO MESTRES-VENTURA • *Institute Anatomy & Cell Biology, University of Saarland, Germany*
REX A. MOATS • *Department of Radiology, Keck School Medicine, University Southern California, Los Angeles, CA, USA*
YOSHINARI MOCHIZUKI • *Department of Gastroenterological Surgery, Aichi Cancer Center Research Institute, Chikusa-ku, Nagoya, Japan*
DAVID E. MODRAK • *Garden State Cancer Center, Belleville, NJ, USA*
ANDRA MOGUET • *Institute Anatomy & Cell Biology, University of Saarland, Germany*
KATHLEEN MURPHY • *Department of Pathology, Johns Hopkins University School of Medicine, Baltimore, MD, USA*
HAYAO NAKANISHI • *Division of Oncological Pathology, Aichi Cancer Center Research Institute, Chikusa-ku, Nagoya, Japan*
MONICA PALLIS • *Academic Haematology, Nottingham City Hospital, Nottingham, UK*
RACHEL A. PAPA • *Children's Cancer Institute Australia for Medical Research, Sydney, Australia*
PAOLA PEREGO •*Istituto Nazionale Tumori, Milan, Italy*
JULIA POLAND • *Institut für Laboratoriumsmedizin und Pathobiochemie, Universitätsklinikum Charite, Berlin, Germany*

# Contributors

JANET E. PRICE • *Department of Cancer Biology, University of Texas M.D. Anderson Cancer Center, Houston, TX, USA*

C. PATRICK REYNOLDS • *USC-CHLA Institute for Pediatric Clinical Research, University of Southern California and Childrens Hospital Los Angeles, Los Angeles, CA, USA*

WERNER SCHMIDT • *Department of Gynecology-Obstetrics, University of Saarland, Germany*

ANETTE SCHOFER • *Institute Anatomy & Cell Biology, University of Saarland, Germany*

NARENDRA P. SINGH • *Department of Bioengineering, University of Washington, Seattle, WA, USA*

PRANAV SINHA • *Institut für Medizinische und Chemische Labordiagnostik, Landeskrankenhaus Klagenfurt, Klagenfurt, Austria*

JOSEPH A. SPERNYAK • *Roswell Park Cancer Institute, Buffalo, NY, USA*

BEE-CHUN SUN • *USC-CHLA Institute for Pediatric Clinical Research, University of Southern California and Childrens Hospital Los Angeles, Los Angeles, CA, USA*

YASUNARI TAKADA • *Department of Experimental Therapeutics, University Texas M.D. Anderson Cancer Center, Houston, TX, USA*

MASAE TATEMUATSU • *Division of Oncological Pathology, Aichi Cancer Center Research Institute, Chikusa-ku, Nagoya, Japan*

ANDREA URBANI • *Zentrale Proteinanalytik, Deutsches Krebsforschungszentrum, Heidelberg, Germany*

SILKE WANDSCHNEIDER • *Zentrale Proteinanalytik, Deutsches Krebsforschungszentrum, Heidelberg, Germany*

ROBERT WIEDER • *University of Medicine & Dentistry of New Jersey, Division Medical Oncology/Hematology, Newark, NJ, USA*

FRANCO ZUNINO • *Istituto Nazionale Tumori, Milan, Italy*

# Contents of Volume 1

Preface .................................................................................................... v
Contributors ........................................................................................... ix
Contents of Volume 2 ............................................................................ xi

**PART I. OVERVIEW**

 1  An Overview of Chemosensitivity Testing
    *Rosalyn D. Blumenthal* ..................................................................... 3

**PART II. IN VITRO MEASURES OF CHEMOSENSITIVITY**

 2  Clonogenic Cell Survival Assay
    *Anupama Munshi, Marvette Hobbs, and Raymond E. Meyn* ............. 21

 3  High-Sensitivity Cytotoxicity Assays for Nonadherent Cells
    *M. Jules Mattes* ............................................................................... 29

 4  Sulforhodamine B Assay and Chemosensitivity
    *Wieland Voight* ............................................................................... 39

 5  Use of the Differential Staining Cytotoxicity
    Assay to Predict Chemosensitivity
    *Gertjan J. L. Kaspers* ....................................................................... 49

 6  Collagen Gel Droplet Culture Method
    to Examine In Vitro Chemosensitivity
    *Hisayuki Kobayashi* ........................................................................ 59

 7  The MTT Assay to Evaluate Chemosensitivity
    *Jack D. Burton* ................................................................................ 69

 8  Histoculture Drug Response Assay to Monitor Chemoresponse
    *Shinji Ohie, Yasuhiro Udagawa, Daisuke Aoki,
    and Shiro Nozawa* ........................................................................... 79

 9  In Vitro Testing of Chemosensitivity in Physiological Hypoxia
    *Rita Grigoryan, Nino Keshelava, Clarke Anderson,
    and C. Patrick Reynolds* .................................................................. 87

10  Chemosensitivity Testing Using Microplate Adenosine
    Triphosphate–Based Luminescence Measurements
    *Christian M. Kurbacher and Ian A. Cree* ...................................... 101

11  High-Throughput Technology:
    Green Fluorescent Protein to Monitor Cell Death
    *Marylène Fortin, Ann-Muriel Steff, and Patrice Hugo* ................... 121

12  DIMSCAN: A Microcomputer Fluorescence-Based Cytotoxicity
    Assay for Preclinical Testing of Combination Chemotherapy
    **Nino Keshelava, Tomáš Frgala, Jiří Krejsa, Ondrej Kalous,
    and C. Patrick Reynolds** ................................................................. 139

13  The ChemoFx® Assay: *An Ex Vivo Cell Culture Assay
    for Predicting Anticancer Drug Responses*
    **Robert L. Ochs, Dennis Burholt, and Paul Kornblith** ................ 155

14  Evaluating Response to Antineoplastic Drug
    Combinations in Tissue Culture Models
    **C. Patrick Reynolds and Barry J. Maurer** ................................... 173

15  Image Analysis Using the Fluochromasia Assay
    to Quantify Tumor Drug Sensitivity
    **John F. Gibbs, Youcef M. Rustum, and Harry K. Slocum** ........ 185

16  Immunohistochemical Detection of Ornithine Decarboxylase
    as a Measure of Chemosensitivity
    **Uriel Bachrach** ............................................................................. 197

17  Immunohistochemistry of p53, Bcl-2 and Ki-67
    as Predictors of Chemosensitivity
    **Mitsuyoshi Itaya, Jiro Yoshimoto, Kuniaki Kojima,
    and Seiji Kawasaki** ....................................................................... 213

Index ................................................................................................... 229

# I

# MEASUREMENTS OF DNA DAMAGE, CELL DEATH, AND REGULATORS OF CYTOTOXICITY

# 1

# In Vitro Micronucleus Technique to Predict Chemosensitivity

## Michael Fenech

### Summary

The study of DNA damage at the chromosome level is an essential part of genetic toxicology because chromosomal mutation is an important event in carcinogenesis. The micronucleus assays have emerged as one of the preferred methods for assessing chromosome damage because they enable both chromosome loss and chromosome breakage to be measured reliably. Because micronuclei can only be expressed in cells that complete nuclear division a special method was developed that identifies such cells by their binucleate appearance when blocked from performing cytokinesis by cytochalasin-B, a microfilament-assembly inhibitor. The *cytokinesis-block micronucleus* (CBMN) *assay* allows better precision because the data obtained are not confounded by altered cell division kinetics caused by cytotoxicity of agents tested or suboptimal cell culture conditions. The method is now applied to various cell types for population monitoring of genetic damage, screening of chemicals for genotoxic potential, and for specific purposes such as prediction of the radiosensitivity of tumors and interindividual variation in radiosensitivity. In its current basic form the CBMN assay can provide, using simple morphological criteria, the following measures of genotoxicity and cytotoxicity: chromosome breakage, chromosome loss, chromosome rearrangement (nucleoplasmic bridges), cell division inhibition, necrosis, and apoptosis. The cytosine-arabinoside modification of the CBMN assay allows for measurement of excision-repairable lesions. The use of molecular probes enables chromosome loss to be distinguished from chromosome breakage and, importantly, nondisjunction in nonmicronucleated binucleated cells can be measured efficiently. The in vitro CBMN technique therefore provides multiple and complimentary measures of genotoxicity and cytotoxicity that can be achieved with relative ease within one system. The basic principles and methods (including detailed scoring criteria for all the genotoxicity and cytotoxicity end points) of the CBMN assay are described and areas for future development identified.

Substantial parts of this chapter were updated from Fenech, M. (2000), The in vitro micronucleus technique, *Mutation Research* **455**, 81–95, with permission from Elsevier Science.

**Key Words**

Micronuclear assay; cytokinesis-block; genome damage; chromosome loss; chromosome breakage.

## 1. Introduction

The observation that chromosome damage can be caused by exposure to ionizing radiation or carcinogenic chemicals was among the first reliable evidence that physical and chemical agents can cause major alterations to the genetic material of eukaryotic cells *(1)*. Although our understanding of chromosome structure is incomplete, evidence suggests that chromosome abnormalities are a direct consequence and manifestation of damage at the DNA level—for example, chromosome breaks may result from unrepaired double-strand breaks in DNA and chromosome rearrangements may result from misrepair of strand breaks in DNA *(2)*. It is also recognized that chromosome loss and malsegregation of chromosomes (nondisjunction) are important events in cancer and aging and that they are probably caused by defects in the spindle, centromere, or as a consequence of undercondensation of chromosome structure before metaphase *(3–5)*.

In the classical cytogenetic techniques, chromosomes are studied directly by observing and counting aberrations in metaphases *(6)*. This approach provides the most detailed analysis, but the complexity and laboriousness of enumerating aberrations in metaphase and the confounding effect of artefactual loss of chromosomes from metaphase preparations has stimulated the development of a simpler system of measuring chromosome damage.

It was proposed independently by Schmid *(7)* and Heddle *(8)* that an alternative and simpler approach to assess chromosome damage in vivo was to measure micronuclei (MNi), also known as Howell–Jolly bodies to hematologists, in dividing cell populations such as the bone marrow. The micronucleus assay in bone marrow and peripheral blood erythrocytes is now one of the best established in vivo cytogenetic assays in the field of genetic toxicology, but it is not a technique that is applicable to other cell populations in vivo or in vitro and methods have since been developed for measuring MNi in a variety of nucleated cells in vitro.

MNi are expressed in dividing cells that either contain chromosome breaks lacking centromeres (acentric fragments) and/or whole chromosomes that are unable to travel to the spindle poles during mitosis. At telophase, a nuclear envelope forms around the lagging chromosomes and fragments, which then uncoil and gradually assume the morphology of an interphase nucleus with the exception that they are smaller than the main nuclei in the cell, hence the term *micronucleus* (**Fig. 1**). MNi, therefore, provide a convenient and reliable

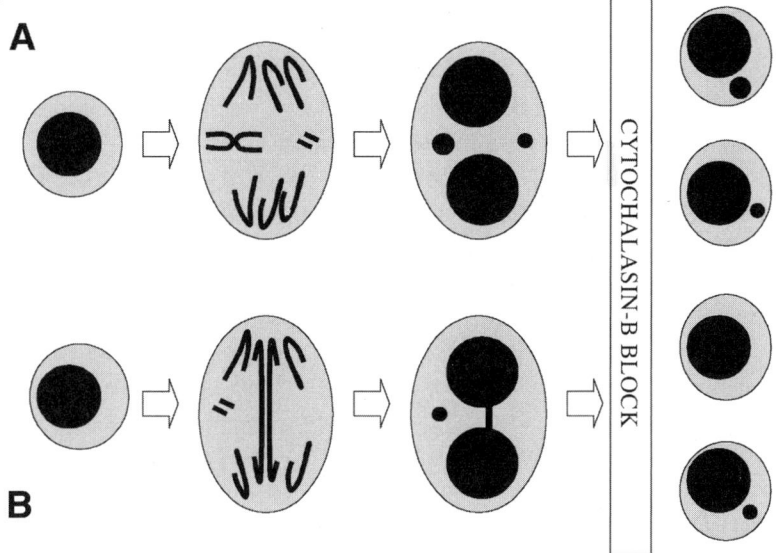

Fig. 1. (**A**) The origin of micronuclei from lagging whole chromosomes and acentric chromosome fragments at anaphase. (**B**) The formation of a nucleoplasmic bridge from a dicentric chromosome in which the centromeres are pulled to opposite poles of the cell; the formation of a micronucleus from the accompanying acentric chromosome fragment is also illustrated. The critical role of cytochalasin-B in blocking dividing cells at the binucleate stage is also indicated in this diagram. The example shown is for a hypothetical cell with two pairs of chromosomes only.

index of both chromosome breakage and chromosome loss. Because MNi are expressed in cells that have completed nuclear division, they are ideally scored in the binucleated stage of the cell cycle *(9,10)*. Occasionally, nucleoplasmic bridges between nuclei in a binucleated cell are observed. These are probably dicentric chromosomes in which the two centromeres were pulled to opposite poles of the cell and the DNA in the resulting bridge covered by nuclear membrane (**Fig. 1**). Thus nucleoplasmic bridges in binucleated cells provide an additional and complementary measure of chromosome rearrangement, which can be scored together with the micronucleus count.

It is evident from the above that MNi can only be expressed in dividing eukaryotic cells. In other words, the assay cannot be used efficiently or quantitatively in nondividing cell populations or in dividing cell populations in which the kinetics of cell division are not well understood or controlled. Consequently, there was a need to develop a method that could distinguish between cells that are not dividing and cells that are undergoing mitosis within a cell population. Furthermore, because of the uncertainty of the fate of MNi following more than one nuclear division, it is important to identify cells that have completed one nuclear division only. These requirements are also necessary because cells divide at different rates in vivo and in vitro depending on the various physiological, genetic, and micronutrient conditions.

Several methods have been proposed based on stathmokinetic, flow cytometric, and DNA labeling approaches, but the method that has found most favor because of its simplicity and lack of uncertainty regarding its effect on baseline genetic damage, is the *cytokinesis-block micronucleus* (CBMN) *assay (9–11)*.

In the CBMN assay, cells that have completed one nuclear division are blocked from performing cytokinesis using cytochalasin-B (Cyt-B) and are consequently readily identified by their binucleated appearance (**Fig. 1**). Cyt-B is an inhibitor of actin polymerization required for the formation of the microfilament ring that constricts the cytoplasm between the daughter nuclei during cytokinesis *(12)*. The use of Cyt-B enables the accumulation of virtually all dividing cells at the binucleate stage in dividing cell populations, regardless of their degree of synchrony and the proportion of dividing cells. MNi are then scored in binucleated cells only, which enables reliable comparisons of chromosome damage between cell populations that may differ in their cell division kinetics. The method was initially developed for use with cultured human lymphocytes *(9,10)* but has now been adapted to various cell types such as solid tumor and bone marrow cells *(13,14)*. Furthermore, new developments have also occurred that allow (1) MNi originating from whole chromosomes to be distinguished from MNi originating from chromosome fragments *(15–20)*, (2) the conversion of excision-repaired sites to MNi within one cell division *(21)*, (3) the use of molecular probes to identify nondisjunction events in binucleated cells *(22–24)*, and (4) the integration of necrotic and apoptotic cells within the CBMN assay *(25,26)*.

It has recently been proposed that the micronucleus assay be used instead of metaphase analysis for genotoxicity testing of new chemicals. A recent special issue of *Mutation Research* has been dedicated to this topic *(27)*. The current methodologies and data for the in vitro micronucleus test were reviewed at the Washington International Workshop on Genotoxicity Test Procedures, which was held in 1999 *(28)*.

The standard CBMN assay and its various modifications are described in detail in the next sections. The methods described are mainly applicable to cultured human lymphocytes; however, modifications of the assay for application to other cell types are included.

## 2. Materials
### 2.1. Cytokinesis-Block Micronucleus Assay

1. Cytochalasin-B stock solution in dimethyl sulfoxide (DMSO) (600 µg/mL).
2. Ficoll Paque.
3. Hank's balanced salt solution (HBSS).
4. RPMI 1640 culture medium + 10–15% heat-inactivated fetal calf serum.
5. Phytohemagglutinin (PHA) (Glaxo Wellcome HA15) stock, 2.25 mg/mL (not required for transformed cell lines or tumor cell cultures).
6. Diff Quik (Lab-Aids, Australia).
7. Depex (DPX) mounting medium.
8. Acridine orange: 40 µg/mL in Sorensen's phosphate buffer, pH 6.9.

### 2.2. Kinetochore Detection in Micronuclei

1. Serum samples from scleroderma patients of the CREST subtype.
2. Rabbit FITC-conjugated secondary antihuman IgG antibody.
3. Peroxidase-labeled rabbit antihuman IgG.
4. Diaminobenzidine (1 mg/mL in Tris-base buffer stock, 60.5 g/L, pH 7.6), 3 mL of Tris-base buffer stock, pH 7.6 (60.5 g/L).
5. $NiCl_2$ solution: 8% solution in Tris-base buffer stock prepared immediately before use.
6. 40 µL of 0.1 $M$ imidazole and 10 µL of 30% hydrogen peroxide solution.
7. Neutral Red (0.1% in distilled water).

## 3. Methods
### 3.1. Standard Cytokinesis-Block Micronucleus Assay for Isolated Human Lymphocytes

In this technique, MNi are scored only in those cells that have completed one nuclear division following PHA stimulation. These cells are recognized by their binucleated appearance after they are blocked from performing cytokinesis by Cyt-B, which should be added before the first mitotic wave. Optimal culture conditions should yield 35–60% or more binucleates as a proportion of viable cells (i.e., all cells excluding necrotic and apoptotic cells) at 72 h after PHA stimulation. All equipment should have biosafety features to protect the operator, and solutions used in this procedure should be filter-sterilized.

#### 3.1.1. Lymphocyte Isolation, Cell Culture, and Cell Harvesting

1. Fresh blood is collected by venipuncture in tubes with heparin as anticoagulant and stored at 22°C for less than 4 h prior to lymphocyte isolation.
2. The blood is then diluted 1:1 with isotonic (0.85%) sterile saline and gently inverted to mix.

3. The diluted blood is overlaid gently on Ficoll Paque (Pharmacia) density gradients using a ratio of approx 1:3 (e.g., 2 mL Ficoll Paque to 6 mL of diluted blood), being very careful not to disturb the interface.
4. The gradient is then spun in a centrifuge at 400$g$ for 25–40 min at 22°C after carefully balancing the tubes.
5. The lymphocyte layer at the interface of Ficoll Paque and diluted plasma is collected with a sterile plugged Pasteur pipet and added to 3–5 times volume of HBSS at 22°C. The resulting cell suspension is centrifuged at 280–400$g$ for 5–10 min depending on the volume.
6. The supernatant is discarded, the cells resuspended in 2–5 times volume HBSS and centrifuged at 180–400$g$ for 5 min depending on the volume.
7. The supernatant is discarded and the cells resuspended in 1 mL RPMI 1640 culture medium.
8. Cell concentration is then measured using a Coulter counter or hemocytometer and the concentration it adjusted by the percentage of viable cells measured using trypan blue exclusion assay.
9. The cells are resuspended in RPMI 1640 medium containing 10–15% heat-inactivated fetal calf serum at 0.5–1.0 × $10^6$ cells/mL and cultured in 0.75–1.0 mL vol in round-bottom tissue culture tubes (10-mm width).
10. Lymphocytes are then stimulated to divide by adding PHA to each culture tube at 10 µL/mL and incubated at 37°C with loose lids in a humidified atmosphere containing 5% $CO_2$. The concentration of PHA used has to be optimized depending on the purity and source of the reagent to ensure maximum number of binucleated cells after cytochalasin-B block.
11. Forty-four hours after PHA stimulation, 4.5 µg Cyt-B is added to each milliliter of culture (*use gloves and fume hood*): a 100-µL aliquot of Cyt-B stock solution is thawed, 900 µL culture medium added and mixed. 75 µL of the mixture is added to each 1 mL of culture to give a final concentration of 4.5 µg Cyt-B/mL (other laboratories have successfully used 6.0 µg Cyt-B/mL in their cultures). Culture tubes are then reincubated with loose lids.
12. Twenty-eight hours after adding Cyt-B, cells are harvested by cytocentrifugation (Shandon Elliot). One hundred microliters of the culture medium is removed without disturbing the cells and then cells are gently resuspended in their tubes; 100–120 µL of cell suspension is transferred to cytocentrifuge cups (Shandon Elliot) and centrifuged to produce two spots per slide (*see* **Note 1**). (Set the cytocentrifuge as follows: time, 5 min; speed, 480$g$). Slides are removed from the cytocentrifuge and allowed to air-dry for 10–12 min *only* and then fixed for 10 min in absolute methanol.
13. The cells can be stained using a variety of techniques that can clearly identify nuclear and cytoplasmic boundaries. In our experience, the use of Diff Quik, a commercial ready-to-use product, provides rapid and optimal results (*see* **Note 1**).
14. After staining, the slides are air-dried and cover slips placed over the cells using Depex (DPX) mounting medium. This procedure is carried out in the fume hood

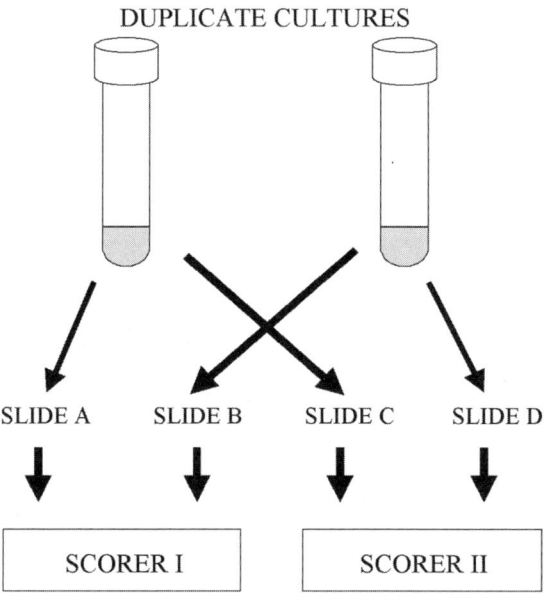

Fig. 2. An optimal sampling schedule for the in vitro micronucleus assay that enables an estimation of experimental variation (results for A + C vs B + D) as well as the effect of scorer bias (results for A + B versus C + D).

and the slides are left to set in the fume hood and then stored indefinitely until required.

Duplicate cultures of control or genotoxin-treated cells should be set up and slides from each culture should be prepared. This is essential to obtain a measure of experimental variation, i.e., coefficient of variation, which should be quoted with each set of duplicate cultures (*see* **Notes 2** and **3**). This experimental design is summarized in **Fig. 2**.

For fluorescence microscopy, staining with acridine orange (40 µg/mL in Sorensen's phosphate buffer pH 6.9) is recommended. If a cytocentrifuge is not available, slides can be prepared using the procedure described below for whole blood cultures.

### 3.1.2. Examination of Slides and Assessment of MN Frequency

Slides are best examined at 1000× magnification using a light or fluorescence microscope. Slides should be coded before analysis so that the scorer is not aware of the identity of the slide. A score should be obtained for slides from each duplicate culture, ideally from two different scorers using identical microscopes (*see* **Notes 4** and **5**). The number of cells scored (*see* **Note 6**) should be determined depending on the level of change in the micronucleus (MN) index that the experiment is intended to detect and the expected standard deviation of the estimate. For each slide, the following information should be obtained:

1. The number of micronuclei (MNi) in at least 1000 binucleate (BN) cells should be scored and the frequency of MNi per 1000 BN cells calculated. The criteria for scoring MNi in BN cells are detailed below.
2. The distribution of BN cells with zero, one, or more MNi; the number of MNi in a single binucleated cell normally ranges from 0 to 3 in lymphocytes of healthy individuals but can be greater than 3 on occasion depending on genotoxin exposure and age.
3. The frequency of micronucleated BN cells in at least 1000 BN cells.
4. The frequency of nucleoplasmic bridges in 1000 BN cells. Scoring criteria for nucleoplasmic bridges are described below.
5. The proportion of mononucleated, binucleated, trinucleated, and tetranucleated cells per 500 cells scored. From this information the Nuclear Division Index (explained below) can be derived.
6. The number of dead or dying cells due to apoptosis or necrosis per 500 cells may also be scored on the same slide (scoring criteria for these cells are detailed below) while scoring the frequency of viable mono-, bi-, and multinucleated cells (*see* **Note 7**).

It is important to note that it is best to skip scoring a cell if one is uncertain on how to classify it. The basic elements of a typical score sheet are listed in **Table 1**.

### 3.1.3. Criteria for Selecting Binucleated Cells and Scoring Micronuclei, Nucleoplasmic Bridges, and Apoptotic and Necrotic Cells

1. *Criteria for selecting binucleated cells.* The cytokinesis-blocked cells that may be scored for MN frequency should have the following characteristics:
   a. The cells should be binucleated.
   b. The two nuclei in a binucleated cell should have intact nuclear membranes and be situated within the same cytoplasmic boundary.
   c. The two nuclei in a binucleated cell should be approximately equal in size, staining pattern, and staining intensity.
   d. The two nuclei within a BN cell may be attached by a fine nucleoplasmic bridge that is no wider than one-fourth the nuclear diameter.
   e. The two main nuclei in a BN cell may touch but ideally should not overlap each other. A cell with two overlapping nuclei can be scored only if the nuclear boundaries of each nucleus are distinguishable.
   f. The cytoplasmic boundary or membrane of a binucleated cell should be intact and clearly distinguishable from the cytoplasmic boundary of adjacent cells.

## Table 1
## Information That Should Be Included on a Score Sheet for the Cytokinesis-Block Micronucleus Assay

1. Code number of each slide
2. Number of BN cells scored
3. Distribution of BN cells with 0, 1, 2, 3, or more MNi in at least 1000 BN cells
4. Total number of MNi in BN cells
5. Frequency of MNi in 1000 BN cells
6. Frequency of micronucleated BN cells in 1000 BN cells
7. Proportion of BN cells with nucleoplasmic bridges
8. Proportion of mono-, bi-, tri-, and tetranucleated cells in 500 viable cells
9. Frequency of BN cells in a total of 500 viable cells
10. Nuclear division index
11. Proportion of cells that are undergoing apoptosis or necrosis in 500 cells
12. Nuclear division cytotoxicity index
13. Coefficient of variation for duplicate estimates of above parameters

BN, binucleate; MNi, micronuclei.

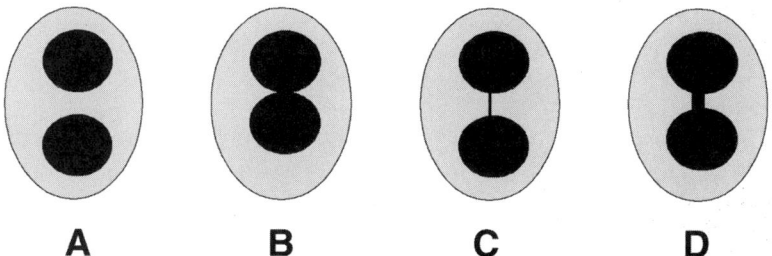

Fig. 3. Criteria for choosing binucleate cells in the cytokinesis-block micronucleus assay: **(A)** ideal binucleate cell; **(B)** binucleate cell with touching nuclei; **(C)** binucleate cell with narrow nucleoplasmic bridge between nuclei; **(D)** binucleate cell with relatively wide nucleoplasmic bridge. Cells with two overlapping nuclei may be considered suitable to score as binucleated cells if the nuclear boundaries are distinguishable. Occasionally, binucleated cells with more than one nucleoplasmic bridge are observed.

Examples of the type of binucleated cells that may or may not be scored are illustrated diagrammatically in **Fig. 3**. The cell types that should not be scored for micronucleus frequency include mono-, tri-, quadri-, and multinucleated cells, and cells that are necrotic or apoptotic (illustrated in **Fig. 4**).

2. *Criteria for scoring micronuclei.* MNi are morphologically identical to but smaller than nuclei. They also have the following characteristics:

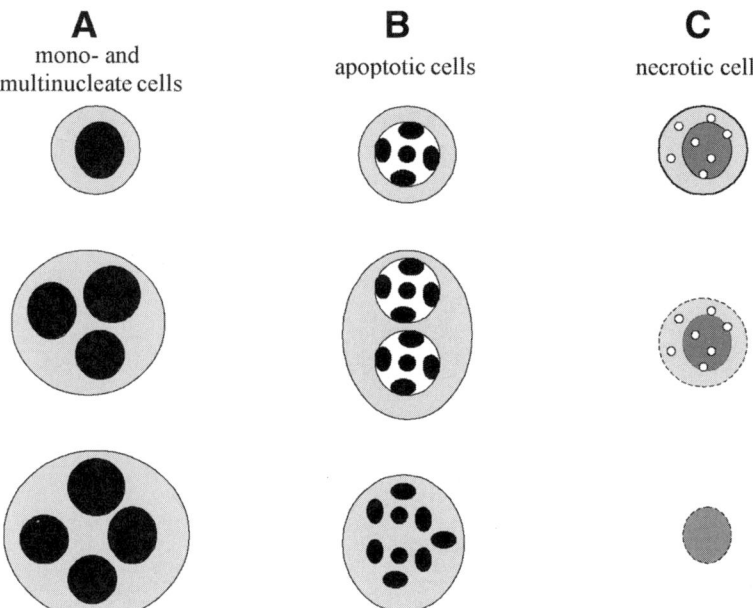

Fig. 4. The various types of cells that may be observed in the in vitro cytokinesis-block micronucleus assay excluding binucleated cells. These cell types shown should not be scored for MN frequency: **(A)** viable mono-, tri-, and quadrinuclear cells; **(B)** mono- and binucleated cells at early stage of apoptosis when chromatin condensation has occurred but nuclear membrane has not disintegrated and late-stage apoptotic cells with intact cytoplasm, no nucleus, and apoptotic chromatin bodies within the cytoplasm; **(C)** cells at the various stages of necrosis including early stages, showing vacuolization, disintegration of cytoplasmic membrane and loss of cytoplasm with an intact nucleus, and late stages in which cytoplasm is partially or completely lost, nuclear membrane is visibly damaged, and nuclear material is commencing to leak from the remnant nucleus.

    a. The diameter of MNi in human lymphocytes usually varies between 1/16th and 1/3rd the mean diameter of the main nuclei, which corresponds to 1/256th and 1/9th of the area of one of the main nuclei in a BN cell, respectively.
    b. MNi are nonrefractile and they can therefore be readily distinguished from artefacts such as staining particles.
    c. MNi are not linked or connected to the main nuclei.
    d. MNi may touch but not overlap the main nuclei, and the micronuclear boundary should be distinguishable from the nuclear boundary.
    e. MNi usually have the same staining intensity as the main nuclei, but occasionally staining may be more intense.

    Examples of typical MNi that meet the criteria set above are shown in **Fig. 5**. Examples of cellular structures that resemble MNi but should not be classified as

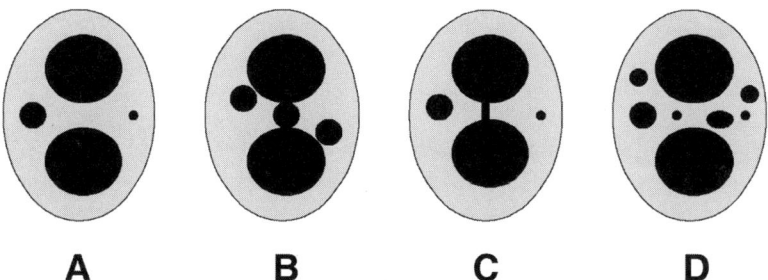

Fig. 5. Typical appearance and relative size of micronuclei in binucleated cells. (**A**) Cell with two micronuclei, one with one-third and the other one-ninth the diameter of one of the main nuclei within the cell. (**B**) Micronuclei touching but not overlapping the main nuclei. (**C**) A binucleated cell with nucleoplasmic bridge between main nuclei and two micronuclei. (**D**) A binucleated cell with six micronuclei of various sizes; this type of cell is rarely seen.

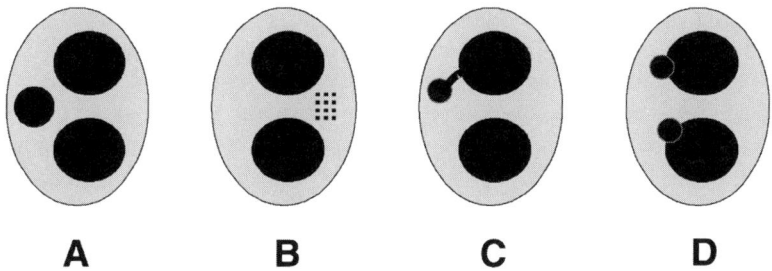

Fig. 6. Occasionally, binucleated cells (or cells that resemble binucleated cells) may contain structures that resemble micronuclei but should not be scored as micronuclei originating from chromosome loss or chromosome breakage. These situations include: (**A**) a trinucleated cell in which one of the nuclei is relatively small but has a diameter greater than one-third the diameter of the other nuclei; (**B**) dense stippling in a specific region of the cytoplasm; (**C**) extruded nuclear material that appears like a micronucleus with a narrow nucleoplasmic connection to the main nucleus; (**D**) nuclear blebs that have an obvious nucleoplasmic connection with the main nucleus.

> MNi originating from chromosome breakage or loss are illustrated in **Fig. 6**. Induction of gene amplification may lead to extrusion of amplified genes into nuclear buds (e.g., **Figs. 6C,D**) during S phase that are eventually detached from the nucleus to form a micronucleus *(70)*; it may be necessary to quantify the frequency of nuclei with nuclear bud formation if gene amplification is suspected (*see* **Note 8**).
> 3. *Criteria for scoring nucleoplasmic bridges.* Nucleoplasmic bridges are sometimes observed in binucleated cells following exposure to clastogens.
>    a. They are a continuous link between the nuclei in a binucleated cell and are thought to be due to dicentric chromosomes in which the centromeres were pulled to opposite poles during anaphase.

b. The width of a nucleoplasmic bridge may vary considerably but usually does not exceed one-fourth of the diameter of the nuclei within the cell.
c. The nucleoplasmic bridge should have the same staining characteristics of the main nuclei.
d. On very rare occasions, more than one nucleoplasmic bridge may be observed within one binucleated cell. A binucleated cell with a nucleoplasmic bridge often contains one or more micronuclei. Examples of binucleated cells with nucleoplasmic bridges are illustrated in **Figs. 1** and **5** (*see* **Note 9**).
4. *Criteria for scoring apoptotic and necrotic cells.* **Figure 7** describes the various pathways and events that may be expected to occur in cultured lymphocytes exposed to a toxic agent. Cytogenetic genotoxicity assays that require hypotonic treatment for the preparation of interphase cells (for whole-blood micronucleus assay) or metaphase plates for chromosome analysis are not usable for cytotoxicity assays because hypotonic treatment may destroy necrotic cells and apoptotic cells, making them unavailable for assay. Inclusion of necrosis and apoptosis is important for the accurate description of mechanism of action and measurement of cellular sensitivity to a chemical or radiation. Isolated lymphocyte culture assay or culture of cell lines does not require hypotonic treatment of cells for slide preparation, thus making it is possible to preserve the morphology of both necrotic and apoptotic cells. The use of cytochalasin-B should make it easier to score apoptotic cells because it is expected to inhibit the disintegration of apoptotic cells into smaller apoptotic bodies. The latter process requires microfilament assembly *(29)* which is readily inhibited by cytochalasin-B *(12)*.

The following guidelines for scoring necrotic and apoptotic cells are recommended:
a. Cells showing chromatin condensation with intact cytoplasmic and nuclear boundaries or cells exhibiting nuclear fragmentation into smaller nuclear bodies within an intact cytoplasm/cytoplasmic membrane are classified as apoptotic.
b. Cells exhibiting a pale cytoplasm with numerous vacuoles and damaged cytoplasmic membrane with a fairly intact nucleus or cells exhibiting loss of cytoplasm and damaged/irregular nuclear membrane with a partially intact nuclear structure are classified as necrotic. These criteria and results for these measures with hydrogen peroxide have been recently reported elsewhere *(26)*.

**Figures 4** and **7** illustrate typical examples of necrotic and apoptotic cells.

## 3.1.4. Calculation of Nuclear Division Index (NDI) and Nuclear Division Cytotoxicity Index (NDCI)

1. NDI is often calculated according to the method of Eastmond and Tucker *(30)*. Five hundred viable cells are scored to determine the frequency of cells with one, two, three, or four nuclei and calculate the NDI using the formula

$$NDI = (M1 + 2 \times M2 + 3 \times M3 + 4 \times M4) / N$$

where M1–M4 represent the number of cells with one to four nuclei and N is the total number of viable cells scored. The NDI and the proportion of binucleated

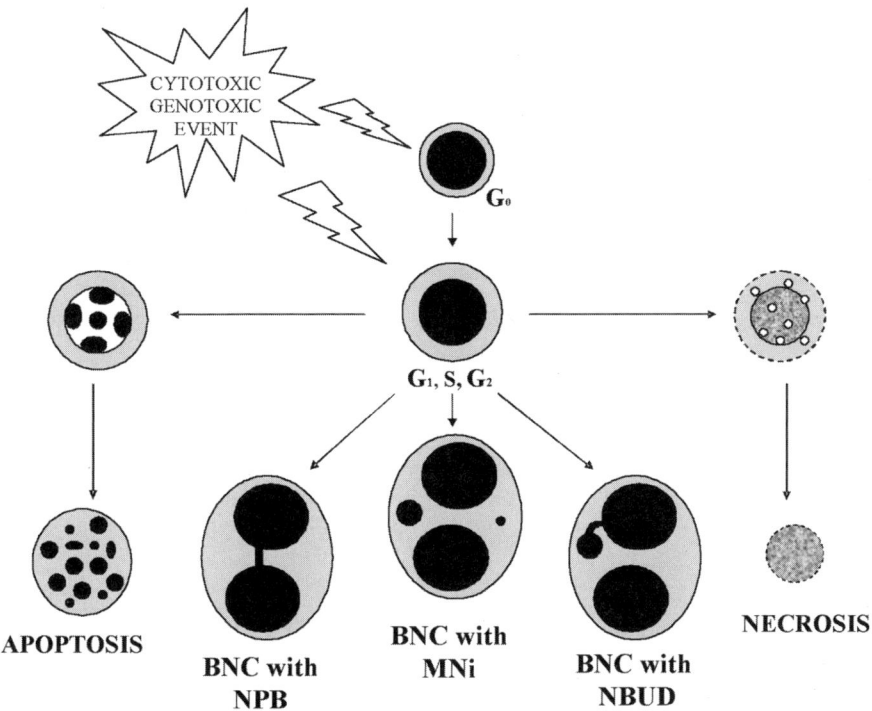

Fig. 7. Genome damage and cell-death biomarkers scored in the comprehensive CBMN assay. The CBMN assay allows the measurement of all possible outcomes following a genome damage event. In this assay a cell with genome damage may either undergo cell death via apoptosis or necrosis or, alternatively, may survive and undergo further nuclear division. In the latter case, dividing cells are recognized as binucleated cells (BNCs) by blocking cytokinesis with cytochalsin-B. BNCs are then scored for the following genome damage events: (a) micronuclei (MNi), which originate from lagging whole chromosomes or broken chromosome fragments and are therefore a marker of chromosome breakage and chromosome loss events, the latter being due to defects in centromere or spindle structure; (b) nucleoplasmic bridges (NPB), which originate from dicentric chromosomes caused by misrepair of chromosome breaks and are therefore a marker of chromosome rearrangement; and (c) nuclear buds (NBUD), which are the mechanism by which the nucleus eliminates amplified DNA resulting from breakage–fusion–bridge cycles generated by NPB. NBUD therefore provide a measure of gene amplification. An increase in MNi, NPB, and NBUD is indicative of an increase in genome instability commonly seen in cancer.

cells are useful parameters for comparing the mitogenic response of lymphocytes and cytostatic effects of agents examined in the assay.
2. A more accurate assessment of nuclear division status is obtained if necrotic and apoptotic cells are included in the total number of cells scored, because at higher

toxic doses of chemicals tested one can expect a very large proportion of cells to become nonviable. It is therefore important to note that both binucleate ratio and the NDI are overestimated if necrotic and apoptotic cells are not included when scoring cells.
3. A more accurate estimate of nuclear division status and cell division kinetics can be obtained using the following modified equation, which takes account of viable as well as necrotic and apoptotic cells:

$$NDCI = (Ap + Nec + M1 + 2 \times M2 + 3 \times M3 + 4 \times M4) / N^*$$

where NDCI = nuclear division cytotoxicity index, Ap = number of apoptotic cells, Nec = number of necrotic cells, M1–M4 = number of viable cells with one, two, three, or four nuclei, and $N^*$ = total number of cells scored (viable and nonviable).

## 3.2. Measurement of Excision-Repaired DNA Lesions in $G_0/G_1$ Human Lymphocytes Using the Cytosine Arabinoside Micronucleus Assay in Human Lymphocytes

After assessing the MN response in human $G_0$ lymphocytes following exposure to a variety of genotoxins, it became evident that the extent of micronucleus formation in relation to cytotoxicity was low for chemicals and ultraviolet radiation, which mainly induce base lesions and adducts on DNA rather than strand breakage or spindle damage *(21)*. We hypothesized that this was due to either efficient repair of the lesions or that such sites, if left unrepaired, do not convert to a double-stranded break in DNA following one round of DNA synthesis. Furthermore, we reasoned that inhibition of excision repair by cytosine arabinoside (ARA) would result in the conversion of such base lesions to a single-stranded break, which would become a double-stranded break following DNA synthesis leading to the production of an acentric fragment, which would then be expressed as a MN within one division cycle *(21,31)*.

1. Using this concept (illustrated in **Fig. 8**), we showed that addition of ARA during the first 16 h of lymphocyte culture (i.e., before DNA synthesis) did result in a dramatic increase (10-fold or greater) in the MN dose response following UV or methylnitroso urea (MNU) treatment. However, the ARA-induced increase following X-ray exposure was only 1.8-fold, as would be expected from the proportion of DNA adducts or base lesions relative to the induction of DNA strand breaks. This method has since been used to identify pesticides that induce excision repair and to distinguish between genotoxic agents that do or do not induce excision repair *(32)*.

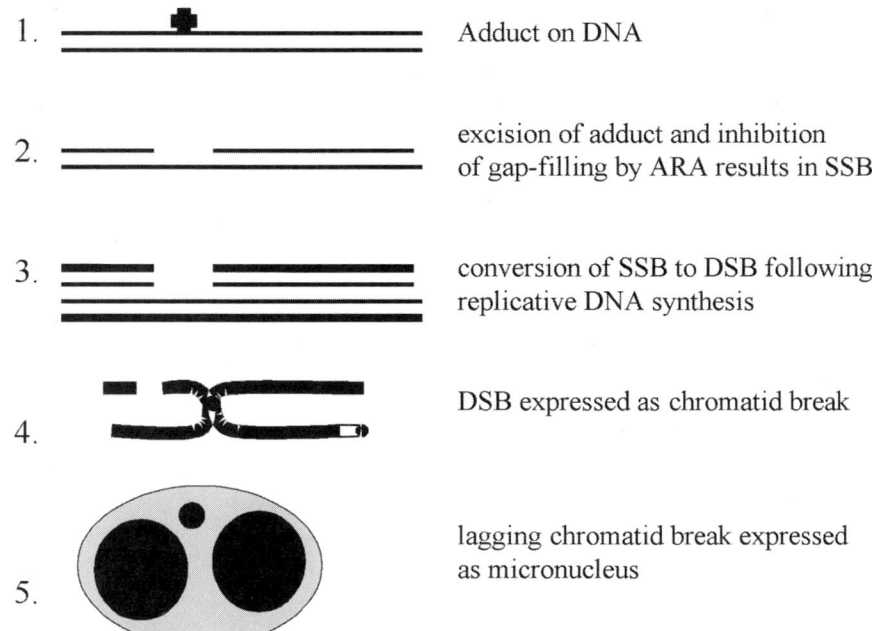

Fig. 8. A schematic diagram explaining the mechanism for the conversion by ARA of an excision-repairable DNA lesion to a micronucleus within one division cycle.

2. The ARA protocol is an important adjunct to the basic CBMN assay and should be attempted particularly if strong cytotoxic effects are observed in conjunction with weak MN induction.
3. Precise measurement of excision-repaired DNA lesions using the ARA method is only possible using the CBMN assay because (a) the conversion of excision-repaired DNA lesions to MN occurs only in cells that have completed nuclear division and (b) the addition of ARA may also result in significantly altered cell division kinetics, which could confound results in MN assays without Cyt-B.
4. ARA inhibition of DNA polymerase may cause DNA strand breaks in cells undergoing replicative DNA synthesis. Therefore, it is only possible to use this method in PHA-stimulated $G_0$ lymphocytes with ARA exposure occurring during the $G_1$ phase and prior to S phase, because excision repair is activated during $G_1$.
5. In practice, this means that cells are cultured in the presence of ARA during the first 16–20 h after PHA stimulation, following which the cells are washed to remove ARA and incubated in culture medium containing deoxycyidine to reverse ARA inhibition of DNA polymerase.
6. After these steps, the standard CBMN protocol (described above) is followed. For more procedure details and typical results, refer to Fenech and Neville *(21)* and Surrales et al. *(32)*.

## 3.3. CBMN Assay in Other Cell Culture Systems

### 3.3.1. Whole Blood Cultures for Human Lymphocytes

1. The CBMN assay in human lymphocytes can also be performed using whole-blood cultures.
2. Typically, 0.4–0.5 mL of whole blood is added to 4.5 mL of culture medium (e.g., RPMI 1640) supplemented with fetal calf serum containing L-glutamine, antibiotics (optional), and PHA.
3. Cyt-B is added at 44 h post-PHA stimulation. The recommended optimal concentration of Cyt-B for accumulating binucleated cells in whole blood cultures is 6 µg/mL *(33)*.
4. The binucleated lymphocytes are harvested 28 h after adding Cyt-B as follows:
5. The cells are centrifuged gently (300$g$) for 5 min and the supernatant culture medium is removed.
6. The cells are hypotonically treated with 7 mL cold (4°C) 0.075 $M$ KCl to lyse red blood cells and centrifuged immediately (300$g$) for 8 min.
7. The supernatant is removed and replaced with 5 mL fixative consisting of methanol/acetic acid (3/1) (the fixative should be added while agitating the cells to prevent clumps forming).
8. The cells are then centrifuged again at 300$g$ for 8 min and washed with two further changes of fixative.
9. The cells are resuspended gently, and the suspension is dropped onto clean glass slides and allowed to dry.

    As an alternative, it is also possible to isolate the binucleated lymphocytes directly from the whole-blood culture using Ficoll gradients and then transfer cells to slides by cytocentrifugation prior to fixation and staining (unpublished observation), which precludes the requirement for hypotonic treatment and enables optimal preservation of the cytoplasm.
10. Staining of cells can be done using either 10% Giemsa in potassium phosphate buffer (pH 7.3) for light microscopy or acridine orange (10 µg/mL in phosphate-buffered saline, pH 6.9) for fluorescence microscopy).

### 3.3.2 Murine Lymphocyte Cultures

1. Lymphocytes are isolated either from the spleen or peripheral blood and cultured according to the procedures described by Fenech et al. *(34)*.
2. Because murine lymphocytes have shorter cell division cycles than human lymphocytes, it is essential to add Cyt-B no later than 18 h after stimulation by mitogen and to harvest the cells 20 h later. Depending on the culture conditions, it is possible to obtain good binucleate ratios even at 72 h post-mitogen stimulation.

### 3.3.3. Other Primary Cell Cultures, Including Tumor Cell Cultures

The CBMN assay can be readily adapted to other primary cell types to assess DNA damage induced in vitro, in vivo, or ex vivo. The most important points to remember are (a) to ensure that MNi are scored in the first nuclear division following the genotoxic insult and (b) to perform preliminary experiments to determine the concentration of Cyt-B and incubation time at which the maximum number of dividing cells will be blocked at the binucleate stage (*see* **Note 10**). It is also important to remember that Cyt-B may take up to 6 h before it starts to exert its cytokinesis-blocking action (unpublished observation).

1. When using established or primary cell lines from dividing cell populations, it is usual to add Cyt-B shortly after exposure to genotoxin to capture all cells undergoing their first nuclear division as binucleated cells—this usually requires an incubation period of about 24–48 h, depending on the cell cycle time, before harvesting the cells.
2. Attached cells can be trypsinized and then prepared by cytocentrifugation as described for human lymphocytes. Specific methods have been described for use with nucleated bone marrow cells *(14)*, lung fibroblasts *(35)*, skin keratinocytes *(36)* and primary tumor cell cultures *(13)*.
3. It is generally more practical to assess in vivo induction of micronuclei by blocking cytokinesis in dividing cells after the cells have been isolated from the animal and placed in culture medium in the presence of Cyt-B; this approach has proven to be successful with a variety of cell types, including fibroblasts, keratinocytes, and nucleated bone marrow cells.

### 3.4. Micronucleus Assay in Cell Lines or Cultured Tumor Cells with or without Cytokinesis Block

1. There is some debate that Cyt-B, used to accumulate binucleated cells, may interfere with the expression of MN *(28)*. Studies with normal cells do not show an induction of MNi by Cyt-B or a dose–response effect of Cyt-B with MN frequency in binucleated cells at doses that are usually used to block cells in cytokinesis *(10,37–39)*. A recent study suggests that MN expression induced by spindle poisons may be less than expected in the cytokinesis-blocked BN cells because of pole-to-pole distance shortening, which may increase the probability of reinclusion of lagging chromosome fragments or whole chromosomes back into a nucleus, but this did not diminish the effectiveness of the CBMN assay *(40)*.
2. There has been an increased interest in exploring further the possibility of performing the in vitro MN assay without Cyt-B to minimize the possible confounding effect of Cyt-B while running the potential risk of obtaining a false negative result because of inadequate control of cell division kinetics; i.e., inhibition of nuclear division inhibits micronucleus expression.
3. While the evidence of obtaining a false positive result with the CBMN assay in normal cells is lacking, there is already adequate evidence that performing the MN assay in a manner that does not account for inhibition of nuclear division can lead to false negative results or an underestimate of MN induction in human lymphocyte cultures *(10,11,41)*, and an example of this defect of MN assays without Cyt-B is shown in **Fig. 9**.

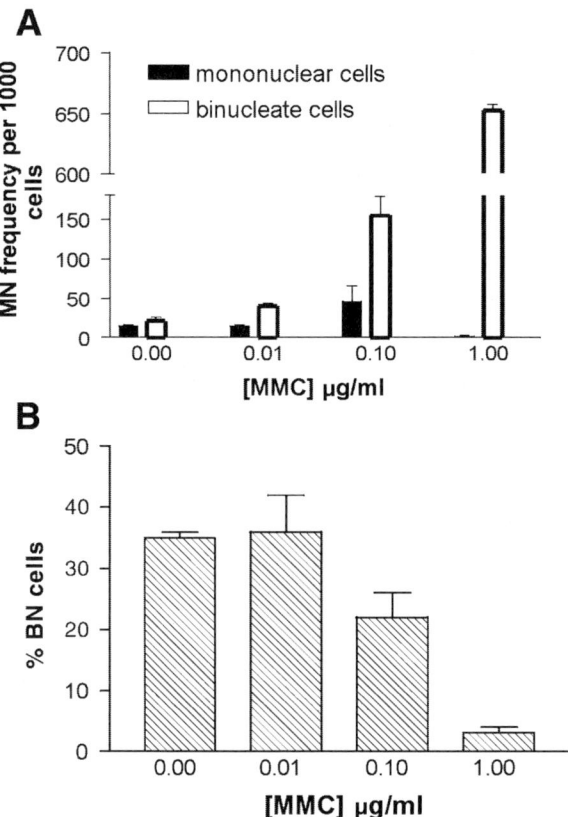

Fig. 9. (**A**) Comparison of the micronucleus dose-response in human lymphocytes exposed in vitro in G1/S/G2 to mitomycin-C (MMC), measured either in mononucleated cells in cultures without Cyt-B (solid black bars) or in binucleated cells in cultures with Cyt-B (white bars). (**B**) The level of dividing cells assessed by measuring the percentage of binucleated cell in the cytokinesis-blocked cultures. It is evident that the assay without Cyt-B underestimates the extent of genetic damage induced by MMC, particularly at doses that inhibit nuclear division. The data represent the mean ± 1 SE of three replicate cultures.

4. Nevertheless, recent studies comparing the micronucleus assay with or without cytochalasin-B suggest that if cell lines with good growth characteristics are used and culture and nuclear division conditions are optimal, it is possible to obtain comparable results between the CBMN assay and the MN assay without Cyt-B when strong clastogens are tested *(42,43)*.
5. A mathematical model of MN expression predicts (a) that scoring MN in BN cells is the most reliable way of determining micronucleus frequency and (b) scoring MN in mononucleated cells in cultures without cytokinesis block is likely to

generate false negative results when nuclear division is significantly inhibited by the chemical tested or the culture conditions do not allow an optimal number of dividing cells *(44)*.
6. Consequently, results for micronucleus frequency obtained by scoring micronuclei in mononucleated cells in cultures without Cyt-B cannot be considered conclusive, and a negative result with this system should be confirmed using the CBMN assay.

## 3.5. Molecular Techniques for Measuring Chromosome Loss in Micronuclei and Nondisjunction

To take full advantage of the ability of the CBMN assay, it is essential to distinguish between MNi originating from whole chromosomes and acentric fragments. This is best achieved by using probes that are specific for the centromeric DNA or antibodies that bind to the kinetochore proteins that are assembled at the centromeric regions of active chromosomes. The use of MN size as a discriminant is not recommended for human cells or other cell types in which the size of chromosomes is heterogenous, because a small MN may contain either a fragment of a large chromosome or a whole small chromosome. The simplest and least expensive technique to use is the antikinetochore antibody method *(45)*, but this approach does not distinguish between unique chromosomes and may not detect chromosome loss occurring due to absence of kinetochores on inactive centromeres *(46)*. The use of *in situ* hybridization (ISH) to identify centromeric regions is more expensive and laborious, but it can provide greater specificity; for example, centromeric probes for unique chromosomes can be used, which also enables the detection of nondisjunctional events (i.e., unequal distribution of homologous chromosomes in daughter nuclei) in binucleated cells *(17)*. In this chapter, only the kinetochore antibody method will be described. For details on the use of centromere detection by ISH, refer to the papers by Farooqi et al. *(17)*, Hando et al. *(18)*, Ehajouji et al. *(23,47)*, and Schuler et al. *(24)*. The types of results that can be expected with the various techniques are illustrated in **Fig. 10**.

### 3.5.1. Kinetochore Detection in MNi in the CBMN Assay

#### 3.5.1.1. SLIDE PREPARATION

1. In this technique, BN cells are accumulated as described in the standard CBMN assay, transferred to a slide using a cytocentrifuge, air-dried for 5 min, fixed in methanol for 10 min, and air-dried again.
2. At this stage, slides may either be processed immediately or stored for a maximum of 3 mo in a sealed desiccated box in a nitrogen atmosphere above liquid nitrogen.
3. For detection of kinetochores, the stored slides are removed from the nitrogen atmosphere and allowed to equilibrate at room temperature within the sealed box.

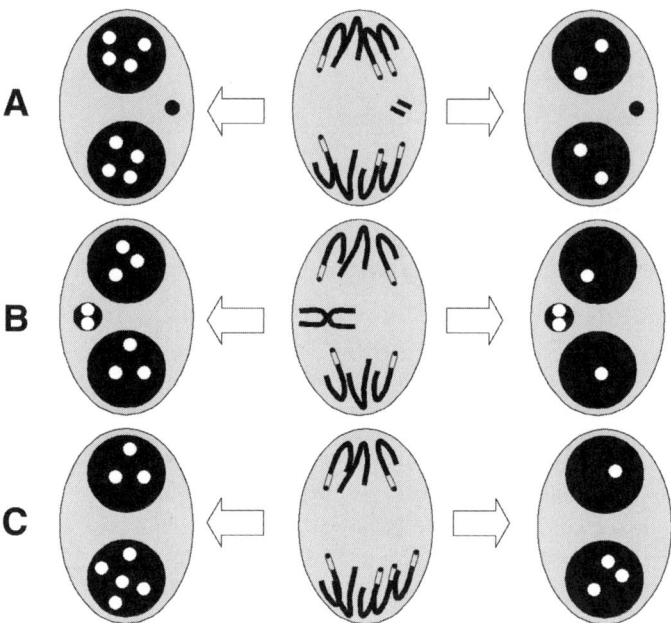

Fig. 10. The use of molecular techniques for identifying (**A**) a micronucleus originating from a lagging acentric chromosome fragment, (**B**) a micronucleus originating from a lagging whole chromosome, and (**C**) nondisjunction of a chromosome leading to aneuploid daughter nuclei. The white spots in the nuclei and micronuclei of the binucleated cells on the left of each panel show the centromeric or kinetochore pattern of staining when pancentromeric probes or kinetochore antibodies are used. The white spots in the nuclei and micronuclei of the binucleated cells on the right of each panel show the pattern of centromic staining when a centromeric probe specific to the chromosomes involved in micronucleus formation or nondisjunction events is used. The example shown is for a hypothetical cell with only two pairs of chromosomes.

3.5.1.2. Kinetochore Detection

1. The antikinetochore sera may be obtained either commercially or from an immunology clinic that has serum samples from scleroderma patients of the CREST subtype *(48)*. Use of the latter sera would require Human Ethics approval and consent from the donor patient.
2. The sera should be tested on slides of metaphase spreads of cultured cells using a rabbit FITC-conjugated secondary antihuman IgG antibody and examined by fluorescence microscopy. Only sera that appear to react exclusively with kinetochores on metaphase chromosomes should be selected for the assay.
3. The use of FITC-conjugated secondary antibody to visualize kinetochores is a direct technique but requires the use of a fluorescence microscope and nonper-

manent slide preparations; the fluorescence technique has been described in detail elsewhere *(45)*. An alternative procedure is to use an immunoperoxidase staining method that allows permanent slide preparations to be obtained *(49)*, which is more practical for routine screening and is described in the next paragraph.

4. In the immunoperoxidase technique, fixed slides are incubated overnight at 20°C in a humidity chamber with the primary antikinetochore antibody diluted 1/40 in Tris-saline buffer, pH 7.6 (6.0 g Tris-base/L saline).
5. Negative control slides are exposed to the diluted serum of a normal healthy individual.
6. The following day, the slides are washed by dipping for 30 s in the same Tris-saline buffer used to dilute the antibody.
7. Slides are then drained without drying, and incubated for 3 h with peroxidase-labeled rabbit antihuman IgG.
8. Again, slides are then drained without drying in preparation for the peroxidase histochemical reaction.
9. The histochemical method that gives best contrast is the nickel chloride/imidazole modification of the standard diaminobenzidine (DAB) reaction, which produces a black precipitate *(50,51)*.
10. The DAB reaction mixture is prepared just before use and applied immediately to slides through a 0.22-μm filter to minimize nonspecific precipitation on the slides.
11. Slides should be stained in batches, including a slide with the negative control serum.
12. The reaction is allowed to proceed for 1 min at 20°C and then stopped by draining the slides and rinsing in water.
13. The slides are then air-dried, counterstained with the nuclear stain Neutral Red (0.1% in distilled water) for 30 s, washed in water, air-dried, and mounted to give permanent preparations.

3.5.1.3. SCORING PROCEDURE

1. Scoring of kinetochore status of MNi is restricted to those binucleated cells in which a minimium of 20 kinetochores within each nucleus is observed.
2. A minimum of 100 MNi should be classified according to whether they contain kinetochores or not, and the number of kinetochores within each MN should be noted.
3. The final value for the proportion of MNi with kinetochores is determined by the formula $[P_s - P_c] / [1 - P_c]$, where $P_c$ is the proportion of MNi that has a positive peroxidase reaction in slides exposed to normal control serum and $P_s$ is the proportion of MNi that have a positive peroxidase reaction in slides exposed to antikinetochore serum.

## *3.6. Treatment Schedules for in Vitro Chemosensitivity Testing*

1. Ideally, each chemical should be tested for its genotoxic potential at the various stages of the cell cycle. Because human peripheral blood lymphocytes are in the $G_0$ phase when collected, they are ideal for assessing damage at this stage.

2. However, cells are expected to be more sensitive to genotoxic effects during S phase, $G_2$ phase, and M phase, and for this purpose it is essential to expose cell cultures when most cells are dividing. Because MN expression requires one nuclear division to be completed, the period between treatment and harvest time has to allow for this.
3. With human peripheral blood lymphocytes treated in $G_0$, it is necessary to accumulate binucleated cells as early as possible and for as long as possible, to ensure that even cells experiencing mitotic delay are examined. Typically, the standard protocol of adding Cyt-B at 44 h and harvesting cells at 72 h should suffice for this purpose. However, it is equally practical to add Cyt-B at 24 h and harvest cells at 96 h, which may maximize the number of late-dividing cells available for analysis.
4. If treatment of cells in S, $G_2$, and M phases is required, as would be the case with tumor cell cultures, then exposure to the chemical should occur during logarithmic growth phase of the culture, followed shortly afterwards with cytochalasin-B to accumulate dividing cells, and cells are then harvested between 6 and 24 h later, depending on the stage of the cell cycle that is being examined.
5. At the very early harvest times, mainly cells exposed in $G_2$ or late S phase are accumulated as binucleated cells, while at the later harvest time cells exposed in all stages of the cell cycle are blocked in the binucleate stage. Thus the harvest time relative to Cyt-B addition would affect the type of cell examined.
6. Typical schedules for use of the CBMN assay for in vitro genotoxicity testing are summarized in **Table 2**.
7. The use of a metabolic activation system such as S9 mix should be considered as an option when testing new chemicals, but this could limit the exposure period because of the possible cytotoxicity of S9 to the target cells. A better option may be the use of metabolically competent cells such as genetically modified MCL-5 cells *(52)*.

### 3.7. Future Developments

It is evident that the in vitro micronucleus assay has evolved into a robust assay for genetic damage with applications in ecotoxicology *(53)*, nutrition *(54)*, radiation sensitivity testing both for cancer risk assessment *(55)* and optimization of radiotherapy *(13,56)*, biomonitoring of human populations *(57)*, and importantly, testing of new pharmaceuticals and agrichemicals *(27,28)*. There is little doubt that there is a need for an automated scoring system for quicker and more reliable data acquisition, which would ideally be based on the scoring of slides also prepared for visual scoring—this should enable consistent results to be obtained that are not influenced by the interindividual and temporal variability of human scorers. For this goal to be achieved it is essential that scoring criteria are well developed and that a robust slide preparation protocol be put in place and that slide preparations be permanent so that they can be reexamined visually if necessary. Currently, image analysis systems have been

## Table 2
## Typical Protocols Used for Testing Micronucleus Inducion by a Chemical or Radiation

| Culture time (h) | Peripheral blood human lymphocytes | | | | Cell lines in log phase[a] |
|---|---|---|---|---|---|
| | CBMN assay $G_0$ exposure | CBMN assay $G_1/S$ exposure | CBMN assay $G_1/S/G_2/M$ exposure | CBMN/ARA assay, $G_0$ exposure | CBMN assay $G_1/S/G_2/M$ exposure |
| −4 | Add test agent | | | | Add test agent |
| 0 | Add PHA | Add PHA | Add PHA | Add test agent (1) Add PHA (2) Add ARA | Add Cyt-B |
| 16 | | | | (1) wash out ARA (2) fresh medium with IL-2 and DC | |
| 20 | | Add test agent | | | |
| 24 | | | | | Harvest cells |
| 44 | Add Cyt-B[b] | Add Cyt-B[b] | Add test agent | Add Cyt-B[b] | Harvest cells |
| 48 | | | Add Cyt-B | | |
| 72 | Harvest cells | Harvest cells | Harvest cells | Harvest cells | |
| 96 | Harvest cells | Harvest cells | Harvest cells | Harvest cells | |

The proposed protocols assume that the test agent is retained in the culture medium even after Cyt-B is added. However, it may also be desirable to remove test chemical by replacing culture medium (1) after a brief exposure period to test chemical or (2) just prior to addition of Cyt-B. In the latter case, IL-2 should be added to fresh medium for lymphocyte cultures. ARA = cytosine arabinoside; Cyt-B = cytochalasin-B; DC = deoxycytidine; IL-2 = interleukin-2; PHA = phytohemagglutinin. [a]This treatment schedule is most appropriate for testing chemosensitivity in tumor cell cultures. [b]Alternatively, Cyt-B could be added at 24 h.

developed for automated scoring of micronuclei in mammalian cells *(58–62)*, but these systems do not take account of other important events such as necrosis, apoptosis, and cytostasis, which are essential for the correct interpretation of the result obtained *(26)*. In the future we should expect to have an automated system that can score reliably the various end points possible with the cytokinesis-block micronucleus assay outlined in this chapter.

Finally, it is also essential to keep abreast of more recent developments in our understanding of micronucleus formation and events that may alter expression of this end point. Some notable examples are (a) the formation of micronuclei as a result of gene amplification in which the cell eliminates excess amplified DNA directly from the nucleus, during S phase, into a micronucleus produced by nuclear budding *(63,64)*; (b) the use of the cytokinesis-block micronucleus assay to measure breakage–fusion–bridge cycles that are the one of the hallmarks of genomic instability in preneoplastic cells and folate deficient cells *(64,65)*, (c) the observation that treatment with specific mitotic spindle inhibitors may cause mitotic slippage leading to polyploid nuclei and micronuclei and therefore implicating that it may be useful to score not only MNi in binucleated cells but also MNi in mononucleated cells in cytokinesis-blocked cultures *(47)*, and (d) the possible elimination of micronucleated cells and micronuclei by apoptosis *(66,67)*. Furthermore, scoring criteria in the cytokinesis-block micronucleus assay are continually being reviewed as part of the activity of the HUMN project (www.humn.org), and a more comprehensive and recommended description of scoring criteria with photomicrographs has been published recently *(68)*.

All of the above points to the fact that the full potential of the in vitro cytokinesis-block micronucleus assay is readily achievable once all the morphological end points of cytotoxicity, cytostasis, and DNA damage are integrated into the system.

## 4. Notes

1. In our experience, most of the problems in the CBMN assay arise during slide preparation and staining. This is because the quality of the score depends on the quality of the slide. Main points to note: (a) avoid cell clumps by gently resuspending cells prior to harvest and transfer to slides; (b) maintain a moderate cell density so that it is relatively easy to identify cytoplasmic boundaries; (c) stain only one slide initially, to ensure that staining is optimal before staining the whole batch.
2. The use of duplicate cultures is critical for producing robust results also because it allows the measurement of the intraexperimental coefficient of variation. Cytogenetic assays should be subject to the same rigor as analytical assays, which typically reject duplicate results with a CV greater than 10%. Because of the visual scoring, greater latitude in the acceptable CV is understandable. In our experience and the results of international interlaboratory scoring comparison *(69)*, CVs greater than 40% are not acceptable for baseline data, and with radiation-exposed cultures in which more than 100 MN per 1000 BN cells are induced, CVs less than 20% are expected.
3. Scores from inexperienced personnel (e.g., students, new staff) should not be relied on until they are able to achieve acceptable CVs (no greater than 40%) for repeat scores of standard control slides.
4. Interscorer variability is one of the key sources of variation in the micronucleus assay *(69)*. It is therefore essential that the same scorers are maintained throughout a single study and ideally two scorers are used, each providing a count from each of the duplicate cultures and their mean values calculated as indicated in **Fig. 2**. An alternative approach is to calibrate scorers by using a common set of

standard slides with "low," "medium," and "high" MN frequencies. The scores of each scorer on the standard slides can then be used to calculate a corrected value. The latter approach is still in development but worth noting as an option, because it can take account of differences in the visual capacity of scorers within the same laboratory and between laboratories.
5. Another important source of variability between scorers and between laboratories is the quality of the microscopes and their optics. In our experience, scoring of nucleoplasmic bridges is influenced by the quality of the microscope, because fine bridges can be missed with low-quality optics. The main issue here is for scorers to avoid switching microscopes during experiments, and for the laboratory manager to upgrade the optics of the microscopes to a uniform and high level whenever possible.
6. One of the most common questions is the number of BN cells to be scored in the CBMN assay. The accepted protocol is to score a minimum of 1000 BN cells per treatment or time point, although reports vary between 500 and 2000 BN cells. An alternative approach is to keep on scoring BN cells until a fixed number of micronuclei are observed (e.g., 45 micronuclei). The latter has the advantage that more BN cells are scored when fewer MNi are induced, thus maintaining similar statistical power across different treatments. The main disadvantage is that more than 2000 cells may have to be scored in cultures with low MN frequency. In our experience, scoring 1000 BN cells from each of the duplicate cultures always yields robust results.
7. With respect to scoring slides, it is best first to score the frequency of mononucleated, binucleated, multinucleated, apoptotic, and necrotic cells to determine the NDI and NDCI indices. Then focus on scoring binucleated cells for the presence of micronuclei, nucleoplasmic bridges, and nuclear buds to determine the genome damage rate.
8. It should be noted that the use of nuclear buds within the CBMN assay is expected to increase because of the consistent significant relationship of this biomarker of gene amplification with nucleoplasmic bridges and micronuclei *(64)*. It is therefore recommended that nuclear buds be scored. In our experience, the expression of this biomarker may be more prevalent following long-term exposure (>3 d) to a genotoxic agent, which is consistent with the notion that it may take three or more nuclear divisions for breakage–fusion–bridge cycles to generate sufficient amplified DNA to be eliminated by nuclear budding.
9. When scoring nucleoplasmic bridges in binucleated cells, it is important to note that the score may depend on the frequency of binucleated cells with nuclei that touch or overlap. This is because nucleoplasmic bridges are more likely to be visible in binucleated cells, in which the nuclei are clearly separated from each other.
10. In maximizing the number of cytokinesis-blocked binucleated cells by increasing exposure time to cytochalasin-B, there is the risk of also increasing the proportion of cytokinesis-blocked multinucleated cells that arise from binucleated cells that attempt another nuclear division while cytokinesis-blocked. Ideally, the proportion of binucleated among cytokinesis-blocked cell should be in excess of 80%. The

proportion of binucleated cells among all cells will depend on the proportion of dividing cells in the culture. The latter depends on the cell line or tumor cells and the culture conditions.

## Acknowledgments

The development of the cytokinesis-block micronucleus assay was the result of research performed at the Medical School of the Flinders University of South Australia in Prof. Alec Morley's laboratory and CSIRO Health Sciences and Nutrition with the support of the Anti-Cancer Foundation of the Universities of South Australia. I would also like to acknowledge the important role of Ms. J. Rinaldi, Ms. C. Aitken, Ms. S. Neville, Ms. J. Turner, Ms. F. Bulman, Ms. C. Salisbury, Mr. P. Thomas, Mr. J.Crott, Ms. S. Brown, and Mr. W. Greenrod, who have contributed significantly to the more recent research effort. Prof. Micheline Kirsch-Volders and Prof. Wushou P. Chang are thanked for critically reading the manuscript and for their constructive suggestions.

## References

1. Evans, H. J. (1977) Molecular mechanisms in the induction of chromosome aberrations, in *Progress in Genetic Toxicology* (Scott, D., Bridges, B. A., and Sobels, F. H., eds.), Elsevier North Holland Biomedical, Amsterdam, pp. 57–74.
2. Savage, J. R. K. (1993) Update on target theory as applied to chromosomal aberrations. *Environ. Mol. Mutagen.* **22**, 198–207.
3. Evans, H. J. (1990) Cytogenetics: overview. *Prog. Clin. Biol. Res.* **340B,** 301–323.
4. Dellarco, V. L., Mavournin, K. H., and Tice, R. R. (1985) Aneuploidy and health risk assessment: current status and future directions. *Environ. Mutagen.* **7,** 405–424.
5. Guttenbach, M. and Schmid, M. (1994) Exclusion of specific human chromosomes into micronuclei by 5-azacytidine treatment of lymphocyte cultures. *Exp. Cell Res.* **211,** 127–132.
6. Natarajan, A. T. and Obe, G. (1982) Mutagenicity testing with cultured mammalian cells: cytogenetic assays, in *Mutagenicity: New Horizons in Genetic Toxicology (Heddle, J. A., ed.), Academic Press, New York, pp. 171–213.*
7. Schmid, W. (1975) The micronucleus test. *Mutation Res.* **31,** 9–15.
8. Heddle, J. A. (1973) A rapid *in vivo* test for chromosome damage. *Mutation Res.* **18,** 187–192.
9. Fenech, M. and Morley, A. A. (1985) Solutions to the kinetic problem in the micronucleus assay. *Cytobios* **43,** 233–246.
10. Fenech, M. and Morley, A. A. (1985) Measurement of micronuclei in lymphocytes. *Mutation Res.* **147,** 29–36.
11. Fenech, M. and Morley, A. A. (1986) Cytokinesis-block micronucleus method in human lymphocytes: effect of *in vivo* ageing and low-dose x-irradiation. *Mutation Res.* **161,** 193–198.

12. Carter, S. B. (1967) Effects of cytochalasins on mammalian cells. *Nature* **213,** 261–264.
13. Masunaga, S., Ono, K., and Abe, M. (1991) A method for the selective measurement of the radiosensitivity of quiescent cells in solid tumors—combination of immunofluorescence staining to BrdU and micronucleus assay. *Radiation Res.* **125,** 243–247.
14. Odagiri, Y., Takemoto, K., and Fenech, M. (1994) Micronucleus induction in cytokinesis-blocked mouse bone-marrow cells *in vitro* following *in vivo* exposure to X-irradiation and cyclophosphamide. *Env. Mol. Mutagen.* **24,** 61–67.
15. Degrassi, F. and Tanzarella, C. (1988) Immunofluorescent staining of kinetochores in micronuclei: a new assay for the detection of aneuploidy. *Mutation Res.* **203,** 339–345.
16. Thompson, E. J. and Perry, P. (1988) The identification of micronucleated chromosomes: a possible assay for aneuploidy. *Mutagenesis* **3,** 415–418.
17. Farooqi, Z., Darroudi, F., and Natarajan, A. T. (1993) Use of fluorescence in situ hybridisation for the detection of aneugens in cytokinesis-blocked mouse splenocytes. *Mutagenesis* **8,** 329–334.
18. Hando, J. C., Nath, J., and Tucker, J. D. (1994) Sex chromosomes, micronuclei and aging in women. *Chromosoma* **103,** 186–192.
19. Parry, E. M., Henderson, L., and Mackay, J. M. (1995) Guidelines for testing of chemicals. Procedures for the detection of chemically induced aneuploidy: recommendations of a UK Environmental Mutagen Society working group. *Mutagenesis* **10(1),** 1–14.
20. Elhajouji, A., Van Hummellen, P., and Kirsch-Volders, M. (1995) Indications for a threshold of chemically induced aneuploidy in vitro in human lymphocytes. *Environ. Mol. Mutagen.* **26,** 292–304.
21. Fenech, M. and Neville, S. (1992) Conversion of excision-repairable DNA lesions to micronuclei within one cell cycle in human lymphocytes. *Environ. Mol. Mutagen.* **19(1),** 27–36.
22. Zijno, A., Marcon, F., Leopardi, P., and Crebelli, R. (1994) Simultaneous detection of X-chromosome loss and non-disjunction in cytokinesis-blocked human lymphocytes by in situ hybridisation with a centromeric DNA probe; implications for the human lymphocyte *in vitro* micronucleus assay using cytochalasin-B. *Mutagenesis* **9(3),** 225–232.
23. Elhajouji, A., Tibaldi, F., and Kirsch-Volders, M. (1997) Indication for thresholds of chromosome non-disjunction versus chromosome lagging induced by spindle inhibitors in vitro in human lymphocytes. *Mutagenesis* **12,** 33–140.
24. Schuler, M., Rupa, D. S., and Eastmond, D. A. (1997) A critical evaluation of centromeric labelling to distinguish micronuclei induced by chromosomal loss and breakage *in vitro*. *Mutation Res.* **392,** 81–5.
25. Kirsch-Volders, M., Elhajouji, A., Cundari, E., and Van Hummelen, P. (1997) The *in vitro* micronucleus test: a multi-end-point assay to detect simultaneously mitotic delay, apoptosis, chromosome breakage, chromosome loss and non-disjunction. *Mutation Res.* **392,** 19–30.

26. Fenech, M., Crott, J., Turner, J., and Brown, S. (1999) Necrosis, apoptosis, cytostasis and DNA damage in human lymphocytes measured simultaneously within the cytokinesis-block micronucleus assay: description of the method and results for hydrogen peroxide. *Mutagenesis* **14(6),** 605–612.
27. Kirsch-Volders, M. (ed.) (1997) The CB *in vitro* micronucleus assay in human lymphocytes. Special Issue. *Mutation Res.* **392(1, 2).**
28. Kirsch-Volders, M., Sofuni, T., Aardema, M., et al. (2000) Report from the *in vitro* micronucleus assay working group, Washington International Workshop on Genotoxicity Test Procedures, 25–26 March 1999.
29. Atencia, R., Garciasanz, M., Perezyarza, G., Asumendi, A., Hilario, E., and Arechaga, J. (1997) A structural analysis of cytoskeletal components during the execution phase of apoptosis. *Protoplasma* **198,** 163–169.
30. Eastmond, D. A. and Tucker, J. D. (1989) Identification of aneuploidy-inducing agents using cytokinesis-blocked human lymphocytes and an antikinetochore antibody. *Environ. Mol. Mutagen.* **13(1),** 34–43.
31. Fenech, M., Rinaldi, J., and Surrales, J. (1994) The origin of micronuclei induced by cytosine arabinoside and its synergistic interaction with hydroxyurea in human lymphocytes. *Mutagenesis* **9(3),** 273–277.
32. Surrales, J., Xamena, N., Creus, A., and Morcos, R. (1995) The suitability of the micronucleus assay in human lymphocytes as a new biomarker of excision repair. *Mutation Res.* **341(1–2),** 43–59.
33. Surralles, J., Carbonell, E., Marcos, R., Degrassi, F., Antoccia, A., and Tanzarella, C. (1992) A collaborative study on the improvement of the micronucleus test in cultured human lymphocytes. *Mutagenesis* **7(6),** 407–410.
34. Fenech, M. F., Dunaiski, V., Osborne, Y., and Morley, A. A. (1991) The cytokinesis-block micronucleus assay as a biological dosimeter in spleen and peripheral blood lymphocytes in the mouse following acute whole body irradiation. *Mutation Res.* **263,** 119–126.
35. Heddle, J. A., Bouch, A., Khan, M. A., and Gingerich, J. D. (1990) Concurrent detection of gene mutations and chromosomal aberrations induced *in vivo* in somatic cells. *Mutagenesis* **5(2),** 179–184.
36. He, S. and Baker, R. S. U. (1989) Initiating carcinogen, triethylenemelamine, induces micronuclei in skin target cells. *Environ. Mol. Mutagen.* **14(1),** 1–5.
37. Wakata, A. and Sasaki, M. S. (1987) Measurement of micronuclei by cytokinesis-block method in cultured Chinese hamster cells: comparison with types and rates of chromosome aberrations. *Mutation Res.* **190,** 51–57.
38. Prosser, J. S., Moquet, J. E., Lloyd, D. C., and Edwards, A. A. (1988) Radiation induction of micronuclei in human lymphocytes. *Mutation Res.* **199,** 37–45.
39. Lindholm, C., Norrpa, H., Hayashi, M., and Sorsa, M. (1991) Induction of micronuclei and anaphase aberrations by cytochalasin-B in human lymphocyte cultures. *Mutation Res.* **260,** 369–375.
40. Minissi, S., Gustavino, B., Degrassi, F., Tanzarella, C., and Rizzoni, M. (1999) Effect of cytochalasin-B on the induction of chromosome missegregation by colchicine at low concentrations in human lymphocytes. *Mutagenesis* **14,** 43–49.

41. Fenech, M. (1997) The advantages and disadvantages of the cytokinesis-block micronucleus method. *Mutation Res.* **392,** 11–18.
42. Kalweit, S., Utesch, D., von der Hude, W., and Madle, S. (1999) Chemically induced micronucleus formation in V79 cells—comparison of three different test procedures. *Mutation Res.* **439(2),** 183–190.
43. Matsushima, T., Hayashi, M., Matsuoka, A., et al. (1999) Validation study of the *in vitro* micronucleus test in a Chinese hamster lung cell line (CHL/IU). *Mutagenesis* **14(6),** 569–580.
44. Fenech, M. (2000) Mathematical model of the *in vitro* micronucleus assay predicts false negative results if micronuclei are not scored specifically in binucleated cells or cells that have completed one nuclear division. *Mutagenesis* **15(4),** 329–336.
45. Vig, B. K. and Swearngin, S. E. (1986) Sequence of centromere separation: kinetochore formation in induced laggards and micronuclei. *Mutagenesis* **1,** 464–465.
46. Earnshaw, W. C. and Migeon, B. R. (1985) Three related centromere proteins are absent from the inactive centromere of a stable dicentric chromosome. *Chromosoma* **92,** 290–296.
47. Elhajouji, A., Cunha, M., and Kirsch-Volders, M. (1998) Spindle poisons can induce polyploidy by mitotic slippage and micronucleate mononucleates in the cytokinesis-block assay. *Mutagenesis* **13(2),** 193–198.
48. Moroi, Y., Hartman, A. L., Nakane, P. K., and Tan, E. M. (1981) Distribution of kinetochore antigen in mammalian cell nuclei. *J. Cell Biol.* **90,** 254–259.
49. Fenech, M. and Morley, A. A. (1989) Kinetochore detection in micronuclei: an alternative method for measuring chromosome loss. *Mutagenesis* **4(2),** 98–104.
50. Straus, W. (1982) Imidazole increases the sensitivity of the cytochemical reaction for peroxidase with diaminobenzidine at neutral pH. *J. Histochem. Cytochem.* **30,** 491–493.
51. Scopsi, I. and Larsson, L. I. (1986) Increased sensitivity in peroxidase immunochemistry. A comparative study of a number of peroxidase visualisation methods employing a model system. *Histochemistry* **84,** 221–230.
52. White, N. H., de Matteis, F., Davies, A., et al. (1992) Genotoxic potential of tamoxifen and analogues in female Fischer F344/n rats, DBA/2 and C57BL/6 mice and in human MCL-5 cells. *Carcinogenesis* **13(12),** 2197–2203.
53. Gauthier, J. M., Dubeau, H., Rassart, E., Jarman, W. M., and Wells, R. S. (1999) Biomarkers of DNA damage in marine mammals. *Mutation Res.* **444(2),** 427–439.
54. Fenech, M. and Rinaldi, J. (1995) A comparison of lymphocyte micronuclei and plasma micronutrients in vegetarians and non-vegetarians. *Carcinogenesis* **16(2),** 223–230
55. Scott, D., Barber, J. P. B., Levine, E. L., Burrill, W., and Roberts, S. A. (1998) Radiation-induced micronucleus induction in lymphocytes identifies a high frequency of radiosensitive cases among breast cancer patients: a test for predisposition? *Br. J. Cancer* **77(4),** 614–620.
56. Shibamoto, Y., Streffer, C., Fuhrmann, C., and Budach, V. (1991) Tumor radiosensitivity prediction by the cytokinesis-block micronucleus assay. *Radiation Res.* **128,** 293–300.

57. Fenech, M., Holland, N., Chang, W. P., Zeiger, E., and Bonassi, S. (1999) The Human MicroNucleus Project—An international collaborative study on the use of the micronucleus technique for measuring DNA damage in humans. *Mutation Res.* **428,** 271–283.
58. Tates, A. N., van Welie, M. T., and Ploem, J. S. (1990) The present state of the automated micronucleus test for lymphocytes. *Int. J. Radiat. Biol.* **58,** 813–825.
59. Castelain, P., Van Hummelen, P., Deleneer, A., and Kirsch-Volders, M. (1993) Automated detection of cytochalasin-B blocked binucleated lymphocytes for scoring micronuclei. *Mutagenesis* **8(4),** 285–293.
60. Bocker, W., Muller, W. U., and Streffer, C. (1995) Image processing algorithms for the automated micronucleus assay in binucleated human lymphocytes. *Cytometry* **19(4),** 283–294.
61. Frieauff, W., Potterlocher, F., Cordier, A., and Suter, W. (1998) Automatic analysis of the *in vitro* micronucleus test on V79 cells. *Mutation Res.* **413(1),** 57–68.
62. Verhaegen, F., Vral, A., Seuntjens, J., Schipper, N. W., de Ridder, L., and Thierens, H. (1994) Scoring of radiation-induced micronuclei in cytokinesis-blocked human lymphocytes by automated image analysis. *Cytometry* **17,** 119–127.
63. Shimizu, N., Itoh, N., Utiyama, H., and Wahl, G. M. (1998) Selective entrapment of extrachromosomally amplified DNA by nuclear budding and micronucleation during S phase. *J. Cell Biol.* **140,** 1307–1320.
64. Fenech, M. and Crott, J. W. (2002) Micronuclei, nucleoplasmic bridges and nuclear buds induced in folic acid deficient human lymphocytes—evidence for breakage-fusion-bridge cycles in the cytokinesis-block micronucleus assay. *Mutation Res.* **504(1–2),** 131–136.
65. Fenech, M. (2002) Chromosomal biomarkers of genomic instability relevant to cancer. *Drug Discovery Today* **7(22),** 1128–1137.
66. Unger, C., Kress, S., Buchmann, A., and Schwarz, M. (1994) Gamma-irradiation-induced micronuclei from mouse hepatoma cells accumulate high levels of the tumor suppressor protein p53. *Cancer Res.* **54(14),** 3651–3655.
67. Sablina, A. A., Ilyinskaya, G. V., Rubtsova, S. N., Agapova, L. S., Chumakov, P. M., and Kopnin, B. P. (1998) Activation of p53-mediated cell cycle checkpoint in reponse to micronuclei formation. *J. Cell Sci.* **111,** 977–984.
68. Fenech, M., Chang, W. P., Kirsch-Volders, M., Holland, N., Bonassi, S., and Zeiger, E. (2003) HUMN project: detailed description of the scoring criteria for the cytokinesis-block micronucleus assay using isolated human lymphocyte cultures. *Mutation Res.* **534(1–2),** 65–75.
69. Fenech, M., Bonassi, S., Turner, J., et al. (2003) Intra- and inter-laboratory variation in the scoring of micronuclei and nucleoplasmic bridges in binucleated human lymphocytes. Results of an international slide-scoring exercise by the HUMN project. *Mutation Res.* **534(1–2),** 45–64.
70. Shimizu, N., Itoh, N., Utiyama, H., and Wahl, G. M. (1988) Selective entrapment of extrachromasomally amplified DNA b, nuclear budding and micronucleation during S phase. *J. Cell Biol.* **140(6),** 1307–1320.

# 2

## Cell Cycle and Drug Sensitivity

### Aslamuzzaman Kazi and Q. Ping Dou

#### Summary

Induction of tumor cell death by chemotherapeutic modalities often occurs in a cell cycle–dependent manner. It has also been observed that several regulatory proteins involved in tumor chemosensitivity and apoptosis are expressed periodically during the cell cycle progression. However, the nature of cancer cellular chemosensitivity and mechanisms of action of anticancer drugs in different phases of the cell cycle still remain unknown. In this chapter we describe two methods (serum deprivation and pharmacological drug treatment) to synchronize human tumor cells in specific phases of the cell cycle, followed by induction of cell death by anticancer drugs. We also descrbi three methods (flow cytometry, Western blot, and DNA fragmentation) to measure the cell cycle-associated cytotoxic effects of chemotherapeutic agents.

#### Key Words

Cell synchronization; serum deprivation; cell cycle; flow cytometry; chemosensitivity; chemotherapeutic agents; apoptosis; cell death.

### 1. Introduction

The cell proliferation process is tightly controlled in normal mammalian cells, but disregulated in cancer cells *(1)*. There are four broad phases of the cell cycle: $G_1$ (and $G_0$) (regulatory phase prior to beginning replication), S (phase of active replication), $G_2$ (regulatory phase prior to beginning mitosis), and M (mitotic phase). Progression of the cell cycle is regulated by interactions of growth-stimulatory and -inhibitory proteins. By working together, these proteins tell the cell when to grow and divide and when to stop *(1)*. The cell cycle regulatory proteins include cyclins, the cyclin-dependent kinases (CDKs), the CDK inhibitors, the tumor suppressor proteins (i.e., the retinoblastoma protein, p53) and transcription factors (i.e., E2F family members).

Cell numbers are regulated by balanced cell proliferation and cell death processes. Indeed, proper cellular regulation requires an accurate coordination, or cross-talk, between these two processes. Disregulated expression of cell cycle proteins can trigger programmed cell death or apoptosis. For example, overexpression of the transcription factor E2F is able to induce inappropriate S-phase entry and subsequent apoptosis (2,3). Disruption of RB function can also lead to a similar demise (4). On the other hand, several cell death–regulatory proteins, such as Bcl-2, Bax, and p53, are expressed in a cell cycle–dependent manner (5–8), indicating that chemosensitivity of tumor cells might be periodic. Consistent with this prediction, many chemotherapeutic agents act in a cell cycle–specific fashion. It has been found that the in vivo sensitivity of some tumor cells to several chemotherapeutic drugs correlated to the size of the S-phase population (9,10). The topoisomerase II inhibitor VP-16 can also block cells in S phase and subsequently induce apoptosis (11). In addition, cancer-preventative agents can also induce apoptosis from S-phase tumor cells (12–14). When S-phase Jurkat T-cells were treated with the green tea polyphenol (–)-epigallocatechin, progression to $G_2/M$ phase was blocked, followed by induction of apoptosis (12). It should be noted that $G_1$ cells could be most sensitive to induction of apoptosis under some experimental conditions (7,15,16). Therefore, knowing how to synchronize tumor cells to various phases of cell cycle is essential for studying the nature of cancer cellular chemosensitivity and mechanisms of action of anticancer drugs. In this chapter we introduce methods for cell synchronization, cell cycle analysis, anticancer drug treatment, and cell death measurement.

## 2. Materials
### 2.1. Cell Culture

1. Appropriate complete tissue culture medium, for example, RPMI-1640, 10% fetal calf serum (FCS), 100-U/mL penicillin, and 100-µg/mL streptomycin (Life Technologies) for human leukemia Jurkat T-cells and prostate cancer LNCaP cells. Store at 4°C.
2. 1× Trypsin-EDTA: 0.05% trypsin, 0.53 m$M$ EDTA.4Na (Life Technologies).
3. 1× phosphate-buffered saline (PBS): 8 g NaCl, 0.2 g KCl, 0.2 g $KH_2PO_4$, and 1.15 g $Na_2HPO_4$ in 1 L double-distilled water (dd$H_2O$). Adjust pH to 7.2, autoclave at 121°C (15 psi) for 15 min, and store at room temperature (see **Note 1**).
4. Tissue culture flasks (e.g., T-25, T-75; Nunc) or dishes (e.g., 100-mm, 60-mm; Nunc).
5. 15-mL and 50-mL conical tubes (Corning).
6. Incubator: 37°C with 5% $CO_2$.

### 2.2. Cell Cycle Synchronization

1. Lovastatin (arrest cells in early $G_1$ phase).
2. Mimosine (arrest cells in late $G_1$ phase).

3. Aphidocolin (arrest cells in $G_1/S$ boundary phase).
4. Hydroxyurea (arrest cells in early S phase).
5. Nocodazole (arrest cells in $G_2$ or M phase).

## 2.3. Cell Cycle Analysis

1. Propidium iodide (PI): 1 mg/mL PI in $ddH_2O$ (called 20X PI solution). Light-sensitive. Store at 4°C.
2. RNase A: 1000 U/mL in $ddH_2O$ (called 10X RNase A). Prepare freshly just before use.
3. Sample buffer: 1 mg/mL glucose in 1X PBS (without $Ca^{2+}$ and $Mg^{2+}$). Store at 4°C.

## 2.4. Protein Extraction and Measurement

1. Whole-cell lysis buffer: 50 m$M$ Tris-HCl (pH 8.0), 5 m$M$ EDTA (pH 8.0), 150 m$M$ NaCl, 0.5% Nonidet P-40, 0.5 m$M$ phenylmethylsulfonyl fluoride (PMSF) (add fresh before use), and 0.5 m$M$ dithiothreitol. Can be store at 4°C for up to 1 mo.
2. 2X sodium dodecyl sulfate (SDS) sample buffer: For example, to prepare 10 mL, you need 1.43 mL of 1 $M$ Tris-HCl (pH 6.8), 4.57 mL of 10% SDS, 2.29 mL of 100% glycerol, 0.11 mL of 1% bromophenol blue, and 1.60 mL of $ddH_2O$. Make aliquots and store at –20°C. Store short-term at 4°C. Add 60 µL of 2-merchaptoethanol β-mercaptoethanol) (Sigma, cat. no. M3148) into 1 mL of 2X SDS sample buffer before use.
3. Protein assay: Bio-Rad Protein Assay Dye Reagent Concentrate (Bio-Rad, cat. no. 500-0006).

## 2.5. SDS-PAGE

1. Acrylamide solution: purchased as a ready-mixed 40% acrylamide/bis (AB) solution, 29:1 (Bio-Rad, cat. no. 161-0146).
2. Ammonium persulfate (AP) (Bio-Rad, cat. no. 161-0700): 10% solution prepared freshly using $ddH_2O$.
3. Running gel: For example, to prepare 18 mL of 15% gel solution, you need 4.75 mL of $ddH_2O$, 6.75 mL of 40% acrylamide/bis solution, 6.50 mL of 1 $M$ Tris-HCl (pH 8.8), 175 µL of 10% SDS, 200 µL of 10% AP, and 20 µL of N,N,N′, N-tetramethyl-ethylenediamine (TEMED) (Bio-Rad, cat. no. 161-0801).
4. Stacking gel: For example, to prepare 8 mL of 3% gel solution, you need 6.2 mL of $ddH_2O$, 0.6 mL of 40% acrylamide/Bis solution, 1.0 mL of 1 $M$ Tris-HCl (pH 6.8), 80 µL of 10% SDS, 100 µL of 10% AP, and 12 µL of TEMED.
5. 5X electrode buffer: 144 g glycine, 30.25 g Tris base and 10 g SDS in 2-liter $ddH_2O$. Dilute to 1X with $ddH_2O$ before use.
6. Semidry transfer buffer: 3.75 mL 10% SDS, 5.82 g Tris base, 2.93 g glycine, 200 mL methanol (analytical grade). Make the volume up to 1 L using $ddH_2O$. Store at room temperature in a sealed container.
7. Protein blotting membrane: Pure nitrocellulose blotting membranes (PALL Life Science). Cut to the size of gels.

8. Filter paper: Whatman 3 MM filter paper, cut to the same size of blotting membranes.
9. Enhanced chemiluminescence (ECL) system (Amersham): The protein bands are visualized with 1:1 ratio of the ECL, according to the manufacturer's instruction.
10. 1X PBS-T: 200 mL 10X PBS, 1798 mL ddH$_2$O, and 2 mL Tween-20.
11. Blocking buffer: 5 g nonfat dry milk in 100 mL 1X PBS-Tween-20.

## 2.6. DNA Extraction and Gel Electrophoresis

1. Lysis buffer: 20 m$M$ Tris-HCl (pH 7.4), 10 m$M$ EDTA (pH 8.0), 0.2% Triton-X.
2. Tris-EDTA (TE) buffer (pH 8.0): 10 m$M$ Tris-HCl (pH 8.0), 1 m$M$ EDTA (pH 8.0), and ddH$_2$O. Autoclave and store at 4°C.
3. 50X TAE buffer (electrophoresis buffer): 242 g Tris base, 57.1 mL glacial acetic acid, 100 mL 0.5 $M$ EDTA (pH 8.0), and make the final volume up to 1 L using ddH$_2$O. Autoclave and preserve at room temperature. Before use, dilute to 1X using ddH$_2$O.
4. Proteinase K (DNase-free) (*see* **Note 2**).
5. RNase A (DNase-free) (*see* **Note 2**).
6. Phenol (molecular-biology grade).
7. Chlorophorm (molecular-biology grade).
8. Isopropanol (molecular-biology grade).
9. 5 $M$ NaCl.
10. 70% ethanol in ddH$_2$O.
11. Ethidium bromide (*see* **Note 3**).
12. Bromophenol blue (BPB) loading buffer (0.25% BPB + 40% sucrose).
13. Agarose (DNA-grade).
14. Lambda DNA marker (available from Promega).

## 2.7. Equipment

1. Spectrophotometer.
2. Hemocytometer.
3. Water bath.
4. Labtop centrifuge machine.
5. Electric heating block with Eppendorf tube adaptor.
6. Vertical and horizontal gel electrophoresis apparatus (Pharmacia Biotech) and power supply (Life Technologies).
7. Blotting apparatus and power supply: e.g., Trans-blot SD Semi-Dry Transfer Cell (Bio-Rad); VWR 570 power supply.
8. Flow cytometer.
9. Gel-application disposable tips.
10. Rocking apparatus.
11. pH meter.
12. Micropipet and disposable tips.
13. Refrigerator and freezer.
14. Biosafety cabinet.

## 3. Methods

### 3.1. Cell Synchronization

To date, various methods have been developed to synchronize cells, such as serum or growth factor deprivation, contact inhibition, use of pharmacological agents, mitotic selection, use of cell cycle mutants, and centrifugal elutriation. Each of these methods has its advantages and disadvantages. Serum deprivation or pharmacological inhibitors are two most commonly used techniques for synchronization of mammalian cells. We therefore describe these two methods here (*see* **Note 4**).

#### 3.1.1. Serum Deprivation

1. Cells are cultured in complete medium to log phase in 25- or 75-cm$^2$ tissue culture flasks (in case of cells growing in suspension) or ~approx 70–80% confluence in 60- or 100-mm tissue culture dishes (in case of attached cells).
2. Remove the medium, and wash cells three times with medium alone (without serum).
3. Reincubate the cells with serum-free media for 48–96 h (*see* **Note 5**).
4. Remove the serum-free (or low-serum-containing) medium and stimulate the cells to proliferate (time 0) by the addition of 10% FBS-containing medium (complete medium) for different hours in order to have synchronized cells in other phases of the cell cycle.

#### 3.1.2. Synchronization by Pharmacological Agents (see **Note 6**)

1. Same as described in **step 1** under **Subheading 3.1.1.**
2. Remove the medium and wash cells once with 1X PBS (pH 7.2).
3. Reincubate the cells with fresh complete medium containing a pharmacological agent at a defined concentration (e.g., 5 µg/mL Aphidicolin for MCF-7 cells) for 24–36 h (under aphidicolin treatment, MCF-7 cells become arrested in $G_1/S$ phase) (*see* **Note 7**).
4. Remove the pharmacological agent-containing medium and wash the cells twice with sterile 1X PBS (pH 7.2) and stimulate the cells to proliferate (time 0) by the addition of fresh complete medium for different hours in order to have synchronized cells in other phases of the cell cycle.

#### 3.1.3. Cell Cycle Analysis by Flow Cytometry

1. Harvest, and count about 2–5 × 10$^6$ cells at each time point. Attached cells will be harvested through trypsinization.
2. Centrifugation at 150*g* for 5 min at 4°C and remove the medium.
3. Wash the cells with 1 mL ice-cold PBS (pH 7.2) twice by centrifugation at 150*g* for 5 min at 4°C.
4. Dissolve the pellet gently and completely with 1 mL of ice-cold PBS (pH 7.2) (*see* **Note 8**).

5. Add the suspended cells dropwise to 5 mL of ice-cold 70% ethanol while vortexing at low speed to avoid clumping.
6. Fix the cells at least 2 h (or overnight) at –20°C. Cells can be kept in cell fixation solution for up to 3 mo at 4°C.
7. Prepare PI staining solution (*see* **Note 9**).
8. Centrifuge the fixed cells at 150*g* for 5 min at 4°C.
9. Carefully remove the supernatant without disturbing the pellet.
10. Dry the pellet by inverting the tube on a sheet of filter paper.
11. Add 1 mL of PI staining solution and dissolve the pellet gently by micropipet. Cells can be kept in PI stain for up to 1 wk at 4°C.
12. Transfer the cell solution into a plastic polystyrene, round-bottom tube (12 × 75 mm) (Becton Dickinson Labware).
13. Incubate the cells at room temperature for 30 min in the dark.
14. Analyze the cells by flow cytometry (within 2 h of staining).

### 3.1.4. Measurement of Cell Cycle Regulatory Proteins by Western Blot Assay

1. Harvest cells at each time point. (Attached cells will be harvested by scraping.)
2. Remove the medium by centrifugation at 200*g* for 5 min at 4°C.
3. Dissolve the pellet gently with 1 mL of ice-cold PBS (pH 7.2), transfer to an Eppendorf tube, and centrifugation at 200*g* for 5 min at 4°C.
4. Remove the supernatant carefully without touching the pellet. This pellet can be preserved at –80°C for a short period of time (e.g., 1 mo).
5. Add 1 vol of lysis buffer to the pellet (*see* **Note 10**).
6. In cold room, vortex (gently) and rock the cell pellet for 30 min.
7. Centrifuge the cell lysate at high speed, 12,000*g*, for 30 min at 4°C, collect the clear supernatant (whole protein extract) in a new sterile Eppendorf tube, and keep on ice until next step.
8. Measure the amount of extracted protein and prepare the protein aliquots (50 µg per aliquot) to run the SDS-PAGE.
9. Resolve equal amounts of protein by SDS-PAGE and transfer to a nitrocellulose membrane using Trans-Blot SD Semi-Dry Transfer Cell (Bio-Rad).
10. Block the membrane with 5% nonfat dry milk for 1 h at room temperature and then incubate 1 h at room temperature (or overnight at 4°) with the specific primary antibody (i.e., to cyclins, CDKs, or CDK inhibitors).
11. Wash the membrane and incubate it with secondary antibody at room temperature for 1 h and then wash the membrane again.
12. Detect the protein bands with the enhanced chemiluminescence system according to manufacturer's instructions.

## 3.2. Treatment of Synchronized Cells with an Anticancer Drug

To test the sensitivity of the cells synchronized in different phases of the cell cycle (*see* **Subheading 3.1.**), at each point, cells can be treated by a

# Cell Cycle and Drug Sensitivity

selected anticancer drug at selected concentration(s) for various hours, followed by measurement of cell death by, for example, sub-$G_1$ cell population, poly(ADP-ribose) polymerase (PARP) cleavage, and DNA ladder formation (*see* **Note 11**).

### 3.2.1. Drug Treatment

1. Treat the cells with a selected anticancer drug at an optimal concentration (should be predetermined) for various hours (*see* **Note 12**).
2. At each time point, total cell populations (or a mixture of detached and attached cells) will be collected and used for determination of cell sensitivity by various assays (see examples below). Attached cells will be collected either by trypsinization or scraping.

### 3.2.2. Sub-$G_1$ Population by Flow Cytometry

During the process of cell death, dead or dying cells will have fragmented DNA, which appears at a sub-$G_1$ population that can be detected by flow cytometry. Therefore, at each time point after drug treatment, cells can be collected for flow cytometry analysis (*see* **Subheading 3.1.3.**).

### 3.2.3. Measurement of PARP Cleavage by Western Blot Assay

At the initiation of apoptotic execution, PARP of 116 kDa can be cleaved by casepase-3 or -7 into a p85 fragment, which can be detected in Western blotting using a specific antibody to PARP. Therefore, at each time point after drug treatment, cells can be collected for Western blot assay (*see* **Subheading 3.1.4.**).

### 3.2.4. Measurement of DNA Fragmentation

DNA ladder formation is another characteristic of apoptosis.

1. As described in **steps 1–4** under **Subheading 3.1.4.**
2. Add 0.5 mL DNA lysis buffer to the pellet and mix gently and thoroughly with a micropipet (*see* **Note 13**).
3. Incubate the sample for 10 min at room temperature.
4. Centrifuge the sample at 10,000g for 10 min at 4°C.
5. Collect the supernatant into a new sterile Eppendorf tube, add 100 µg/mL proteinase K, and incubate the sample mixture overnight at 50°C.
6. Add 1 vol of phenol/chloroform (1/1) and mix gently by vortexing at low speed for a few seconds (*see* **Note 14**).
7. Centrifuge the sample at 10,000g for 5 min at room temperature.
8. Carefully collect the upper aqueous phase using a micropipet, without taking the organic phase (*see* **Note 15**).
9. Add 1 vol of isopropanol and 500 m$M$ NaCl to the collected aqueous phase and incubate at –20°C for overnight to precipitate the DNA.

10. Centrifuge the sample at 14,000g for 30 min at 4°C. A white pellet of DNA should be observed at the bottom of the tube.
11. Aspirate the supernatant carefully without touching the DNA pellet. If there is a small amount of DNA, you may not see the pellet.
12. Wash the pellet once with 200 µL of 70% ethanol. Suspend the pellet gently with a micropipet to wash the pellet. Over pipetting may shear the DNA.
13. Centrifuge the sample at high speed, 14,000g, for 10 min at 4°C and aspirate the supernatant carefully.
14. Dry the pellet using a vacuum air dryer (*see* **Note 16**).
15. Dissolve the DNA in 25 µL TE buffer for 1 h at 37°C with 1 µg/mL RNase-A.
16. Measure the DNA concentration using optical density (OD) at 260 nm.
17. Make 2% agarose gel with 0.1% SDS (e.g., 1 g agarose + 0.5 mL 10% SDS + 50 mL 1X TAE). Remember, add 10% SDS only after melting the agarose.
18. Take 5 µL DNA (0.5–1 µg) sample solution and mix with 1 µL 6X BPB dye, heat the sample mixture at 65°C for 10 min and then apply to agarose gel electrophoresis. For lambda DNA marker, take 1 µL of 6X BPB dye + 1 µL lambda DNA marker + 4 µL TE buffer in a tube, mix, and apply to agarose gel electrophorsis.
19. Run the DNA gel at 100 V for 1 h with 1X TAE.
20. Stain the gel with 0.5 µg/mL ethidium bromide for 10 min. Use ddH$_2$O to prepare the gel staining solution.
21. Rinse the gel with water, and visualize the DNA by UV transilluminator (e.g., Gel Doc 2000, Bio-Rad).
22. Take picture of the DNA gel.

## 4. Notes

1. If PBS (pH 7.2) is used for cell culture, it should be filtered after autoclaving by using a 0.2-µm filter to avoid the microbial contamination.
2. Make up fresh immediately before use. It can be made as a stock of 10 mg/mL in ddH$_2$O and stored in aliquots at −20°C.
3. Prepare stock concentration of 10 mg/mL and cover the container with aluminum foil to protect from light. Preserve at room temperature. This is a highly carcinogenic agent. Wear gloves while handling this chemical.
4. Serum starvation or treatment with a pharmacological agent for too long might cause cell death, while too short may not synchronize cells completely. Optimal conditions should be empirically determined.
5. Depending on cell types, sometimes you may need to use 0.2–0.5% FBS-containing medium instead of serum-free medium. Furthermore, the accumulation of the majority of cells in $G_0/G_1$ phase requires different time periods in serum-free (or reduced-serum) conditions, depending on cell types. For example, 0.2% serum for 24 h will be needed for NIH3T3 cells to be synchronized in $G_0/G_1$ phase, while 0.5% serum for 48 h will be needed for synchronization of HL-60RG cells in $G_0/G_1$ phase.

6. Better cell synchronization can be achieved by using two different pharmacological agents in combination. For example, first use lovastatin to synchronize most of the cells in early $G_1$ phase, followed by release. Then change to fresh medium containing aphidicolin for the second block at the $G_1/S$ boundary.
7. Different types of cells have different growth patterns. Depending on cell type, the treatment times may vary for synchronization of the majority of cells in a specific phase of the cell cycle.
8. The number of apoptotic cells may be very low. Therefore, if you vigorously pipetted the cells, the apoptotic cells may break down.
9. To prepare 10 mL of PI solution, 0.5 mL of 20X PI solution (1 mg/mL) is mixed with 1 mL of 10X RNase A (1000 U) and 8.5 mL of sample buffer (1 mg/mL glucose in 1X PBS). The 1X PI solution contains 50 µg/mL of PI and 100 U/mL of RNase A.
10. When you preserve the pellets at –80°C, they must be thawed first before adding lysis buffer. Keep the sample cold (4°C) at all times when you are handling it.
11. Keep in mind that some cells in S phase are highly sensitive to apoptosis induction, while other cells are not. Various apoptosis stimuli may also play a role in the determination of cell cycle-dependent sensitivity.
12. After synchronization, cells become more sensitive to any cytotoxic agents. Therefore, conditions for posttreatment with an anticancer drug should be carefully determined (e.g., drug concentrations, treatment hours, etc.). The conditions for synchronization and posttreatment with anticancer drugs may vary from cell line to cell line.
13. When you preserve the cell pellet at –20°C, it must be thawed first at 37°C or at room temperature before adding the lysis buffer.
14. High-speed vortex may shear the DNA and you may see a smear band instead of distinct separate bands when you visualize under the UV transilluminator.
15. After centrifugation, two phases will be observed in the sample tube. The top aqueous phase contains the DNA and the bottom organic phase contains the proteins and other cellular debris.
16. Instead of vacuum air drying, simple air drying of the pellet is also fine. An overdried pellet will require longer time to dissolve completely.

## Acknowledgments

We thank Mr. Kenyon Daniel for critical reading of the manuscript. This work was supported in part by research grants from the National Cancer Institute—National Institutes of Health, the United States Army Medical Research and Material Commend, and H. Lee Moffitt Cancer Center & Research Institute (to Q. P. D.).

## References

1. Pardee, A. B., Dubrow, R., Hamlin, J. L., and Kletzien, R. F. (1978) Animal Cell Cycle. *Annu. Rev. Biochem.* **47,** 715–750.

2. Kowalik, T. F., DeGregori, J., Schwarz, J. K., and Nevins, J. R. (1995) E2F1 overexpression in quiescent fibroblasts leads to induction of cellular DNA synthesis and apoptosis. *J. Virol.* **69,** 2491–2500.
3. Shan, B., Durfee, T., and Lee, W. H. (1996) Disruption of RB/E2F-1 interaction by single point mutations in E2F-1 enhances S-phase entry and apoptosis. *Proc. Natl. Acad. Sci. USA* **2,** 679–684.
4. Almasan, A., Yin, Y., Kelly, R. E., et al. (1995) Deficiency of retinoblastoma protein leads to inappropriate S-phase entry, activation of E2F-responsive genes, and apoptosis. *Proc. Natl. Acad. Sci. USA* **12,** 5436–5440.
5. Vairo, G., Soos, T. J., Upton, T. M., et al. (2000) Bcl-2 retards cell cycle entry through p27(Kip1), pRB relative p130, and altered E2F regulation. *Mol. Cell Biol.* **13,** 4745–4753.
6. Brady, H. J., Gil-Gomez, G., Kirberg, J., and Berns, A. J. (1996) Bax alpha perturbs T cell development and affects cell cycle entry of T cells. *EMBO J.* **24,** 6991–7001.
7. Yonish-Rouach, E., Grunwald, D., Wilder, S., et al. (1993) p53-mediated cell death: relationship to cell cycle control. *Mol. Cell Biol.* **3,** 1415–1423.
8. North, S. and Hainaut, P. (2000) p53 and cell-cycle control: a finger in every pie. *Pathol. Biol. (Paris)* **3,** 255–270.
9. Poot, M., Gollahon, K. A., and Rabinovitch, P. S. (1999) Werner syndrome lymphoblastoid cells are sensitive to camptothecin- induced apoptosis in S-phase. *Hum. Genet.* **1,** 10–14.
10. Fukuoka, K., Nishio, K., Fukumoto, H., et al. (2000) Ectopic p16(ink4) expression enhances CPT-11-induced apoptosis through increased delay in S-phase progression in human non-small-cell-lung-cancer cells. *Int. J. Cancer* **2,** 197–203.
11. Solary, E., Bertrand, R., and Pommier, Y. (1994) Apoptosis induced by DNA topoisomerase I and II inhibitors in human leukemic HL-60 cells. *Leuk. Lymphoma* **1–2,** 21–32.
12. Smith, D. M. and Dou, Q. P. (2001) Green tea polyphenol epigallocatechin inhibits DNA replication and consequently induces leukemia cell apoptosis. *Int. J. Mol. Med.* **7,** 645–652.
13. Shinomiya, N., Takemura, T., Iwamoto, K., and Rokutanda, M. (1997) Caffeine induces S-phase apoptosis in *cis*-diamminedichloroplatinum-treated cells, whereas *cis*-diamminedichloroplatinum induces a block in $G_2$/M. *Cytometry* **4,** 365–373.
14. Liang, J. Y., Fontana, J. A., Rao, J. N., et al. (1999) Synthetic retinoid CD437 induces S-phase arrest and apoptosis in human prostate cancer cells LNCaP and PC-3. *Prostate* **3,** 228–236.
15. Wang, H., Grand, R. J., Milner, A. E., Armitage, R. J., Gordon, J., and Gregory, C. D. (1996) Repression of apoptosis in human B-lymphoma cells by CD40-ligand and Bcl-2: relationship to the cell-cycle and role of the retinoblastoma protein. *Oncogene* **2,** 373–379.
16. Ryan, J. J., Danish, R., Gottlieb, C. A., and Clarke, M. F. (1993) Cell cycle analysis of p53-induced cell death in murine erythroleukemia cells. *Mol. Cell Biol.* **1,** 711–719.

# 3

# TUNEL Assay as a Measure of Chemotherapy-Induced Apoptosis

## Robert Wieder

### Summary

Chemotherapy induces injury to tumor cells, which subsequently die by a number of processes. One of those processes is apoptosis, and its measurement can be a useful tool to understanding the mechanisms of action of chemotherapy agents, drug resistance, and tumor biology. Cells undergoing apoptosis eventually cleave their DNA with nucleases in a characteristic pattern that leaves free 3'OH ends. This permits the identification of cells undergoing apoptosis by transfer of fluorescence-labeled dUTP to the free 3'OH ends using the enzyme terminal deoxynucleotidyl transferase (TdT) in a process termed terminal deoxynucleotidyl transferase dUTP-mediated nick end labeling (TUNEL). This chapter outlines the concepts governing the measurement of apoptosis following chemotherapy by TUNEL in cells in culture and in tissue biopsied from patients or laboratory animals that received chemotherapy. It lists the reagents, procedures for cell and tissue handling, labeling techniques, caveats, and appropriate controls for labeling 3'OH termini with TdT and quantifying the results.

### Key Words

3'OH termini; apoptosis; cell death; chemotherapy; necrosis; terminal deoxynucleotidyl transferase; TUNEL.

## 1. Introduction

Chemotherapy is the prime mode of treatment for unresectable cancers and leukemias *(1)*. It is also used in treating other hyperproliferative diseases, including rheumatoid arthritis *(2)*. Dozens of chemotherapy drugs with different mechanisms of action, along with a growing number of novel agents that target molecular functions of progressively greater specificity, are being used in therapy or in clinical and preclinical investigations *(3)*. The common effect among the agents is the killing of tumor cells, although additional functions such as inhibition of tumor cell proliferation, migration, invasion, and induction of differentiation are also achieved. Agents can also inhibit migration and proliferation and induce apoptosis in vascular endothelial cells *(4,5)* in a process that targets tumor angiogenesis. Measuring the effects of chemotherapy on cell death is important in studying the agent's mechanisms of action or the mechanisms responsible for drug resistance. In vivo, measurements of cell death can be correlated with the molecular characteristics of the tumor, its response to therapy, and ultimately, the effect on patient survival.

Cells die from chemotherapy by several means, including reproductive death *(6,7)*, necrosis *(8,9)*, and apoptosis *(10–12)*. These mechanisms are not mutually exclusive and can occur simultaneously or sequentially in the same cell *(13,14)*, depending on the timing and intensity of the insult *(8,15)*, the availability of ATP *(16)*, and the integrity of the apoptotic pathway *(17)* in the particular cell line or tumor being queried. Low doses of chemotherapy may induce reproductive death and also initiate apoptosis by activating cell death-signaling pathways *(18)*. Cell death may begin by apoptosis but can devolve to necrosis if conditions such as low oxygen tension, lack of caspase 3 expression prevail, or if a fragmented cell is not phagocytosed in a timely manner, for example *(11,16,19)*. Higher, rapidly administered concentrations of toxic stimuli may induce toxic cell death that results in a process characteristic of necrosis *(20)*. The divide between apoptosis and necrosis is not as clear as initially described by morphological criteria *(8)* for many reasons, and measurements of apoptosis need to be done using more than one assay to obtain a relatively accurate representation of actuality. The timing and selection of a technique for measuring cell death due to a particular cytotoxic agent is crucial in determining the extent of the measured cell death.

Apoptosis is necessary for organogenesis in the fetus *(21)* and for maintenance of the differentiated organ, and every eukaryotic cell harbors the program *(22,23)*. The process can be initiated by several described signal pathways *(24)*. These converge on the Bcl-2 family of proteins that reside on the mitochondrial membrane *(25)*. Modulation of the Bcl-2 proteins affects mitochondrial membrane transition through channels formed by Bax and other death-related factors *(26)* that result in release of cytochrome C *(25)*. Bax, however can initiate both apoptosis and necrosis *(14)*. The step appears to be the irreversible event in apoptosis, and in the absence of sufficient ATP, cells will die by necrosis *(17)*. Cytochrome C activates caspases, initially Apaf 1, caspase 9, then caspase 3 and capases 6 and 7 *(27)*. Alternate activation by chemotherapy involves death receptor–initiated pathways through caspase 8 that activate caspase 3, 7, and 6 *(28)*. Active caspases in turn activate proteases and nucleases that disrupt the membrane, cleave DNA at the sites of attachment in the nuclear scaffolding, and result in DNA fragments with 3′OH ends of initially 700-,

300-, and 50-kb lengths *(29–31)*. Additional nucleases then cleave the DNA in the internucleosomal spaces resulting in fragments of lengths equivalent to multiples of 180 bp that give a characteristic ladder appearance on an agarose gel *(32)*. A number of enzymes that cleave DNA resulting in 3′OH ends have been described and are reviewed by Lecoeur *(33)*. Apoptosis can be quantified by determining the extent of 3′OH DNA end cleavage. As a cautionary note, caspase-initiated apoptosis can devolve into necrosis *(8)*.

The 3′OH ends of apoptosis-derived DNA fragments can be labeled with fluorescent dUTP using the enzyme terminal deoxynucleotidyl transferase (TdT) in a process termed terminal deoxynucleotidyl transferase dUTP-mediated nick end labeling (TUNEL) *(34)*. Blunt ends, 3′OH overhangs, and recessed ends, including sites of DNA excision repair, can be labeled by TUNEL, but blunt ends and overhangs are much more efficiently labeled than recessed ends *(35,36)*. While there are roughly 50 times as many internucleosomal fragments as large molecules *(33)*, because the genome has on the order of $10^{10}$ base pairs, these larger fragments can be detected by TUNEL. Similarly, a cell that dies by necrosis results in breakup of the DNA into random fragments, some of which have 3′OH ends and are thus labeled by TUNEL *(37)*. In addition, DNA undergoing repair has 3′OH ends that can be accessed by TdT, albeit less efficiently than 3′OH overhangs *(38)*. For these and other reasons, although TUNEL has become a reference assay for apoptosis, there are a number of caveats and cautionary points to be considered when using it to assay apoptosis.

Measuring the effects of chemotherapy agents on apoptosis by TUNEL assay can be carried out in cells growing in tissue culture and in tissue biopsies. This chapter delineates the TUNEL procedures for assaying cytotoxic therapy–induced apoptosis in cultured cells by immunofluorescence microscopy and flow cytometry. It also outlines the steps for labeling tissue specimens obtained from animal tumors or patients receiving cytotoxic therapy. The methods stress the careful attention that must be paid to the handling and preparation of samples, incubation of cells or tissue with terminal deoxynucleotidyl transferase at the appropriate conditions in a buffer containing ATP, potassium cacodylate, and cobalt chloride, the transfer of fluorochrome-tagged dUTP to available 3′OH ends, and quantifying the amount of fluorescence by determining the percentage of positive fluorescent cells. Because of the nature of the TdT enzyme, the most efficient transfer occurs to DNA that has 3′OH overhangs and blunt ends and less efficiently to recessed 3′OH ends that include nicked DNA undergoing repair. The percent positive cells can be quantified by manual counts of both cultured cells and cells in tissue biopsies or by flow cytometry of cultured cells above a threshold established by experimental conditions, taking into account a number of variables that can result in false positives and false negatives.

## 2. Materials

The following reagents will be needed for the labeling procedures. Special storage conditions are indicated. Solutions without annotation can be kept at room temperature.

### 2.1. Tissue Culture

#### 2.1.1. Flow Cytometry

1. Phosphate-buffered saline (PBS).
2. Trypsin 0.05%/EDTA 0.53 m$M$ (store at –20°C).
3. PBS/2% fetal calf serum (FCS) (store at 4°C).
4. 0.1% paraformaldehyde in PBS.
5. Permeabilization solution: 0.1% Triton X-100, 0.1% Na-citrate in PBS.
6. TdT/FITC solution (store at –20°C in the dark): 5 µL 5X TdT buffer: 1 $M$ potassium cacodylate, 125 m$M$ Tris-HCl, 1.25 mg/mL bovine serum albumin (BSA), pH 6.6, at 25°C + 5 µL 25 n$M$ CoCl$_2$ + 0.03 µL dATP 100 nmol/µL (3 nmol) + 0.5 µL TdT (12.5 U) + 0.3 mL dUTP-FITC 1 nmol/µL (0.3 nmol) + 39.2 µL H$_2$O = 50.0 µL total volume.

#### 2.1.2. Immunofluorescence Microscopy

1. Acetone/methanol 1/1 (store at –20°C).
2. 3.7% formaldehyde (alternate fixative).
3. 1% paraformaldehyde (alternate fixative).
4. 0.1% Triton X-100, 0.1% Na-citrate.
5. Antifade reagent (available form several biotech suppliers) (store at –20°C in the dark).

### 2.2. Paraffin-Embedded Tissue

1. Xylene.
2. 100% ethanol.
3. Proteinase K, 20 µg/mL in 10 m$M$ Tris-HCl, pH 7.4 (store at –20°C).
4. DNAse I, 1 U/mL (store at –20°C).

## 3. Methods

### 3.1. Tissue Culture

Determining the proapoptotic effects of chemotherapy agents or other toxic interventions on cells in tissue culture as measured by TUNEL assay must be approached with careful planning and an understanding of the variables that can affect the data. These include:

1. Dose of the drug (see **Note 1**).
2. Timing of assay (see **Note 2**).

3. Cell type—each cell type will have its own spectrum of response to each agent.
4. Adherent or suspension cells. Measurement of adherent cells by TUNEL immunofluorescence on slides underestimates apoptosis because dying cells detach either spontaneously or preferentially with serial washes. Both suspension cells and trypsinized adherent cells prepared for flow cytometric analysis undergo multiple washes and centrifugations that can lyse dying cells preferentially.

In addition to standardizing the time, dose, and conditions for TUNEL measurements, because of these potentially confounding factors, additional methods of cell death measurements must be carried out in parallel to validate the results obtained with TUNEL.

### 3.1.1. Flow Cytometry

Most of the reagents listed are available in kits. There are a number of kits available commercially, and they have all been perfected to provide fidelity in labeling if the instructions are followed. The methods presented here serve to ensure correct handling of the cells in order to obtain meaningful biological data from experiments. The flow cytometry acquisition and the fine-tuning of the instrument and analysis of output data require specialized training and experience in the technical aspects of flow cytometry and should be handled by someone with that training and experience.

#### 3.1.1.1. ADHERENT CELLS

1. Culture cells in log phase.
2. Treat the cells with the chemotherapy agent with variable doses in each of triplicate 10-cm-diameter plates for each point in standard medium. Set up sufficient number of plates to allow for analysis on at least three time points after treatment.
3. Remove medium from 10-cm-diameter plate (7 mL) and transfer to 15-mL conical tube.
4. Wash cells with 3 mL PBS and add the wash to the medium in the 15-mL conical tube (*see* **Note 3**).
5. Add 1 mL trypsin to adherent cells and incubate at 37°C for 1–3 min. Keep checking every minute and tap plate with lateral force to dislodge cells until they deadhere.
6. Triturate cells to obtain single-cell suspension (*see* **Note 4**). Check status of cells with respect to dispersal in an inverted phase-contrast microscope to ensure single-cell nature before proceeding.
7. Add 3 mL medium with 10% FCS to trypsinized cells and triturate well. Transfer to 15-mL conical tube with the previously removed medium.
8. Centrifuge cells at $87g$ (800 rpm in a Beckman model T-J6 refrigerated centrifuge) for 10 min at 4°C (*see* **Note 5**).
9. Resuspend cell pellet with gentle trituration in 5 mL PBS/2% FCS.

10. Repeat centrifugation at 87g for 10 min.
11. Fix cells by adding 5 mL 0.1% paraformaldehyde/PBS, triturate lightly to resuspend, and keep on ice for 10 min.
12. Centrifuge at 87g for 10 min at 4°C.
13. Remove supernatant, wash once by resuspending in PBS/2% FCS and centrifuging, as before. Remove supernatant.
14. Permeabilize cells adding 5 mL 0.1% Triton X-100, 0.1% Na-citrate in PBS. Gently triturate the cell pellet to resuspend and leave on ice for 10 min.
15. Centrifuge at 87g for 10 min.
16. Remove supernatant, wash once by resuspending in PBS/2% FCS and centrifuging, as before. Remove supernatant by decanting as much liquid as possible.
17. Add 50 µL premixed TdT/FITC solution and resuspend pellet with the micropipet. (As a negative control, incubate slides with TdT/FITC solution without TdT enzyme.)
18. Incubate 37°C for 1 h.
19. Wash twice with PBS/2% BSA, as before and resuspend pellet in 1 mL PBS/2%BSA.
20. Assay with flow cytometer within 24 h.

3.1.1.2. CELLS GROWING IN SUSPENSION

Begin procedure with **step 8** above and continue as outlined for adherent cells.

### 3.1.2. Immunofluorescence Microscopy

1. Culture cells on sterilized microscope slide cover slips placed at the bottom of 6-cm-diameter tissue culture dishes. Treat with chemotherapy time and dose variations as above.
2. Remove medium and wash once gently with PBS/2% FCS (*see* **Note 6**).
3. Fix cells by adding acetone/methanol 1/1 at –20°C. Keep the plate in –20°C freezer for 2 min (*see* **Note 7**).
4. Aspirate fixative and wash gently once with PBS/2% FCS.
5. Permeabilize cells by incubating with permeabilization solution for 2 min on ice.
6. Wash twice with PBS.
7. Dry area around sample by blotting.
8. Add 50 µL TUNEL reaction mixture to sample and incubate slide in humidified chamber for 60 min at 37°C in the dark.
9. Wash slide three times with PBS.
10. Add antifade and apply a cover slip. Keep in dark.
11. Visualize using an immunofluorescence microscope with a 420–500-nm filter.
12. Photograph at least five fields containing at least 100 cells on each slide. Count the number of TUNEL positive cells present in the total number of cells counted and obtain the ratio. Average the value from at least three slides per point and calculate the standard deviation.

# TUNEL Assay as a Measure of Apoptosis

## 3.2. Paraffin-Embedded Tissue

The measurement of tumor apoptosis following in vivo administration of chemotherapy is confounded by a great number of variables. These include:

1. Tumor type (*see* **Note 8**).
2. Site of tumor (*see* **Note 9**).
3. Extent of intrinsic necrosis and oxygen tension, dependent on tumor vascularity, rate of tumor growth, and its relationship to rate of neovascularization (*see* **Note 10**).
4. Interpatient variability of tumor (*see* **Note 11**).
5. Sample size (*see* **Note 12**).
6. Type of drug, route of administration, rate, and dose (*see* **Note 13**).
7. Time after chemotherapy administration that specimen was obtained (*see* **Note 14**).
8. Length of time between obtaining of sample and processing (*see* **Note 15**).
9. Specimen cut thickness, cutting artifact (*see* **Note 16**).

Taking all of these factors into account, a reasonable correlation between chemotherapy and resulting apoptosis can be measured by TUNEL. Additional means of cell death measurement are strongly encouraged to correlate with the results of TUNEL measurements because of the very high probability of artifactual positive and negative TUNEL data. The following is an outline of the methods.

### 3.2.1. Dewaxing and Rehydration

1. Heat slides at 70°C for 10 min.
2. Transfer slides serially in "coupling jars" in the following sequence:
   a. Xylene—5 min
   b. Xylene—5 min
   c. 96% ethanol—3 min
   d. 96% ethanol—3 min
   e. 90% ethanol—3 min
   f. 80% ethanol—3 min
   g. Distilled water—3 min
   h. Distilled water—3 min
   i. Distilled water—3 min
   After this point, the specimen should be kept moist at all times.

### 3.2.2. Proteinase K Treatment

1. Add 100 µL of 20-µg/mL proteinase K in 10 m$M$ Tris-HCl, pH 7.4, to specimen, place a cover slip on it and incubate for 15–30 min at room temperature.
2. Wash four times with double-distilled water.

### 3.2.3. TUNEL Labeling

1. Drain the slide, dry around the specimen using a Kimwipe (*see* **Note 17**).
2. Incubate an additional slide obtained from a tumor biopsy before treatment with DNAse I, 1 U mL, for 30 min at 37°C as a positive control (*see* **Note 18**).

3. Place 50 µL of TUNEL mixture on specimen, place a cover slip on it, incubate at 37°C for 1 h (or overnight at 4°C) in the dark. As a negative control, incubate an additional slide with TdT/FITC solution without TdT enzyme.
4. Wash three times with PBS.
5. Place 10 µL of antifade, cover with a cover slip, and store in the dark at 4°C.
6. Photograph at least five representative areas at 400X magnification of each slide and count all of the cells in the photographed fields for a total of at least 100 cells. Determine the percent apoptotic cells in the count, including the positive (DNAse I-treated) and negative (pretreatment sample) controls.

## 4. Notes

1. Different means of cell death can occur at different concentrations of a toxin. At low concentrations, cells may suffer reproductive death, that is, lose the ability to form clones or proliferate, but do not yet undergo cell death *per se*. At very high concentrations of a toxin, cells may undergo cell death by necrosis, while at concentrations below that, the apoptotic pathways are likely activated. A careful dose-finding study needs to be performed with a viability assay using trypan blue, MTT, or any number of available assays to determine the linear range where apoptosis is likely to have a role. This will then determine where TUNEL measurements should be carried out.
2. Timing of the TUNEL assay is critical. TUNEL measures a very late event in apoptosis, and a number of events can influence the prevalence of cells with a predictable number of DNA fragments with available 3′OH ends for assay by TUNEL. These include the devolution of apoptosis to necrosis at a number of sites, including at the level of Bax, mitochondria in the absence of sufficient ATP generation in hypoxic conditions, caspases, including the absence of caspase 3 in some cells that prevent the conversion of large DNA fragments to those of internucleosomal length, the presence of some 3′OH ends in necrosis-generated random DNA fragments that react in the TUNEL assay, the loss of small DNA fragments with time resulting in a hypodiploid cell measurable by PI analysis but simultaneously dimming the TUNEL signal, and the fragmentation of apoptotic cells that can devolve into necrosis in the late stages of apoptosis. DNA fragmentation can occur from 6 to 24 h following an insult, but if the chemotherapy agent is left in the medium, additional cells can begin the process in a continuous process. The measurement of apoptosis must be standardized in each cell type, with each concentration of each agent with respect to time. It is imperative to understand that the measured rate is not cumulative of all dead cells, but only a "freeze frame" of the fraction of TUNEL positive cells sampled at a given time.
3. Attached cells undergoing apoptosis curl up and begin to detach from tissue culture plates. Cells that have not yet detached but are undergoing apoptosis have decreased adherence to the tissue culture coated plastic. With any assay measuring apoptosis, it is absolutely crucial to collect detached cells floating in the

medium and ones that are dislodged by a PBS wash prior to trypsinization; otherwise the assay will significantly underestimate the rate of apoptosis, signaling, or other process being quantified.
4. Do not handle cells too roughly or force liquid from pipet to impact the plate with too great a force, because cells undergoing apoptosis are more fragile and will lyse and be lost to assay.
5. There are multiple centrifugation steps in this procedure that will damage and lyse apoptotic cells if the cumulative $g$ forces are higher than specified. At the speed and time indicated, there should be no cells in the supernatant after a spin.
6. This procedure underestimates the percentage of cells undergoing apoptosis because washes remove dying cells or cells that have entered the apoptotic process that have decreased adhesion.
7. Alternative methods for fixation are adding either 1% paraformaldehyde or 3.7% formaldehyde to the cells for 30 min at room temperature.
8. Intrinsic apoptosis, necrosis, and response to specific chemotherapy agents varies with tumor types. Baseline apoptosis in well-perfused parts of the tumor, positive controls with DNAse I digestion, and extent of necrosis by histological examination of H&E stains are all necessary for standardization.
9. Primary tumors at different sites may have an intrinsic variability as well as variability to therapy. In addition, metastatic tumors may be inherently different from primary tumors from both genetic as well as microenvironmentally induced aspects and vascularity. Consequently, the response to chemotherapy may vary drastically. This necessitates standardization of the protocol for obtaining tissue from specific sites for measurement of apoptosis.
10. Apoptosis must be quantitated at tumor sites that are well vascularized and away from areas of necrosis, as much as possible. Pretreatment tumor samples from analogous areas as posttreatment biopsies must be assayed for baseline TUNEL staining to determine the increase in labeling as a result of chemotherapy. Positive controls of pretreatment slides with DNAse I treatment should be performed to determine the efficiency of the TUNEL labeling procedure.
11. Tumor types must be confirmed by a pathologist and patients with identical histological diagnoses compared. This is not an issue in animal studies with xenograft tumors.
12. Statistical calculation must be incorporated in protocols during design to permit data to achieve statistical significance. The percentage of cells in a solid tumor that is positive for apoptosis by TUNEL in response to chemotherapy is typically small, often in the single digits. In addition, endogenous endonucleases and DNA repair may render a percentage of cells in untreated tissue positive by TUNEL at baseline. Sufficient numbers of specimen slides and cells from each slide must be counted to obtain statistical significance.
13. The effects of chemotherapy on a tumor type vary with the drug, dose, and route of administration. The effects on apoptosis will have to be measured in tumor specimens from hosts who received chemotherapy on a standardized regimen, keeping these issues constant.

14. The effects of chemotherapy result in the induction of apoptosis from 6 to 24 h later, with variable sequelae such as subsequent devolution into necrosis. The time for tumor biopsy following administration of chemotherapy must be standardized.
15. Surgical samples frequently sit at room temperature for variable times following resection, yielding variable result when such tissue is prepared for analysis. The investigator must be present at the time of biopsy to ensure proper handling of specimens and equal timing between biopsy and processing.
16. Specimens must be cut to ≤5-μm thickness. Thicker sections can result in nonspecific artifactual staining. Cutting artifacts can result in necrosis at the edges, making it imperative to measure apoptosis in areas inward from the edge.
17. All procedures should be done in a relatively dark room.
18. TUNEL staining needs to be optimized for each set of slides assayed, for results to be meaningful. As a positive control, an additional pretreatment slide should be treated with DNAse I to determine the efficiency of the TUNEL procedure. Pre- and posttreatment samples and the DNAse I-treated pretreatment sample should be stained at the same time.

## References

1. DeVita, V. T. Jr., Hellman, S., and Rosenberg, S. A. (eds.) (2001) *Cancer Principles & Practice of Oncology.* Lippincot Williams & Wilkins, Philadelphia.
2. Saravanan, V. and Hamilton, J. (2002) Advances in the treatment of rheumatoid arthritis: old versus new therapies. *Expert Opin. Pharmacoth.* **3,** 845–856.
3. Szekeres, T. and Novotny. L. (2002) New targets and drugs in cancer chemotherapy. *Med. Principles Practice* **11,** 117–125.
4. Bocci, G., Nicolaou, K. C., and Kerbel, R. S. (2002) Protracted low-dose effects on human endothelial cell proliferation and survival in vitro reveal a selective antiangiogenic window for various chemotherapeutic drugs. *Cancer Res.* **62,** 6938–6943.
5. McCrudden, K. W., Yokoi, A., Thosani, et al. (2002) Topotecan is anti-angiogenic in experimental hepatoblastoma. *J. Pediatr. Surg.* **37,** 857–861.
6. Brunet, C. L., Gunby, R. H., Benson, R.S., Hickman, J. A., Watson, A. J., and Brady, G. (1998) Commitment to cell death measured by loss of clonogenicity is separable from the appearance of apoptotic markers. *Cell Death Different.* **5,** 107–115.
7. Tannock, I. F. and Lee, C. (2001) Evidence against apoptosis as a major mechanism for reproductive cell death following treatment of cell lines with anti-cancer drugs. *Br. J. Cancer* **84,** 100–105.
8. Green, D. R. and Reed, J. C. (1998) Mitochondria and apoptosis. *Science* **281,** 1309–1312.
9. Matsuo, A., Watanabe, A., Takahashi, T., et al. (2001) A simple method for classification of cell death by use of thin layer collagen gel for the detection of apoptosis and/or necrosis after cancer chemotherapy. *Jpn. J. Cancer Res.* **92,** 813–819.

10. Kaufmann, S. H. and Earnshaw, W. C. (2000) Induction of apoptosis by cancer chemotherapy. *Exp. Cell Res.* **256,** 42–49.
11. Oyaizu, H., Adachi, Y., Taketani, S., Tokunaga, R., Fukuhara, S., and Ikehara, S. (1999) A crucial role of caspase 3 and caspase 8 in paclitaxel-induced apoptosis. *Mol. Cell Biol. Res. Commun.* **2,** 36–41.
12. Milner, A. E., Palmer, D. H., Hodgkin, E. A., et al. (2002) Induction of apoptosis by chemotherapeutic drugs: the role of FADD in activation of caspase-8 and synergy with death receptor ligands in ovarian carcinoma cells. *Cell Death Different.* **9,** 287–300.
13. Kerr, J. F. R., Wyllie, A. H., and Currie, A. R. (1972) Apoptosis: a basic biological phenomenon with wide-ranging implications in tissue kinetics. *Br. J. Cancer* **26,** 239–257.
14. Xiang, J., Chao, D. T., and Korsmeyer, S. J. (1996) BAX-induced cell death may not require interleukin 1 beta-converting enzyme-like proteases. *Proc. Natl. Acad. Sci. USA* **93,** 14,559–14,563.
15. Kumi-Diaka, J. (2002) Chemosensitivity of human prostate cancer cells PC3 and LNCaP to genistein isoflavone and β-lapachone. *Biol. Cell* **94,** 37–44.
16. Leist, M., Single, B., Castoldi, A. F., Kühnle, S., and Nicotera, P. (1997) Intracellular adenosine triphosphate (ATP) concentration: a switch in the decision between apoptosis and necrosis. *J. Exp. Med.* **185,** 1481–1486.
17. Hirsch, T., Marchetti, P., Susin, S. A., et al. (1997) The apoptosis–necrosis paradox. Apoptogenic proteases activated after mitochondrial permeability transition determine the mode of cell death. *Oncogene* **15,** 1573–1581.
18. Wang, Q., Yang, W., Uytingco, M. S., Christakos, S., and Wieder, R. (2000) 1,25(OH)$_2$ vitamin D3 and all-*trans* retinoic acid sensitize breast cancer cells to chemotherapy-induced cell death. *Cancer Res.* **60,** 2040–2048.
19. Kerr, J. F. R., Winterford, C. M., and Harmon, B. V. (1994) Apoptosis: its significance in cancer and cancer therapy. *Cancer* **73,** 2013–2026.
20. Bonfoco, E., Krainc, D., Ankarcrona, M., Nicotera, P., and Lipton, S. A. (1995) Apoptosis and necrosis: two distinct events induced respectively by mild and intense insults with NMDA or nitric oxide/superoxide in cortical cell cultures. *Proc. Natl. Acad. Sci. USA* **92,** 7162–7166.
21. Kuan, C. Y., Yang, D. D., Samanta Roy, D. R., Davis, R. J., Rakic, P., and Flavell, R. A. (1999) The Jnk1 and Jnk2 protein kinases are required for regional specific apoptosis during early brain development. *Neuron* **22,** 667–676.
22. Kawase, Y., Takemura, G., Hayakawa, K., et al. (2002) Abundant apoptosis in nutmeg liver of cardiomyopathic hamsters. Apoptotic cell death as a possible mechanism of hepatic remodeling by congestion. *Pathol. Res. Practice* **198,** 291–298.
23. Swynghedauw, B. (1999) Molecular mechanisms of myocardial remodeling. *Physiolog. Rev.* **79,** 215–262.
24. Kim, R., Tanabe, K., Uchida, Y., Emi, M., Inoue, H., and Toge, T. (2002) Current status of the molecular mechanisms of anticancer drug-induced apoptosis. The

contribution of molecular-level analysis to cancer chemotherapy. *Cancer Chemother. Pharmacol.* **50,** 343–352.
25. Kluck, R. M., Bossy-Wetzel, E., Green, D. R., and Newmeyer, D. D. (1997) The release of cytochrome c from mitochondria: a primary site for Bcl-2 regulation of apoptosis. *Science* **275,** 1132–1136.
26. Desagher, S., Osen-Sand, A., Nichols, A., et al. (1999) Bid-induced conformational change of Bax is responsible for mitochondrial cytochrome C release during apoptosis. *J. Cell Biol.* **144,** 891–901.
27. Li, P., Nijhawan, D., Budihardjo, I., et al. (1997) Cytochrome C and dATP-dependent formation of Apaf-1/caspase-9 complex initiates an apoptotic protease cascade. *Cell* **91,** 479–489.
28. Earnshaw, W. C., Martins, L. M., and Kaufmann, S. H. (1999) Mammalian caspases: structure, activation, substrates, and functions during apoptosis. *Ann. Rev. Biochem.* **68,** 383–424.
29. Oberhammer, F., Wilson, W. W., Dive, C., et al. (1993) Apoptotic death in epithelial cells: cleavage of DNA to 300 and/or 50 Kb fragments prior to or in the absence of internucleosomal fragmentation. *EMBO J.* **12,** 3679–3684.
30. Brown, D. G., Sun, X. M., and Cohen, G. M. (1992) Dexamethasone-induced apoptosis involves cleavage of DNA to large fragments prior to internucleosomal fragmentation. *J. Biol. Chem.* **268,** 3037–3039.
31. Huang, P., Robertson, L. E., Wright, S., and Plunkett, W. (1995) High molecular weight DNA fragmentation: a critical event in nucleotide analogue-induced apoptosis in leukaemia cells. *Clin. Cancer Res.* **1,** 1005–1013.
32. Wyllie, A. H. (1980) Glucocorticoid-induced thymocyte apoptosis is associated with endogenous endonuclease activation. *Nature* **284,** 555–556.
33. Lecoeur, H. (2002) Nuclear apoptosis detection by flow cytometry: influence of endogenous endonucleases. *Exp. Cell Res.* **277,** 1–14.
34. Gavrieli, Y., Sherman, Y., and Ben-Sasson, S. A. (1992) Identification of programmed cell death in situ via specific of nuclear DNA fragmentation. *J. Cell Biol.* **119,** 493–501.
35. McKenna, S. L., Hoy, T. Holmes, J. A., Whittaker, J. A., Jackson, H., and Padua, R. A. (1998) Flow cytometric apoptosis assays indicate different types of endonuclease activity in haematopoietic cells and suggest a cautionary approach to their quantitiative use. *Cytometry* **31,** 130–136.
36. Jin, K., Chen, J., Nagayama, T., et al. (1999) In situ detection of neuronal DNA strand breaks using the Klenow fragment of DNA polymerase I reveals different mechanisms of neuron death after global cerebral ischemia. *J. Neurochem.* **72,** 1204–1214.
37. Collins, R. J., Harmon, B, V., Gobe, G. C., and Kerr, J. F. (1992) Internucleosomal DNA cleavage should not be the sole criterion for identifying apoptosis. *Intl. J. Rad. Biol.* **61,** 451–453.
38. Kanoh, M., Takemura, G., Misao, J., et al. (1999) Significance of myocytes with positive DNA in situ nick end-labeling (TUNEL) in hearts with dilated cardiomyopathy. Not apoptosis but DNA repair. *Circulation* **99,** 2757–2764.

# 4

## Apoptosis Assessment by the DNA Diffusion Assay

Narendra P. Singh

### Summary

A simple, sensitive, and reliable DNA diffusion assay for quantification of apoptosis is based on the principle that nuclear DNA of apoptotic cells have abundant alkali-labile sites and under alkaline conditions small pieces of DNA thus generated diffuse in agarose, giving the appearance of a halo if stained with a sensitive fluorescent dye such as YOYO-1. The protocol for detection of apoptosis described here is tested for estimation of apoptosis in human leukocytes (mostly neutrophils) incubated at 37°C for 24 h. Cells were mixed with agarose, microgels were made, and cells were lysed in a solution of high salt, detergents, and alkali. DNA was precipitated in microgels by ethanol and spermine. Staining of DNA was done with an intense fluorescent dye, YOYO-1. Apoptotic cells show a circular gradient of granular DNA with a dense central zone and a lighter and hazy outer zone, giving the overall appearance of a halo.

### Key Words

DNA diffusion assay; apoptosis; necrosis.

## 1. Introduction

Apoptosis (Greek, meaning "dropping off") is programmed cell death in the tissues of an organism. Unlike necrosis (Greek, meaning "dead"), apoptosis is not associated with inflammation or scarring. Apoptosis seems to be induced by mild genotoxic stimuli, and as the strength of the stimuli increases, the cell death mode shifts to necrosis. This seems to be due to the fact that intense genotoxic stimuli often damage the proteins (or the genes that are making those proteins) and other cellular macromolecules that may be required for apoptosis. Apoptosis is a normal, often inevitable event, occurring continually both during and after development. Apoptosis plays an important role in the remodeling of tissues during development and aging *(1,2)*. However, apoptosis may also occur in response to cell injury (such as exposure to toxic agents) or disease (e.g., it is a crucial process for eliminating cancer cells). Research on apoptosis and elucidation of apoptotic mechanisms has been recognized as vitally important. Apoptosis is considered a feature of diseases such as Alzheimer's, Parkinson's, HIV/AIDS, and cancer *(3–9)*. Agents of bioterrorism, including anthrax *(10)*, can also trigger apoptotic pathways. Additionally, apoptosis has been increasingly recognized as critically important to research on aging and age-related diseases *(11–13)*.

The biological significance of this phenomenon underscores the need for a highly sensitive and simple method for apoptosis assessment. Currently, the commonly used techniques for the estimation of apoptosis are as follows. Agarose gel electrophoresis *(14)* is used to demonstrate the ladder pattern of DNA (a hallmark of apoptosis), which is generated by endonucleolytic cleavage of genomic DNA into nucleosomal size. This method usually involves a DNA isolation procedure from millions of cells, and results cannot be quantified. Caspase-3 quantification *(15)* is used for the estimation of apoptosis in cell lysates. Both of the above assays require large numbers of apoptotic cells and thus are relatively insensitive for the detection of low levels of apoptosis. TUNEL (TdT-mediated dUTP nick-end labeling) assay *(16)* or *in situ* nick translation is the established method for detecting apoptosis. Although it is sensitive, this method is associated with a number of artifacts, as it labels DNA strand breaks from any insult, in both apoptotic and nonapoptotic cells *(17)*. Also, loss of frail apoptotic cells during processing is common with this method. Morphological estimation for apoptosis *(18)* is based on cell characteristics such as chromatin condensation, formation of apoptotic bodies from one cell (each having a fragmented piece of nucleus surrounded by a viable cell membrane), shrinkage of cytoplasm, and blebbing of plasma membrane with an irregular outline *(1)*. However, in this assay, because of the size of apoptotic cells, a light microscope may not detect late apoptotic cells *(1)*. Also, early apoptotic cells may not show classical morphological features of apoptosis. Antibodies against annexin V, labeled with fluorescein isothiocyanate, are used for rapid cytoflurometric analysis *(19,20)* of apoptosis. Annexin V is a protein that possesses a strong affinity for phosphatidylserine *(21)*, which is externalized onto the cell surface in the very early stages of cell death. As phosphatidylserine is present in normal cells (inside of the cell membrane), this assay can provide false positive results when membranes are damaged *(22)*.

The DNA diffusion assay described here is a simple, sensitive, and rapid method for estimating apoptosis in single cells *(23)*. The assay involves mixing cells with agarose and making a microgel on a microscopic slide, then lysing the embedded cells with salt and detergents (to allow the diffusion of small-molecular-weight DNA in agarose), and finally visualizing the DNA by a sensitive fluorescent dye, YOYO-1. The present procedure makes it possible to detect virtually all of early, typical, and late apoptotic cells. The method may also be used to distinguish apoptosis from necrosis. Apoptotic cell nuclei have a hazy or undefined outline without any clear boundary due to nucleosomal-sized DNA diffusing into agarose. Necrotic cell nuclei are bigger and are poorly defined. They have a clear, defined outer boundary of the DNA and a relatively homogeneous appearance. Cells with only damaged DNA (not necrotic or apoptotic cells), on the other hand, are clearly defined and nuclei have a larger size with a projection of DNA all around. To reveal all apoptotic cells, it is critical to use lysis and alkaline treatment. Enhancement in sensitivity due to alkaline treatment may be due to numerous alkali-labile sites present in the DNA of apoptotic cells. Alkaline treatment may also be essential in degrading RNA (which may interferes in identification of apoptotic cells). The DNA diffusion assay has been used previously to evaluate efficacy of anticancer strategies (various chemical and physical agents) in vitro *(22)*. Aside from apoptosis assessment in whole blood, also included here are methodologies for estimation of apoptosis in sperm and cells from soft solid tissue. Though the DNA diffusion assay can be adapted for a variety of desired cell types, the importance of apoptosis assessment in sperm and cells from soft solid tissue, such as the brain, justified their inclusion in this work *(23,24)*.

## 2. Materials

All chemicals were purchased from Sigma Chemical (St. Louis, MO) unless mentioned otherwise.

1. Heparinized 1.5-mL microfuge tubes (Kew Scientific, Columbus, OH).
2. MGE slides (Erie Scientific, Portsmouth, NH, cat. no. ES 370 or Blue Label Scientifics Pvt. Ltd., Mumbai, India).
3. Agarose 3:1, high resolution (Amresco, Solon, OH).
4. Agarose SFR (Amresco, Solon, OH).
5. 24 × 50-mm$^2$ #1 cover glass (Corning Glass Works, Corning, NY).
6. Slide tray (Ellard instrumentation, Monroe, WA).
7. YOYO-1 (Molecular Probe, Eugene, OR).
8. Tissue press (BioSpec Product, Bartlesville, OK).
9. Phosphate-buffered saline (PBS) 10X stock: 80 g NaCl, 2 g KCl, 2 g $KH_2PO_4$, 11.5 g anhydrous $Na_2HPO_4$ or 29 g $Na_2HPO_4 \cdot 7H_2O$, 32 g trizma hydrochloride (FW = 157.6), pH 7.4 (phosphoric acid). Autoclave and adjust volume to 1 L, dispense in 10-mL aliquots.
10. Lysis and denaturing solution (can be prepared in advance and stored for up to 1 yr): 1.25 $M$ NaCl, 1 m$M$ tetrasodium EDTA, 0.01% sodium lauroyl sarcosine, 5 m$M$ Tris. The following *must* be added *fresh* to this solution: 0.2% dimethyl sulfoxide (DMSO), final concentration; 0.3 $N$ NaOH, pH > 13.5, added fresh in final concentration from a stock of 10 $N$ NaOH.

11. Neutralizing and DNA precipitating solution (can be prepared in advance and stored for up to 1 yr): 40 m$M$ Tris-HCl, pH 7.4 (50 mL) (final concentration 20 m$M$), 200 proof ethanol (50 mL) (final concentration 50%). The following *must* be added *fresh* to this solution: 100 mg spermine (final concentration 1 mg/mL).
12. YOYO-1: 1 µ$M$ YOYO-1 (Molecular Probe, Eugene, OR) in 2.5% DMSO and 0.5% sucrose is needed. Stock solution of YOYO is 1 m$M$; take 1 µL of it and add to 1 mL of DMSO sucrose solution mentioned below.
13. DMSO sucrose solution. For year-long storage of sucrose the following procedure is used: Fill a 100-mL bottle with 35 mL of distilled water, then dissolve 10 g of sucrose in the bottle. Raise the volume to 50 mL by adding distilled water. Add 50 mL of DMSO. Use 50 µL of above to 1 ml (2.5% DMSO and 0.5% sucrose).

## 3. Methods (see Note 1)

All experiments were done in indirect incandescent light.

### 3.1. DNA Diffusion Assay for Apoptosis in Leukocytes

As a model for standardizing the DNA diffusion assay for apoptosis, experiments can be conducted to induce apoptosis in whole-blood leukocytes. This is based on the principle that leukocytes undergo spontaneous apoptosis at 37°C in vitro. Percent apoptotic cells should be approx 3–20% in 24 h and 30–60% at 48 h, depending on the age and nutrition status of the individual from whom the blood is collected.

#### 3.1.1. Collection of Blood (see **Note 2**)

Twenty to 100 µL of blood from a healthy volunteer is drawn using a fingerprick and collected in a 1.5-mL heparinized microfuge tube.

#### 3.1.2. Preparation of Agarose

Making agarose is a critical step. If agarose is not prepared properly, it will not adhere to the glass slide. All types of agarose should be made 24 h in advance and stored at 55°C, for better adherence and resolution. To make 0.6% agarose:

1. Sixty milligrams of 3:1 high-resolution agarose are suspended in 9 mL distilled water in an 80- or 100-mL glass beaker and microwaved until just boiling.
2. To heat agarose uniformly, the boiling step is repeated twice more.
3. One milliliter of 10X PBS is added to the agarose solution and mixed by swirling the beaker.
4. After adjusting the final volume to 10 mL using distilled water, the agarose solution is boiled once more.
5. As a general rule, when 10 mL of solution are boiled in a microwave, 1 mL of the volume is lost by evaporation. Assuming this, 60 mg of agarose could be suspended in 10 mL distilled water and adding 1 mL of 10X PBS volume should compensate for lost volume.

## DNA Diffusion Assay for Apoptosis

6. Dispense this agarose in microfuge tubes and maintain at 55°C in a heat block.
7. 2% SFR agarose is made in a similar manner as PBS. Making 2% agarose, however, requires thorough and constant swirling while hot, as it has a tendency to stick to the walls of beaker, after the first, second, and third boiling. Alternately, agarose can be boiled on a hot plate with a magnetic stirrer.
8. The agarose solution is dispensed into microfuge tubes and maintained at 55°C in a heat block.
9. The final agarose solution is the 1% 3:1 high-resolution agarose prepared with 20 m$M$ Tris (pH7) in distilled water, for making the first dried layer of microgel. Making 1% agarose (to be used for making the first layer of microgel, which has to be dried) in 20 m$M$ Tris avoids a dried and precipitated phosphates-mediated (phosphates are present in PBS) background with YOYO dye.

### 3.1.3. Making Microgels

Microgels should be prepared on custom-made MGE slides (*see* Materials). These slides provide a clear nonfrosted area in the center (1 × 3 cm$^2$) for better visualization of DNA and a surrounding frosted area for the attachment of agarose. Agarose precoated slides are made as follows (*see* **Note 3**).

1. Spread 50 µL of 1% (3:1 high-resolution agarose) in distilled water on each slide and air-dry. This dried layer of agarose provides a better substrate for attachment of subsequent layers.
2. Five microliters of blood (approx 50,000 nucleated cells) are then mixed with 50 µL of 0.6% agarose in PBS. Although the current experiment involves leukocytes from whole blood, appropriate number of cells can be used from other desired sources.
3. Microgels are made on these agarose-precoated slides by pipetting a mixture of cell and agarose onto the slide. This agarose is immediately covered with a 24 × 50-mm$^2$ #1 cover glass and allowed to solidify for 5 min at room temperature (23°C).
4. The cover glasses are removed from the second layer of microgel, and 200 µL of 2% agarose (SFR, Amresco, Solon, OH) solution is layered as before to make a third layer. After 2 min, cover glasses are removed and slides are placed in a slide-holding tray (described in detail in **ref. 25**).

### 3.1.4. Lysis of Cell and Alkaline Denaturation of DNA (see **Note 4**)

Slides are immersed at room temperature for 10 min in a freshly made lysing and denaturing solution in a plastic container. Use of the plastic tray and container for alkaline treatment and ethanol precipitation *(25)* ensures uniform fluorescent background from slide to slide.

### 3.1.5. Neutralization and DNA Precipitation

Slides are then immersed in neutralizing and DNA-precipitating solution for 30 min. This step must be repeated (30 min) to remove salts, detergents, and cel-

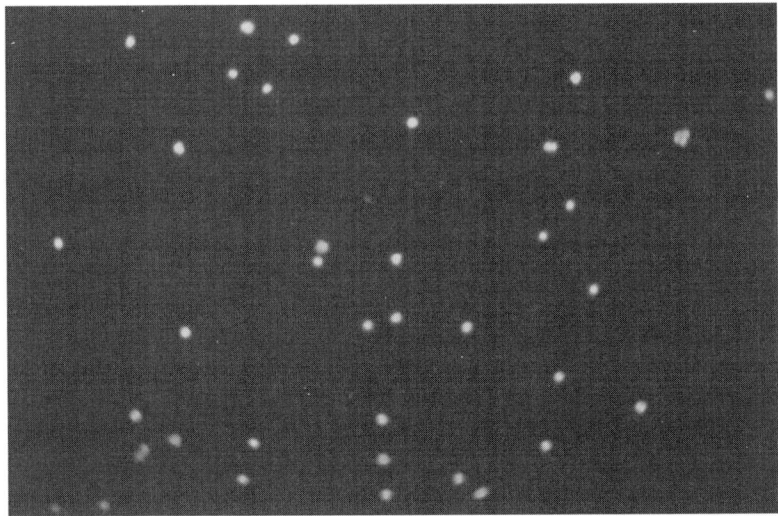

Fig. 1. A photomicrograph of leukocytes from whole blood processed for the DNA diffusion assay. No apoptotic cells are seen in this figure, although the incidence of apoptosis detected using this assay is 0.1–0.2% in fresh whole-blood leukocytes. Magnification 100×. Dye YOYO-1.

lular macromolecules, while retaining DNA in agarose. Slides are then air-dried and stored at room temperature.

### 3.1.6. Staining of Slides with YOYO and Analysis

1. Slides are stained with 50 µL of 2.5% DMSO, 0.5% sucrose having 1 µ$M$ YOYO-1.
2. An individual apoptotic cell shows a circular gradient of granular DNA with a dense central zone and a lighter and hazy outer zone, giving the overall appearance of a halo.
3. The percentage of apoptotic cells is calculated usually from a total of 1000 cells (*see* **Note 5**). **Figure 1** is a photomicrograph of normal leukocytes without any apoptosis after 0 h of incubation of whole blood at 37°C. **Figure 2** is a photomicrograph of five apoptotic and numerous normal leukocytes after 24 h of incubation of whole blood at 37°C. **Figure 3** is a photomicrograph of six apoptotic and 14 normal leukocytes after 48 h of incubation of whole blood at 37°C. **Figure 4** shows one apoptotic and two normal leukocytes from the 48-h sample at a higher magnification (400×). Dye: YOYO-1.
4. In contrast, necrotic cells show an unusually large homogeneous nucleus with a clearly defined boundary. **Figure 5** is a photomicrograph showing one necrotic

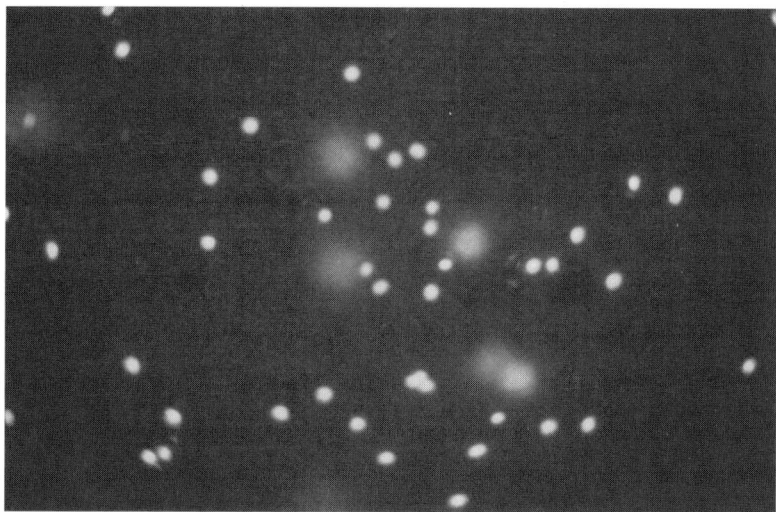

Fig. 2. A photomicrograph showing five apoptotic and numerous normal leukocytes. Whole blood was incubated for 24 h at 37°C and processed for the DNA diffusion assay. Magnification 100×. Dye YOYO-1.

and five normal leukocytes from whole blood incubated at 42°C for 1 h. Normal range for apoptosis in human blood is 0.1–0.2%. However, rates of apoptosis may vary significantly from person to person (*see* **Notes 6** and **7**).

### *3.2. DNA Diffusion Assay for Apoptosis in Human Sperm*

The methodology is similar to that described under **Subheading 3.1.**

1. A fresh semen sample from a healthy donor containing approx 10,000–500,000 sperm cells is diluted with 10 µL of PBS and mixed with 50 µL of 0.6% high-resolution 3:1 agarose.
2. Thus agarose is immediately covered with a cover glass and allowed to solidify for 5 min at room temperature (23°C).
3. The cover glasses are removed, and 200 µL of 2% agarose solution is layered as before to make a third layer.
4. After 2 min, cover glasses are removed and slides are placed in a slide-holding tray.
5. The slides are processed further as described under **Subheadings 3.1.3.–3.1.6.** **Figure 6** is a photomicrograph of two apoptotic sperm (one in the early stages and one late stage) and one normal sperm. Normal range for apoptosis in human sperm is 4–25%. However, rates of apoptosis may vary significantly from person to person.

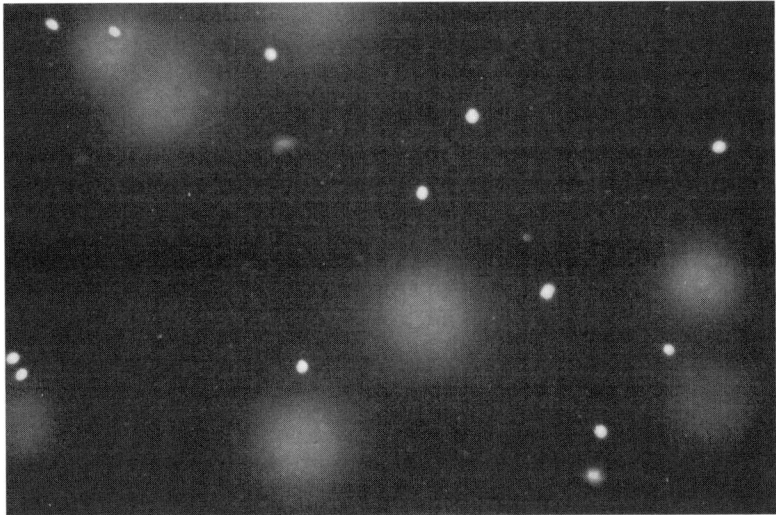

Fig. 3. A photomicrograph showing six apoptotic and 14 normal leukocytes. Whole blood was incubated for 48 h at 37°C and processed for the DNA diffusion assay. Magnification 100×. Dye YOYO-1.

## 3.3. DNA Diffusion Assay for Apoptosis in Soft Solid Tissue (Such as Thymus and Brain Cells) in Rats (see Note 8)

### 3.3.1. Isolation of Cells from Soft Solid Tissue (Such as Thymus and Brain) in Rats

1. All steps must be conducted in dim and indirect light.
2. The rat thymus and brain are dissected out and immediately washed three times in an excess of ice-cold PBS (phosphate-buffered saline without calcium and magnesium, having 200 µmol of N-1-butyl-α-phenynitrone, PBN, and 5% sucrose) to remove blood cells.
3. A tissue press is used to disperse thymus and brain tissue into a single-cell suspension (26). Tissue is placed on the wire screen of an ice-cold tissue press. This screen is supported by a supporting plate and screw-on cap. The device is then assembled and the lower end of the device with tissue is immersed in 20 mL of cold PBS in a beaker (this minimizes the contact of tissue with air). The piston is brought down by rotation. This provides pressure on the tissue, which can then be squeezed through the wire screen into the beaker.
4. Tissue pieces (which settle very quickly to the bottom of a 50-mL polypropylene tube without centrifugation) are then washed with cold PBS.
5. These smaller tissue pieces are dispersed into single-cell suspension in 5 mL of cold PBS using a 5-mL pipetman.

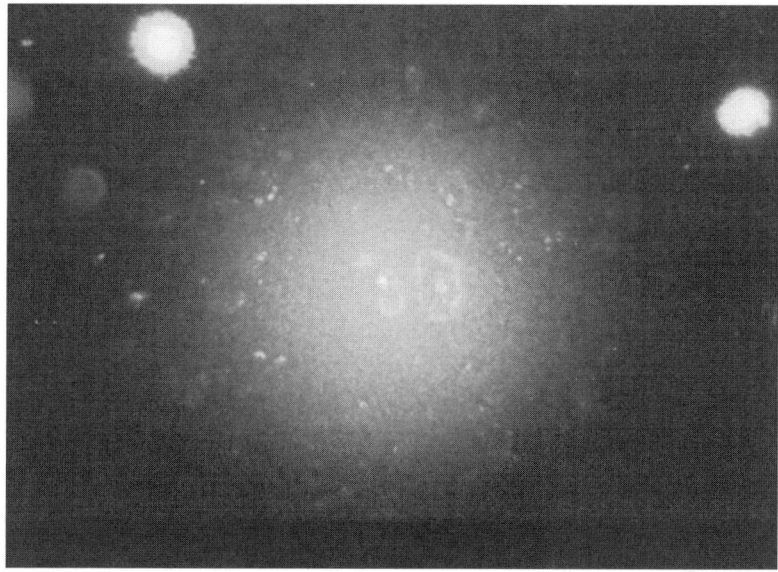

Fig. 4. A photomicrograph showing one apoptotic and two normal leukocytes. Whole blood was incubated for 48 h at 37°C and processed for the DNA diffusion assay. Magnification 400×. Dye YOYO-1.

6. Ten microliters of this cell suspension is mixed with 50 µL of agarose, and 50 µL of this mixture are used to make a second layer of microgels as described under **Subheading 3.1.2.**
7. Slides for DNA diffusion assay are processed as described under **Subheading 3.1.3.–3.1.5.** (*see* **Note 9**).

## 4. Notes

1. All the solutions can be prepared and stored at room temperature for up to 1 yr prior to experiments, unless mentioned otherwise. The preparation of solutions takes about 1 h. The assay procedure can be broken down into the following time scale:
    30 min—slide preparation (making eight slides)
    10 min—lysing and denaturing (mostly waiting time)
    30 min—neutralization and precipitation of DNA (mostly waiting time)
    30 min—neutralization and precipitation of DNA (mostly waiting time)
    30 min—air drying of slides (mostly waiting time) *or* drying can be enhanced by placing slides on a hot plate set at 70°C
    15 min/slide—screening and scoring for apoptosis
2. Whole blood can also be collected in microfuge tubes containing 1 m$M$ tetrasodium EDTA (final concentration) as an anticoagulant, if heparanized tubes are not available.

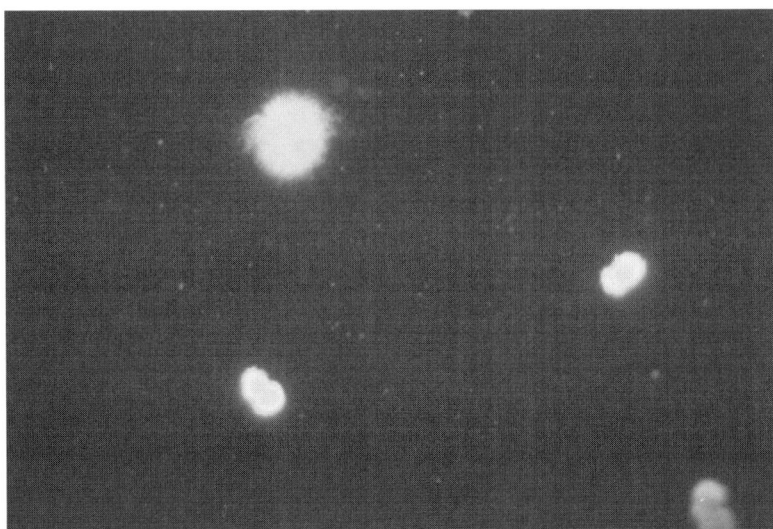

Fig. 5. A photomicrograph showing one necrotic and five normal leukocytes. Whole blood was incubated at 42°C for 1 h and processed using the DNA diffusion assay. Magnification 400×. Dye YOYO-1.

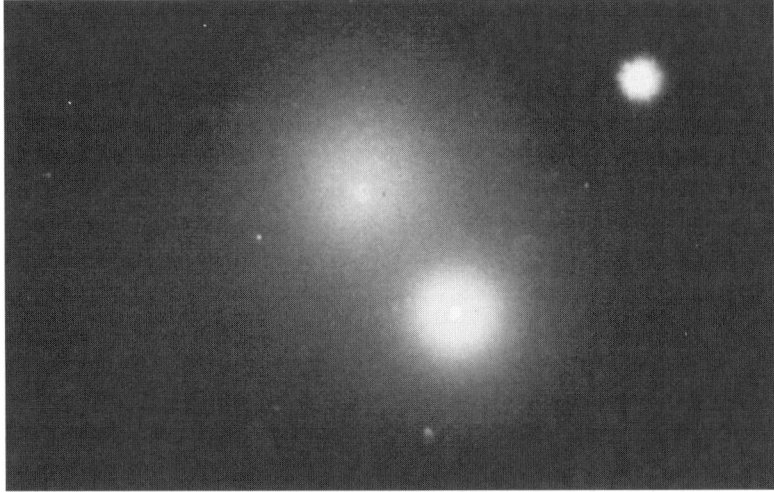

Fig. 6. A photomicrograph of sperm processed for the DNA diffusion assay. Two apoptotic cells (one in the early stages and one late stage) and one normal cell are seen in this figure. Magnification 400×. Dye YOYO-1.

3. If performed correctly with uniform proper layering of agarose, the assay will detect 98.2% of the apoptotic cells, as shown previously *(23)*. Variations in sensitivity may be observed due to variations in thickness of the top layer of agarose. If the agarose in the top layer is too thick, then background will increase and slides will require more time in spermine and ethanol solution. If the top layer is too thin, then some of the apoptotic cells will be lost.
4. Slides can also be placed in Coplin jars during processing when there are very few slides or when researchers do not have access to a slide tray.
5. High background, which may make scoring of apoptotic cells difficult, is observed for several reasons. The most common factor accounting for high background is a failure to use fresh solutions. This problem may also be encountered when the YOYO used is not fresh. In addition, insufficient time in spermine ethanol solution and use of too-thick third layer of agarose may produce the same problem. In order to prevent such problems, avoid reusing the neutralizing and DNA-precipitating solutions, and use fresh YOYO dye. Additionally, ensure that slides remain in the spermine ethanol solution for an adequate time (1 h) and apply a uniform thickness of third-layer agarose. To remove high background due to any reason mentioned above, immerse slides in 1 mg/mL spermine in distilled water for 10 min. Dry them and restain them with YOYO.
6. Although two modes of death can be identified easily, sometimes early apoptosis and late necrosis may be difficult to distinguish because of extensive DNA degradation occurring in late necrotic cell nuclei at their periphery. Thus, late necrotic cells with degraded DNA at the periphery may be mistaken for an early apoptotic cell. Experience with the technique and careful scoring may clarify this complexity. However, such indistinguishable cells are rare and can be categorized separately during scoring. This difficulty in differentiating between early apoptotic and late necrotic cells has been previously reported using the TUNEL assay *(17)*.
7. Procedural damage to the DNA (excessive light, excessive time spent in processing samples particularly during solidification of agarose) may degrade the DNA to such a degree that even a normal cell may show necrotic or apoptotic morphology, depending on the degree of DNA damage.
8. Some of the apoptotic cells are broken into apoptotic bodies during dispersion of solid tissue into single cells. Although these pieces are recognizably apoptotic, quantification of total apoptotic cells becomes difficult, as it is impossible to determine into how many pieces the original cell fragmented. This problem can be minimized by gentle handling during the solid tissue dispersion process.
9. The DNA diffusion assay for apoptosis is extremely versatile and can be applied for estimation of apoptotic cells from a variety of sources, including urine, sputum, nasal secretions, and tissue biopsies. This technique is a valuable tool for exploring the effects of nutrition, aging, and various environmental insults to humans and other living organisms. The technique may also prove useful for monitoring the efficacy of cancer treatment *(27)* and observing apoptosis during development in different organs.

## References

1. Searle, J., Kerr, J. F. R., and Bishop, C. J. (1982) Necrosis and apoptosis: distinct modes of cell death with fundamentally different significance. *Pathol. Ann.* **17,** 229–259.
2. von Wangenheim, K. H., and Peterson, H. P. (1998) Control of cell proliferation by progress in differentiation: clues to mechanisms of aging, cancer causation and therapy. *J. Theor. Biol.* **193,** 663–678.
3. Guchelaar, H. J., Vermes, A., Vermes, I., and Haanen, C., (1997) Apoptosis: molecular mechanisms and implications for cancer chemotherapy. *Pharm. World Sci.* **19,** 119–125.
4. Orrenius, S. (1995) Apoptosis: molecular mechanisms and implications for human disease. *J. Intern. Med.* **237,** 529–536.
5. Roshal, M., Zhu, Y., and Planelles, V. (2001) Apoptosis in AIDS. *Apoptosis* **6,** 103–116.
6. Temlett, J. A. (1996) Parkinson's disease: biology and aetiology. *Curr. Opin. Neurol.* **9,** 303–307.
7. Gorman, A. M., McGowan, A., O'Neill, C., and Cotter, T. (1996) Oxidative stress and apoptosis in neurodegeneration. *J. Neurol. Sci.* **139 (Suppl.),** 45–52.
8. Aguila, M. B., Mandarim de Lacerda, C. A., and Apfel, M. I. (1998) Stereology of the myocardium in young and aged rats. *Arq. Bras. Cardiol.* **70,** 105–109.
9. Sabbah, H. N. and Sharov, V. G. (1998) Apoptosis in heart failure. *Prog. Cardiovasc. Dis.* **40,** 549–562.
10. Popov, S. G., Villasmil, R., Bernardi, J., et al. (2002) Effect of *Bacillus anthracis* lethal toxin on human peripheral blood mononuclear cells. *FEBS Lett.* **527,** 211–215.
11. Warner, H. R., Hodes, R. J., and Pocinki, K. (1997) What does cell death have to do with aging? *J. Am. Geriatr. Soc.* **45,** 1140–1146.
12. Tomei, L. D. and Umansky, S. R. (1998) Aging and apoptosis control. *Neurol. Clin.* **16,** 735–745.
13. Aggarwal, S. and Gupta, S. (1998) Increased apoptosis of T cell subsets in aging humans: altered expression of Fas (CD95), Fas ligand, Bcl-2, and Bax. *J. Immunol.* **160,** 1627–1637.
14. Wyllie, A. H., Kerr, J. F. R., and Currie, A.R. (1980) Cell death: the significance of apoptosis. *Int. Rev. Cytol.* **68,** 251–306.
15. Nicholson, D. W., All, A., Thornberry, N. A., et al. (1995) Identification and inhibition of ICE/CED-3 protease necessary for mammalian apoptosis. *Nature* **376,** 37–43.
16. Gavrieli, Y., Sherman, Y., and Ben-Sasson, S. A. (1992) Identification of programmed cell death in situ via specific labeling of nuclear DNA fragmentation. *J. Cell Biol.* **119,** 493–501.
17. Kockx, M. M, Muhring, J., Knaapen, M. W., and de Meyer, G. R. (1998) RNA synthesis and splicing interferes with DNA in situ end labeling techniques used to detect apoptosis. *Am. J. Pathol.* **152,** 885–888.
18. Kerr, J. F. R., Wyllie, A. H., and Currie, A. R. (1972) Apoptosis: basic biological phenomenon with wide-ranging applications in tissue kinetics. *Br. J. Cancer* **26,** 239–257.

19. Koopman, G., Reutelingsperger, C. P., Kuiiten, G. A., Keehnen, R. M., and Pals, S. T. (1994) Annexin V for flow cytometiric detection of phosphatidylserine expression on B cells undergoing apoptosis. *Blood* **85,** 332–340.
20. Vincent, A. M., and Maiese K. (1999) Direct temporal analysis of apoptosis induction in living adherent neurons. *J. Histochem. Cytochem.* **47,** 661–671.
21. Andree, H. A., Reutelingsperger, C. P., Hauptmann R., Hemker, H. C., Hermens, W.T. and Willems, G.M. (1990) Binding of vascular anticoagulant alpha (VAC alpha) to planar phospholipid bilayers. *J. Biol. Chem.* **265,** 4923–4928.
22. Koester, S. K. and Bolton, W. E., (1999) Differentiation and assessment of cell death. *Clin. Chem. Lab. Med.* **37,** 311–317.
23. Singh, N. P. (2000) A simple method for accurate estimation of apoptotic cells. *Exp. Cell Res.* **256,** 328–237.
24. Singh, N. P., Muller, C. E., and Berger, R. E. (2003) Effects of age on DNA double strand breaks and apoptosis in human sperm. *Fertil. Steril.* **80,** 1420–1430.
25. Singh, N. P. (1997) Sodium ascorbate induced DNA strand breaks in human cell in vitro. *Mutat. Res.* **375,** 195–203.
26. Singh, N. P. (1998) A rapid method for the preparation of single-cell suspensions from solid tissues. *Cytometry* **31,** 229–232.
27. Singh, N. P. and Lai H. (2004) Artemisinin induces apoptosis in human cancer cells. *AntiCancer Res.* **24,** 2277–2280.

# 5

## PARP Cleavage and Caspase Activity to Assess Chemosensitivity

### Alok C. Bharti, Yasunari Takada, and Bharat B. Aggarwal

#### Summary

The ultimate aim of cancer therapeutics is to eradicate tumor cells. Upon lethal exposure to chemotherapeutic agents, cells undergo apoptosis—an active, energy-requiring, programmed cell death. Apoptosis follows a well-orchestrated activation of cysteine proteases, known as caspases. In normal conditions, all the caspases exist as inactive procaspases; they require proteolytic cleavage for activation. A variety of methods are currently used to detect procaspases and caspases and their activity. Immunodetection and fluorescent substrates are widely accepted methods that are utilized for this purpose. These methods are described in detail in this chapter.

#### Key Words

Apoptosis; PARP; caspases; chemosensitivity; fluorescent caspase inhibitors.

### 1. Introduction

Chemosensitivity testing is an ex vivo means of determining the cytotoxic (or cytostatic) activity of potential chemotherapeutic agents on either cancer cell lines or malignant cells isolated from tumors or biopsy specimens. Recent achievements put this type of test in a promising position in oncology. A number of them test chemosensitivity, including MTT assay of overall mitochondrial activity and $^3$H-thymidine incorporation to measure DNA synthesis. However, these methods are insufficient to differentiate cytotoxicity from cytostasis or to reveal the mechanism of action of the drug. New methods under development rely on analysis of poly(ADP-ribose) polymerase (PARP) cleavage and caspase activation, the hallmark features of cytotoxicity mediated through apoptosis to assess chemosensitivity *(1,2)*.

From: *Methods in Molecular Medicine, vol. 111: Chemosensitivity:*
*Vol. 2: In Vivo Models, Imaging, and Molecular Regulators*
Edited by: R. D. Blumenthal © Humana Press Inc., Totowa, NJ

Caspases are the main executers of apoptosis. To date, 14 members of this family have been identified *(3–6)*. This group of cysteine proteases exist within the cell as inactive proforms or zymogens. These zymogens can be cleaved to form active enzymes following the induction of apoptosis. Caspase enzymes specifically recognize a four-amino-acid sequence (on their substrate) that necessarily includes an aspartic acid residue. This residue is the target for the cleavage reaction, which occurs at the carbonyl end of the aspartic acid residue *(7)*.

Caspases can be detected via immunoprecipitation, immunoblot analysis using caspase-specific antibodies, or assays employing fluorogenic substrates that become fluorescent upon cleavage by the caspase. One of the latest approaches is based on carboxyfluorescein (FAM)-labeled fluoromethyl ketone (FMK)-peptide inhibitors of caspases *(8–10)*. These inhibitors are cell-permeable and noncytotoxic. Once inside the cell, the inhibitor binds covalently to the active caspase *(11)*. Cells that contain bound inhibitor can be analyzed by fluorescence microscopy. FAM-VAD-FMK, a FAM analog of benzyloxycarbonylvalylalanylaspartic acid FMK (zVAD-FMK), is one such agent. Because FAM gives a green fluorescence, it can be combined with vital fluorescent dyes such as propidium iodide (PI), which specifically stains dead cells. The FAM-VAD-FMK enters the cell and irreversibly binds to activated caspases (caspase-1, -2, -3, -4, -5, -6, -7, -8, and -9) and indicates the cells that are undergoing apoptosis. In addition, proteolysis of individual caspases can be demonstrated by Western blot analysis using specific antibodies.

Caspase-3 acts as the central executer of apoptosis and is responsible for proteolysis of several key proteins *(12)* (**Table 1**). PARP is the first substrate of caspase-3 to be studied extensively *(13)*. Although many caspases, including caspase-2, -4, -6, -8, -9, and -10, can cleave PARP in vitro when added at high concentrations, it appears that caspase-3 and -7 are primarily responsible for PARP cleavage during apoptosis. Assay of PARP cleavage is the preferred biochemical method for checking the induction of caspase -3 and -7 and the induction of apoptosis. During apoptosis, PARP, a 116-kDa protein, gets degraded to characteristic 89-kDa and 24-kDa fragments. This degradation of PARP can be very beautifully shown by Western blot analysis. Antibodies can detect either both intact and cleaved PARP or just the cleaved fragment. Both types of antibodies are readily available from various suppliers.

These methods detect activated caspases in cell lysates, but they provide little information on which caspases are activated in apoptotic cells. If it is necessary to characterize the specific protease activated in vivo by a given apoptotic stimulus, it is necessary to immunoblot the total cell lysate using antibodies recognizing individual caspases. Because caspases are activated by auto- or heteroproteolysis of the proenzyme, the appearance of bands with lower molecular weight corresponding to the subunit of the active enzymes

## Table 1
## Caspases and Their Substrates

| Caspase | Alternate name | Molecular weight of intact and spliced form[a] | Substrates |
|---|---|---|---|
| Caspase-1 | ICE | 45 (p), 33 (i), 20 (a), 10 (a) | Pre-interleukin-1β, interleukin-18, lamins |
| Caspase-2 | Ich-1 (human), Nedd2 (rat, mouse) | 48 (p), 35 (a) | Golgin-160, lamins |
| Caspase-3 | CPP32, Yama, apopain | 32 (p), 17 (a), 12 (a) | PARP, SREBs, gelsolin, caspase-6, caspase-7, caspase-9, DNA-PK, MDM2, Gas2, fodrin, β-catenin, lamins, NuMA, HnRNP proteins, topoisomerase I, FAK, calpastatin, p21Waf1, presenelin2, ICAD, SP-1, bid, NF-κB, Rb, Bcl-2, actin, PKC, TRAF1, PAK2, gelsolin |
| Caspase-4 | Ich-2, ICErel-II, TX | 43 (p) | Caspase-1 |
| Caspase-5 | ICErel-III, TY | 20 (a), 10 (a) | — |
| Caspase-6 | Mch2 | 34 (p), 18 (a), 10 (a) | Lamins, NuMA, FAK, caspase-3, keratin-18 |
| Caspase-7 | Mch3, ICE-LAP3, CMH-1 | 35 (p), 17 (a), 11 (a) | PARP, Gas2, SREB1, EMAP II, FAK, calpastatin, p21Waf1 |
| Caspase-8 | FLICE, MACH, Mch5 | 55 (p), 40 (a), 23 (a), 18 (a), 10 (a) | Caspase-3, caspase-4, caspase-6, caspase-7, caspase-9, caspase-10, caspase-13, bid |
| Caspase-9 | Apaf-33, ICE-LAP6, Mch6 | 46–48 (p), 35 (a), 10 (a) | Caspase-3, caspase-7, caspase-9 |
| Caspase-10 | FLICE-2, Mch4 | 55 (p), 23 (a), 17 (a), 12 (a) | Caspase-3, caspase-4, caspase-6, caspase-7, caspase-8, caspase-9 |
| Caspase-11 | Ich-3, ICE-B | | ? |
| Caspase-12 | ICE-C | 55 (p), 42 (a) | ? |
| Caspase-13 | ERICE | | ? |
| Caspase-14 | MICE | | ? |

[a]Human caspases. (p) precursor, (a) processed fragments, (i) intermediate.

indicates their activation. With the same method it is possible to analyze individual substrates cleaved in vivo by caspases. The same membrane can be reused to be tested with different antibodies, specific for other caspases or substrates, by stripping and reblotting. Most of the antibodies for caspases and their substrates are readily available commercially. We describe both PARP cleavage and immunodetection methods below.

## 2. Materials
### 2.1. PARP Cleavage

1. Lysis buffer: 20 m$M$ HEPES, pH 7.4, 2 m$M$ EDTA, 250 m$M$ NaCl, 0.1% NP-40, 2-μg/mL leupeptin, 2-μg/mL aprotinin, 1 m$M$ PMSF, 0.5 μg/mL benzamidine, 1 m$M$ dithiothreitol (DTT) (*see* **Note 1**).
2. 6X sodium dodecyl sulfate (SDS) sample buffer: 100 m$M$ Tris-HCl, pH 6.8, 1% SDS, 3% glycerol, 0.093 g/mL DTT, 0.12-mg/mL bromophenol blue.
3. Molecular-weight maker.
4. Transfer buffer: 192 m$M$ glycine, 25 m$M$ Tris, 20% v/v aqueous methanol (store at 4°C).
5. PBST: Phosphate-buffered saline (PBS) with 0.5% Tween-20 (prepare fresh from 10X PBS stock).
6. Blocking buffer: 5% nonfat dry milk in PBST (prepare fresh).
7. Antibody dilution buffer: 3% bovine serum albumin (BSA) in PBST (prepare fresh).
8. Stripping solution: 100 m$M$ 2-β-mercaptoethanol, 2% SDS, 62.5 m$M$ Tris-HCl, pH 6.8.
9. Primary antibody (against cleaved protein, or one that detects both intact and cleaved protein).
10. Corresponding secondary antibody conjugated with horseradish peroxidase (HRP).
11. Enhanced chemiluminescence (ECL) reagent.
12. X-ray film.
13. Nitrocellulose membrane.
14. *Apparatus:* Vertical SDS-PAGE unit, gel-transfer unit, membrane-washing trays and X-ray exposure cassette, X-ray film developing solutions.

### 2.2. In Situ Activated Caspase Detection Using FAM-VAD-FMK

1. ApoLogix FAM-VAD-FMK (FAM100-1) (Cell Technology, Minneapolis, MN).
2. PBS.
3. Dimethyl sulfoxide (DMSO).
4. PI solution (50 μg/mL; PBS) (*see* **Note 2**).
5. Working dilution of FAM-VAD-FMK.
    a. Reconstitute lyophilized FAM-peptide-FMK with DMSO to a 150X concentration. Keep FAM-labeled inhibitors protected from light at all times.
    b. Mix contents at room temperature until completely dissolved. Aliquots should be made and stored frozen at –20°C until ready to use (*see* **Note 3**).

c. Prior to use, make 30X working dilution as per requirement. Dilute the 150X solution 1:5 in PBS, pH 7.4 (1 part 150X FAM-VAD-FMK and 4 parts PBS). Mix the vial contents thoroughly to assure that a homogeneous solution is obtained.

d. Use diluted FAM-VAD-FMK solution immediately for best results. Protect from light at all times.

4. *Apparatus:* Fluorescence microscope with appropriate filters (488-nm excitation filter and emission filter range 520–535 nm), slides, and cover slips.

## 3. Methods
### 3.1. PARP Cleavage

1. Two million cells should be taken per sample. Treat them as required (*see* **Note 4**).
2. After completion of the treatment, put the cells on ice and centrifuge at 350*g* for 5 min at 4°C. Aspirate the medium and wash the cells with chilled PBS twice. Lyse the cells in 300 µL of lysis buffer for 30 min on ice with intermittent vortexing.
3. Centrifuge the lysate at 15000*g* for 10 min at 4°C. Collect the supernatant. Estimate proteins in the sample. The Bradford reagent can be used for protein estimation.
4. Aliquot 50 µg of protein for PARP estimation from each sample into tubes. Remaining lysates can be frozen at −70°C for assay at a later time. Add 1:5 vol of 6X SDS sample buffer and boil the sample for 5 min. Pulse-spin and run on a 7.5% SDS-PAGE at a constant current of 35 mA/minigel. Also run molecular-weight standards in one lane of the same gel to confirm the molecular weight of the protein of interest.
5. Stop electrophoresis when the dye front reaches the bottom. Carefully remove the gel and cut off the stacking gel.
6. Put the gel for transfer of proteins to the nitrocellulose membrane for 12–14 h at constant 40 V in cold room.
7. After transfer, remove the membrane, wash once with PBST, and incubate in blocking buffer for 2 h at room temperature.
8. Dilute anti-PARP antibody in antibody dilution buffer. Incubate the membrane in the diluted primary antibody overnight at 4°C. (*see* **Note 5**).
9. Wash the membrane in PBST four times for 10 min with gentle shaking. Dilute HRP-conjugated secondary antibody (1:3000) in blocking buffer. Incubate the membrane in diluted secondary antibody for 1 h at room temperature. Wash the membrane four times with PBST for 10 min with gentle shaking.
10. Develop the membrane with ECL solution for detection of proteins. Expose the X-ray film for 30 s, 1 min, and 5 min, depending on the intensity of the signal (*see* **Note 6**).
11. For the results of PARP-immunodetection, indicating one slow-moving band of 118 kDa, which is intact PARP, or a fast-migrating band of 89 kDa. However, the small 24-kDa cleavage product cannot be detected in a 7.5% acrylamide gel. Appcarance of 89-kDa fragment is an indication of caspase-3 activity in the cells (**Fig. 1**) (*see* **Note 7**).

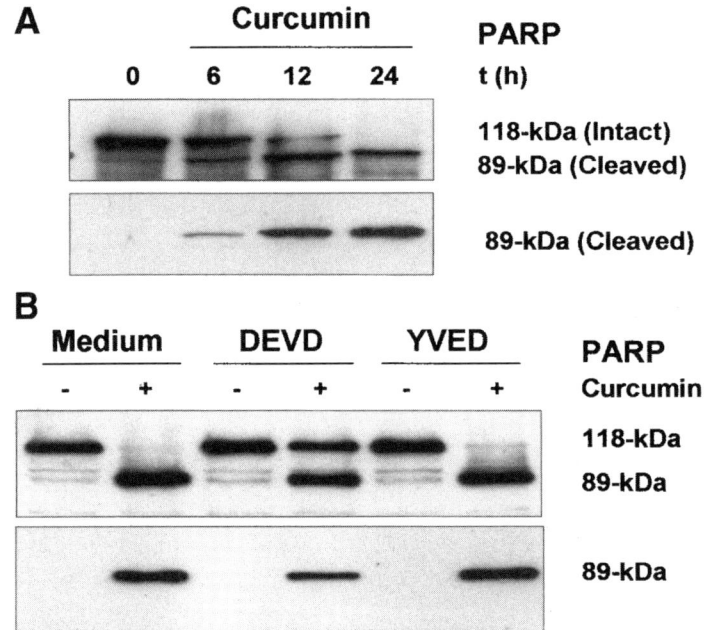

Fig. 1. PARP cleavage by Western blot analysis. (**A**) U266 cells ($2 \times 10^6$ cells/mL) were incubated in the absence or presence of curcumin (50 µ$M$) for indicated times. The cells were washed and total proteins were extracted by lysing the cells. Sixty micrograms of extracts were resolved on 7.5% SDS-PAGE gel, electrotransferred to a nitrocellulose membrane, and probed with anti-PARP (upper panel) or anticleaved PARP (lower penal) antibodies. (**B**) Suppression of curcumin-induced PARP cleavage by caspase-3 inhibitor. U266 cells ($2 \times 10^6$ cells/mL) were preincubated with Ac-DEVD-CHO (10 µ$M$), a specific caspase-3 inhibitor, or Ac-YVAD-CHO (10 µ$M$), a specific caspase-1 inhibitor, for 2 h and then treated with curcumin (50 µ$M$) for 24 h. Thereafter, cell extracts were prepared and analyzed for PARP cleavage by using either anti-PARP antibody (upper panel) or anticleaved PARP (lower penal) antibodies.

### 3.2. In Situ *Caspase Activation Assay–Staining with FAM-VAD-FMK*

1. Cells: Treat cells with potential chemotherapeutic agent at desired time points. Take untreated cells as negative control samples. Cells in suspension can be cultured in a tissue culture plate or culture tube. Culture 100–300 µL volume at a maximum density of $1 \times 10^6$ cells/mL (*see* **Note 8**).
2. Cell labeling: Add 3.3–10 µL 30X working dilution FAM-peptide-FMK directly to the cell suspension. Slightly flicking the tissue culture plates or culture tubes sufficiently mixes the cells. Incubate cells for 1 h at 37°C under 5% $CO_2$, protecting the tubes from light.

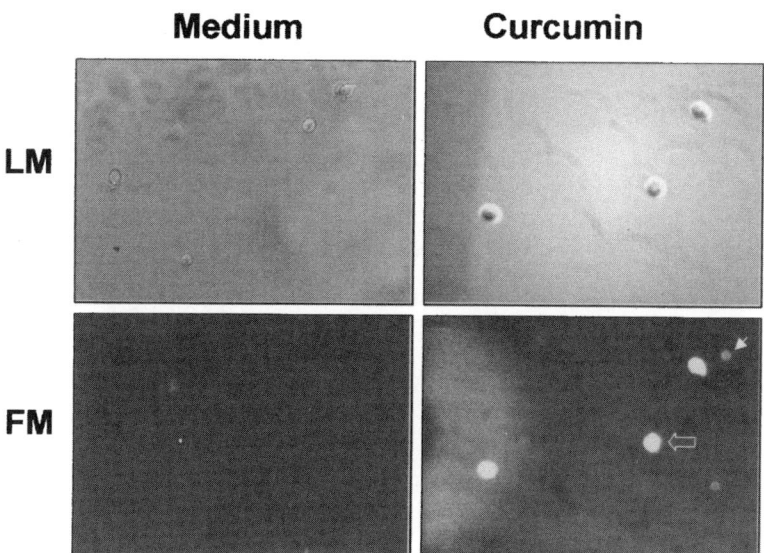

Fig. 2. Detection of caspase activation *in situ* by using fluorogenic substrate FAM-VAD-FMK. Untreated or U266 cells treated with curcumin (50 μ$M$) for 12 h were examined for caspase activation by ApoLogix FAM-VAD-FMK. Cells were analyzed under light microscopy (LM) and by fluorescence microscopy (FM). Green fluorescence indicates activated caspases (empty arrow). Red fluorescence of PI indicates DNA of dead cells with compromised cell membrane (small solid arrow). Original magnification 200×.

3. Washings: Add PBS in cultures with labeled cells to bring the volume to 1.5 mL. Gently mix and transfer to 1.7-mL microfuge tube. Spin down the cells at 350$g$ for 5 min at room temperature. Decant supernatant. To disrupt cell-to-cell clumping, gently vortex the cell pellet. Resuspend the cell pellet in 1.5 mL PBS, followed by a second centrifugation step. Repeat washing twice. Resuspend the cell pellet in 50 μL of PBS. Add 50 μL of PI. Leave at room temperature for 15 min and then put samples on ice.
4. Analysis: Take a drop of cell suspension on a clean slide and put cover slip over it. Now analyze under the light microscope with fluorescence attachments using a bandpass filter (excitation 488 nm, emission 520–535 nm) to view green fluorescence for cells with activated caspases and red fluorescence for dead cells. Live cells can be localized using light microscopy, as they do not fluoresce at the indicated excitation wavelength **(Fig. 2)**.

### *3.3. Analysis of Activation of Specific Caspase by Western Blot Analysis*

The cell lysate used for PARP cleavage can be used for analysis of individual caspases and their activation.

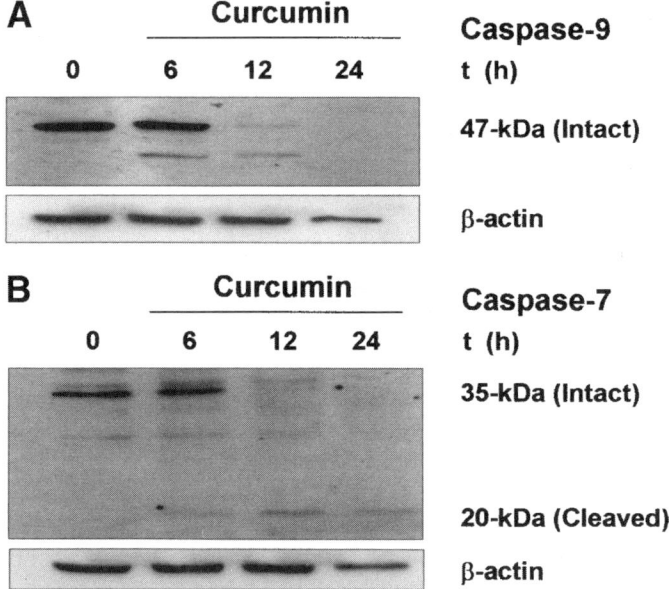

Fig. 3. Caspase-7 and caspase-9 activation by Western blot analysis. U266 cells ($2 \times 10^6$ cells/mL) were incubated in the absence or presence of curcumin (50 μ$M$) for indicated times. The cells were washed and total proteins were extracted by lysing the cells. Sixty micrograms of extracts were resolved on 10% SDS-PAGE gel, electrotransferred to a nitrocellulose membrane, and probed with **A**, anti-caspase-9 or **B**, anti-caspase-7 antibodies.

1. Run the lysates on 10–15% SDS-PAGE gel.
2. Perform Western blot analysis as indicated under **Subheading 3.1.**
3. Immunodetect specific caspases using corresponding antibodies (**Fig. 3**).

### 3.4. Stripping and Reblotting

1. Incubate immunoblotted membrane to protect it from drying up, with prewarmed stripping solution at 50°C for 30 min.
2. Wash membrane 5X with PBST for 15 min.
3. Perform Western blot analysis starting from membrane blocking.

## 4. Notes

1. It is preferable to make fresh lysis buffer from the stock solutions just before use.
2. PI is a potential mutagen. Use of gloves, protective clothing, and eyewear, as well as safe laboratory protocol, is strongly recommended.

3. Reconstituted FAM-labeled inhibitors (150X) may be aliquoted and stored at –20°C, protected from light, for up to 6 mo from date of reconstitution. avoid multiple freeze–thaw cycles.
4. Cells should be acclimatized for about 2 h before treatment in the $CO_2$ incubator for a reproducible result. In order to visualize PARP cleavage, the cells should be treated for 12–24 h.
5. A 1:3000–1:5000 dilution of Santa Cruz Biotech (Santa Cruz, CA) anti-PARP antibody is sufficient to get a good signal, whereas, 1:1000 dilution is required for Transduction Lab (Lexington, KY) antibody that specifically detects cleaved PARP.
6. The chemiluminescence lasts for 30–45 min only, so the membrane should be processed quickly to get crisp results.
7. Troubleshooting problems in Western blot analysis:
   a. Do not see anything on the film: Check all the ECL reagents and their expiration dates.
   b. Cannot see any band recognized by your antibody: Your antibody may not be good; use the specific purified protein as control proteins. In your cell lysate may not be enough, use more lysate-desired protein may be expressed at low levels in your cells.
   c. Do not see any cleavage product: Make sure your cells are apoptotic by morphological examination under microscope at 40× objective. (Apoptotic cells show cell shrinkage, nuclear condensation, and plasma membrane blebbing.)
8. FAM inhibitors can also be used with adherent cells. Add 10 µL 30X working dilution FAM-peptide-FMK per 300 µL medium. Mix well. Remove the medium and wash cells twice with 2 mL PBS. Add PI solution for 15 min and analyze under fluorescence microscope.

## Acknowledgments

This work was supported by the Clayton Foundation for Research (to BBA), Department of Defense US Army Breast Cancer Research Program grant (BC010610, to BBA), a PO1 grant (CA91844) from the National Institutes of Health on lung chemoprevention (to BBA), and a P50 Head and Neck SPORE grant from the National Institutes of Health (to BBA).

## References

1. Bharti, A. C., Donato, N., Singh, S., and Aggarwal, B. B. (2003) Curcumin (diferuloylmethane) down-regulates the constitutive activation of nuclear factor-kappa B and IkappaBalpha kinase in human multiple myeloma cells, leading to suppression of proliferation and induction of apoptosis. *Blood* **101**, 1053–1062.
2. Fulda, S., Scaffidi, C., Pietsch, T., Krammer, P. H., Peter, M. E., and Debatin, K. M. (1998) Activation of the CD95 (APO-1/Fas) pathway in drug- and gamma-irradiation-induced apoptosis of brain tumor cells. *Cell Death Differ.* **5**, 884–893.

3. Hu, S., Snipas, S. J., Vincenz, C., Salvesen, G., and Dixit, V. M. (1998) Caspase-14 is a novel developmentally regulated protease. *J. Biol. Chem.* **273,** 29,648–29,653.
4. Salvesen, G. S. (2002) Caspases and apoptosis. *Essays Biochem.* **38,** 9–19.
5. Nicholson, D. W. and Thornberry, N. A. (2003) Apoptosis. Life and death decisions. *Science* **299,** 214–215.
6. Beauparlant, P. and Shore, G. C. (2003) Therapeutic activation of caspases in cancer: a question of selectivity. *Curr. Opin. Drug Discov. Devel.* **6,** 179–187.
7. Thornberry, N. A., Rano, T. A., Peterson, E. P., et al. (1997) A combinatorial approach defines specificities of members of the caspase family and granzyme B. Functional relationships established for key mediators of apoptosis. *J. Biol. Chem.* **272,** 17,907–17,911.
8. Amstad, P. A., Yu, G., Johnson, G. L., Lee, B. W., Dhawan, S., and Phelps, D. J. (2001) Detection of caspase activation in situ by fluorochrome-labeled caspase inhibitors. *Biotechniques* **31,** 608–610, 612, 614, passim.
9. Bedner, E., Smolewski, P., Amstad, P., and Darzynkiewicz, Z. (2000) Activation of caspases measured in situ by binding of fluorochrome-labeled inhibitors of caspases (FLICA): correlation with DNA fragmentation. *Exp. Cell Res.* **259,** 308–313.
10. Smolewski, P., Bedner, E., Du, L., et al. (2001) Detection of caspases activation by fluorochrome-labeled inhibitors: Multiparameter analysis by laser scanning cytometry. *Cytometry* **44,** 73–82.
11. Ekert, P. G., Silke, J., and Vaux, D. L. (1999) Caspase inhibitors. *Cell Death Differ.* **6,** 1081–1086.
12. Tewari, M., Quan, L. T., O'Rourke, K., et al. (1995) Yama/CPP32 beta, a mammalian homolog of CED-3, is a CrmA-inhibitable protease that cleaves the death substrate poly(ADP-ribose) polymerase. *Cell* **81,** 801–809.
13. Lazebnik, Y. A., Kaufmann, S. H., Desnoyers, S., Poirier, G. G., and Earnshaw, W. C. (1994) Clevage of poly(ADP-ribose) polymerase by a proteinase with properties like ICE. *Nature* **371,** 346–347.

# 6

## Diphenylamine Assay of DNA Fragmentation for Chemosensitivity Testing

### Cicek Gercel-Taylor

#### Summary

Apoptosis is a distinct morphological and biochemical entity resulting in cell death, which occurs because of a variety of pathological and physiological stimuli. Chemotherapeutic agents, at least in part, result in cell death by inducing apoptosis. Quantitation of this process enables the study of differential cellular responses to chemotherapy and potentially clinical sensitivity. Apoptotic process results in cytoskeletal disruption, cell shrinkage, membrane blebbing, nuclear condensation, and internucleosomal DNA fragmentation. A variety of methods exist to determine apoptosis along this pathway. Diphenylamine assay enables the quantitation of degraded DNA. The protocol is simple and allows manipulation of all types of cell cultures. Resulting colorimetric reaction is easily quantitated, and the assay is highly reproducible.

#### Key Words

Diphenylamine assay; apoptosis; tumor cells.

## 1. Introduction

The diphenylamine assay is a very useful method for measuring apoptosis by determining the percentage of fragmentation of DNA into oligosomal-sized fragments. Measure of soluble DNA released from apoptotic nuclei into the cytoplasm constitutes a quantitative measure of cellular response. Another advantage of the diphenylamine assay is that apoptotic DNA fragmentation can be analyzed in both adherent and floating cells following treatment with chemotherapeutic or other agents. Data obtained from the experiment are expressed as a percentage relative to uninduced or untreated controls. Quantitation of DNA with this method was first described by Dische *(1,2)* in the 1930s and later modified by Burton *(3)* in the mid-1950s. These modifications have resulted in

From: *Methods in Molecular Medicine, vol. 111: Chemosensitivity:*
*Vol. 2: In Vivo Models, Imaging, and Molecular Regulators*
Edited by: R. D. Blumenthal © Humana Press Inc., Totowa, NJ

enhanced sensitivity of up to fivefold by adding sulfuric acid and acetaldehyde, and by allowing the colorimetric reaction to develop overnight at room temperature. These changes have also resulted in the reduction of interference from other substances that were an initial drawback with the originally described method, further enhancing the sensitivity of the assay. The diphenylamine reaction takes advantage of the bonds between purines and deoxyribose, which are very labile. Once these bonds are broken, inorganic phosphates are liberated from the DNA and provide the substrate, which is measured by the reaction. The overall preparation time is approx 3 h for 30 samples, with incubation occurring overnight for 12–16 h. Reading of the results takes approx 1 min per sample. We have used this method to quantitate apoptosis in ovarian cancer cells treated with various chemotherapeutic agents *(4,5)*. Other investigators have utilized this method in a variety of systems alone or in combination with other methods in the demonstration of apoptotic cell death *(6–10)*.

## 2. Materials

1. Phosphate-buffered saline (PBS): 10 m$M$ sodium phosphate, 150 m$M$ NaCl, pH 7.4.
2. Trichloroacetic acid (TCA): 10% and 5% solutions in double-distilled water (dd$H_2$O).
3. Lysis buffer: 5 m$M$ Tris-HCl, 20 m$M$ ethylenediaminetetraacetic acid (EDTA), pH 8.0, 0.5% (v/v) Triton X-100 (added immediately before use).
4. TE buffer: 1 m$M$ EDTA, 10 m$M$ Tris, pH 8.0.
5. Diphenylamine reagent: 1.5 g diphenylamine in 100 mL of acetic acid and 1.5 mL $H_2SO_4$ (stored in the dark). This reagent is stable without acetaldehyde for at least 3 mo at 4°C (*see* **Note 1**). Immediately before use, acetaldehyde is added in the cold room to a final concentration of 16 μg/mL (*see* **Note 2**).

## 3. Methods

1. Harvest monolayer cultures by scraping cells into the medium with a rubber policeman (or directly into centrifuge tubes for suspension cultures) and centrifuge (300*g*) at 4°C for 10 min to pellet the cells (*see* **Note 3**).
2. Resuspend the cell pellet in 0.8 mL of 10 m$M$ PBS, pH 7.4, and 0.7 mL of ice-cold lysis buffer.
3. Transfer the cell lysate to microfuge tubes and incubate on ice for 15 min (*see* **Note 4**).
4. Centrifuge the lysate (13,000*g*) at 4°C for 15 min to separate fragmented DNA from high-molecular-weight DNA.
5. Transfer the entire supernatant (about 1.5 mL containing fragmented DNA) to a 5-mL glass tube (*see* **Note 5**).
6. Resuspend the pellet containing intact DNA in 1.5 mL TE, and again transfer to another 5-mL glass tube.

7. Add 1.5 mL of 10% TCA to each tube and incubate for 10 min at room temperature.
8. Centrifuge (500$g$) at 4°C for 15 min and discard the supernatant.
9. Resuspend the 10% TCA precipitates in 0.7 mL of 5% TCA, boil (100°C) for 15 min (*see* **Note 6**), cool to room temperature, and centrifuge (300$g$) at 4°C for 15 min.
10. Transfer 0.5 mL of the supernatant without disturbing the precipitate to a new glass tube.
11. Add 1 mL of the diphenylamine reagent, and incubate overnight at 30°C (*see* **Note 7**).
12. Measure the absorbance at 600 nm.
13. Percentage of DNA fragmentation = $OD_{600}$ of the supernatant/[$OD_{600}$ of the supernatant + $OD_{600}$ of the pellet] × 100.

## 4. Notes

1. If the diphenylamine reagent has any trace of blue discoloration, we recommend that a new reagent be made because this can influence the $OD_{600}$ reading and affect your calculations in an uncontrolled fashion.
2. When mixing the acetic acid and sulfuric acid together, wear protective gloves, as these substances are irritating and caustic. Also note that a cold room is a designated place to add the diphenylamine so that the vapors are kept to a minimum.
3. We recommend a minimum of $2.5 \times 10^6$ cells for determination of DNA fragmentation; however, two times this amount ($5.0 \times 10^6$) is preferable.
4. Suspension created after lysis needs to be homogeneous prior to centrifugation to ensure adequate separation of the fragmented from intact DNA.
5. It is very important not to disturb the precipitate formed in **step 4** because this can interfere with subsequent readings used in the quantitation of the fragmented and intact DNA. The use of a micropipet is recommended.
6. A water bath at 100°C ready prior to processing the samples is most suitable.
7. The time of incubation may be prolonged past 16 h if the colorimetric reaction is weak.

## References

1. Dische, Z. (1930) *Mikrochemise* **8,** 4.
2. Dische, Z. (1955) *The Nucleic Acids* (Chargraff, E. and Davidson, J. N., eds.), Academic, New York.
3. Burton, K. (1956) A study of the conditions and mechanisms of the diphenylamine reaction for the colorimetric estimation of deoxyribonucleic acid. *Biochem. J.* **62,** 315–323.
4. Gercel-Taylor, C., Ackermann M. A., and Taylor, D. D. (2001) Evaluation of cell proliferation and cell death based assays in chemosensitivity testing. *Anticancer Res.* **21,** 2761–2768.
5. Gibb, R. K., Taylor, D. D., Wan, T., O'Connor, D. M., Doering, D. L., and Gercel-Taylor, C. (1997) Apoptosis as a measure of chemosensitivity to cisplatin and taxol therapy in ovarian cancer cell lines. *Gynecol. Oncol.* **65,** 13–22.

6. Messmer, U. K., Winkel, G., Briner, V. A., and Pfeilschifter, J. (2000) Suppression of apoptosis by glucocorticoids in glomerular endothelial cells:effects on proapoptotic pathways. *Br. J. Pharm.* **129,** 1673–1683.
7. Ponnathpur, V., Ibrado, A. M., Reed, J. C., et al. (1995) Effects of modulators of protein kinases on Taxol-induced apoptosis of human leukemic cells possessing disparate levels of p26BCL-2 protein. *Clin. Cancer Res.* **1,** 1399–1406.
8. Sun, Y., Clinkenbeard K. D., Clarke, C., Cudd, L., Highlander, S. K., and Dabo, S. M. (1999) *Pasteurella haemolytica* leukotoxin induced apoptosis of bovine lymphocytes involves DNA fragmentation. *Vet. Microbiology* **65,** 153–166.
9. Trachtman, H., Futterweit, S., Mermelstein, A., Metzger, S., Pettei, M. (2000) Anti-apoptotic effect of L-arginine in cultured rat mesangial cells. *Int. J. Mol. Med.* **6,** 485–489.
10. von Knethen, A., and Brüne, B. (2000) Attenuation of macrophage apoptosis by the cAMP-signalling system. *Mol. Cell. Biochem.* **212,** 35–43.

# 7
## Immunodetecting Members of the Bcl-2 Family of Proteins

### Richard B. Lock and Kathleen M. Murphy

#### Summary
The Bcl-2 family of proteins centrally regulates the cellular commitment to apoptosis (programmed cell death). Apoptosis, in turn, is critical for the development and homeostasis of multicellular organisms, and defects in apoptosis contribute to a broad range of human diseases and disorders. Consequently, studying the regulation of Bcl-2 and its homologs has significant implications for biomedical research. The mechanisms by which Bcl-2 family members regulate apoptosis are complex, and include variations in intracellular protein levels, direct protein–protein interactions, conformational changes, and subcellular redistribution. Therefore, all of these factors should be considered when assessing how one, or a group, of these proteins contributes to a cell's commitment to apoptosis. The methods described in this chapter will allow the researcher to gain a greater understanding of how intracellular levels of multiple members of the Bcl-2 protein family can be analyzed simultaneously by immunoblotting and how protein–protein interactions can be studied using immunoprecipitation techniques. In addition, the methodology describes how conformational changes can be observed by immunofluorescence and immunoprecipitation, and how subcellular redistribution of Bcl-2 homologs can be followed.

#### Key Words
Apoptosis; immunoblotting; immunoprecipitation; immunofluorescence; subcellular; conformation; Bcl-2; Bax; Bcl-X; Bid; Bim; Bak.

### 1. Introduction

Apoptosis is a genetically programmed form of physiological cell death essential for survival of all multicellular organisms, and plays a critical role in development, homeostasis, and protection *(1)*. Dysregulation or malfunction of apoptosis leads to disorders of homeostasis and contributes to the pathogenesis of a number of human diseases *(1,2)*. Unregulated excessive apoptosis has been implicated as the cause of a number of diseases characterized by an increased loss of normal cells, such as neurodegenerative disorders, AIDS, ischemic injury, and osteoporosis. Conversely, inappropriately low rates of apoptosis result in the accumulation of cells. Increasing evidence suggests that the failure of cells to undergo apoptosis is important in the pathogenesis of a number of diseases that were once thought to be proliferative disorders, such as autoimmune diseases, viral infections, and cancer.

Apoptosis can be triggered through a wide variety of extrinsic and intrinsic stimuli, including developmental signals, cellular stress, disruption of cell cycle, and DNA damage *(3)*. Although the capacity to carry out apoptosis appears to be inherent to all cells, the susceptibility to apoptosis varies markedly and is influenced by both external and intrinsic factors. Because of the involvement of apoptosis in such a variety of human diseases, much attention has been focused on defining its molecular mechanisms of regulation. One of the major apoptosis-regulatory protein families is represented by Bcl-2 and its homologs.

Bcl-2 was originally discovered as the protooncogene involved in the t(14:18) chromosomal translocation found in the majority of follicular B-cell lymphomas (reviewed in **ref. 4**). When identified, Bcl-2 had no significant amino acid homology with any other protein whose biochemical mechanism of action was known. Its function remained a mystery until Vaux et al. introduced the gene into interleukin-3-dependent cell lines and demonstrated that overexpression of Bcl-2 abolished dependency on the cytokine (reviewed in **ref. 3**). Thus, *bcl-2* defined a novel class of oncogenes that exerted their effects, not by positively regulating cell growth, but rather by inhibiting cell death.

Subsequent to the discovery of Bcl-2, a growing family of Bcl-2-related proteins has been identified, of which there are at least 16 in humans *(5)*. The family consists of members that inhibit apoptosis (including Bcl-2, Bcl-xL, Mcl-1, and Bcl-w), as well as proteins that promote apoptosis (including Bax, Bak, Bad, Bik, Bcl-xS, Bim, and Bid). Bax was the first proapoptotic member of the family identified and was discovered based on its coimmunoprecipitation with Bcl-2 *(6)*. Bax is capable of forming homodimers as well as heterodimers with Bcl-2 *(6)*. Additionally, Bax and Bcl-2 can mutually antagonize each other when coexpressed in the same cells *(6)*. These findings have led to the hypothesis that the ratio of antiapoptotic molecules, such as Bcl-2, to proapoptotic molecules, such as Bax, dictates the relative sensitivity or resistance of cells to apoptosis *(7)*. Other members of the Bcl-2 family of proteins can also interact with each other, forming homo- and heterodimers *(6,8,9)*. Dimerization among family members provides an important mechanism for controlling their activity.

Bcl-2–related proteins all share homology in at least one of four regions designated the Bcl-2 homology domains BH1-4, with the BH3 domain being common to all family members, both pro- and antiapoptotic. Many of the members contain a C-terminal hydrophobic domain, which putatively functions to target and anchor proteins to intracellular membranes. Despite the presence of a C-terminal hydrophobic domain, Bax is a cytosolic protein in unstressed cells *(10–12)*. Members of the family such as Bad and Bid, which lack a hydrophobic sequence at the C-terminus, also exhibit a predominantly cytoplasmic distribution in the absence of a death signal *(13–15)*. During apoptosis, proapoptotic proteins such as Bax and Bak undergo conformational changes and translocate from the cytosol to intracellular membrane compartments *(10,16–18)*. Translocation of Bax to mitochondria results in loss of mitochondrial transmembrane potential and the release of at least two apoptogenic factors from the mitochondria: cytochrome *c* and apoptosis-inducing factor (AIF) *(19,20)*. Cytosolic cytochrome c plays an active role in the apoptotic process by acting in concert with Apaf-1 and ATP/dATP to activate caspase-9, initiating the caspase cascade of proteolytic cleavages that result in disassembly of the cell *(21)*.

The evidence cited above indicates that regulation of the Bcl-2 family of proteins includes (but is not restricted to): (1) levels of protein expression; (2) heterodimerization between family members; (3) conformational changes; and (4) subcellular redistribution. Over the past 8 yr we have optimized the methodology to analyze all of these parameters and, while this has been restricted to human Bcl-2, Bax, Bcl-xL, Bcl-xS, Bak, Bid, BimEL, BimL, and BimS, it is likely that it can be applied to additional members of the Bcl-2 family. Finally, we have assumed that the reader has a basic knowledge of laboratory technical and safety procedures, including sodium dodecyl sulfate (SDS)-polyacrylamide gel electrophoresis, Western transfer, and immunoblotting.

## 2. Materials

### 2.1. Immunodetection of Bcl-2, Bax, Bcl-xL/S, Bak, Bim, and Bid

1. NP-40 lysis buffer: 50 m$M$ Tris-HCl, pH 7.4, 150 m$M$ NaCl, 0.2% NP-40, 50 m$M$ NaF, 5 m$M$ EDTA, 0.1 m$M$ orthovanadate. This buffer can be stored at 4°C for at least 1 mo, although protease inhibitors (Sigma P8340) should be added immediately prior to use from a concentrated stock stored at –20°C. BCA (bicinchoninic acid) protein assay kit (Pierce Biotechnology).
2. Heating block.
3. 2X SDS sample buffer: 100 m$M$ Tris-HCl, pH 6.8, 4% SDS, 0.2% bromophenol blue, 20% glycerol, 10% 2-mercaptoethanol. This buffer can be stored at 4°C for at least 1 mo, although the 2-mercaptoethanol should be added immediately prior to use.
4. Standard vertical gel electrophoresis apparatus (e.g., Bio-Rad Protean IIxi) and power pack.
5. Standard transfer apparatus (e.g., Bio-Rad Trans-Blot Cell).
6. Polyvinylidene difluoride (PVDF) membrane (Millipore).
7. Ponceau S stain.
8. TBS: 20 m$M$ Tris-HCl, pH 7.5, 500 m$M$ NaCl, 0.02% Na-azide.

**Table 1**
**Antibodies Used for Immunoblotting**

| Specificity | Description | Supplier | Cat. no. | Dilution |
|---|---|---|---|---|
| Actin | Rabbit polyclonal | Sigma | A2066 | 1:2,000 |
| Bak | Rabbit polyclonal | BD PharMingen | 556396 | 1:2,000 |
| Bax | Rabbit polyclonal | BD PharMingen | 554104 | 1:2,000 |
| Bcl-2 | Rabbit polyclonal | BD PharMingen | 554160 | 1:2,000 |
| Bcl-X | Rabbit polyclonal | BD PharMingen | 551269 | 1:1,000 |
| Bid | Goat polyclonal | Santa Cruz | sc-6538 | 1:2,000 |
| Bim | Rabbit polyclonal | Sigma | B7929 | 1:500 |
| Goat IgG | HRP conjugated secondary | Santa Cruz | sc-2020 | 1:5,000 |
| Mouse IgG | HRP conjugated secondary | Amersham Biosciences | NA931 | 1:10,000 |
| Rabbit IgG | HRP conjugated secondary | Amersham Biosciences | NA934 | 1:10,000 |

9. TTBS: 20 m$M$ Tris-HCl, pH 7.5, 500 m$M$ NaCl, 0.05% Tween-20.
10. Nonfat dry milk (available at your local supermarket).
11. Primary and secondary antibodies (*see* **Table 1**): SuperSignal Ultra Chemiluminescence Substrate (Pierce); standard autoradiographic film; chemiluminescence imaging system (e.g., Bio-Rad VersaDoc or equivalent); prestained protein molecular-weight standards (Pierce); stripping buffer, 0.2 $M$ glycine, pH 2.5, 0.05% Tween-20.

*Note:* 2-Mercaptoethanol is toxic and volatile, and should only be handled in a fume hood; Na-azide is also toxic and should be handled appropriately.

### 2.2. Immunoprecipitation of Bcl-2 Homologs

1. Hamster antihuman Bcl-2 monoclonal (clone 6C8, cat. no. 551051, BD PharMingen).
2. Rabbit antihuman Bax and Bcl-X polyclonal antibodies (*see* **Table 1**).
3. Protein A-sepharose (Pierce) and protein G-agarose (Pierce or Santa Cruz Biotechnology).
4. Materials for immunoblotting as described under **Subheading 2.1.**

### 2.3. Conformational Changes in Proapoptotic Bcl-2 Protein Family Members

#### 2.3.1. Immunoprecipitation Using Conformation-Specific Antibodies

1. CHAPS, 3-[(3-cholamidopropyl)dimethylammonio]-1-propanesulfonic acid lysis buffer: 10 m$M$ HEPES, pH 7.4, 150 m$M$ NaCl, 1% CHAPS. This buffer can be

stored at 4°C for at least 1 mo, although protease inhibitors (Sigma P8340) should be added immediately prior to use from a concentrated stock stored at –20°C.
2. BCA (bicinchoninic acid) protein assay kit (Pierce).
3. N-terminal conformation-specific anti-Bax monoclonal antibody (clone YTH-6A7, cat. no. 2281-MC-100, Trevigen).
4. Protein G-agarose (Pierce or Santa Cruz).
5. Materials for immunoblotting as described under **Subheading 2.1.**

### 2.3.2. Immunofluorescence to Detect Conformational Changes in Bax

1. No. 1 glass cover slips.
2. 3% Paraformaldehyde in PBS.
3. N-terminal conformation-specific anti-Bax monoclonal antibody (clone YTH-6A7).
4. FITC-goat antimouse IgG (Zymed Laboratories).
5. ProLong Antifade mounting reagent (Molecular Probes).
6. Zeiss Axioskop 20 fluorescence microscope and Bio-Rad MRC 1024 Laser Scanning Confocal Imaging System (or equivalent systems).

*Note:* Paraformaldehyde is toxic and should be dissolved in phosphate-buffered saline (PBS) by warming in a safety hood.

## 2.4. Subcellular Redistribution of Bax

### 2.4.1. Separation of Subcellular Cytosolic and Nuclear/Membrane Fractions

1. Extraction buffer: 50 m$M$ PIPES, pH 7.0, 50 m$M$ KCl, 5 m$M$ MgCl$_2$, 5 m$M$ EGTA, 1 m$M$ phenylmethylsulfonyl fluoride, 10 µg/mL leupeptin, 10 µg/mL pepstatin A.
2. Trypan blue.
3. Ultracentrifuge.
4. Anticytochrome oxidase subunit VIc (clone 3G5-F7-G3, Molecular Probes).
5. Lactate dehydrogenase assay kit (Sigma).

*Note:* Phenylmethylsulfonyl fluoride is toxic and should be handled with caution. Add from a 100 m$M$ stock solution in methanol prepared immediately prior to use.

### 2.4.2. Immunofluorescence Detection of Bax Subcellular Distribution

1. Triton X-100.
2. Bovine serum albumin (BSA).
3. Rabbit anti-Bax polyclonal antibody 06-499 (Upstate Biotechnology).
4. Mouse monoclonal anticytochrome $c$ 6H2.B4 (BD PharMingen).
5. FluoroLink Cy 2-labeled goat antirabbit IgG and FluoroLink Cy 3-labeled goat antimouse IgG (Amersham Biosciences).
6. Rabbit IgG (Sigma).

## 3. Methods
### 3.1. Immunodetection of Bcl-2, Bax, Bcl-xL/S, Bak, Bim, and Bid

One of the most straightforward methods to assess intracellular levels of Bcl-2 protein family members, and ratios thereof, is by immunoblotting. With the appropriate optimization it is possible to simultaneously probe for multiple proteins on the same membrane, thus conserving the use of cell lysates, secondary antibodies, and chemiluminescence reagents. The following procedures have been optimized for detecting Bcl-2, Bax, Bcl-xL/S, Bak, Bim, and Bid, but could readily be adapted for additional Bcl-2 homologs.

1. Prepare whole-cell extracts by lysing $1–5 \times 10^7$ cells in 1 mL of NP-40 lysis buffer plus protease inhibitor cocktail on ice for 30 min with occasional vortexing. Centrifuge the crude lysate at 10,000$g$ for 10 min at 4°C and retain the supernatant, which can be stored at –80°C for subsequent analysis. Estimate the protein concentration by the bicinchoninic assay method using BSA standard (*see* **Note 1**).
2. Denature equal amounts of protein (at least 25 µg) by the addition of an equal volume of 2X SDS sample buffer to the cell lysate, and heating to 95°C for 5 min in a heating block. Separate proteins by electrophoresis through an SDS-polyacrylamide gel (4% stacking, 12.5% resolving) at constant current (45 mA per gel) for approx 4 h, or until the dye front reaches the bottom of the gel (*see* **Note 2**). Equilibrate the gel and PVDF membrane in transfer buffer for 20 min. Transfer proteins to PVDF membrane at constant voltage (30 V) at 4°C overnight (*see* **Note 3**). Following transfer, verify equal loading and transfer of proteins by staining the gel with Ponceau S. Following image capture, remove the Ponceau S with $H_2O$ and a 10-min wash in TBS. Block nonspecific binding sites with 10% (w/v) nonfat dry milk in TTBS for 1 h followed by two 5-min washes in TTBS.
3. Incubate membranes with primary antibody diluted in TTBS as indicated in **Table 1** for 1 h (monoclonal antibodies) or 3 h (polyclonal antibodies) at room temperature with rocking (*see* **Note 4**). Remove the primary antibody solution (*see* **Note 5**) and wash the membrane three times for 5 min in TTBS. Incubate the membrane with secondary antibodies, as indicated in **Table 1**, for 1 h at room temperature with rocking, followed by five washes for 5 min each with TTBS.
4. Generate chemiluminescence signals by the addition of SuperSignal Ultra Chemiluminescence Substrate, and visually detect on radiographic film and quantify by chemiluminescence analysis (*see* **Notes 6** and **7**). Estimate the molecular mass of proteins by comparison to a prestained protein standard (*see* **Note 8**). The signal intensity of Bcl-2 homologs should be normalized to that of actin.
5. In order to reprobe, incubate the membrane in stripping buffer for 1 h at 80°C. Repeat, and wash the membrane five times for 5 min in TTBS (*see* **Note 9**). Block nonspecific binding sites as in **step 2**. The membrane can then be stored in TTBS at 4°C until reprobed.

## 3.2. Immunoprecipitation of Bcl-2 Homologs

While intracellular levels of Bcl-2 and related proteins are important in the control of apoptosis, these proteins are also known to interact directly as part of the regulatory process. Immunoprecipitation is a relatively simple technique that can be used to study these interactions, and the following describes a reliable experimental protocol.

1. Prepare whole-cell extracts and quantify protein concentration as described under **Subheading 3.1.**
2. Use equal amounts of protein for immunoprecipitation reactions (at least 500 µg, ideally 1 mg), and adjust all tubes to an equal volume with lysis buffer (usually 500 µL). Add an appropriate amount of antibody to each tube (*see* **Notes 10 and 11**). Rotate the mixture for 2 h at 4°C.
3. Centrifuge the tubes in a microfuge at 10,000g for 10 s, place the tubes on ice, then add either protein A-sepharose or protein G-agarose (*see* **Note 12**). Rotate the tubes for at least 30 min at 4°C.
4. Spin down the protein A- or protein G- bound complexes (20 s in microfuge at room temperature). Place the tubes on ice. Remove the supernatant using a 1-mL micropipet (*see* **Notes 13 and 14**).
5. Add 1 mL of ice-cold lysis buffer to each tube. Cap and shake tubes. Spin in the microfuge (20 s), and place the tubes back on ice.
6. Remove the supernatant using a 200-µL micropipet tip attached to suction tubing (*see* **Note 14**) and repeat for a total of 3X 1-mL washes.
7. After the final wash, centrifuge the tubes, place on ice, and remove the supernatant as close as possible to the pellet. Add an appropriate amount of 2X SDS sample buffer to each tube (if running duplicate gels, add 250 µL and load 120 µL per gel; if one gel, add 120 µL and load it all on one gel). Vortex the tubes, spin in microfuge for 20 s and heat to 95°C for 5 min. After allowing to cool to room temperature, vortex, spin again, and immediately analyze by immunoblotting as described under **Subheading 3.1.** (*see* **Note 15**). Alternatively, the samples can be stored at −80°C until required. If doing so, thaw the samples and warm to 37°C prior to loading on the gel.

## 3.3. Conformational Changes in Proapoptotic Bcl-2 Protein Family Members

In response to apoptotic stimuli, proapoptotic members of the Bcl-2 family are known to undergo conformational changes that appear to facilitate their insertion into intracellular membranes, leading to acceleration of the apoptotic process *(12,18,22,23)*. Conformation-specific antibodies are available to study this process *(12,17)*, and the following protocols, while having been optimized to assess conformational changes in the N-terminus of Bax *(23)*, could also be applied to additional Bcl-2 homologs.

### 3.3.1. Immunoprecipitation Using Conformation-Specific Antibodies

1. Prepare whole-cell extracts and quantify protein concentration as described under **Subheading 3.1.**, substituting CHAPS lysis buffer for NP-40 lysis buffer (*see* **Note 16**).
2. Use equal amounts of protein (1 mg) for each immunoprecipitation reaction, and normalize all samples to an equivalent volume (500 µL). Add 6 µg of the N-terminal conformation-specific anti-Bax monoclonal antibody (clone YTH-6A7) to the samples and rotate for 2 h at 4°C (*see* **Notes 11**, **17**, and **18**).
3. Centrifuge the tubes in a microfuge at 10,000*g* for 10 s, place the tubes on ice, then add 50 µL of a 50% slurry of protein G-agarose (*see* **Note 12**). Rotate the tubes for 2 h at 4°C.
4. The remainder of the procedure is exactly as described in **steps 4–7** under **Subheading 3.2.**, substituting CHAPS lysis buffer for NP-40 lysis buffer.

### 3.3.2. Immunofluorescence to Detect Conformational Changes in Bax

1. Grow cells on No. 1 glass cover slips and expose to apoptotic stimuli (*see* **Note 19**). At appropriate time points, wash the cells twice in PBS and fix for 30 min using 3% paraformaldehyde in PBS. Permeabilize the cells for 2 min with 0.2% CHAPS and wash four times with PBS. Block nonspecific binding by incubating with 5% BSA in PBS for 1 h.
2. Incubate the cells with mouse anti-Bax YTH-6A7 monoclonal antibody diluted 1:300 in 3% BSA/PBS for 1 h at 37°C in a humidified chamber (*see* **Note 20**).
3. Remove excess antibody by washing the cover slips six times with PBS. Incubate the cells with the secondary antibody, FITC-goat antimouse IgG diluted 1:20 in 3% BSA/PBS, for 1 h protected from light.
4. After washing six times with PBS, mount the cover slips onto microscope slides using ProLong Antifade mounting reagent. Stain control slides with secondary antibody alone.
5. View cells under a Zeiss Axioskop 20 fluorescence microscope, and image using the Bio-Rad MRC 1024 Laser Scanning Confocal Imaging System, or equivalent of both systems. For each time point, count at least 300 cells.

## 3.4. Subcellular Redistribution of Bax

Bcl-2 homologs, in particular the proapoptotic members of the family, are known to undergo subcellular redistribution that contributes to a cell's commitment to undergo apoptosis *(10,16,18,24)*. The following protocols have been optimized to document Bax translocation from cytosol to cellular membrane fractions by subcellular fractionation followed by immunoblotting *(23,25–27)* or by immunofluorescence *(26,27)*. The latter method includes dual staining for cytochrome *c*.

### 3.4.1. Separation of Subcellular Cytosolic and Nuclear/Membrane Fractions

1. Wash $10^7$ cells twice with cold PBS and suspend in 1 mL of extraction buffer. Lyse cells by five cycles of freezing in liquid nitrogen and thawing at 37°C. Verify by microscopic examination with trypan blue that >95% cells have lysed, and centrifuge the crude lysate at 100,000$g$ for 1 h at 4°C.
2. Separate the resulting supernatant, which consists of the cytosol, from the pellet that contains the cellular membrane and organelles. Wash the pellet once with extraction buffer and suspend in 1 mL of extraction buffer.
3. Verify lack of cross-contamination of fractions by immunoblotting for proteins specifically localized to the nucleus (e.g., DNA topoisomerase I) *(27)* and mitochondria (e.g., cytochrome oxidase subunit VIc) *(23,26,27)*. In addition, lactate dehydrogenase activity should be measured as a cytosolic marker, and experiments should only be deemed valid if >95% of the total lactate dehydrogenase activity is detected in the cytosolic fractions.
4. Denature equal volumes of cytosolic and membrane fractions by the addition of an equal volume of 2X SDS sample buffer, and heating to 95°C for 5 min, then analyze by immunoblotting as described in **steps 2–5** under **Subheading 3.1.**

### 3.4.2. Immunofluorescence Detection of Bax Subcellular Distribution

1. Grow cells on No. 1 glass cover slips and expose to apoptotic stimuli (*see* **Note 19**). At appropriate time points, wash the cells twice in PBS and fix for 30 min using 3% formaldehyde in PBS. Permeabilize the cells for 2 min with 0.2% Triton X-100 in PBS and wash four times with PBS. Block nonspecific binding by incubating with 5% BSA in PBS for 1 h.
2. Incubate the cells with rabbit anti-Bax polyclonal antibody 06-499 and mouse monoclonal anti-cytochrome *c* 6H2.B4 diluted 1:50 in 3% BSA/PBS for 1 h at 37°C in a humidified chamber (*see* **Notes 20** and **21**).
3. Remove excess antibody by washing the cover slips four times with PBS. Incubate the cells for 1 h protected from light with the secondary antibodies; FluoroLink Cy 2-labeled goat antirabbit IgG and FluoroLink Cy 3-labeled goat antimouse IgG, diluted 1:1000 in 3% BSA/PBS. Stain control slides with nonspecific rabbit IgG and both secondary antibodies.
4. After washing four times with PBS, mount the cover slips onto microscope slides using ProLong Antifade mounting reagent. View and image slides as described in **step 5** under **Subheading 3.3.2.**

## 4. Notes

1. Cells should be washed at least twice in ice-cold PBS to prevent proteins in the serum added to tissue culture media interfering with the protein assay. NP-40 is also compatible with other commercially available protein assays (e.g., Bradford). However, compatibility should be verified prior to using other detergents for cell lysis (e.g., SDS).

2. The conditions for detecting Bcl-2 protein homologs were optimized using the Protean IIxi vertical gel electrophoresis system (Bio-Rad), which resulted in overall less background compared to smaller gel formats (e.g., the Bio-Rad Mini Protean System or Hoeffer Mighty Small System). Further optimization should be performed when using the small gel format.
3. Conditions for protein transfer were optimized using the Trans-Blot Cell (Bio-Rad). Proteins can also be transferred at 100 V for 2 h at 4°C.
4. We have been able to combine up to four primary antibodies (e.g., rabbit polyclonal antibodies raised against Bax, Bcl-2, Bcl-X, and actin) in a single incubation *(25–27)*. It is recommended that conditions be optimized in a preliminary experiment using replicate strips of membrane probed with each antibody individually and then all in combination.
5. We have reused diluted antibody up to five times. However, when doing so, the signal strength should be carefully monitored. We recommend adding sodium azide to a final concentration of 0.02% prior to storing the antibody at 4°C to prevent contamination. Despite the known inhibitory effects of azide on horseradish peroxidase, in our experience we have not found this to interfere with secondary antibodies, probably due to its removal during washing. However, if in doubt, merthiolate can be substituted for azide.
6. ECL Plus detection reagent (Amersham) can also be used to generate chemiluminescence signals.
7. Chemiluminescence signals should be quantified using commercially available instrumentation. If this is not available, it is possible to quantify signals scanned from photographic film, but only if the film has been brought to its linear range (to an $OD_{540}$ of 0.15) by the procedure known as "preflashing" *(28)*.
8. The proteins migrate corresponding to the following molecular weights: actin, 42 kDa; Bak, 24 kDa; Bax, 21 kDa; Bcl-2, 26 kDa; Bcl-xL, 29 kDa; Bcl-xS, 17 kDa; Bid, 22 kDa; BimEL, 23kDa; BimL, 17 kDa; BimS, 13 kDa. In addition, proteolytic cleavage of actin, Bax and Bid have been observed during apoptosis *(13,23,25,26,29)*.
9. Despite several methods being available for removing primary and secondary antibodies from membranes for reprobing, we have only been consistently successful using the method outlined.
10. Each antibody should be tested for its ability to immunoprecipitate, as considerable variation has been experienced between different antibodies. Consistent success has been achieved using the following antibodies: hamster antihuman Bcl-2 monoclonal (clone 6C8, cat. no. 551051, BD PharMingen); rabbit antihuman Bax polyclonal (*see* **Table 1**); and rabbit antihuman Bcl-X polyclonal (*see* **Table 1**). While the latter antibody is not sold on the basis that it will immunoprecipitate, we have been successful but only using the NP-40 lysis buffer described. Other buffers containing higher NaCl concentrations or stronger detergents did not allow immunoprecipitation with this anti-Bcl-X antibody. Each batch of antibody should then be titered to determine the minimum amount necessary to immunoprecipitate

100% of the target protein from a constant amount of cell lysate (e.g., 500 µg or 1 mg) used in each reaction.
11. Control tubes should be included that contain antibody and lysis buffer, but no cell lysate. These will assist in the identification of contaminating antibody chains in the subsequent immunoblots. Additional control lanes on the immunoblots should include whole cell lysates (25–100 µg protein).
12. Protein A should be used to bind rabbit polyclonal and hamster monoclonal immunoglobulins, although it has little affinity for mouse IgG1, and protein G is more appropriate. Fifty microliters of a 50% slurry of protein A-sepharose or protein G-agarose should suffice, although the amount should be optimized for each batch.
13. An aliquot of the supernatant should be retained and analyzed by immunoblotting alongside the respective immunoprecipitate to determine the bound vs free proportions of each protein of interest. Mix an aliquot 1:1 with 2X SDS sample buffer, heat to 95°C for 5 min, cool to room temperature, and load on the gel. If the supernatant is too dilute, concentrate the proteins by precipitation, as follows: (1) add 5 vol of ice-cold acetone to the sample, and incubate at –20°C for 30 min; (2) centrifuge at 10,000*g* for 5 min at 4°C; (3) remove supernatant and repeat acetone wash and centrifugation; (4) remove supernatant and dry pellet under vacuum; (5) dissolve pellet in 1X SDS sample buffer, heat to 95°C for 5 min, cool to room temperature, and load onto gel.
14. At this stage it is not necessary to remove the supernatant too close to the pellet (i.e., leave 25–50 µL of buffer above the pellet). The subsequent washes are sufficient to remove any unbound proteins.
15. If background becomes a problem, cell lysates can be precleared with the protein A-sepharose or protein G-agarose prior to immunoprecipitation.
16. Certain detergents, including NP-40, have been shown to induce the N-terminal conformational change in Bax *(12)*. Extracts of cells lysed in buffers containing NP-40 can therefore serve as useful controls for the immunoprecipitation reaction *(23)*. CHAPS detergent does not induce the N-terminal conformational change *(12,23)*.
17. Additional control immunoprecipitation reactions should be included using an antibody that recognizes all conformations of Bax, such as that described under **Subheading 3.2.**, to immunoprecipitate total Bax from the lysate.
18. Bellosillo et al. have recently described a flow cytometry based assay to quantify Bax N-terminal conformational change in intact cells using the same monoclonal antibody *(30)*, which has the advantages of using fewer cells and being more rapid.
19. For suspension cell cultures, spin cells onto slides using a Cytospin apparatus (Shandon Southern Products, Runcorn, England) and then follow the staining procedure. Alternatively, cells can be stained first, suspended in Vectashield mounting medium (Vector Laboratories) and then pipetted dropwise onto a glass slide *(17)*. For some experiments it may be desirable to label cells with organelle-specific dyes. For example, cells can be labeled with Mitotracker Red CM-H$_2$XRos (Molecular Probes), which localizes to mitochondria, prior to exposure to apop-

totic stimuli. In our experience it is necessary to optimize the concentration and labeling time for each cell type studied.
20. A simple humidified chamber can be made by placing gauze or paper towels in the bottom of a Petri dish and moistening with $H_2O$. Two glass or wooden rods can be placed on the gauze/paper towels on which the cover slips can rest. Incubate with lid closed.
21. In our experience, the anti-Bax polyclonal from Upstate Biotechnology has proven the most reliable for immunofluorescence detection of total Bax *(26,27)*.

## Acknowledgments

The Children's Cancer Institute Australia for Medical Research is affiliated with the University of New South Wales and Sydney Children's Hospital.

## References

1. Steller, H. (1995) Mechanisms and genes of cellular suicide. *Science* **267**, 1445–1449.
2. Thompson, C. B. (1995) Apoptosis in the pathogenesis and treatment of disease. *Science* **267**, 1456–1462.
3. Vaux, D. L. and Strasser, A. (1996) The molecular biology of apoptosis. *Proc. Natl. Acad. Sci. USA* **93**, 2239–2244.
4. Kroemer, G. (1997) The proto-oncogene Bcl-2 and its role in regulating apoptosis. *Nature Med.* **3**, 614–620.
5. Reed, J. C. (1998) Bcl-2 family proteins. *Oncogene* **17**, 3225–3236.
6. Oltvai, Z., Milliman, C., and Korsmeyer, S. J. (1993) Bcl-2 heterodimerizes in vivo with a conserved homolog, Bax, that accelerates programmed cell death. *Cell* **74**, 609–619.
7. Yang, E. and Korsmeyer, S. J. (1996) Molecular thanatopsis: a discourse on the BCL2 family and cell death. *Blood* **88**, 386–401.
8. Sedlak, T. W., Oltvai, Z. N., Yang, E., et al. (1995) Multiple Bcl-2 family members demonstrate selective dimerizations with Bax. *Proc. Natl. Acad. Sci. USA* **92**, 7834–7838.
9. Reed, J. C. (1994) Bcl-2 and the regulation of programmed cell death. *J. Cell Biol.* **124**, 1–6.
10. Wolter, K. G., Hsu, Y.-T., Smith, C. L., Nechushtan, A., Xi, X.-G., and Youle, R. J. (1997) Movement of Bax from the cytosol to mitochondria during apoptosis. *J. Cell Biol.* **139**, 1281–1292.
11. Hsu, Y.-T. and Youle, R. J. (1997) Nonionic detergents induce dimerization among members of the Bcl-2 family. *J. Biol. Chem.* **272**, 13,829–13,834.
12. Hsu, Y.-T. and Youle, R. J. (1998) Bax in murine thymus is a soluble monomeric protein that displays differential detergent-induced conformations. *J. Biol. Chem.* **273**, 10,777–10,783.
13. Gross, A., Yin, X.-M., Wang, K., et al. (1999) Caspase cleaved BID targets mitochondria and is required for cytochrome *c* release, while BCL-$X_L$ prevents this release but not tumor necrosis factor-R1/Fas death. *J. Biol. Chem.* **274**, 1156–1163.

14. Kluck, R. M., Esposti, M. D., Perkins, G., et al. (1999) The pro-apoptotic proteins, Bid and Bax cause a limited permeabilization of the mitochondrial outer membrane that is enhanced by cytosol. *J. Cell Biol.* **147,** 809–822.
15. Gross, A., McDonnell, J. M., and Korsmeyer, S. J. (1999) BCL-2 family members and the mitochondria in apoptosis. *Genes Dev.* **13,** 1899–1911.
16. Hsu, Y.-T., Wolter, K. G., and Youle, R. J. (1997). Cytosol-to-membrane redistribution of Bax and Bcl-X(L) during apoptosis. *Proc. Natl. Acad. Sci. USA* **94,** 3668–3672.
17. Griffiths, G. J., Dubrez, L., Morgan, C. P., et al. (1999) Cell damage-induced conformational changes of the pro-apoptotic protein Bak in vivo precede the onset of apoptosis. *J. Cell Biol.* **144,** 903–914.
18. Desagher, S., Osen-Sand, A., Nichols, A., et al. (1999) Bid-induced conformational change of Bax is responsible for mitochondrial cytochrome c release during apoptosis. *J. Cell Biol.* **144,** 891–901.
19. Susin, S. A., Zamzami, N., Castedo, M., et al. (1996) Bcl-2 inhibits the mitochondrial release of an apoptogenic protease. *J. Exp. Med.* **184,** 1331–1341.
20. Kluck, R. M., Bossy-Wetzel, E., Green, D. R., and Newmeyer, D. D. (1997) The release of cytochrome *c* from mitochondria: a primary site for Bcl-2 regulation of apoptosis. *Science* **275,** 1132–1136.
21. Li, P., Nijhawan, D., Budihardjo, I., et al. (1997) Cytochrome *c* and dATP-dependent formation of Apaf-1/caspase-9 complex initiates an apoptosis protease cascade. *Cell* **91,** 479–489.
22. Nechushtan, A., Smith, C. L., Hsu, Y.-T. and Youle, R. J. (1999) Conformation of the Bax C-terminus regulates subcellular location and cell death. *EMBO J.* **18,** 2330–2341.
23. Murphy, K. M., Streips, U. N., and Lock, R. B. (2000) Bcl-2 inhibits a Fas-induced conformational change in the Bax N-terminus and Bax mitochondrial translocation. *J. Biol. Chem.* **275,** 17,225–17,228.
24. Gross, A., Jockel, J., Wei, M. C., and Korsmeyer, S. J. (1998) Enforced dimerization of BAX results in its translocation, mitochondrial dysfunction and apoptosis. *EMBO J.* **17,** 3878–3885.
25. Elliott, M. J., Murphy, K. M., Stribinskiene, L., et al. (1999) Bcl-2 inhibits early apoptotic events and reveals post-mitotic multinucleation without affecting cell cycle arrest in human epithelial tumor cells exposed to etoposide. *Cancer Chemother. Pharmacol.* **44,** 1–11.
26. Murphy, K. M., Streips, U. N., and Lock, R. B. (1999) Bax membrane insertion during Fas(CD95)-induced apoptosis precedes cytochrome c release and is inhibited by Bcl-2. *Oncogene* **18,** 5991–5999.
27. Murphy, K. M., Ranganathan, V., Farnsworth, M. L., Kavallaris, M., and Lock, R. B. (2000) Bcl-2 inhibits Bax translocation from ctyosol to mitochondria during drug-induced apoptosis of human tumor cells. *Cell Death Differ.* **7,** 102–111.
28. Laskey, R. A. and Mills, A. D. (1975) Quantitative film detection of $^3$H and $^{14}$C in polyacrylamide gels by fluorography. *Eur. J. Biochem.* **56,** 335–341.

29. Luo, X., Budihardjo, I., Zou, H., Slaughter, C., and Wang, X. (1998) Bid, a Bcl2 interacting protein, mediates cytochrome c releasee from mitochondria in response to activation of cell surface death receptors. *Cell* **94,** 481–490.
30. Bellosillo, B., Villamor, N., Lopez-Guillermo, A., et al. (2002) Spontaneous and drug-induced apoptosis is mediated by conformational changes of Bax and Bak in B-cell chronic lymphocytic leukemia. *Blood* **100,** 1810–1816.

# 8

## Correlation of Telomerase Activity and Telomere Length to Chemosensitivity

### Yasuhiko Kiyozuka

#### Summary

Telomerase, which is selectively expressed in germline or cancer cells, is a ribonucleoprotein polymerase that contains an integral RNA with a short template element that can compensate telomeric loss by synthesizing TTAGGG repeats at chromosome ends. Telomeres appear to be critical for the integrity of chromosomes, stabilizing them from exonucleolytic degradation, preventing chromosome-to-chromosome fusions, and determining the maximum replicative capacity of cells. During the past decade, the roles of telomere length and telomerase activity have been investigated extensively in a variety of benign and malignant tumors of human origin, and stronger telomerase activity has been observed in more advanced tumors. Generally, the acquisition of telomerase activity in cancer cells is rather universal, which suggests that telomerase inhibition as a novel and potentially selective target for therapeutic intervention. Although a telomerase-specific inhibitor has not been found yet, the possible effect of anticancer agents on telomerase inhibition or the alteration of telomere length has been proposed. Recent development of TRAP assay not only increased the sensitivity but also allowed fast and efficient detection of telomerase activity. Technical aspects of this assay using self-established internal standard and nonradioisotopic detection method are addressed in this report. In addition, an overview of how to determine the telomere length is described.

#### Key Words

TRAP assay; TRF assay; telomerase; telomere; chemosensitivity; anticancer agent; cancer therapy.

### 1. Introduction

Telomerase is a ribonucleoprotein that adds repeated units of TTAGGG to the ends of telomeres. Telomerase activity has been found in almost all human tumors, but not in adjacent normal cells (*1*). This correlation has led to the hypothesis that telomerase is necessary for tumor cells to sustain their proliferation and that telomerase is an exceptional target for a class of chemotherapeutic agents *(2)*. Discovery of the potential of telomerase as target for human therapy requires development of potent and selective synthetic inhibitors and their testing inside cells.

Recently, large-scale surveys of telomerase activity in human cancer cells and tissues have been made since the development of a sensitive polymerase chain reaction (PCR)–based telomerase activity detection method, TRAP (Telomeric Repeats Amplification Protocol) assay *(1)*. TRAP assay is highly sensitive and convenient for the detection and quantification of telomerase activities in cancer cells. This TRAP assay uses a single-tube reaction and is performed in two steps. In the first step of the reaction, telomerase adds a number of telomeric repeats onto the 3′-end of a substrate oligonucleotide (TS primer). In the second step, the extended products are amplified by PCR using the TS and (reverse) CX primers **(Fig. 1)**. Incorporation of the internal positive control to the assay makes it possible to quantitate telomerase activity and to identify false negative samples that contain Taq polymerase inhibitors.

The first report to propose the possible effect of anticancer agents on telomerase inhibition was presented by Burger et al., regarding testicular cancer *(3)*. However, the opposite observation was presented by Ku et al., who found no effect of anticancer agents on the telomerase regulation of nasopharyngeal cancer *(4)*. In a previous report, we observed that alkylating agents (cisplatin, cyclophosphamide, and Ifomide [ifosfamide]) and topoisomerase inhibitors (etoposide and camptothecin) may have the potential to influence the structural alteration of telomerase RNA and telomeres and thus the downregulation of the telomerase activity in ovarian cancer cells *(5)*. More information about the relation between the sensitivities of currently used anticancer agents and telomere-related factors is essential to establish the effect, if any, of anticancer agents on telomerase regulation.

It is a general understanding that cancer cells treated with anticancer agents undergo apoptosis, a possible mechanism of therapy effect. The interaction between telomere function and apoptosis has been examined. The first experimental evidence, by the serum starvation method, showed that maintenance of telomere stability is associated with cellular resistance to apoptosis *(6)*. In various cell types, inhibition of telomere shortening below a critical length results in apoptosis, while resistance to apoptosis was induced with induction of telomerase activity *(7)*. A recent report by Ramirez et al. demonstrated dynamic telomere loss in peripheral blood lymphocytes and HL60 leukemia cells during DNA damage–induced apoptosis with camptothecin and etoposide treatment in vitro *(8)*.

The telomere length is usually expressed as mean length of the terminal restriction fragment (TRF) determined by the TRF assay. The TRF assay is

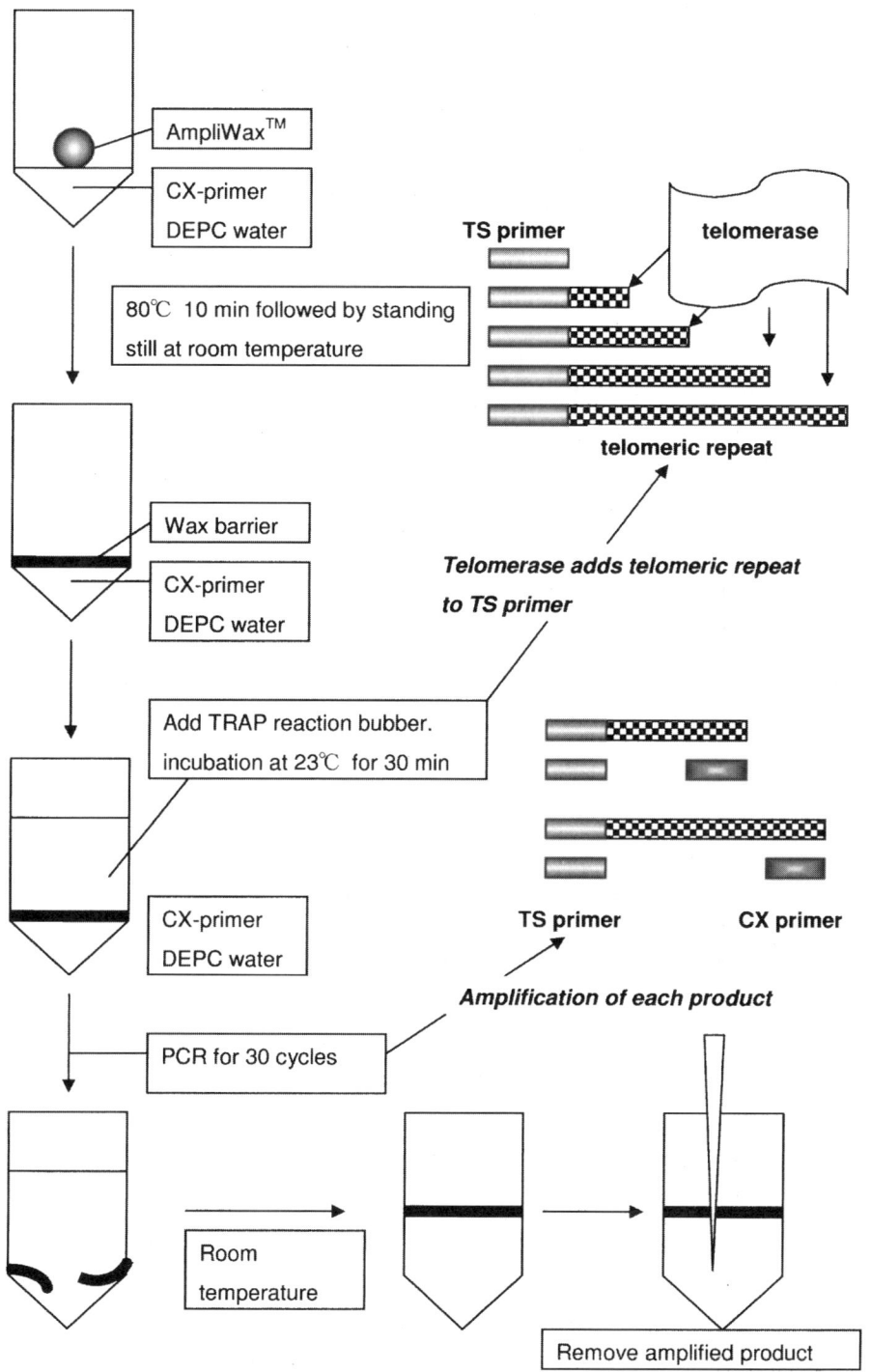

Fig. 1. Schematic flow chart of the TRAP assay.

composed mainly of three steps. In the first step, extraction of genomic DNA is followed by digestion with restriction enzyme(s). Gel electrophoresis and genomic blotting is performed in the second step. Finally, the distribution of telomere is visualized by probe hybridization.

Although the precise mechanisms are still to be elucidated, to study the relation of chemotherapy-induced apoptosis and the alteration of telomere length in cancer cells has not only biological but also clinical relevance for estimating the therapy effect.

Thus, both factors of telomerase activity and telomere length have the possibility of being a useful surrogate marker for representing the chemotherapeutic effect in cancer cells. In this chapter, we describe the experimental procedure to detect telomerase activity by TRAP assay and to determine telomere length by TRF assay.

## 2. Materials

1. TS and CX oligonucleotides (primers). TS primer: 5'-AATCCGTCGAGCAGA GTT-3'. CX primer: 5'-CCCTTACCCTTACCCTTACCCTAA-3'. Oligonucleotides are synthesized at 50 ng/µL in TE buffer, and stored at −20°C.
2. TS and CX overlap primers. TS-overlap primer: 5'-**AATCCGTCGAGCAGAG TT**GACGACATGGAGAAGATCTGG-3'. CX-overlap primer: 5'-**CCCTTACCC TTACCCTTACCCTAA**TGTGGTGGTGAAGCTGTAGC-3' (TS [18 bases] and CX [24 bases] sequences are in bold type here, and the mouse β-actin sequences [21 or 20 bases] are underlined.)
3. GlassMAX DNA isolation matrix system (Invitrogen, Carlesbad, CA).
4. Cell strainer, 70 µm nylon (BD Falcon, MA).
5. Cell washing buffer: 10 m$M$ HEPES-KOH (pH 7.5), 1.5 m$M$ MgCl$_2$, 10 m$M$ KCl, 1 m$M$ dithiothreitol (DTT) (Sigma), DEPC water (DEPC from Nakarai, Kyoto, Japan).
6. Cell lysis buffer: 10 mM Tris-HCl (pH 7.5), 1 m$M$ MgCl$_2$, 1 m$M$ EGTA, 0.1 m$M$ PMSF (Boehringer Mannheim; in EtOH—*see* **Note 5**), 5 m$M$ β-mercaptoethanol (*see* **Note 5**), 0.5% CHAPS (Sigma), 10% glycerol, DEPC water.
7. Bio-Rad Protein Assay Kit (Bio-Rad, Hercules, CA).
8. Ampli WAX PCR Gem 50 (Perkin Elmer, Vaterstetten, Germany).
9. TRAP reaction mixture for one assay: 10 µL of 100 m$M$ Tris-HCl (pH 8.3), 2.0 µL of 37.5 m$M$ MgCl$_2$, 2.0 µL of 1.575 $M$ KCl, 2.0 µL of 1.25 m$M$ dNTPs, 2.0 µL of 0.125% Tween-20 (Nakari, Kyoto, Japan), 2.0 µL of 25 m$M$ EGTA, 1.0 µL of 1 mg/mL T4g32 protein (Boehringer, Mannheim), 2.0 µL of 2.5-mg/mL bovine serum albumin (BSA), 0.4 µL of 5-U/mL Taq DNA polymerase (Takara, Kyoto, Japan), 2.0 µL of 50 ng/mL TS primer, 1.0 µL Ac-ITAS, 2.0 µL CHAPS cell lysates, 11.6 µL DEPC water = 40 µL.
10. 5X loading dye: 3.0 mL deionized water, 0.5 mL 1% bromophenol blue, 1.25 mL glycerol, 0.25 mL of 0.5 $M$ EDTA (pH 8.0) = 5.0 mL.

11. 5X Tris-borate buffer (TBE): 54 g Tris base, 27.5 g boric acid, 20 mL 0.5 $M$ EDTA (pH 8.0); (make up to 1 L with distilled water).
12. 2D-Silver Stain II "Daiichi" (Daiichi Pure Chemicals, Tokyo), PlusOne DNA Silver Staining Kit (Amersham Pharmacia Biotech, NJ), etc.
13. SYBR Green I nucleic acid gel stain (FMC Bioproducts, Rockland, ME).
14. GeneScreen Plus (NEN Research Products, Boston, MA).
15. $^{32}$P-labeled dCTP (Amersham, Buckinghamshire, UK).
16. Bca BEST (Takara, Otsu).
17. 1X SSC: 0.15 $M$ NaCl plus 0.015 $M$ sodium citrate.

## 3. Methods
### 3.1. TRAP Assay Protocol
*3.1.1. Preparation of Internal Standard*

An internal standard (ITAS) for the TRAP assay should be prepared considering the length as long (or short) enough not to interfere with the visualization of the telomere ladder *(9)*. Any genes are available for the preparation of ITAS so far as their sequences are known. For example, we introduce a way to prepare ITAS from mouse β-actin (Ac-ITAS) (**Fig. 2**).

1. Synthesize TS and CX oligonucleotides that contained an additional 20 or 21 bases at their 3′-ends that overlap with sequences encoding 160–531 bp of mouse β-actin. They are designated as the TS-overlap primer and CX-overlap primer.
2. Perform the first PCR (*see* **Note 1**) in the presence of TS- and CX-overlap primers. The amplification of mouse β-actin DNA by PCR with these primers generates a 414-bp product.
3. Perform the second PCR (*see* **Note 1**) using the first PCR product as a template in the presence of TS and CX primers used in the standard TRAP assay.
4. After gel electrophoresis, cut the band corresponding to 414 bp and extract DNA using a silica matrix (*see* **Note 2**). For the use of Ac-ITAS in TRAP, the product must be denatured to a single strand.

*3.1.2. Preparation of Cell Extract*

Cell extract containing telomerase activity must be prepared from viable cells (*see* **Note 3**).

1. Prepare single cells (*see* **Note 4**) in PBS from tissue homogenate or cultured cells with trypsin treatment, followed by centrifugation at 800*g* for 3 min at 4°C.
2. Suspend the pellet in ice-cold washing buffer, then centrifuge at 800*g* for 3 min at 4°C. Repeat twice.
3. Resuspend the pellet (composed of $10^4$–$10^6$ cells) in 200 µL of ice-cold lysis buffer (*see* **Note 5**), followed by incubation on ice for 30 min and centrifugation at 18,000*g* for 30 min at 4°C.
4. Aliquot the supernatant into fresh tubes, and store at –80°C (*see* **Note 6**).

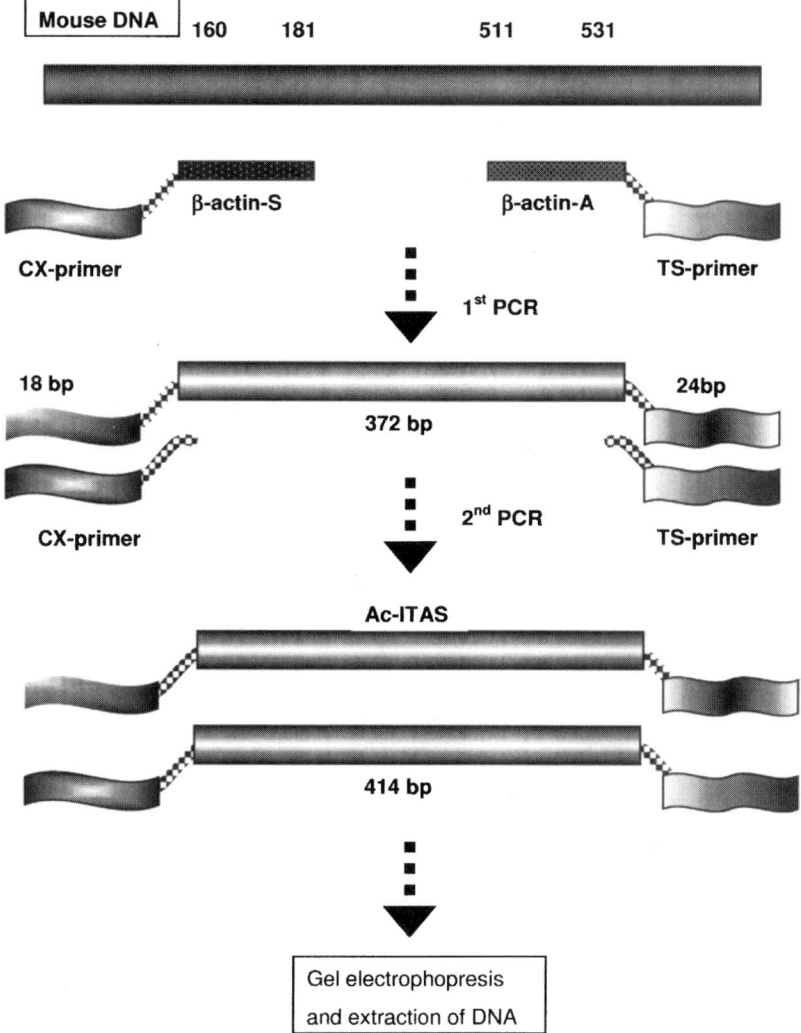

Fig. 2. Schematic explanation for establishing ITAS from mouse β-actin. In addition to TS and CX primers, TS- and CX-overlap primers must be synthesized.

5. The protein concentration is determined by the Bradford assay. The protein concentrations are generally 50–200 mg/mL.

### 3.1.3. TRAP Assay

Prior to starting the TRAP assay, RNase-free clean area of the laboratory must be prepared (**Fig. 1**).

1. Adjust the protein concentrations of each sample (cell extract) to 20 mg/mL.
2. Pipette 2-μL aliquots of CX primer plus 8 μL of water to the bottom of PCR tubes containing one piece of wax gem. Heat the tube at 80°C for 10 min, followed by standing still at room temperature to seal the CX primer under the wax barrier.
3. Aliquot 40 μL of TRAP reaction mixtures on the wax barrier.
4. Incubate at 23°C for 30 min for the telomerase mediated extension of the TS primer.
5. Heat the tube at 90°C for 90 s to inactivate telomerase activity and combine CX primer and TRAP reaction mixture above the wax barrier.
6. Amplify the reaction products by PCR in the presence of 70 attogram of Ac-ITAS (*see* **Note 7**).

### 3.1.4. Polyacrylamide Gel Electrophoresis of TRAP Products

1. Add 5 μL of 5X loading dye to 20 μL of TRAP product.
2. Load and run 25 μL of this on 15% nondenaturing, 1.5-mm-thick polyacrylamide gels (10 × 7 cm) in 0.5X TBE buffer.
3. Run time: Start at 80 V for 15 min, followed by 200 V, constant voltage setting, for about 45 min until the bromophenol blue just runs off the gel on ice (*see* **Note 8**).

### 3.1.5. Visualization of TRAP Products

There are some variations in visualizing the TRAP products run on PAGE. If the TS primer is end-labeled with $^{32}P$ and used in TRAP assay, TRAP products in the gel are visualized by PhosphorImager™ or by autoradiography. In this chapter, we introduce nonisotopic variations that utilize direct staining of the TRAP products with silver, SYBER™ Green I, or ethidium bromide. Although the precise methods for the silver staining are described elsewhere *(10)*, the use of some commercially available silver staining kit is recommended.

Gel is dried by using the gel drier. Dried gels are capable to apply to the usual computer scanner (**Fig. 3**). The intensity of the bands was quantified with the NIH Image 1.47 processing and analysis computer software program. The relative telomerase activities were quantified by taking the ratio of the Ac-ITAS to the entire telomerase ladder in each lane.

Staining of DNA by SYBR Green I is done for 45 min in 50 m$M$ Tris-HCl (pH 8.0) with 10,000X diluted stock in dimethyl sulfoxide (DMSO) (*see* **Note 9**). The gels are photographed with a Polaroid or CCD camera using a SYBR Green filter (yellow) and a 254-nm UV transilluminator (**Fig. 4**) (*see* **Note 10**).

### 3.1.6. Negative and Positive Control Reactions

Because TRAP assay is based on PCR, conventional positive and negative amplification controls in a routine PCR procedure are required. Except for this, both positive and negative controls for TRAP assay must be prepared. As an

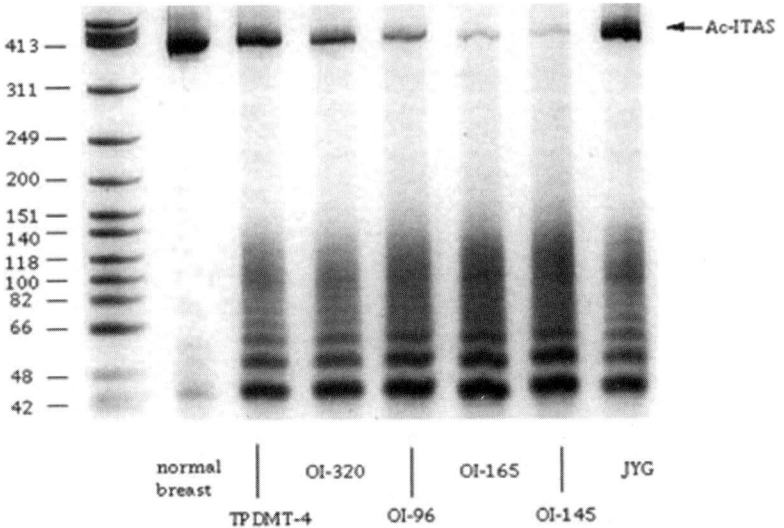

Fig. 3. Telomerase activities of a pregnancy-dependent mouse mammary tumor (TPDMT-4) and its four autonomous sublines (OI-320, nonmetastatic; OI-96, OI-165, and OI-145, artificial metastatic) of DDD/1 mouse origin, and an autonomous growing mammary tumor (JYG) showing spontaneous lung metastasis developed in BALB/c mice were compared to that of normal breast tissue. An internal control (Ac-ITAS) (70 ag) was utilized for standardization. A *Hin*fI digest of ϕX174 DNA was used as a marker. The TRAP products were visualized by silver staining.

internal RNA template is contained in telomerase, RNase-treated sample can be used for negative control for TRAP assay.

1. Negative control: Incubate cell extracts with one-fifth vol of 1 mg/mL RNase for 20 min at room temperature. A 2-µL aliquot of RNase-treated extract is used for the TRAP assay.
2. Positive control: We used the cell extracts from human ovarian cancer cell lines as positive controls *(5)* (*see* **Note 11**).

### *3.2. TRF Assay*

Telomere length is determined by TRF Southern blot analysis (**Fig. 5**) *(11)*. Digested genomic DNA by restriction enzyme, not interfering with telomeric sequence, is applied.

1. Extract genomic DNA from cells or tissues using phenol–chloroform treatment.
2. Digest genomic DNA (5–10 µg) for 16 h with HinfI (Takara, Kyoto) at 37°C.
3. Equal aliquots (10 µg sample/lane) of restricted DNA is electrophoresed in 0.8% agarose gels (when the TRF is less than 10 kb) in 45 m$M$ TBE buffer (pH 8.0) for a total of 660–700 V/h (*see* **Note 12**).

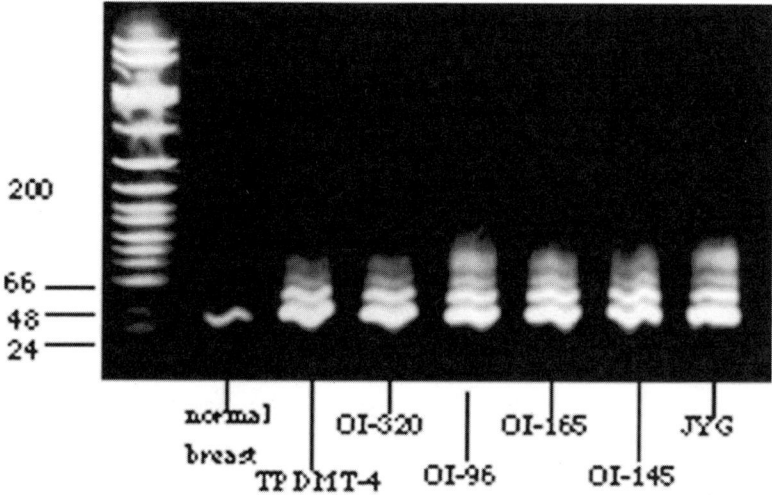

Fig. 4. The TRAP products (of **Fig. 3**) were stained with SYBR Green I and visualized with CCD camera using a yellow filter and a 254-nm UV transilluminator.

4. The separated DNA fragments were then transferred to nylon membranes by alkaline transfer using 0.4 $N$ NaOH in place of the traditional high-salt solution according to the Southern protocol *(12)*.
5. An oligonucleotide of 800 bp TTAGGG repeats inserted in the pSP73 plasmid (a kind gift from Dr. Titia de Lange, Rockefeller University) was cut with EcoRI and isolated with a DNA isolation kit according to the manufacturer's recommendation (*see* **Note 13**). For a standard reaction, 20 ng of this oligonucleotide as a probe for the telomere sequence was labeled in the presence of 1.85 MBq of $^{32}$P-labeled dCTP using a random-priming DNA labeling kit in the recommended buffer. Hybridization was carried out as described previously at 65°C *(13)*. The filters were washed in 4X SSC–0.1% SDS at 65°C prior to exposure to autoradiographic film. TRFs were determined following scanning with a digital scanner, with the center of the peak taken as the TRF.

## 4. Notes

1. PCR for 30 cycles (94°C, 30 s; 60°C, 30 s; 72°C, 1.5 min).
2. In the presence of the chaotropic agent, sodium iodide, DNA will bind to a silica matrix. The DNA–silica complex is purified by washing away non-DNA impurities. The purified DNA is then eluted in TE buffer.
3. The TRAP assay requires enzymatically active cell or tissue samples. Because telomerase is a ribonucleoprotein, RNase-free condition must be maintained even in the preparation of cell extract.
4. When the tissue sample is applied, a few grams of tissue fragment are homogenated by a dounce homogenizer in PBS. Single cells are prepared by filtrating

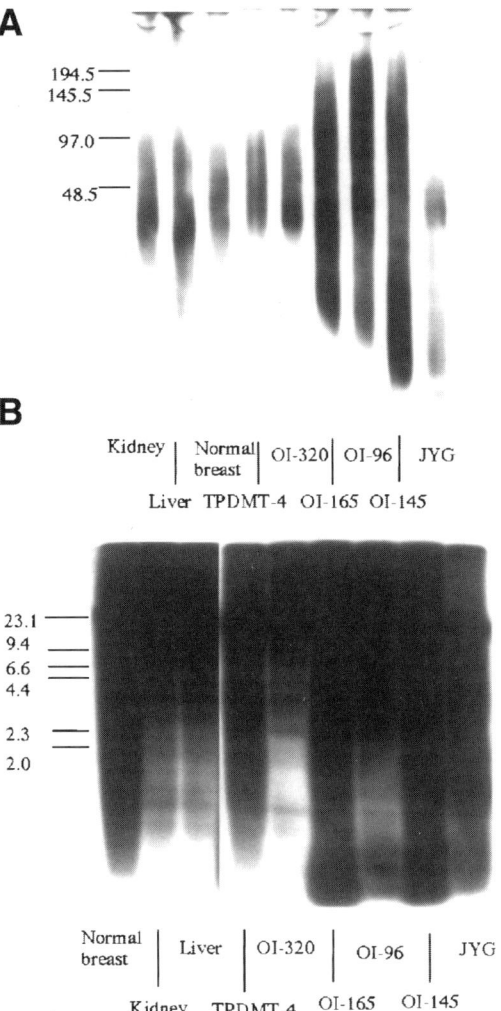

Fig. 5. (**A**) Telomere length determined by TRF assay among a pregnancy-dependent mouse mammary tumor (TPDMT-4) and its four autonomous sublines (OI-320, nonmetastatic; OI-96, OI-165, and OI-145; artificial metastatic) of DDD/1 mouse origin, and an autonomous growing mammary tumor (JYG) showing spontaneous lung metastasis developed in BALB/c mice were compared to those of normal liver and breast tissue using pulse-field gel electrophoresis system. (**B**) The same digested DNA samples were applied to a conventional 0.8% agarose gel electrophoresis. DNA digests more than 10 kb were distributed in void fraction, which makes it impossible to determine the center of the peaks taken as the TRFs.

homogenates through nylon membrane. Prior to cell washing, hemolysis of erythrocytes by hypotonic treatment using 0.3% NaCl is required, to avoid the influence of hemoglobin on the TRAP assay.
5. Combine just before use.
6. The extract is stable for at least 6 mo at −80°C. Aliquots should be freeze-thawed no more than 10 times to avoid loss of telomerase activity.
7. 30 cycles (94°C, 30 s; 50°C, 30 s; 72°C, 45 s).
8. Xylene cyanol is also included in the loading dye in the original method. However, the running marker of only bromophenol blue is sufficient in the TRAP assay.
9. In the SYBR Green I staining, manufacture's construction recommends the thickness of gel be less than 1 mm.
10. This procedure gives slightly less sensitivity compared to silver staining.
11. Generally, an acquisition of telomerase activity is a characteristic aspect for cancer cells, extracts from cancer cells can be used for positive control in TRAP assay.
12. If the sample contains DNA of large sizes (>10–20 kb), pulse-field gel electrophoresis system (PFGE) (Gene Path, Bio-Rad) is required in a 0.8% agarose gel, run in 0.5X TAE buffer (0.8 $M$ Tris, 0.4 $M$ NaOAc, 0.02 $M$ EDTA) (pH 8.2) at 6 V/cm, using a 5-s pulse time at 10°C for 12.7 h.
13. If the oligonucleotide is synthesized for the probe, a use of $(TTAGGG)_3$ oligonucleotide is long enough for the hybridization at 42°C for 3–18 h according to the previous report *(14)*.

## References

1. Kim, N. W,, Piatyszek, M. A., Prowse, K. R., et al. (1994) Specific association of human telomerase activity with immortal cells and cancer. *Science* **266**, 2011–2015.
2. Autexier, C. and Greider, C. W. (1996) Telomerase and cancer: revisiting the telomere hypothesis. *Trends Biol. Sci.* **21**, 387–391.
3. Burger, A. M., Double, J. A., and Newell, D. R. (1997) Inhibition of telomerase activity by cisplatin in human testicular cancer cells. *Eur. J. Cancer* **33**, 638–644.
4. Ku, W. C., Cheng, A. J., and Wang, T. C. V. (1997) Inhibition of telomerase activity by PKC inhibitors in human nasopharyngeal cancer cells in culture. *Biochem. Biophys. Res. Commu.* **241**, 730–736.
5. Kiyozuka, Y., Yamamoto, D., Yang, J., et al. (2000) Correlation of chemosensitivity to anticancer drugs and telomere length, telomerase activity and telomerase RNA expression in human ovarian cancer cells. *Anticancer Res.* **20**, 203–212.
6. Holt, S. E., Glinsky, V. V., Ivanova, A. B., and Glinsly, G. V. (1999) Resistance to apoptosis in human cells conferred by telomerase function and telomere stability. *Mol. Carcinog.* **24**, 241–248.
7. Herbert, B., Pitts, A. E., Baker, S. I., et al. (1999) Inhibition of human telomeres in immortal human cells leads to progressive telomere shortning and cell death. *Proc. Natl. Acad. Sci. USA* **96**, 14,276–14,281.
8. Ramirez, R., Carracedo, J., Jimenez, R., et al. (2003) Massive telomere loss is an early event of DNA damage-induced apoptosis. *J. Biol. Chem.* **278**, 836–842.

9. Wright, W. E., Shay, J. W., and Piatyzek, M. A.(1995) Modification of a telomeric repeat amplification protocol (TRAP) result in increased reliability, lineality and sensitivity. *Nucleic Acids Res.* **23,** 3794–3795.
10. Bassam, B. J., Caetano-Anolles, G., and Gresshoff, P. M. (1991) Fast and sensitive silver staining of DNA in polyacrylamide gels. *Anal. Biochem.* **196,** 80–83.
11. Landsdorp, P. M. (1995) Telomere length and proliferation potential of hematopoietic stem cells. *J. Cell Sci.* **108,** 1–6.
12. Southern, E. M. (1975) Detection of specific sequences among DNA fragments separated by gel electrophoresis. *J. Mol. Biol.* **98,** 503–517.
13. Kipling, D., Wilson, H. E., Thomson, I. J., and Cooke, H. J. (1995) YAC cloning *Mus musculus* telomeric DNA; physical, genetic, in situ and STS markers for the distal telomeres of chromosome 10. *Hum. Mol. Genet.* **4,** 1007–1014.
14. Strahl, C. and Blackburn, E. H. (1996) Effects of reverse transcriptase inhibitors on telomere length and telomerase activity in two immortalized human cell line. *Mol. Cell Biol.* **16,** 53–65.

# 9

## Application of Silicon Sensor Technologies to Tumor Tissue In Vitro

*Detection of Metabolic Correlates of Chemosensitivity*

Pedro Mestres-Ventura, Andrea Morguet, Anette Schofer, Michael Laue, and Werner Schmidt

### Summary

Silicon sensor technologies, developed during the 1990s, allow measurement of extracellular chemical changes related to cell metabolism. Exposition of tumor cells in vitro to anticancer drugs modifies cell metabolism, making it possible to detect on-line with sensor chips patterns of metabolic activity, which depend on drug sensitivity, or drug resistance of the cells. Sensor devices are composed of an incubation chamber with a sensor chip and a fluidic system for medium supply. Basically, two sensor types are available: (1) monosensor systems to detect extracellular acidification; and (2) multisensor arrays for many parameters such as pH, oxygen consumption, and impedance. Two companies have developed such systems: Molecular Devices (USA) and Bionas (Germany). In this chapter, in addition to operation of the sensor devices, we describe techniques for tissue (tumor and non-tumor) preparation. Basically, three procedures are described: (1) tissue dissociation and further cultivation on the sensor chip or on Transwell inserts; (2) preparation of tissue slices (300 μm thick) and attachment to the sensor chip or to inserts, and (3) cultivation of cells in dialysis tubes, a procedure necessary for nonadherent cells and cell suspensions to avoid their washing away. Evaluation of results and selection of controls are also discussed.

### Key Words

Chemosensitivity; tumor slices; culture methods; multisensor arrays; silicon sensors; cell metabolism; microphysiometry; cytotoxicity; cell adhesion; impedance; metabolomics.

### 1. Introduction

The vulnerability of tumor cells to anticancer drugs depends on the degree of sensitivity or resistance. The effects of such drugs can be very distinct, ranging from the arrest of the cell cycle to the induction of cell death. In other cases the tumor cells are resistant, i.e., no drugs are able to kill them; in such cases we speak of multidrug resistance. A common feature in all of these situations is an energetic or metabolic component accompanying the reactions of the treated cells. For these reasons, a sensitive measurement of the metabolic activity of the tumor in vitro could be helpful toward understanding the particular vulnerability (chemosensitivity assays) of a tumor and the effects of the drugs (screening assays).

Many of the metabolic analysis methods, such as tetrazolium (MTT) colorimetric assays, ATP bioluminiscence assays, etc., are limited in their assessment of the temporal effects of drugs. The main problem is that they are end-point tests, i.e., the tissue will be destroyed after measurement. Nevertheless, the idea of predicting ex vivo the response of cancer to drug therapy continues to receive broad support *(1–5)*. The development of silicon sensor chip devices has contributed largely to the creation of an alternative technology able to circumvent these difficulties. Probably the more remarkable advantage lies in the fact that silicon sensors allow on-line measurement during relative long periods and without damage to the tissue; i.e., these methods are no longer end-point tests.

Silicon sensors are transducers, which transform minimal chemical changes in measurable electrical signals. With silicon sensors it is possible to measure several cellular parameters related to adhesion and motility as well as to energy metabolism and respiration.

The grade of cell adhesion to a substrate in which the sensor is integrated can be measured and expressed in terms of impedance *(6,7)*. A high adhesion with formation of large areas of contact with the substrate corresponds to high impedance values. Conversely, when cells round up and become detached—for instance, if they die or display lesions—the area of contact with the sensor diminishes and also the impedance value decreases *(8)*.

Cell metabolism represents a complex network of enzymatic reactions in which energy is produced and, at the same time, catabolized *(9)*. In order to maintain the homeostatic equilibrium in the cells, a number of metabolic end products are eliminated or extruded outside the cell. Some of these substances are already ionically dissociated when they cross the cell membrane or become so when they reach the extracellular space. Examples of such substances are lactic and carbonic acids, which may cause a rise in proton concentration and a corresponding lowering of pH in the extreme pericellular area. Biochemical studies have shown that glycolysis and anaerobic oxidation of glucose are the main sources of protons and, therefore, pericellular acidification reflects the grade of activity of such pathways *(10)*. In view of the fact that extracellular protons originate from several metabolic pathways, the pericellular acidification can be seen as a global parameter. However, it is possible to achieve more accurate information about determined proton sources, for instance, with pharmacological inhibition of key enzymes of corresponding pathways *(10)*.

Over the past decades several types of sensors have been designed for detection of "pericellular acidification." In very early studies the so-called chemically sensitive field-effect transistors were used *(11)*. However, years later the introduction of a light addressable potentiometric sensor (LAPS) was an important innovation, opening new possibilities for systematic measurement of pericellular acidification *(12)*. On the basis of this sensor, the company Molecular Devices constructed and has, since 1990, been marketing an instrument called Cytosensor®, able to measure minimal changes of pericellular pH *(13)*. This instrument, originally developed to measure changes of cell metabolism related to ligand–receptor interactions, has also been successfully applied to the study of metabolic patterns of tumor cell lines and tumor primary cultures under the influence of anticancer drugs *(14–18)*. Because of their biological stability, cell lines are considered to be very useful objects, particularly for drug screening, and even as controls for chemosensitivity testing *(14)*. An important advantage of this technology is the possibility of being able to continuously monitor the metabolic state of tumor tissue exposure to drugs. This "on-line" monitoring enables the determination of points in time of critical events and also when tumor viability declines to an irreversible state, by allowing recovery under drug-free conditions.

During the last decade sensor technology has developed rapidly, particularly with regard to chip manufacturing. These developments have enabled the construction of a new type of chip, the so-called multisensor array, in which sensors for pH, oxygen, and impedance measurements are integrated on the same chip *(19–21)*. Measurements of the relative oxygen concentration in the incubation medium together with the level of pericellular acidification give a wider picture of the metabolic status and its evolution in cultivated cells. This concept, called a "physiocontrol microsystem" (PCM), has been recently adopted and improved by Bionas in a commercially available new device called Mehrfachtester (Bionas 2500 Device). The silicon sensor devices are composed of a chamber in which the sensor chip is integrated, a fluidic system for supplying the chamber with culture medium, and a control unit for the fluidic system (pumps and valves) and for processing of data (**Figs. 1** and **2**). The cells or tissue can be maintained in the chamber at the required temperature. The volume of the chamber is rather small, in the range of a few microliters (**Fig. 2**). With the aid of spacers, i.e., plastic rings 125 µm thick, it is possible to increase the chamber volume (hole diameter of spacer: 5 mm). The waste can be usually directed to a recipient, where it is possible to collect the fluids of each chamber or modules separately for additional analytical purposes.

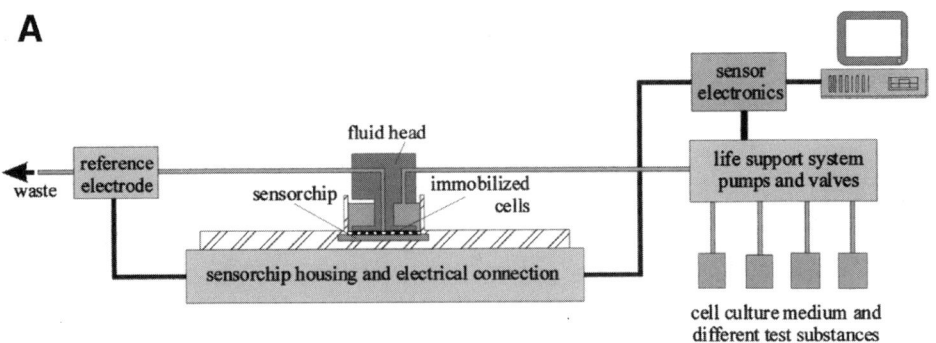

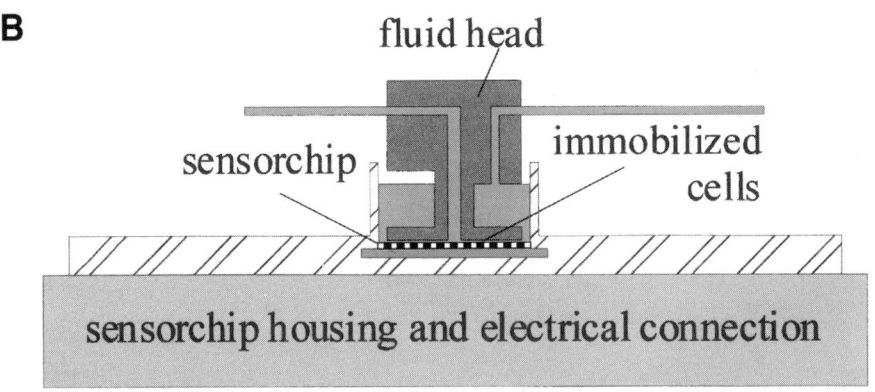

Fig. 1. Diagram of the Bionas multisensor apparatus (Bionas 2500), showing the arrangement of the different components. The apparatus is composed of six sensor chambers. Each chamber is connected with the pump and control unit. The medium or drug-containing fluids first flow to and then through the chamber and are then directed to the waste collector. The reference electrode is installed in the fluidic pathway behind the sensor chamber. The cells or slices are placed into the chamber between the chip and the fluidic head.

As an example, **Fig. 3** displays the data obtained during an experiment in which cells were exposed to cytochalasin B, a drug that alters the function of microfilaments *(22)*. These measurements were performed with the multiple-sensor device of Bionas. The decrease in acidification indicates a diminution of metabolic activity. The increase in the oxygen level in the medium signifies a minor consumption, and this correlates with the reduced metabolic activity.

In the application of this technique a considerable problem is the handling of the tumor tissue, which reacts very sensitively to manipulations linked with the preparation. In general, the most common procedure is to prepare cell suspen-

# Application of Silicon Sensor Technologies

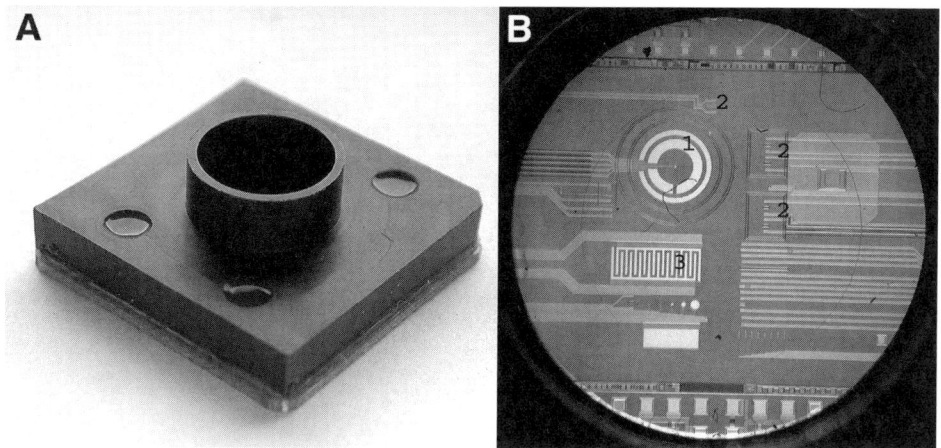

Fig. 2. Sensor chamber and design of the multiple-sensor chip. (**A**) sensor chamber with the opening at the top, which is closed by the introduction of the fluidic head. The sensor chip is located at the bottom. The electronic contacts are placed at the borders of the square-shaped basis. (**B**) Micrograph of the chip showing the sensor arrangement (diameter of chip 10 mm). 1, Oxygen sensor, after Clark; 2, five ISFETs (ionic-sensitive field-effect transistors) for detection of acidification; and 3, IDES (interdigitated electrode sensors) for impedance measurements.

sions by enzymatic dissociation of the tumor specimen. However, in the dissociation of tissue a certain degree of cell loss seems inevitable, with consequent change in the cell populations and the ratio of cancer to noncancer cells. Basically, however, the problem is that dissociation strongly modifies the receptor status of the cells, consequently changing the chemosensitivity *(23)*.

Moreover, with tissue dissociation, we relinquish the three-dimensional arrangement of cancer and stroma cells existing in the original specimen. Despite the presence of cancerous and noncancerous cells in a monolayer, they do not constitute the "original tumor." Considering that stroma and supporting structures (blood vessels, etc.) may be involved in a different manner in the mechanism of anticancer drugs, it appears important to design preparation protocols covering the three-dimensional structure of the sample.

In order, as far as possible, to maintain the relationship between stroma and tumor cells as in the original, we recommend the use of tumor slices. The slice technique is actually a routine approach in neuroscience *(24,25)*, but meanwhile, the tissue slices also play an important role in other areas of research, such as, for instance, in hepatology *(26)*. Slices offer the possibility of examining determined anatomical areas of the brain or other organs in such a way that the cellular elements maintain the arrangement as in the original in vivo. In tumor biology this technique has received only scarce attention up to now.

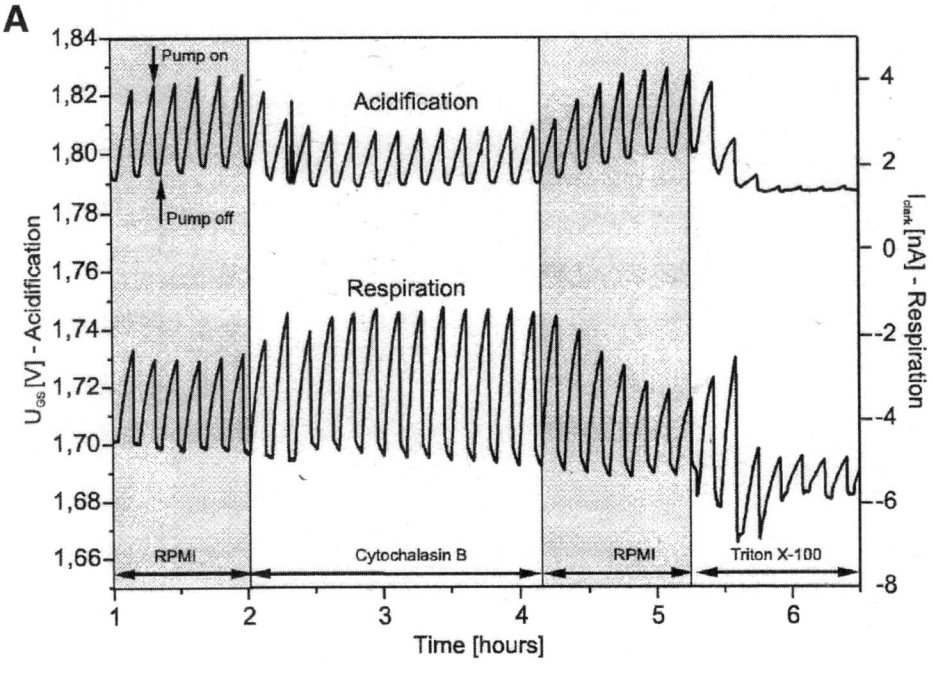
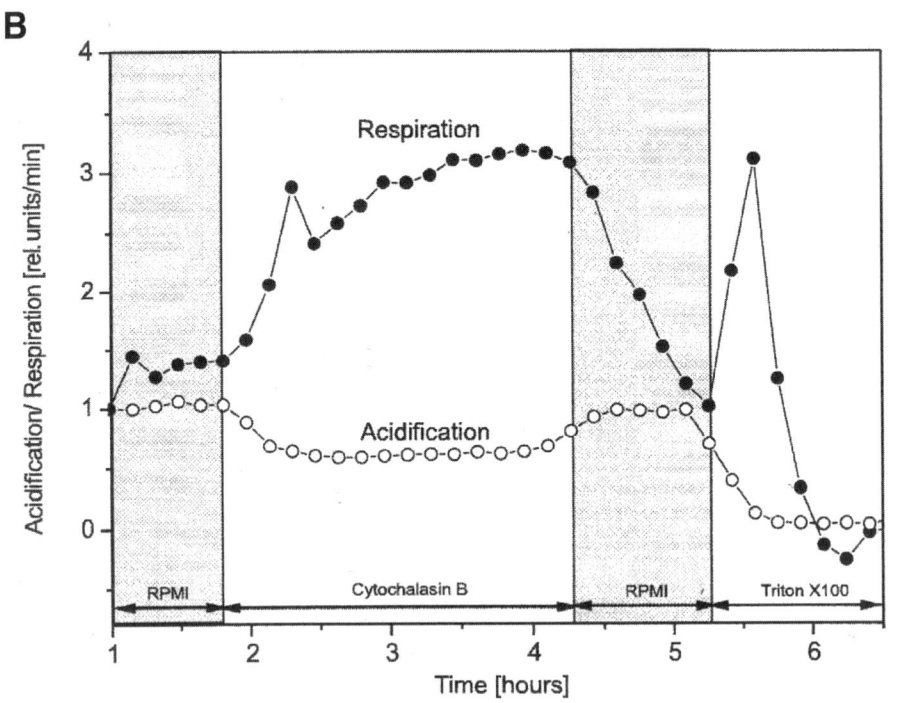

Because of the preservation of the inner histological patterns in the case of slices, we can speak of a "microtumor." Tumor slices are cut to a thickness of 0.2–0.5 mm and a few millimeter in side length. The thickness allows sufficient diffusion of medium and additives, enabling the cells to preserve their viability for a long time. Although the preparation of the slices represents a stress that should not be understimated, suitable medium composition and a preincubation period of a few hours can considerably aid sample recovery (**Fig. 4**). The most important difference is that the gene and protein expression patterns of tumor tissue are clearly less altered after slice production than after dissociation *(27,28)*. The production of slices is quickly carried out and, even with an incubation time for tissue recovery, one can soon start the measurements and obtain useful results within a few hours. Thus, sensor testing is much faster than other techniques, which require days.

In the case of cancer forms with nonadherent cells, such as leukemia, the investigation of metabolic activity with a silicon sensor device could be difficult because the cells can be washed away from the sensor chamber. A common strategy to retain the cells in the chamber is to embed them, for example, in agar-agar (low-melting-point). An alternative is to place the cells in a dialysis tube *(29)*, taking several small segments of these tubes for further measurements with the sensor devices.

In **Fig. 5** a flow diagram shows the interconnections between the preparation methods. The cultivation of slices and monolayers on inserts or cell suspensions in dialysis tubes are technical approaches that give the whole method more technical flexibility, as it is possible to alternate phases of measurement in the silicon sensor devices with periods of cultivation in the incubator for recovery after individual experiments.

The aim of this chapter is to describe methods of preparing solid tumors, nonadherent cancer cells, as well as cell lines for measurement of the metabolic activity (metabolomics) using a silicon sensor device. In our experiments the following objects were mostly used: breast and ovarian carcinoma, the cell lines CHO (expressing acetylcholine receptor) and MCF-7. The schedules

---

Fig. 3. *(see opposite page)* Measurements of metabolic activity of LS 174T cells, a line of a human colon adenocarcinoma, treated with cytochalasin. (**A**) raw data. (**B**) The same data after normalization. The effects of cytochalasin B are characterized by a lowering of the acidification curve. The oxygen curve becomes elevated. These results indicate that metabolic activity is reduced under the influence of cytochalasin B. The pump off and on phases are indicated. The sensor carries out the measurements during the stop phase.

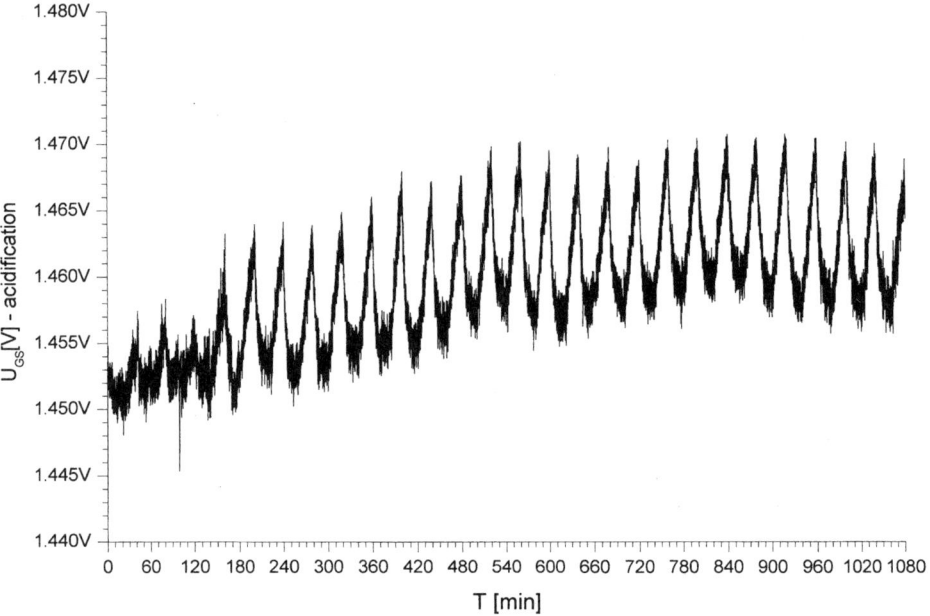

Fig. 4. Measurements of the metabolic activity of a breast carcinoma slice. The curve shows the acidification rate during nearly 24 h. The first 2 h are characterized by an unusual noice and a low acification rate. Later the rhythm of acidification is regular, indicating normal metabolic activity and consequently giving information on slice vitality. No drugs were used in this experiment.

described can be applied to every other tumor case with only minimal adaptation, which can be determined empirically.

## 2. Materials
### 2.1. Transport of Specimens to the Laboratory

1. Fifty milliliter tubes as tissue containers.
2. Culture medium for transport: sterile DMEM / F12 (Invitrogen) with 20 U/mL penicillin, 20 U/mL streptomycin, and without fetal calf serum (FCS) or additives.
3. Cooler box with ice for tissue transport.

### 2.2. Tissue Dissociation

1. Sterile instruments: scalpel, fine tweezers, scissors.
2. Sterile Falcon culture flasks.
3. Sterile Petri dishes.
4. Sterile Pasteur pipets.
5. Sterile complete medium: DMEM/F12 (Invitrogen), supplemented with 1–10% FCS, 10 ng/mL EGF, 2 m$M$ glutamine, 20-U/mL each penicillin/streptomycin,

*Application of Silicon Sensor Technologies* 117

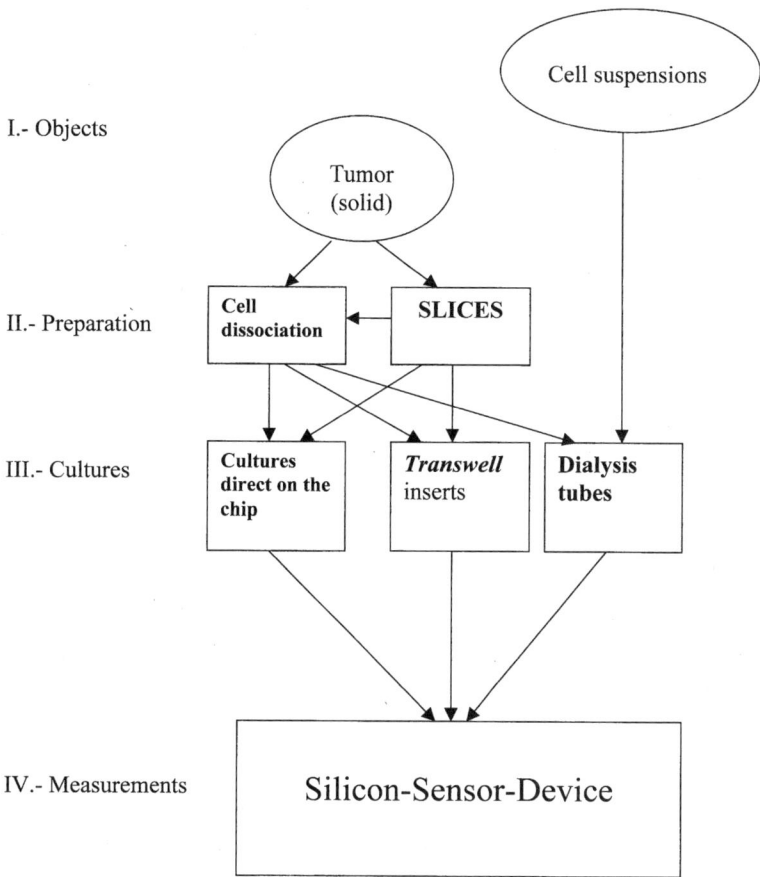

Fig. 5. Flow diagram with the methods to prepare the tissues for measurements in a silicon sensor device.

100X NEA (Invitrogen) 1.0%, 10 µg/mL hydrocortisone, 10–20 µg/mL insulin, bicarbonate or HEPES buffer.
6. 0.2-µm sterile filter (Sarstedt).
7. 100-U/mL collagenase I in complete medium; 1000 U ≈ 5, 18 mg.
8. 40-µm nylon cell strainer (Becton & Dickinson).
9. 0.26% Trypsin.
10. Sterile phosphage-buffered saline (PBS) (Boehringer Mannheim).

## 2.3. Acute Preparation and Cultivation of Tumor Slices

1. Special equipment: Tissue chopper (Sorvall, McIllwain) and stereomicroscope to assess slices and to complete dissection.
2. Small instruments and accessories for microchopper (Shick razor blades, fine tweezers, scissors, small scalpels, Teflon plates to bind the tissue for sectioning).

3. Complete medium as in **Subheading 2.2**.
4. Tissue adhesive: Histoacryl (Braun-Melsungen).
5. Ice bath.
6. Large Petri dishes (10-cm diameter).
7. 24-well plates (Corning).
8. Plasmaclot (purified fibrinogen and purified human thrombin [Sigma]).
9. Transwell® inserts, 6.5-mm diameter and 3.0-µm pore size (Costar).

## 2.4. Cultivation of Cells Directly on the Chip (Bionas Mehrfachtester).

1. Sterile complete medium.
2. Sterile incomplete medium without buffer (Invitrogen).
3. Multisensor chip (Bionas) and LAPS sensor (Molecular Devices).
4. Small Petri dishes.
5. Larger Petri dishes to make a humidity chamber for incubation at 37°C.
6. Special forceps to pack the chips.
7. Sterile Pasteur pipets.

## 2.5. Cultivation in Dialysis Tubes

1. Capillary dialyzer with Hemophan membrane GFS Plus 20 (kD) (Gambro).
2. Complete medium as in **Subheading 2.2**.
3. Incomplete medium (*see* **Subheading 2.4.**).
4. Sterile Petri dishes.
5. 24-well plates.
6. Small instruments as above (*see* **Subheading 2.3.**).

## 2.6. Measurements with the Silicon Sensor Devices

1. Incomplete medium (*see* **Subheading 2.4.**).
2. Cleaning silicon sensor device with Na-hypochlorite (Cytosensor Sterilant Kit, cat. no. R 8012, Molecular Devices).
3. Multisensor chips and spacers (Bionas, Rostock, Germany).
4. LAPS is the sensor working in the cytosensor and can usually provide life-long functioning.
5. Anticancer drugs depending on experimental design or tissue to be analyzed.

## 3. Methods

## 3.1. Transport of Samples to the Laboratory (see Note 1)

1. The specimens are transported to the laboratory in 50-mL tubes filled with sterile medium for transport and maintained at a low temperature (about 4°C).
2. Immediately after extirpation, the tissue blocks are placed in the sterile tube and closed with a screw cap.
3. Transport to the laboratory is carried out in a styrofoam container with ice.
4. Under sterile conditions (laminar flow), the specimen is examined and repeatedly washed with fresh culture medium for transport before dissection.

5. During dissection, tissue warming can be avoided by cooling the dish where preparation is to take place with ice.

## 3.2. Cell Dissociation (see Note 2)

1. In order to obtain single-cell suspensions, tissue specimens are cut into small particles with a sharp scissors and further digested enzymatically by collagenase or trypsin. Slices can be used for these purposes as well.
2. Small tissue particles or slides are placed in a centrifuge tube or Petri dish covered with trypsin (0.25% in sterile PBS) or collagenase I (100-U/mL complete medium) solution.
3. The samples in trypsin are incubated overnight at 4°C and, before further preparation, transferred to an incubator at 37°C for 30 min. The samples to be dissociated with collagenase are incubated overnight at 37°C.
4. After enzymatic treatment the samples are filtered through a cell strainer (40-μm Nylon, Becton & Dickinson).
5. The filtrate is collected in a tube and centrifuged at 250$g$ for 4 min.
6. The pellet is resuspended and seeded in complete medium.
7. Before seeding, cells treated with trypsin have to be incubated with a medium and 10% FCS for enzyme inactivation.
8. The addition of 2.2 m$M$ EDTA (0.1%) may improve the results of enzymatic digestion with trypsin.

## 3.3. Preparation of Acute Tumor Slices (see Note 3)

1. Examine the tissue block under the stereomicroscope for the purpose of estimating the size and the presence of tumor tissue (solid tumor).
2. Cover the specimen completely with medium to liberate trivial tissue elements (subcutaneous and fatty tissue) with the aid of fine instruments, taking care to avoid compression of tissue.
3. The tissue chopper can cut samples with a maximum height of approx 5 mm; therefore, the size of the tissue block may have to be reduced.
4. All these manipulations are done in a medium precooled at +4°C. The blocks can be placed in abundant fresh medium, taking out one block each time for sectioning.
5. The block is glued to a Teflon plate with Histoacryl and immediately covered with medium. Because of the surface properties of Teflon, the medium forms a conspicuous meniscus, covering the bonded tissue block completely.
6. The sample on the Teflon plate is transferred to the tissue chopper, which has been previously adjusted to cut slices 250–300 μm thick. Usually, the automatic cutting mode can be used.
7. Because of the Histoacryl present between the sample and the Teflon surface, the slices have to be separated from the Teflon plate carefully with a sharp scalpel and quickly transferred to a Petri dish with fresh medium.
8. The single slices are examined under the stereomicroscope and, if necessary, remaining Histoacryl can be eliminated.

9. In order to reduce the trauma of preparation and to neutralize the intracellular substances released from lesioned cells, it is advisable to operate with abundant medium, enriched with FCS, changing it frequently. This step should last at least 2–3 h; in some cases it is better to incubate the slices overnight (*see* **Note 4**).
10. At this stage it is possible to evaluate the quality of the slices so that those areas containing no tumor cells can be excluded. Because of the variable presence of connective tissue, it is difficult to give general rules for this step. Usually, areas of necrosis or bleeding can be easily identified and dissected out.
11. As indicated in **Fig. 5**, slices can be cultivated, bonded to an appropriate substrate by Plasmaclot (well plates, Transwell inserts, or sensor chip) or dissociated enzymatically in accordance with the protocol described under **Subheading 3.2.**
12. In addition to tumors, slices of other tissues such as brain and liver can be collected using similar procedures. The media and their composition are adjusted to the requirements of these tissues. This is a very important point in order to minimize the grade of sublethal metabolic stress that arises from the situation after dissection and cutting with the tissue chopper.

### *3.4. Cultivation on Transwell Inserts*

Both cell suspensions and slices can be cultivated on Transwell inserts. Adherent cells become attached within a short time (a few hours). It is necessary to immobilize the slices, because otherwise the cells suffer extreme stress. It is therefore recommended to adhere the slices with Plasmaclot (*see* **Note 5**) *(30)*.

1. The slices are immersed in 1 mL complete medium (*see* **Subheading 2.2.**) with 280-µg/mL $CaCl_2$, 0.1 mL of 0.2% (wt/vol) purified fibrinogen (Sigma), resuspended in PBS, and 0.1 mL of 0.2 U/mL purified human thrombin (95%; Sigma) in PBS. The rate of growth is controlled with the microscope.
2. It is also possible to cut the membrane of the insert, separating it from the frame. The membrane is 5 mm in diameter, with cells growing only on one side. The gap between the sensors and the cells can be greatly reduced by placing the membrane with the cells facing the chip. In the same way, the slices on the Transwell membrane can be cultivated, adhering the tissue with a Plasmaclot and cutting out the membrane for further operation in the sensor device as described above (*see* **Note 6**).

### *3.5. Cultivation of Cell Suspensions in Dialysis Tubes (D-tubes)*

1. The cell number of the suspension is controlled with a hemocytometer (Neubauer-type chamber).
2. The cell suspension is placed in an Eppendorf reaction vial or in a small Petri dish. 3. The cells are moved into the D-tubes by capillary forces. The tubes used in our experiments are of the Hemophan membrane 20-kDa type. There are other materials with different permeability specifications (more or less than 20 kDa). It is important to take into consideration that, for microscopic controls, it is better if the tube wall is transparent.

4. The tubes are cut with a sharp scissors, avoiding any strong deformation or compression, because otherwise the openings may become obstructed. The length of the segment tube should be approx 2 or 3 cm.
5. The tube is introduced into the cell suspension with a fine tweezers and, if this is done under the microscope, the ascent of the cells in the tube can be observed.
6. Because of the size of the sensor chamber, the tubes should be cut into segments shorter than 1 cm. Both ends of the tube are cut with the tweezer and closed at the same time. Press the tube firmly in order to ensure that the tube is closed.
7. The small segments are placed in 24-well plates filled with complete medium and cultivated as usual. If measurement in the silicon sensor device is planned, it is advisable to fill the tubes with cells previously resuspended in an incomplete medium (*see* **Subheading 2.4.**).

## *3.6. Measurement with a Silicon Sensor Device (see Notes 7 and 8)*

The description of the operation with a silicon sensor device applies primarily to the Bionas Mehrfachtester, but because of the similarity of the technical principles, it can be applied to the operation of a Cytosensor® as well. The procedure is outlined in the following steps.

1. Start the processor by loading the software, selecting the parameters, and setting the values for the experiment: (a) pump speed: in general, 50–100 µL/min; (b) total time of experiment: hours or days; (c) pump cycle: the stop phase in which the measurements take place is in general shorter than the perfusion phase in which the medium of the sensor chamber is renewed, and a general rule of thumb is to select the perfusion phase to last three times longer than the stop phase. It has been empirically established that long "go" phases are necessary in order to eliminate all drug residuals, etc. Moreover, it is important to reach the baseline again after each stop phase. However, these guidelines must not necessarily be adhered to, and other procedures can be adopted. For instance, 5 min stop/5 min perfusion has also rendered good results.
2. Install the sensor chip (*see* **Fig. 2**) and close the chamber. The device is then desinfected with pure ethanol 70% (many pump cycles) and subsequently washed with sterile PBS (several pump cycles).
3. The system is perfused with incomplete medium enriched with FCS (1–10%). This treatment is important in order to condition the surfaces of the conducting tubes and chamber for the next steps. Place this medium in the tubes for chamber supply. Replace the tubes, putting in one the fresh medium as required and in the other the medium with the drugs to be used. Take into consideration that two supply tubes per chamber are available (*see* **Note 9**).
4. The sample is then introduced into the sensor chamber. Depending on previous preparation, the samples are on inserts, in dialysis tubes, or in direct contact with the chip. The inserts fit the chamber dimensions exactly. The segments of dialysis tubes are approx 1 cm long and are placed directly on the sensor chip with a

spacer (125 μm thick) to separate them from the fluidic head. After positioning of the sample the fluid head is lowered, simultaneously closing the chamber.
5. Initiate the measurements or experiments by starting the software (or program). The data will be stored automatically, being accessible only at the end of the session.
6. Cleaning of the sensor device. After each session the system should be washed with a solution of PBS containing 0,1% Tween-20, followed by distilled water. Use the pump to air-dry the system. It is important to clean the system at least once per week with a sodium hypochloride solution, followed by the same program as described above (*see* **Note 10**).
7. Raw data can be automatically normalized by the Cytosensor software. The data of the Bionas device are normalized as follows. The signal changes during the stop phase are used as a measurement category. Each single value collected during experiments is divided through the value of the first stop phase The resulting values express the relative change in acidification or oxygen consumption. For this step we use the Origin 7.0 software. It is important that, after the application of Triton, the zero line is registered, indicating that all the cells have died and that the device is operating correctly.

After each experiment or session, the state of the sample may be additionally evaluated with cytological methods. The metabolic situation can be determined with WST-1 (Roche Diagnostic, Germany) or the alamar blue test (Biosource International, USA). The live/dead test (Molecular Probes) or dye exclusion test with Trypan blue provides data on cell viability and, in addition, cell cultures and slices can be prepared for histology or electron microscopy.

## 4. Notes

1. The preparation of the media, the packing, and maintaince at a low temperature (+4°C)—which also applies to storage in the hospital—are measures that contribute to improvement of sterility. Transfer to the laboratory generally takes less than 30 min. In addition, repeated washing of the tissue blocks before preparation is very important to reduce contamination of the sample surface.
2. For tumor cell suspensions and slices, it is important to carry out cell typing to determine fractions of genuine tumor cells and noncancer cells. For this purpose a current immunocytochemical procedure with specific markers (data exchange with the pathologist required) could be implemented.
3. Assessment of tumor slices is important, with the aim of examining the ratio between tumor and nontumor areas. This evaluation can be made with a stereomicroscope equipped with appropriate illumination. As already mentioned, areas of necrosis and bleeding can be identified to a certain degree. Therefore, examination of the sections under the stereomicrosocpe can help to select relevant sections.
4. The cutting of slices represents considerable stress for the cells. In our experience, the cultivation of slices in complete medium (with FCS) overnight contributes to a

quick recovery of the cells. If measurements are performed immediately, the slices can be incubated in complete medium with 10% FCS, changing the solution every hour. FCS, in particular, helps to neutralize the effects of enzymes released from cells opened by sectioning. In order to minimize changes of the milieu, we have also used the serum of patients (tumor and serum of the same patient), with the same results as FCS. The final composition of the culture medium must be defined according to the requirements of the tumor type. Relevant bibliography should be consulted.

5. The slices must be fixed to the substrate with Plasmaclot, otherwise metabolic patterns may be altered and turbulences negatively influence the operation of the sensors.
6. Transwell inserts can also be used to maintain contact of the slices with the chip, if a bonding with Plasmaclot is not desired.
7. Sensor chip types can be checked by running a simple program of measurement with PBS at two different pH values. The multisensor array chips (Bionas) are one-way chips. The LAPS sensor (Molecular Devices) is designed for long-life use or at least for many years, if the recommendations of the manufacturers with regard to cleaning and storage are observed.
8. One serious problem with silicon sensor devices is the formation of bubbles within the system during the measurements. Bubbles arise from the interaction between the fluids (medium, etc.) and the different surfaces with which they come into contact, i.e., the tubes connecting the pumps and the sensor chamber and the chip surface. The systems are, in general, endowed with a debubbler, but their efficiency varies. The presence of bubbles in the system can be observed in changes in the registration curves of the corresponding sensor chamber. If the bubbles are in the tube segment between the pump and the chamber, the noise is increased. Air bubbles that develop directly on the chip very often generate irregular and noninterpretable curves with considerable changes in amplitude. This is not easy to correct. In some case it is possible to eliminate the bubbles located on the chip with fine rubber, by using the stop phase. Then it is possible to open the chamber, move the fluidic head, and inspect the bottom of the chamber. If the bubbles are located elsewhere, no intervention is possible, but often the bubbles can be removed and transported away, enabling continuation of effective measurement. For this reason, practically permanent survey of the apparatus during measurements is recommended.The incidence of bubbles is more frequent after long periods in which the apparatus has not been used.
9. Controls can be of two types: (a) one of the chambers will be perfused with a medium without drugs, and (b) in the case of a study concerning a certain drug, then a cell line that is sensitive to it should be used or, in the case of multidrug resistence, a resistent cell line.
10. Contamination by bacteria is possible. In such cases, control of the media under the microscope is indicated. A thorough cleaning of the system is required, followed by measurements without cells, with media containing high doses of antibiotics and long enough to exclude any possible residual contamination.

## Acknowledgments

The authors are indebted to Dr. Ralf Ehret and Bionas GmbH for the support received in many of the experiments and handling of the Mehrfachtester and to Mrs. Ann Soether for proofreading the manuscript. This work was generously supported by grants from the Federal Ministery for Education and Research (BMBF) and by the Saving Bank Union of Saarland (SV Saar), both to P.M.V.

## References

1. Weisenthal, L. M. (1981) In vitro assays in preclinical antineoplastic drug screening. *Semin. Oncol.* **8**, 362–376.
2. Bellamy, W. T. (1992) Prediction of response to drugs therapy of cancer. A review of in vitro assays. *Drugs* **44**, 690–708.
3. Cree, I. A., Kurbacher, C. M., Untch, M., et al. (1996) Correlation of the clinical response to chemotherapy in breats cancer with ex vivo chemosensitivity. *Anticancer Drugs* **7**, 630–635.
4. Kurbacher, Ch. M., Janát, M. M., Brenne, U., et al. (2000) Chemosensitivitätstestung beim Mammakarzinom, in *Diagnostik und Therapie des Mammakarzinoms—State of the Art* (Untch, M., Konecny, G., Sittek, H., Kessler, M., Reiser, M., and Hepp, H., eds.), W. Zuckschwerdt, Munich, Bern, Wien, New York, pp. 388–398.
5. Krasna, L., Natikova, I., Chaloupkova, A., et al. (2003) Assessment of in vitro drug resistance of human breast cancer cells subcultured from biopsy specimens. *Anticancer Res.* **23**, 2593–2599.
6. Giaever, I. and Keese, C. R. (1984) Monitoring fibroblast behaviour with an applied electric field. *Proc. Natl. Acad. Sci. USA* **81**, 3761–3764.
7. Giaever, I. and Keese, Ch. R. (1991) Micromotion of mammalian cells measured electrically. *Proc. Natl. Acad. Sci. USA* **88**, 7896–7900.
8. Mitra, P., Keese, C. R., and Giaever, I. (1991) Electric measurements can be used to monitor the attachment and spreading of cell in tissue culture. *Biotechniques* **11**, 504–511.
9. Mandel, L. (1986) Energy metabolism of cellular activation, growth and transformation. *Curr. Topics Membr. Transport* **27**, 261–291.
10. Hafner, F. (2000) Cytosensor microphysiometer: technology and recent applications. *Biosensors Bioelectron.* **15**, 149–158.
11. Bergveld, P. (1970) Development of an ion-sensitive solid state device for neurophysiological measurements. *IEEE Trans. Biomed. Eng.* **19**, 70.
12. Wada, H. G., Owicki, J. C., and Parce, J. W. (1991) Cells on silicon: bioassays with a microphysiometer. *Clin. Chem.* **37**, 600–601.
13. Owicki, J. C. and Parce, J. W. (1992) Biosensors based on the energy metabolismof living cells: the physical chemistry and cell biology of extracellular acidification. *Biosensors Bioelectron.* **7**, 255–272.
14. Ekelund, S., Nygren, P., and Larsson, R. (1998) Microphysiometry: new technology for evaluation of anticancer drug activity in human tumor cells in vitro. *Anti-cancer Drugs* **9**, 531–538.

15. Ekelund, S., Sjöholm, A., Nygren, P., Binderup, L., and Larsson, R. (2001) Cellular pharmacodynamics of the cytotoxic guanidino-containing drug CHS 828. Comparison with nethylglyoxal-bis(guanylhydrazone). *Eur. J. Pharmacol.* **418,** 39–45.
16. Mestres-Ventura, P. (2003) Chemosensitivity testing of human tumors using Si-sensor chips. *Recent Results Cancer Res.* **161,** 26–38.
17. Metzger, R., Deglmann, C. J., Hoerrlein, S., Zapf, S., and Hilfrich, J. (2001) Towards in-vitro prediction of an in-vivo cytostatoc response of human tumor cells with a fast chemosensitivity assay. *Toxicology* **166,** 97–108.
18. Waldenmaier, D. S., Babarina, A., and Kischkel, F. C. (2003) Rapid in vitro chemosensitivity analysis of human colon tumor cell lines. *Toxicol. Appl. Pharmacol.* **192,** 237–245.
19. Wolf, B., Brischwein, M., Baumann, W., Ehret, R., and Kraus, M. (1998) Monitoring of cellular signaling and metabolism with modular sensor-tecnique. The PhysioControl-Microsystem (PCM®). *Biosensors Bioelectron.* **13,** 501–509.
20. Wolf, B., Brischwein, M., Baumann, W., et al. (1998) Microsensor-aided measurements of cellular signaling and metabolism on tumor cells (Cell Monitoring System (CMS©). *Tumor Biol.* **19,** 374–383.
21. Otto, A. M., Brischwein, M., Niendorf, A., Henning T., Motrescu, E., and Wolf, B. (2003) Microphysiological testing for chemosensitivity of living tumor cells with multiparametric microsensor chips. *Cancer Detect. Prevent.* **27,** 291–296.
22. Tillmann, U. and Bereiter-Hahn, J. (1986) Relation of actin fibrils to energy metabolism of endothelial cells. *Cell Tissue Res.* **243,** 579–585.
23. Jing, Y., Xu, X. C., Lotan, R., Waxman, S., and Mira y Lopez, R. (1996) Human breast carcinoma slice cultures retain retinoic acid sensitivity. *Braz. J. Med. Biol. Res.* **29,** 1105–1108.
24. Ajilore, O. A. and Sapolsky, R. M. (1997) Application of silicon microphysiometry to tissue slices: detection of metabolic correlates of selective vulnerability. *Brain Res.* **752,** 99–106.
25. Thiébaud, P., Rooij, N. F., Koudelka-Hepp, M., and Stoppini, L. (1997) Microelectrode arrays for electrophysiological monitoring of hippocampal organotypic slice cultures. *IEEE Trans. Biomed. Eng.* **44,** 1159–1163.
26. Martin, H., Bournique, B., Sarsat, J. P., Albadalajo, V., and Lerche-Langrand, C. (2000) Cryopreserved rat liver slices: a critical evaluation of cell viability, histological integrity, and drug-metabolizing enzymes. *Cryobiol.* **41,** 135–144.
27. Mira y Lopez, R. and Ossowski, L. (1990) Preservation of steroid hormone receptors in organ cultures of human breats carcinomas. *Cancer Res.* **50,** 78–83.
28. Jing, Y., Zhang, J., Bleiweiss, I. J., Waxman, S., Zelent, A., and Mira y Lopez, R. (1996) Defective expression of cellular retinol binding protein type I and retinoic acid receptors α2, β2 and γ2 in human breats cancer cells. *FASEB J.* **10,** 1064–1070.
29. Hohenberg, H., Mannweiler, K., and Müller, M. (1994) High-pressure freezing of cell suspensions in cellulose capillary tubes. *J. Microsc.* **175,** 34–43.
30. Zauli, G., Furlini, G., Vitale, M., et al. (1994) A subset of human CD34+ hematopoietic progenitors express low levels of CD4, the high-affinity receptor for human immunodeficiency virus-type 1. *Blood* **84,** 1896–1905.

# 10

## Overview of Tumor Cell Chemoresistance Mechanisms

### Laura Gatti and Franco Zunino

#### Summary

Drug resistance of tumor cells is recognized as the primary cause of failure of chemotherapeutic treatment of most human tumors. Although pharmacological factors—including inadequate drug concentration at the tumor site—can contribute to clinical resistance, cellular factors play a major role in chemoresistance of several tumors. Although manifestations of resistance are conventionally referred to as acquired or intrinsic on the basis of the initial response to the first therapy, a common feature is the development of a phenotype resistant to a variety of structurally and functionally distinct agents. In both manifestations, drug resistance is a multifactorial phenomenon involving multiple interrelated or independent mechanisms. A heterogeneous expression of involved mechanisms may characterize tumors of the same type or cells of the same tumor and may at least in part reflect tumor progression. The relevant mechanisms that can contribute to cellular resistance include: increased expression of defense factors involved in reducing intracellular drug concentration; alterations in drug–target interaction; and changes in cellular response, in particular increased cell ability to repair DNA damage or tolerate stress conditions, and defects in apoptotic pathways. This chapter presents an overview of the drug resistance mechanisms.

#### Key Words

Drug resistance; defense factors; cellular response; antitumor drugs; apoptosis.

### 1. Introduction

Resistance of tumor cells to chemotherapy is a common phenomenon in human tumors, most evident in advanced metastatic disease. Although two distinct manifestations of drug resistance, i.e., acquired and intrinsic (or natural), are known, it is likely that a common cellular basis exists. Indeed, in both manifestations, resistant cells tend to develop simultaneous resistance to a number of structurally and functionally diverse antitumor agents. Clinical resistance is a major obstacle in effective treatment of human tumors. Therapeutic approaches

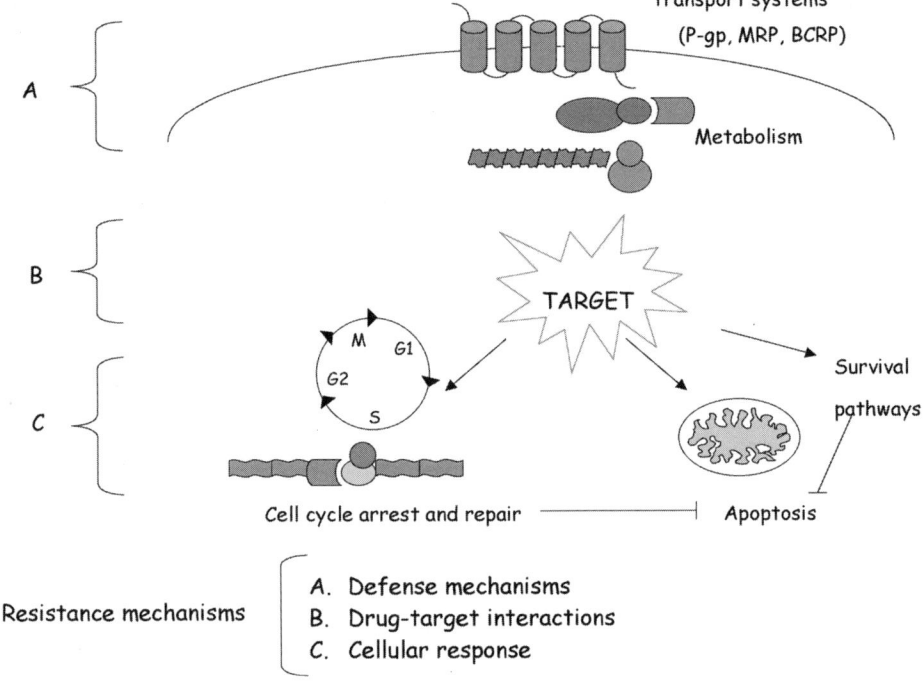

Fig. 1. The main chemoresistance mechanisms.

aimed to overcome a single resistance mechanism have been unsuccessful because the phenomenon is multifactorial, with a variable espression of interrelated or independent mechanisms among different tumor types or patients. Given the adaptability and genomic instability of tumor cells, it seems likely that drug resistance will continue to be an important clinical problem even in the age of targeted therapeutics and tailored treatment approaches. The main mechanisms for chemoresistance of tumor cells can be grouped in three varieties (**Fig. 1**): (1) decrease of active drug concentration at target level due to activation of transporter proteins or detoxification mechanisms within the cell; (2) alterations affecting drug–target interactions; (3) factors influencing cellular response that affect tumor cell survival *(1–3)*.

## 2. Intracellular Defense Factors
### 2.1. Drug Transporters

A decrease of intracellular drug accumulation may result both from decrease of drug influx as well as increase of efflux from the cells. Because most chemotherapeutic drugs enter cells by passive diffusion through the plasma membrane, changes in drug influx can be connected with alterations in the cell membrane structures. Many cytotoxins found in nature and used in chemotherapy as natural drugs enter cells by passive diffusion. These amphipathic drugs are hydrophobic enough to diffuse through a lipid bilayer, but they are also hydrophilic enough to be water-soluble and to reach their target. Because these drugs (i.e., doxorubicin) do not require a transport system to enter the cell, organisms cannot defend themselves against those compounds by altering an import protein. The latter strategy is effective to keep out water-soluble drugs, such as methotrexate, which is dependent on the reduced folate carrier for rapid cellular uptake *(4)*. The mechanism of impaired cisplatin accumulation is unknown, and also the mechanism by which it enters or exits from cells remains poorly defined. Data concerning alterations of drug uptake by cells are scarce, so drug efflux is considered to be the main mechanism implicated in decreased drug accumulation in tumor cells *(5)*.

The primary cause of the multidrug resistance (MDR) phenotype is attributed to the overexpression by tumor cells of some members of a highly conserved family of transmembrane proteins characterized by an ATP-binding cassette or domain, and therefore called the ABC superfamily of transporters *(6)*. Many chemotherapeutic agents can act as substrates for such efflux pumps, designed to export toxins derived from natural products or processes *(7)*.

The prototypical representative of this family, the 170-kDa P-glycoprotein (P-gp), was first characterized in the plasma membrane of Chinese hamster ovary cells and identified as being encoded by the *MDR1* gene *(8)*. P-gp can transport a large variety of different molecules, including cytostatic drugs and endogenous substrates (steroid hormones, cytokines), and is able to bind and transport drugs against a drug concentration gradient at the expense of ATP hydrolysis *(4,6)*. One of the most popular hypotheses proposes that the drug molecule binds to a specific site of P-gp within the lipid bilayer of the cell plasma membrane, and by means of the energy of ATP hydrolysis is transported out of the cell *(5)*. Another study suggests that P-gp may function as a flipase that moves bound substances to the external membrane layer or outside the cell *(9)*. P-gp functional activity mediates cellular resistance to diverse antitumor drugs (anthracycline antibiotics, plant alkaloids, epipodophyllotoxins, taxanes) and to numerous other substances *(5,10)*. P-gp-mediated MDR has been linked to an increased human *MDR1* mRNA level that can be due to gene amplification and/or increased gene transcription *(11)*. Several genes and signaling pathways have been implicated in the regulation of P-gp activity and expression and include p53, EGR1, *ras, raf, RARα/β, c-fos, c-jun*, PKC, PKA, and NF-κB *(5,11)*. The evidence for multiple regulators of *MDR1*/P-gp transcription/activity supports a critical relevance of this defense system to remove toxic exogenous agents. The problem of P-gp reversal is complex in both experimental and clinical testing, probably due to the fact that MDR is caused by the activity of several proteins. The difficulties encountered with several generations of these products in modulating the MDR phenotype may be counterbalanced by the search for an adequately specific target in the regulatory structures of the h*MDR1* promoter *(11)*. Recent studies indicate that small interfering RNA-induced suppression of h*MDR1* gene restores sensitivity in MDR preclinical models *(12)*.

Another subfamily of the ABC transporter family, the human multidrug resistance-associated proteins (MRPs), includes at least seven members that are *MRP*-related genes and have an established role in multidrug transport, particularly glutathione (GSH)-conjugated derivatives of several toxic compounds (the so-called GS-X pumps) *(13)*. MRPs are transport systems that recognize anionic drugs (i.e., methotrexate) and neutral drugs conjugated to acidic ligands, such as GSH, glucuronate, or sulfate, whereas P-gp has a low affinity for negatively charged compounds *(14)*. However, MRP1, MRP2, and MRP3 can be implicated in resistance to neutral organic drugs, which are not known to be conjugated to acidic ligands, by transporting these drugs together with free GSH *(15)*. MRP1 can even confer resistance to arsenite and MRP2 to cisplatin, again probably by transporting these compounds in complexes with GSH *(16)*. The spectrum of drug resistance induced by MRP2 (vincristine, vinblastin, doxorubicin, etoposide, mitoxantrone, CPT11, SN38) may eventually turn out to be similar to that shown for MRP1, except for cisplatin resistance, which has been related only to MRP2 overexpression *(4,17)*. Although MRP1 has been detected in almost every tumor type examined, no strong association has emerged between MRP1 levels and clinical resistance *(15)*. A close relation between MRP2 expression and cisplatin resistance has been experimentally observed using hammerhead ribozymes *(18)* and also in patients *(19)*. MRP4 overexpression is associated with high-level resistance to nucleoside analogs used as antihuman immunodeficiency virus drugs *(4)*. What makes the MRP family so remarkable is the range of anticancer drugs handled by its members. Whereas P-gp has become famous for transporting a wide range of neutral or slightly basic organic compounds, the current members of the MRP family are even more versatile. Transport by MRPs therefore affects a wide range of anticancer drugs and provides a link between transporters and the GSH system *(4)*. The potential involvement of MRP proteins in clinical drug resistance has led to a search for compounds that can be used to inhibit these transporters in cancer patients. Attempts to find inhibitors for MRPs have concentrated mainly on MRP1 and MRP2. Substrates for MRP1 and MRP2 are organic anions with a substantial hydrophobic moiety and at least one, but preferably two, negative charge(s) *(4)*. Other inhibitors for MRP1 are organic acids that were originally developed to inhibit transport of uric acid. Since charged compounds do not readily enter cells, they do not provide obvious lead compounds for drug development. Good inhibitors probably have to be made as prodrugs in which the charged moiety is shielded *(4)*. However, in the absence of effective and specific MRPs inhibitors, it is impossible to analyze the contribution of MRPs to resistance by intervention approaches in which anticancer drugs recognized by MRPs are combined with inhibitors *(4)*.

Unlike P-gp and MRPs, the protein LRP (lung resistance-related protein, molecular weight 110 kDa) is found not on the cell membrane, but in the cytoplasm. It is expressed by the cells of normal epithelium and cells of tissues that are exposed to toxic substances, and unlike the ABC transporters, does not contain an ATP-binding cassette. LRP has been found to be identical to the human major vault protein (MVP), which is the main component of "vaults" *(20,21)*. These highly conserved organelles are multimeric complexes of ribonucleoprotein particles exhibiting an octagonal barrel-shaped structure, with protruding caps and an invaginated waist. Their physiological role in normal tissue and in intrinsic or acquired drug resistance is yet to be defined *(22)*. Vaults are located mainly within the cytoplasm, while a minor fraction concurs to the formation of nuclear pore complexes and is associated with vesicles and lysosomes; therefore, they have been implicated in vesicular and nucleocytoplasmic transport of drugs and xenobiotics *(20)*. It is likely that these molecules are extruded either through a vesicle-mediated exocytosis or efflux by conventional ABC transporters *(6)*. Moreover, the entrapment of drugs into vesicular compartments and decreased nuclear/cytoplasmic ratios have been observed in some MDR cell lines that overexpress LRP *(23,24)*. Thereby, LRP alters the intracellular drug localization, keeping the drug away from its target. The range of drugs associated with LRP-mediated resistance is broader than that associated with P-gp and MRPs, and encompasses nonclassical MDR substrates such as melphalan and platinum compounds *(25)*. Overexpression of LRP was originally observed in a NSCLC cell line selected for doxorubicin resistance and then detected in other cell lines of different histotype, and therefore it has been proposed to play a major role in MDR phenotype *(22)*. There are data suggesting that LRP may cause MDR in patients with ovarian cancer and acute myeloid leukemia *(26,27)*. The current clinical data on LRP/MVP detection indicate that expression of this protein may have predictive value in the response to chemotherapy of several tumor types, including testicular germ cell tumors, breast cancer, and soft tissue sarcomas *(21,25,28,29)*.

The most recent ABC transporter identified with a role in the MDR phenotype is BCRP (breast cancer resistance-related protein, also known as MXR, ABCP, and ABCG2) *(30,31)*. This is the only half-transporter recognized in drug resistance, and whether it homo- or heterodimerizes to form a fully functional ABC transporter is not known *(32)*. BCRP is a 72-kDa protein that may be overexpressed through gene amplification or gene rearrangement *(33)* and localizes to the plasma membrane. In normal tissues, it is abundantly expressed in placenta, liver (bile canalicular membrane), intestinal mucosa, brain endothelium, and stem cells *(34)*. In fact, BCRP may serve a protective function by preventing toxins from entering cells as well as potentially playing a role in regulating stem cell differentiation *(35)*. This membrane-localized half-transporter was initially found to cause mitoxantrone resistance *(31,36)*, and has subsequently also been associated with resistance to camptothecins (topotecan and SN-38) *(37)*, anthracyclines, methotrexate *(38)*, and etoposide *(37)*. Interestingly, a novel 7-modified camptothecin analog has been shown to overcome BCRP-associated resistance in a mitoxantrone-selected cell line exhibiting cross-resistance to topotecan and SN38 *(39)*, thus suggesting a recognition of functional groups in some chemotypes rather than chemotype itself. BCRP shares various features with P-gp in terms of range of recognized drugs and pattern of expression by normal tissues. However, the multidrug-resistant phenotype related to BCRP expression is overlapping with, but dinstinct from, that due to P-gp *(31)*.

## 2.2. The GSH-Dependent System

The GSH system is a critical component of cellular detoxification. GSH and GSH-dependent enzymes play a central role in cellular defense against toxic environmental agents, in particular electrophilic agents (e.g., alkylating agents). Modulation of cellular GSH homeostasis can also have a profound effect on the sensitivity of cancer cells to a wide range of cytotoxic drugs. These effects mediated by the GSH system involve inactivation of toxic electrophiles by conjugation, modulation of cellular redox state, activation of drug transporter systems, and regulation of cell signaling and repair pathways *(40)*. The cellular stress response involves changes in thiol content, as a consequence of activation of protective pathways *(41)*. The sulfur-containing tripeptide GSH is the most abundant nonprotein thiol on cells (being found in the millimolar range in most tissues), and is a major component of the process for defense against the toxicity of xenobiotics and oxidants. The major pathways for GSH metabolism in defense of the cell are reduction of $H_2O_2$ and lipid hydroperoxides by GSH peroxidases. GSH forms conjugates with a large variety of reactive electrophilic compounds nonenzymatically, or more often through the reactions catalyzed by GSH S-transferases (GST) *(41)*. Conjugation with GSH is an essential aspect of both xenobiotic and normal physiological metabolism. The water-soluble conjugate is removed from the cell with the participation of transporter proteins named GS-X (including MRPs) *(6)*. Increased levels of GSH were found in cell lines resistant to alkylating agents *(42)*. Also, cisplatin resistance has been correlated with elevated GSH concentrations in several tumor cell lines *(43–46)*, although this relation is not a general observation *(47,48)*. Reactions with other cysteine-rich peptides, such as metallothioneine (MT), that may be overexpressed in resistant cells, are likely to inactivate platinum drugs. Recently, it has been shown that detoxification by GSH is an effective resistance mechanism also against multinuclear platinum compounds, although such complexes are less sensitive toward detoxification compared to cisplatin. This is probably because of the rapid binding of dinuclear cationic complexes to DNA, which reduces the drug exposure to GSH in the cytosol *(49)*. Enzymes that catalyze GSH synthesis have been implicated in drug resistance, but their role in this phenomenon is still unclear *(5)*. GSH is synthesized via two ATP-requiring steps catalyzed by γ-glutamylcysteine synthetase (γ-GCS), a rate-limiting enzyme for the synthesis of GSH, and GSH synthetase. It has been reported that the γ-GCS subunits are concomitantly expressed in response to cisplatin in human cancer cells *(46)*, and more recently it has been observed that hammerhead ribozyme against γ-GCS sensitizes human cancer cells to cisplatin by downregulating both the GSH synthesis and the expression of MDR proteins *(50)*.

Resistance of tumor cells to drugs associated with the MDR phenotype can also be connected with alterations of the GSH system *(42,51)*. Introduction into mammalian cells of the cDNA of various GSTs resulted in a slight increase of the level of resistance to alkylating agents *(42)*. Several chemical inhibitors of GSTs have been studied for their role in potentiating anticancer drugs. However, as a consequence of lack of specificity *(52–54)*, these agents are not suitable for the clinical modulation of drug resistance *(55)*. The peptidomimetic drug TER199, an analog of GSH designed to be an isozyme-specific inhibitor of GSTπ *(56)*, has been shown to be an effective inhibitor of MRP1-mediated drug resistance *(55)*. More recently, a novel GSTπ-activated prodrug (TLK286) has been suggested for use in the clinical modulation of cisplatin resistance of ovarian cancer *(57)*. A novel strategy to overcome MDR in cancer cells involves treatment with a combination of alkylating agents and nontoxic reversing antimalarial drugs, with the aim of inhibiting GSTs *(58)*. BSO (buthioninesulfoximine) is a GSH-depleting agent and thereby overcomes resistance of tumor cell lines to alkylating agents *(42,59)* and to etoposide *(60)*. The clinical usefulness of GSH depletion in heavily pretreated patients with drug-resistant ovarian cancer *(61)* remains questionable, because, as in the case of P-gp, alterations of the GSH system cannot completely explain drug resistance. It is likely that several defense systems are activated simultaneously in the tumor, and this can provide grounds for further selection of MDR cells *(5)*.

## 2.3. Alteration in Metabolism and/or Subcellular Distribution

Antimetabolite drugs work by inhibiting key enzymes of nucleic acid metabolism, or by being incorporated into macromolecules and inhibiting their normal function *(62)*. The mechanism of cytotoxicity of the anticancer agent 5-fluorouracil (5-FU), widely used for the treatment of colorectal cancer, has been ascribed to the misincorporation of fluoronucleotides into RNA and DNA and to inhibition of the essential enzyme thymidylate synthase (TS). 5-FU rapidly enters the cell using the same facilitated transport mechanism as uracil, and it is then converted to active metabolites. The rate-limiting enzyme in 5-FU catabolism is dihydropyrimidine dehydrogenase (DPD): alterations in DPD may therefore explain failure of 5-FU response and the development of resistance. In this case, as well as in all other examples of alteration in metabolism and/or subcellular distribution of anticancer agents, an analysis of relevant enzymes and other factors involved in modulation of drug activity and toxicity are required, with the aim of eventually selecting eligible patients and better predicting the response to chemotherapy *(63,64)*.

## 3. Alterations of the Target

The efficacy of a cytotoxic agent may be critically influenced by the content (or activity) of the target molecules. The drug targets often implicated as determinants of drug activity are enzymes of DNA functions or proteins of the cellular replication apparatus. These alterations may be quantitative (e.g., level of expression) or qualitative (e.g., mutation). In the case of antimetabolites that interfere with various steps in nucleic acid metabolism through inhibition of key enzymes (thymidylate synthase, dihydrofolate reductase, ribonucleotide reductase, DNA polymerase), an increased content of the target enzyme may result in drug resistance. An example is fluorouracil resistance due to increased level of thymidilate synthase *(62,64)*. By contrast, because the genotoxic damage caused by DNA topoisomerase inhibitors is mediated by the target enzyme, downregulation of the DNA topoisomerase is expected to decrease sensitivity to important antitumor agents, including anthracyclines and camptothecins *(65)*. However, drug resistance to DNA topoisomerase inhibitors is likely to be multifactorial, and no unequivocal relation was observed between expression or activity of the topoisomerase genes and clinical response to chemotherapy *(66)*. Resistance to taxol can be also associated with multiple alterations of its intracellular target, including modification of tubulin levels, altered electrophoretic mobility of $\alpha$- or $\beta$-tubulin isoforms, and acetylation of $\alpha$-tubulin *(10)*. The contribution of these alterations to the paclitaxel-resistant phenotype has not yet been elucidated. Indeed, both reduced and increased tubulin levels have been found in paclitaxel-resistant cell lines *(67,68)*.

## 4. Cellular Response

Treatment with cytotoxic drugs activates several distinct cellular responses. Activation of DNA repair processes is considered to be the first and most frequent response to genotoxic damage. However, the biological response to genotoxic insult embraces more than the repair and tolerance of DNA damage *(69)*. The exposure of cells to cytotoxic agents results in the transcriptional modulation of a large number of genes, the precise function(s) of many of which remains to be established. Additionally, cells have evolved complex signaling pathways to arrest the progression of the cell cycle in the presence of DNA damage, thus allowing DNA repair *(70)*. Finally, when the burden of cellular insult exceeds cell ability to repair, programmed cell death (apoptosis) can be induced *(71)*.

### 4.1. DNA Repair and Tolerance

Upregulation of DNA repair mechanisms, which is necessary for maintenance of the genetic stability of the cell *(72)*, has been associated with resistance to genotoxic drugs including alkylating agents, platinum compounds, and topoisomerase inhibitors *(73)*. DNA repair of different types of DNA lesions involves multiple distinct mechanisms for excising damaged bases, termed nucleotide excision repair (NER), base excision repair (BER), and mismatch repair (MMR) *(69)*. In all three mechanisms of repair the process involves recognition of the damage, splicing out the lesion, and inserting new bases to fill the gap, followed by ligation of the repaired strand(s).

The process of NER involves as many as 30 distinct proteins in human cells that function as a large complex, called the nucleotide excision repairosome. This "repair machine" facilitates the excision of damaged nucleotides by generating bimodal incisions in the flanking regions and removing a fragment of about 30 nucleotides in length *(74)*. Several NER genes in this pathway including XPB, XPA, and ERCC1, have been implicated in anticancer drug resistance in human tumor cells *(75)*. In mammalian cells, this repair pathway is the only known mechanism for the removal of bulky, helix-distorting DNA adducts, such as those generated by certain chemotherapeutic agents, and it serves as a backup repair system for the removal of other lesions from DNA *(76)*. Indeed, the NER pathway is a major mechanism contributing to resistance to platinum compounds *(77)*, because this repair mechanism removes the intrastrand crosslinks between adjacent purines that are the main adducts introduced by cisplatin *(78)*. Recently, it has been shown that it is possible to substantially enhance the cisplatin cytotoxicity by disturbing the NER pathway in cisplatin-resistant cell lines *(79)*. DNA interstrand cross-links (ICLs) between the two complementary strands of the double helix are produced by effective antitumor agents. ICL-inducing agents, such as platinum compounds and nitrogen mustards, are thought to exert their cytotoxic effect by preventing efficient DNA replication and transcription *(73)*. The ability of cells to repair DNA ICLs is a critical determinant of sensitivity, and recent clinical studies indicate that

DNA repair capacity is strongly implicated in both inherent tumor sensitivity and acquired drug resistance. DNA repair of ICLs is a complex challenge because of the involvement of both DNA strands *(80)*. Eukaryotic cells eliminate ICLs through the coordinate action of several DNA repair pathways *(80)*. In mammalian cells, it has been suggested that ICLs repair occurs via the activity of the NER endonuclease (ERCC1/XPF) as well as the nonhomologous DNA end-joining (NHEJ) and also the Rad51-related homologous recombination repair (HRR) *(81)*. Recently, it has been shown that among different NER proteins only the XPD protein levels correlate with resistance to alkylating agents in human tumor cells, suggesting that XPD plays an important role in the development of this resistance *(75,82)*.

Damaged bases that are not recognized by the NER machinery are corrected by BER, whereby the bases are excised from the genome as free bases by a different set of repair enzymes. After removal of base substrates by a DNA glycosilase, an AP (apurinic/apyrimidinic)-endonuclease initiates repair of the lesion *(83)*. The activity of the major human AP endonuclease (APE1/Ref1) has been shown to contribute to human glioma cell resistance to alkylating agents *(84)*. The BER pathway is essential for the repair of damaged DNA induced by oxidizing and alkylating agents. The importance of this pathway in processing DNA damage makes its members potential targets for novel chemotherapeutic agents *(83)*.

The MMR is a postreplicative DNA repair process involved in maintaining genomic stability, through the correction of single-base mispairs and mismatched loops incorporated as a result of mistakes during DNA replication or drug exposure *(85)*. Tumors with defects in MMR system exhibit marked resistance to alkylating agents and a variety of anticancer agents that modify DNA to create substrates for the MMR system. The analysis of involvement of the MMR in the response to platinum compounds highlights differences among drugs *(86)*. In fact, several studies have suggested a role for the MMR pathway in cellular sensitivity to platinum drugs, and the loss of MMR is associated with a relative resistance to cisplatin *(87,88)*. In this regard, it has been proposed that resistance is a consequence of the lack of a system coupling DNA damage recognition with cell death, as a result of futile repair cycling or replication stalling *(87)*. This does not appear to be the case of oxaliplatin that seems to cause DNA distortions that prevent binding of the MMR complex *(89)*. The MMR pathway is instead absolutely required for signaling the initiation of apoptosis in response to other alkylating agents *(90)*. Although the loss of MMR function clearly contributes to the resistance of tumor cells to methylating O6-alkylating agents, such loss happens only sporadically in most cancers. The main factor in resistance of tumors to nitrosoureas and triazenes is the ATase protein (O6-alkylguanine-DNA alkyltransferase), also known as MGMT or OGAT, which recognizes and removes alkyl adducts from potentially cytotoxic lesions generated in DNA by such agents *(91)*. Its inactivation can reverse resistance to the above-mentioned agents. Moreover, MGMT has been implicated as a determinant of camptothecin sensitivity and may play some role in the topo I-mediated DNA damage/repair *(92)*.

Reactive oxygen species and ionizing radiation are prevalent sources of DNA strand breaks, which must be repaired in order to maintain genomic integrity. Several mechanisms for the repair of double strand breaks (DSBs) have been elucidated. One of these involves swapping equivalent regions of DNA between homologous chromosomes (recombination). It can be used to repair a damaged site on a DNA strand by using information located on the undamaged homologous chromosome. An alternative mechanism for the repair of DSBs, called nonhomologous end joining (NHEJ; see above), also requires a multiprotein complex, and essentially joins broken chromosome ends in a manner that does not depend on sequence homology and may not be error-free *(69)*. Translesion DNA synthesis is instead a damage-tolerance mechanism that involves the replication machinery bypassing sites of base damage, allowing normal DNA replication and gene expression to proceed downstream of the (unrepaired) lesion *(93)*. To overcome the DNA lesions, specialized low-fidelity DNA polymerases add nucleotides to the replicating strand opposing the DNA lesion, thus allowing replication to continue, but nevertheless introducing mutations into the newly synthesized sequence *(93)*.

Understanding DNA repair pathways is expected to identify factors that confer resistance to anticancer drugs and to develop strategies for modulating repair capacity as a means of overcoming resistance or enhancing sensitivity to DNA-damaging agents. Different pathways perform the repair of different forms of DNA damage, and it is difficult to inhibit all of these. Nevertheless, inhibition of DNA repair is currently exploited to resensitize tumors to chemotherapy.

## *4.2. Cell Cycle and Drug Resistance*

Cells respond to DNA damage by activating checkpoints pathways that ultimately block the activity of CDKs and consequently cause an arrest in cell cycle progression. Current models predict that sensor molecules, which detect DNA damage or incompletely replicated DNA, initiate checkpoint responses to halt cell cycle progression. Eukaryotic cells activate an evolutionarily conserved set of checkpoint proteins that rapidly induce cell cycle arrest to prevent replication or segregation of damaged DNA before repair is completed. The G1 checkpoint ensures that the cell does not begin DNA replication unless the molecular machinery for DNA synthesis is ready and DNA is undamaged. The replication checkpoint blocks the cell cycle in S-phase in response to either depletion of deoxynucleotides or DNA damage that would stall replication forks

*(94)*. Furthermore, insults to DNA integrity during G2 normally lead to arrest of cell cycle progression to ensure that DNA replication is complete and ready for mitosis *(95)*. Finally, DNA damage that occurs in methaphase activates spindle checkpoint pathways that generate cell cycle arrest in preanaphase *(96)*.

Cell cycle–mediated drug resistance is best described as a relative insensitivity to a phase-specific agent. For instance, the camptothecins are considered to be S-phase-specific, thereby implicating that cancer cells that are not actively replicating DNA could be unaffected by the drug *(97)*. This phenomenon is relevant in combination chemotherapy. The best example demonstrating the relevance of the cell cycle in combination chemotherapy includes those combinations that involve taxanes, the prototypical class of phase-specific cytotoxic agents. In view of the fact that paclitaxel is predominately an M-phase-specific drug, one would hypothesize that agents that arrest cells before they enter M-phase would antagonize paclitaxel effects *(98)*. This issue is of clinical importance because cell cycle inhibitors are entering clinical trials in combination with chemotherapy, in particular with paclitaxel *(98)*. Indeed, it has been shown that the combination of two novel antineoplastic CDK inhibitors (flavopiridol or bryostatin-1) with paclitaxel resulted in cell cycle-mediated drug resistance *(99,100)*, a phenomenon that may be overcome by appropriate sequencing of the drug combination. Cell cycle-mediated drug resistance also plays an important role in combination therapies that do not include specific cell cycle modulators, as in the case of combination between cisplatin and taxanes. The combination of conventional chemotherapeutic agents may result in cell cycle-mediated drug resistance, as documented when cisplatin exposure precedes paclitaxel, whereas a synergistic effect was observed using inverse drug sequencing *(98)*. An understanding of the mechanisms by which anticancer agents influence the cell cycle may offer insights into strategies for sensitizing cancer cells to current therapeutics and can also provide a rationale for the administration of combinations of drugs *(94)*.

### 4.3. Apoptosis and the Response to Anticancer Therapy

Because anticancer treatments act, at least in part, by inducing apoptosis, antiapoptotic mechanisms or defects in the pathways involved in apoptosis have been postulated to play a role in drug resistance *(101,102)*. Understanding of cell death processes after cytotoxic damage would allow the development of a more rational approach to overcoming the problem of drug resistance *(103)*. Many of the biochemical and morphological features of apoptotic cells result from the selective cleavage of a subset of cellular polypeptides, mediated by caspases *(104)*. Two major intracellular caspase cascades, one activated predominately by death-receptor ligands and the other triggered by various cellular stresses, including DNA damage and microtubule disruption, have been described *(105)*. Activation of these protease cascades is tightly regulated by a number of factors, including Bcl-2 family members, inhibitor of apoptosis proteins, and several protein kinases *(105)*. Signaling through the death-receptor pathway (also called the extrinsic pathway) begins with ligation of specialized cell surface receptors (e.g., Fas/CD95, TNF-R, TRAIL-R), inducing caspase activation *(106)*. The mitochondrial pathway (also called the intrinsic pathway) is initiated by release of cytochrome-*c* and other polypeptides (e.g., AIF, Smac/DIABLO, endonuclease G, Omi/HtrA2) from the mitochondrial intermembrane space *(107)*. This process involves mitochondrial permeability transition as well as the trafficking of certain Bcl-2 family members from the cytoplasm to the outer mitochondrial membranes *(108,109)*. The overall survival threshold is probably determined by the balance of interactions between proapoptotic and antiapoptotic members of the Bcl-2 family *(103)*. There is considerable cross-talk between the extrinsic and intrinsic pathways. For example, caspase-8 (extrinsic pathway), can proteolitically activate Bid, which can then facilitate cytochrome-*c* release *(110)*. Conversely, activators of the intrinsic pathway can sensitize the cell to extrinsic death ligands.

A variety of chemotherapeutic agents induce common apoptotic pathways in susceptible cell types *(111,112)*. Thus, various defects that disable apoptosis can produce multidrug resistance. Among the various factors regulating apoptosis, the p53 tumor-suppressor protein seems to have a major role, because emerging evidence suggests that both induced and repressed target genes are required for the programmed cell death pathways *(113)*. Thus, mutations in *p53* or in the *p53* pathway can produce resistance to DNA-damaging agents *(114)*. However, *p53* status is not a universal predictor of treatment response, in part because not all drugs require p53 for activation of apoptosis *(115)* and, in some settings, p53 loss can enhance drug-induced cell death *(116)*. Also, mutations or altered expression of Bcl-2-related proteins can drastically alter drug sensitivity in experimental models *(101,117,118)*, and are associated with multidrug resistance in human cancers *(101)*. Although the contribution of postmitochondrial events to cellular outcome is less well defined, defects at this level can also promote drug resistance. For example, epigenetic inactivation of *Apaf-1* in malignant melanoma, or increases in IAP and HSP expression in various tumors, are associated with drug resistance *(119–121)*. The role of the death-receptor pathway in drug-induced cell death is controversial *(115)*. It has been argued that certain cell types require both the death-receptor and mitochondrial pathways for drug-induced apoptosis, while others require only the mitochondrial pathway *(122)*. In some cases, the same stimulus that induces apoptosis also initiates an antagonistic antiapoptotic program (e.g., TNF/NF-kB pathway) *(2,123)*. The potentially lethal lesion initiates a complex cascade of signaling pathways that have either proapoptotic or protective functions *(115)*.

Apoptosis seems to be induced if damage exceeds the capacity of repair. This presumably allows life-and-death decisions to be tightly regulated.

The overall contribution of apoptosis in antitumor drug efficacy and of defects in apoptosis pathways to clinical multidrug resistance is still matter of debate *(2,124)*. Other drug-induced effects, such as cytostasis, may result in mitotic catastrophe and can augment apoptosis. Moreover, the relative contribution of each activated pathway and resistance mechanism to clinical multidrug resistance is likely to depend on the mechanism of drug action, as well as the tissue origin and genetic background of the tumor *(2)*. The similarity between physiological and drug-induced apoptotic programs establishes a clear link between tumor development and intrinsic resistance to anticancer treatment, and thus provides a biological basis for how tumor genotype can determine treatment outcome. Besides, the fact that defects in apoptosis can promote drug resistance downstream of the drug–target interaction raises the possibility that genotoxic agents may induce further genetic mutations owing to "damage without death" *(2)*.

## 5. Conclusions

It is now evident that cellular drug resistance is a complex multifactorial phenomenon. Clinical drug resistance may involve additional physiological mechanisms mediated by tumor–host interactions. A common resistance mechanism observed in preclinical systems selected with various cytotoxic agents (vinca alkaloids, anthracyclines) is the overexpression of drug efflux proteins (Pgp, MPR, BCRP). Although these defence mechanisms could contribute to the drug resistance of some tumor types, the available evidence supports that cellular response to genotoxic stress plays a primary role in determining the sensitivity or resistance status of tumor cells. Potentially lethal damage caused by most conventional agents activates diverse signaling pathways that may have proapoptotic or protective functions. The type and extent of damage and biological context could critically influence the cellular outcome following treatment. Activation of cell death programs could be the result of cell inability to efficiently repair or tolerate DNA damage. Defects in cellular processes controlling apoptosis or overexpression of signaling pathways promoting survival could be the basis for tumor cell insensitivity to a wide variety of antitumor agents. A detailed understanding of regulation of apoptosis, growth arrest and DNA repair, and identification of defects in death pathways is expected to provide insight into relevant mechanisms of drug resistance with clinical implications.

## References

1. Johnstone, R. W., Ruefli, A. A., and Smyth, M. J. (2000) Multiple physiological functions for multidrug transporter P-glycoprotein? *Trends Biochem. Sci.* **25,** 1–6.

2. Johnstone, R. W., Ruefli, A. A., and Lowe, S. W. (2002) Apoptosis: a link between cancer genetics and chemotherapy. *Cell* **108,** 153–164.
3. Volm, M. (1998) Multidrug resistance and its reversal. *Anticancer Res.* **18,** 2905–2917.
4. Borst, P., Evers, R., Kool, M., and Wijnholds, J. (2000) A family of drug transporters: the multidrug resistance-associated proteins. *J. Natl. Cancer Inst.* **92,** 1295–1302.
5. Stavrovskaya, A. A. (2000) Cellular mechanisms of multidrug resistance of tumor cells. *Biochemistry* **65,** 95–106.
6. Bush, J. A. and Li, G. (2002) Cancer chemoresistance: the relationship between p53 and multidrug transporters. *Int. J. Cancer* **98,** 323–330.
7. Guminski, A. D., Harnett, P. R., and de Fazio, A. (2002) Scientists and clinicians test their metal-back to the future with platinum compounds. *Lancet* **3,** 312–318.
8. Juliano, R. L. and Ling, V. (1976) A surface glycoprotein modulating drug permeability in Chinese hamster ovary cell mutants. *Biochim. Biophys. Acta* **455,** 152–162.
9. Higgins, C. F., Callaghan, R., Linton, K. J., Rosenberg, M. F., and Ford, R. C. (1997) Structure of the multidrug resistance P-glycoprotein. *Semin. Cancer Biol.* **8,** 135–142.
10. Zunino, F., Cassinelli, G., Polizzi, D., and Perego, P. (1999) Molecular mechanisms of resistance to taxanes and therapeutic implications. *Drug Resist. Updates* **2,** 351–357.
11. Labialle, S., Gayet, L., Marthinet, E., Rigal, D., and Baggetto, L.G. (2002) Transcriptional regulators of the human multidrug resistance 1 gene: recent views. *Biochem. Pharmacol.* **64,** 943–948.
12. Wu, H., Hait, W. N., and Yang, J. M. (2003) Small interfering RNA-induced suppression of MDR1 (P-glycoprotein) restores sensitivity to multidrug-resistant cancer cells. *Cancer Res.* **63,** 1515–1519.
13. Ishikawa, T., Kuo, M. T., Furuta, K., and Suzuki, M. (2000) The human multidrug resistance-associated protein (MRP) gene family: from biological function to drug molecular design. *Clin. Chem. Lab. Med.* **38,** 893–897.
14. Jedlitschky, G., Leier, I., Buchholz, U., Barnouin, K., Kurz, G., and Keppler, D. (1996) Transport of glutathione, glucuronate, and sulfate conjugates by the MRP gene-encoded conjugate export pump. *Cancer Res.* **56,** 988–994.
15. Hipfner, D. R., Deeley, R. G., and Cole, S. P. (1999) Structural, mechanistic and clinical aspects of MRP1. Biochim. Biophys. Acta 1461, 359–376.
16. Konig, J., Nies, A. T., Cui, Y., Leier, I., and Keppler, D. (1999) Conjugate export pumps of the multidrug resistance protein (MRP) family: localization, substrate specificity, and MRP2-mediated drug resistance. *Biochim. Biophys. Acta* **1461,** 377–394.
17. Cui, Y., Konig, J., Buchholz, J. K., Spring, H., Leier, I., and Keppler, D. (1999) Drug resistance and ATP-dependent conjugate transport mediated by the apical multidrug resistance protein, MRP2, permanently expressed in human and canine cells. *Mol. Pharmacol.* **55,** 929–937.

18. Materna, V., Holm, P. S., Dietel, M., and Lage, H. (2001) Kinetic characterization of ribozymes directed against the cisplatin resistance-associated ABC transporter cMOAT/MRP2/ABCC2. *Cancer Gene Ther.* **8,** 176–184.
19. Hinoshita, E., Uchiumi, T., Taguchi, K., et al. (2000) Increased expression of an ATP-binding cassette superfamily transporter, multidrug resistance protein 2, in human colorectal carcinomas. *Clin. Cancer Res.* **6,** 2401–2407.
20. Scheffer, G. L., Wijngaard, P. L., Flens, M. J., et al. (1995) The drug resistance-related protein LRP is the human major vault protein. *Nat. Med.* **1,** 578–582.
21. Scheffer, G. L., Chhroeijers, A. B., Izquierdo, M. A., Wiemer, E. A., and Scheper, R. (2000) Lung resistance-related protein/major vault protein and vau in multidrug-resistant cancer. *Curr. Opin. Oncol.* **12,** 550–556.
22. Meschini, S., Marra, M., Calcabrini, A., et al. (2002) Role of the lung resistance-related protein (LRP) in the drug sensitivity of cultured tumor cells. *Toxicol. in Vitro* **16,** 389–398.
23. Dietel, M., Arps, H., Lage, H., and Niendorf, A. (1990) Membrane vesicle formation due to acquired mitoxantrone resistance in human gastric carcinoma cell line PG85-257. *Cancer Res.* **50,** 6100–6106.
24. Schuurhuis, G. J., Broxterman, H. J., de Lange, J. H. M., et al. (1991) Early multidrug resistance, defined by changes in intracellular doxorubicin distribution, independent of P-glycoprotein. *Br. J. Cancer* **64,** 857–861.
25. Komdeur, R., Plaat, B. E. C., van der Graaf, W. T. A., et al. (2003) Expression of multidrug resistance proteins, P-gp, MRP1 and LEP, in soft tissue sarcoma analysed according to their histological type and grade. *Eur. J. Cancer* **39,** 909–916.
26. Izquierdo, M. A., van der Zee, A. G., Vermorken, J. B., et al. (1995) Drug resistance-associated marker Lrp for prediction of response to chemotherapy and prognoses in advanced ovarian carcinoma. *J. Natl. Cancer Inst.* **87,** 1230–1237.
27. List, A. F., Spier, C. S., Grogan, T. M., et al. (1996) Overexpression of the major vault transporter protein lung-resistance protein predicts treatment outcome in acute myel leukemia. *Blood* **87,** 2464–2469.
28. Zurita, A. J., Diestra, J. E., Condom, E., et al. (2003) Lung resistance-related protein as a predictor of clinical outcome in advanced testicular germ-cell tumours. *Br. J. Cancer* **88,** 879–886.
29. Burger, H., Foekens, J. A., Look, M. P., et al. (2003) RNA expression of breast cancer resistance protein, lung resistance-related protein, multidrug resistance-associated proteins 1 and 2, and multidrug resistance gene 1 in breast cancer: correlation with chemotherapeutic response. *Clin. Cancer Res.* **9,** 827–836.
30. Doyle, L.A., Yang, W., Abruzzo, L. E., et al. (1998) A multidrug resistance transporter from human MCF-7 breast cancer cells. *Proc. Natl. Acad. Sci. USA* **95,** 15,665–15,670.
31. Litman, T., Brangi, M., Hudson, E., et al. (2000) The multidrug-resistant phenotype associated with overexpression of the new ABC half-transporter, MXR (ABCG2). *J. Cell Sci.* **113,** 2011–2021.
32. Kowalski, P., Wichert, A., Holm, P. S., Dietel, M., and Lage, H. (2001) Selection and characterization of a high-activity ribozyme directed against the antineoplas-

tic drug resistance-associate ABC transporter BCRP/MXR/ABCG2. *Cancer Gene Ther.* **8,** 185–192.
33. Bates, S. E., Robey, R., Miyake, K., Rao, K., Ross, D. D., and Litman, T. (2001) The role of half-transporters in multidrug resistance. *J. Bioenerg. Biomembr.* **33,** 503–511.
34. Allen, J. D. and Schinkel, A. H. (2002) Multidrug resistance and pharmacological protection mediated by the breast cancer resistance protein (BCRP/ABCG2). *Mol. Cancer Ther.* **1,** 427–434.
35. Ejendal, K. F. and Hrycyna, C. A. (2002) Multidrug resistance and cancer: the role of the human ABC transporter ABCG2. *Curr. Protein Peptide Sci.* **3,** 503–511.
36. Ross, D. D., Yang, W., Abruzzo, L. V., et al. (1999) Atypical multidrug resistance: breast cancer resistance protein messenger RNA expression in mitoxantrone-selected cell lines. *J. Natl. Cancer Inst.* **91,** 429–433.
37. Allen, J. D., van Dort, S. C., Buitelaar, M., van Tellingen, O., and Schinkel, A. H. (2003) Mouse breast cancer resistance protein (Bcrp1/Abcg2) mediates etoposide resistance and transport, but etoposide oral availability is limited primarily by P-glycoprotein. *Cancer Res.* **63,** 1339–1344.
38. Volk, E. L., Farley, K. M., Wu, Y., Li, F., Robey, R. W., and Schneider, E. (2002) Overexpression of wild-type breast cancer resistance protein mediates methotrexate resistance. *Cancer Res.* **62,** 5035–5040.
39. Perego, P., De Cesare, M., De Isabella, P., et al. (2001) A novel 7-modified camptothecin analog overcomes breast cancer resistance protein-associated resistance in a mitoxantrone-selected colon carcinoma cell line. *Cancer Res.* **61,** 6034–6037.
40. McLellam, L. I. and Wolf, C. R. (1999) Glutathione and glutathione-dependent enzymes in cancer drug resistance. *Drug Resist. Updates* **2,** 153–164.
41. Dickinson, D. A. and Forman, H. J. (2002) Cellular glutathione and thiols metabolism. *Biochem. Pharmacol.* **64,** 1019–1026.
42. Tew, K. D. (1994) Glutathione-associated enzymes in anticancer drug resistance. Perspectives in cancer research. *Cancer Res.* **54,** 4313–4320.
43. Andrews, P. A., Schiefer, M. A., Murphy, M. P., and Howell, S. B. (1988) Enhanced potentiation of cisplatin cytotoxicity in human ovarian carcinoma cells by prolonged glutathione depletion. *Chem. Biol. Interact.* **65,** 51–58.
44. Ishikawa, T. and Ali-Osman, F. (1993) Glutathione-associated cis-diamminedichloroplatinum(II) metabolism and ATP-dependent efflux from leukaemia cells. Molecular characterization of glutathione-platinum complex and its biological significance. *J. Biol. Chem.* **268,** 20,116–20,125.
45. Goto, S., Yoshida, K., Morikawa, T., Urata, Y., Suzuki, K., and Kondo, T. (1995) Augmentation of transport for cisplatin-glutathione adduct in cisplatin-resistant cancer cells. *Cancer Res.* **55,** 4297–4301.
46. Iida, M., Doi, H., Asamoto, S., et al. (1999) Effect of glutathione-modulating compounds on platinum compounds-induced cytotoxicity in human glioma cell lines. *Anticancer Res.* **19,** 5383–5384.
47. Mistry, P., Kelland, L. R., Abel, G., Sdhar, S., and Harrap, K. R. (1991) The relationships between glutathione, glutathione-S-transferase and cytotoxicity of

platinum drugs and melphalan in eight human ovarian carcinoma cell lines. *Br. J. Cancer* **64**, 215–220.
48. Timmer-Bosscha, H., Mulder, N. H., and De Vries, E. G. E. (1992) Modulation of cis-diamminedichloroplatinum(II) resistance: review. *Br. J. Cancer* **66**, 227–238.
49. Jansen, B. A. J., Brouwer, J., and Reedijk, J. (2002) Glutathione induces cellular resistance against cationic dinuclear platinum anticancer drugs. *J. Inorg. Biochem.* **89**, 197–202.
50. Iida, T., Kijima, H., Urata, Y., et al. (2001) Hammerhead ribozyme against γ-glutamylcysteine synthetase sensitizes human colonic cancer cells to cisplatin by down-regulating both the glutathione synthesis and the expression of multidrug resistance proteins. *Cancer Gene Ther.* **8**, 803–814.
51. Sinha, B. K., Trush, M. A., Kennedy, K. A., and Mimnaugh, E. G. (1984) Enzymatic activation and binding of adriamycin to nuclear DNA. *Cancer Res.* **44**, 2892–2896.
52. Tew, K. D., Bomber, A. M., and Hoffman, S. J. (1988) Ethacrynic acid and piriprost as enhancers of cytotoxicity in drug resistant and sensitive cell lines. *Cancer Res.* **48**, 3622.
53. Shen, H., Kauvar, L., and Tew, K. D. (1997) Importance of glutathione and associated enzymes in drug response. *Oncol. Res.* **9**, 295–302.
54. Burg, D. and Mulder, G. J. (2002) Glutathione conjugates and their synthetic derivatives as inhibitors of glutathione-dependent enzymes involved in cancer and drug resistance. *Drug. Metab. Rev.* **34**, 821–863.
55. O'Brien, M. L., Vulevic, B., Freer, S., Boyd, J., Shen, H., and Tew, K. D. (1999) Glutathione peptidomimetic drug modulator of multidrug resistance-associated protein. *J. Pharmacol. Exp. Ther.* **291**, 1348–1355.
56. Morgan, A. S., Ciaccio, P. J., Tew, K. D., and Kauvar, L. M. (1996) Isozyme-specific glutathione S-transferase inhibitors potentiate drug sensitivity in cultured human tumor cell lines. *Cancer Chemother. Pharmacol.* **37**, 363–370.
57. Townsend, D. M., Shen, H., Staros, A. L., Gate, L., and Tew, K. D. (2002) Efficacy of a glutathione S-transferase pi-activated prodrug in platinum-resistant ovarian cancer cells. *Mol. Cancer Ther.* **1**, 1089–1095.
58. Mukanganyama, S., Widersten, M., Naik, Y. S., Mannervik, B., and Hasler, J. A. (2002) Inhibition of glutathione S-transferases by antimalarial drug possible implications for circumventing anticancer drug resistance. *Int. J. Cancer* **97**, 700–705.
59. Schnelldorfer, T., Gansauge, S., Gansauge, F., Schlosser, S., Berger, H. G., and Nussler, A. K. (2000) Glutathione depletion causes cell growth inhibition and enhanced apoptosis in pancreatic cancer cells. *Cancer* **89**, 1440–1447.
60. Grech, K. V., Davey, R. A., and Davey, M. W. (1998) The relationship between modulation of MDR and glutathione in MRP-overexpressing human leukemia cells. *Biochem. Pharmacol.* **55**, 1283–1289.
61. Lewandowicz, G. M., Britt, P., Elgie, A. W., Williamson, C. J., Coley, H. M., and Sargent, J. M. (2002) Cellular glutathione content, in vitro chemoresponse, and therapeutic effect of BSO modulation in samples derived from patients with advanced ovarian cancer. *Gynecol. Oncol.* **85**, 298–404.

62. Longley, D. B., Harkin, D. P., and Johnston, P. G. (2003) 5-fluorouracil: mechanisms of action and clinical strategies. *Nature* **3,** 330–338.
63. Katsumata, K., Tomioka, H., Sumi, T., et al. (2003) Correlation between clinicopathologic factors and kinetics of metabolic enzymes for 5-fluorouracil given to patients with colon carcinoma by two different dosage regimens. *Cancer Chemother. Pharmacol.* **51,** 155–160.
64. Banerjee, D., Mayer-Kuckuk, P., Capiaux, G., Budak-Alpdogan, T., Gorlick, R., and Bertino, J. R. (2002) Novel aspects of resistance to drugs targeted to dihydrofolate reductase and thymidylate synthase. *Biochim. Biophys. Acta* **1587,** 164–173.
65. Larsen, A. K. and Skladanowski, A. (1998) Cellular resistance to topoisomerase-target drugs: from drug uptake to cell death. *Biochim. Biophys. Acta* **1400,** 257–274.
66. Dingemans, A. M., Pinedo, H. M., and Giaccone, G. (1998) Clinical resistance to topoisomerase-targeted drugs. *Biochim. Biophys. Acta* **1400,** 275–288.
67. Dumontet, C. and Sikic, B. I. (1999) Mechanisms of action of and resistance to antitubulin agents: microtubule dynamics, drug transport and cell death. *J. Clin. Oncol.* **17,** 1061–1070.
68. Nishio, K. and Saijo, N. (1999) Cytoskeletons and antimitotic agents developed in Japan. *Anti-Cancer Drug Design* **14,** 133–141.
69. Friedberg, E. C. (2003) DNA damage and repair. *Nature* **421,** 436–440.
70. Zhou, B.-B. S. and Elledge, S. J. (2000) The DNA damage response: putting checkpoints in perspective. *Nature* **408,** 433–439.
71. Cory, S. and Adams, J. M. (2002) The Bcl2 family: regulators of the cellular life-or-death switch. *Nature Rev. Cancer* **2,** 647–656.
72. Hoeijmakers, J. H. (2001) Genome maintenance mechanisms for preventing cancer. *Nature* **411,** 366–374.
73. Chaney, S. G. and Sancar, A. (1996) DNA repair: enzymatic mechanisms and relevance to drug response. *J. Natl. Cancer Inst.* **88,** 1346–1360.
74. Friedberg, E. C., Walker, G. C., and Siede, W. (1995) *DNA Repair and Mutagenesis.* American Society of Microbiology Press, Washington, D.C.
75. Xu, Z., Chen, Z. P., Malapetsa, A., et al. (2002) DNA repair protein levels vis-a-vis anticancer drug resistance in the human tumor cell lines of the National Cancer Institute drug screening program. *Anticancer Drugs* **13,** 511–519.
76. Reardon, J. T. and Sancar, A. (1998) Molecular mechanism of nucleotide excision repair in mammalian cells, in *Advances in DNA Damage and Repair* (Dizdaroglu, M. and Karakaya, A., eds.), Plenum, New York, pp. 377–393.
77. Reardon, J. T., Vaisman, A., Chaney, S. G., and Sancar, A. (1999) Efficient nucleotide excision repair of cisplatin, oxaliplatin, and bis-aceto-ammine-dichlorocyclohexylamine-platinum(IV) (JM216) platinum intrastrand DNA diadducts. *Cancer Res.* **59,** 3968–3971.
78. Petit, C. and Sancar, A. (1999) Nucleotide excision repair: from *E. coli* to man. *Biochimie* **81,** 15–25.
79. Selvakumaran, M., Pisarcik, D. A., Bao, R., Yeung, A. T., and Hamilton, T. C. (2003) Enhanced cisplatin cytotoxicity by distributing the nucleotide excision repair pathway in ovarian cancer cell lines. *Cancer Res.* **63,** 1311–1316.

80. McHugh, P. J., Spanswick, V. J., and Hartley, J. A. (2001) Repair of DNA interstrand crosslinks: molecular mechanism and clinical relevance. *Lancet Oncol.* **2**, 483–490.
81. Panasci, L., Xu, Z. Y., Bello, V., and Aloyz, R. (2002) The role of DNA repair in nitrogen mustard drug resistance. *Anticancer Drugs* **13**, 211–220.
82. Chen, Z. P., Malapetsa, A., Monks, A., et al. (2002) Nucleotide excision repair protein levels vis-à-vis anticancer drug resistance in 60 human tumor cell lines. *Ai Zheng* **21**, 233–239.
83. Kelley, M. R., Kow, Y. W., and Wilson, D. M. (2003) Disparity between DNA base excision repair in yeast and mammals: translational implications. *Cancer Res.* **63**, 549–554.
84. Silber, J. R., Bobola, M. S., Blank, A., et al. (2002) The apurinic/apyrimidinic endonuclease activity of Ape1/Ref contributes to human glioma cell resistance to alkylating agents and is elevated by oxidative stress. *Clin. Cancer Res.* **8**, 3008–3018.
85. Fishel, R. and Kolodner, R. D. (1995) Identification of mismatch repair genes and their role in the development of cancer. *Curr. Opin. Gent. Dev.* **5**, 382–395.
86. Manic, S., Gatti L., Carenini, N., Fumagalli, G., Zunino, F., and Perego, P. (2003) Mechanisms controllino sensitività to platinum complexes: role of p53 and DNA mismatch repair. *Curr. Cancer Drug Targets* **3**, 21–29.
87. Aebi, S., Kurdi-Haidar, B., Gordon, R., et al. (1996) Loss of DNA mismatch repair in acquired resistance to cisplatin. *Cancer Res.* **56**, 3087–3090.
88. Anthoney, D. A., Mcilwrath, A. J., Gallagher, W. M., Edlin, A. R., and Brown, R. (1996) Microsatellite instability, apoptosis, and loss of p53 function in drug-resistant tumor cells. *Cancer Res.* **56**, 1374–1381.
89. Arnauld, S., Hennebelle, I., Canal, P., Bugat, R., and Guichard, S. (2003) Cellular determinants of oxaliplatin sensitivity in colon cancer cell lines. *Eur. J. Cancer* **39**, 112–119.
90. Hickman, M. J. and Samson, L. D. (1999) Role of DNA mismatch repair and p53 in signalling induction of apoptosis by alkylating agents. *Proc. Natl. Acad. Sci. USA* **96**, 10,764–10,769.
91. Middleton, M. R. and Margison, G. P. (2003) Improvement of chemotherapy efficacy by inactivation of a DNA-repair pathway. *Lancet* **4**, 37–44.
92. Okamoto, R., Takano, H., and Okamura, T. (2002) O(6)-methylguanine-DNA methyltransferase (MGMT) as a determinant of resistance to camptothecin derivatives. *Jpn. J. Cancer Res.* **93**, 93–102.
93. Goodman, M. F. (2002) Error-prone repair DNA polymerases in prokaryotes and eukaryotes. *Annu. Rev. Biochem.* **71**, 17–50.
94. Sampath, D. and Plunkett, W. (2001) Design of new anticancer therapies targeting cell cycle checkpoint pathways. *Curr. Opin. Oncol.* **13**, 484–490.
95. Hartwell, L. H. and Weinert, T. A. (1989) Checkpoints: controls that ensure the order of cell cycle events. *Science* **46**, 629–634.
96. Wang, H., Liu, D., Wang, Y., Qin, J., and Elledge, S. J. (2001) Pds1 phosphorylation in response to DNA damage is essential for its DNA damage checkpoint function. *Genes Dev.* **15**, 1361–1372.

97. Feeney, G. P., Errington, R. J., Wiltshire, M., Marquez, N., Chappell, S. C., and Smith, P. J. (2003) Tracking the cell cycle origins for escape from topotecan action by breast cancer cells. *Br. J. Cancer* **88,** 1310–1317.
98. Shah, M. A. and Schwartz, G. K. (2001) Cell cycle-mediated drug resistance: an emerging concept in cancer therapy. *Clin. Cancer Res.* **7,** 2168–2181.
99. Motwani, M., Delohery, T. M., and Schwartz, G. K. (1999) Sequential dependent enhancement of caspase activation and apoptosis by flavopiridol on paclitaxel-treated human gastric and breast cancer cells. *Clin. Cancer Res.* **5,** 1876–1883.
100. Kaubisch, A., Kelsen, D. P., Saltz, L., et al. (1999) A phase I trial of weekly sequential bryostatin (Bryo) and paclitaxel in patients with advanced solid tumors. *Proc. Am. Soc. Clin. Oncol.* **18,** 166a.
101. Reed, J. C. (1999) Dysregulation of apoptosis in cancer. *J. Clin. Oncol.* **17,** 2941–2953.
102. Zunino, F., Perego, P., Pilotti, S., Pratesi, G., Supino, R., and Arcamone, F. (1997) Role of apoptotic response in cellular resistance to cytotoxic agents. *Pharmacol. Ther.* **76,** 177–185.
103. Makin, G. and Dive, C. (2001) Modulating sensitivity to drug-induced apoptosis: the future for chemotherapy? *Breast Cancer Res.* **3,** 150–153.
104. Enari, M., Sakahira, H., Yokoyama, H., Okawa, K., Iwamatsu, A., and Nagata, H. (1998) A caspase-actived DNase that degrades DNA during apoptosis, and its inhibitor ICAD. *Nature* **391,** 43–50.
105. Mow, B. M. F., Blajeski, A. L., Chandra, J., and Kaufmann, S. H. (2001) Apoptosis and the response to anticancer therapy. *Curr. Opin. Oncol.* **13,** 453–462.
106. Siegel, R. M., Martin, D. A., Zheng, L., et al. (1998) Death-effector filaments: novel cytoplasmic structures that recruit caspases and trigger apoptosis. *J. Cell Biol.* **141,** 1243–1253.
107. van Loo, G., Saelens, X., van Gurp, M., MacFarlane, M., Martin, S. J., and Vandenabeele, P. (2002) The role of mitochondrial factors in apoptosis: a Russian roulette with more than one bullet. *Cell Death Diff.* **9,** 1031–1042.
108. Green, D. R. and Reed, J. C. (1998) Mitochondria and apoptosis. *Science* **281,** 1309–1312.
109. Kroemer, G. and Reed, J. C. (2000) Mitochondrial control of cell death. *Nat. Med.* **6,** 513–519.
110. Green, D. R. (2000) Apoptotic pathways: paper wraps stone blunts scissors. *Cell* **102,** 1–4.
111. Kaufmann, S. H. and Earnshaw, W. C. (2000) Induction of apoptosis by cancer chemotherapy. *Exp. Cell Res.* **256,** 42–49.
112. Lowe, S. W. and Lin, A. W. (2000) Apoptosis in cancer. *Carcinogenesis* **21,** 485–495.
113. Weber, J. D. and Zambetti, G. P. (2003) Renewing the debate over the p53 apoptotic response. *Cell Death Differ.* **10,** 409–412.
114. Wallace-Brodeur, R. R. and Lowe, S. W. (1999) Clinical implications of p53 mutations. *Cell. Mol. Life Sci.* **55,** 64–75.

115. Herr, I. and Debatin, K. M. (2001) Cellular stress response and apoptosis in cancer therapy. *Blood* **98,** 2603–2614.
116. Bunz, F., Hwang, P. M., Torrance, C., et al. (1999) Disruption of p53 in human cancer cells alters the responses to therapeutic agents. *J. Clin. Invest.* **104,** 263–269.
117. Wei, M. C., Zong, W. X., Cheng, E. H., et al. (2001) Proapoptotic BAX and BAK: a requisite gateway to mitochondrial dysfunction and death. *Science* **292,** 727–730.
118. Zhang, L., Yu, J., Park, B. H., Kinzler, K. W., and Vogelstein, B. (2000) Role of BAX in the apoptotic response to anticancer agents. *Science* **290,** 989–992.
119. Creagh, E. M., Sheehan, D., and Cotter, T. G. (2000) Heat shock proteins—modulators of apoptosis in tumour cells. *Leukemia* **14,** 1161–1173.
120. Deveraux, Q. L. and Reed, J. C. (1999) IAP family proteins—suppressors of apoptosis. *Genes Dev.* **13,** 239–252.
121. Soengas, M. S., Capodieci, P., Polsky, D., et al. (2001) Inactivation of the apoptosis effector Apaf-1 in malignant melanoma. *Nature* **409,** 207–211.
122. Fulda, S., Meyer, E., Friesen, C., Susin, S. A., Kroemer, G., and Debatin, K. M. (2001) Cell type specific involvement of death receptor and mitochondrial pathways in drug-induced apoptosis. *Oncogene* **20,** 1063–1075.
123. Baldwin, A. S. (2001) Control of oncogenesis and cancer therapy resistance by the transcription factor NF-kB. *J. Clin. Invest.* **107,** 241–246.
124. Brown, J. M. and Wouters, B. G. (1999) Apoptosis, p53, and tumour cell sensitivity to anticancer agents. *Cancer Res.* **59,** 1391–1399.x

# 11

## Flow Cytometric Monitoring of Fluorescent Drug Retention and Efflux

### Awtar Krishan and Ronald M. Hamelik

### Summary

Laser flow cytometry has been used for monitoring cellular retention of fluorescent drugs such as fluorescent anticancer antibiotics (e.g., doxorubicin) and fluorochromes used for the detection of cellular drug efflux and resistance (e.g., rhodamine 123, Hoechst 33342). Multiparametric flow cytometry can be used for identification of tumor cell subpopulations based on their drug retention profiles with or without the presence of an efflux blocker. This rapid procedure can be used for identification of tumor cells with the drug-resistance phenotype based on drug efflux as well as for efflux blockers that may block efflux of a chemotherapeutic agent and thus increase cellular retention and sensitivity. It has been reported recently that some of the bone marrow stem cells (SP cells) efflux the Hoechst 33342 fluorochrome and thus can be rapidly identified by comparing red vs blue fluorescence in the presence or absence of an efflux blocker such as verapamil. The present chapter discusses some of the flow cytometric methods used for the study of cellular drug retention and the artifacts that may arise in such analysis.

### Key Words

Drug efflux; drug fluorescence; drug resistance; drug retention; drug transport; flow cytometry; multiple drug resistance (MDR).

### 1. Introduction

Flow cytometric monitoring of drug retention and efflux is a useful technique for the study of drug resistance. Most published work has focused on laser excitation of cellular fluorescent drug content and its modulation by efflux blockers. In multiparametric flow analysis, data on drug fluorescence can be correlated with other parameters such as cell size or expression of different cellular markers. Two major uses of this methodology have been for identification of agents that block drug efflux and increase intracellular drug retention and for the rapid identification of cells that have drug efflux as a phenotypic characteristic. A

From: *Methods in Molecular Medicine, vol. 111: Chemosensitivity:*
*Vol. 2: In Vivo Models, Imaging, and Molecular Regulators*
Edited by: R. D. Blumenthal © Humana Press Inc., Totowa, NJ

more recent and important use of flow cytometry has been for the rapid identification of a subset of stem cells (SP) characterized by reduced retention and efflux of Hoechst 33342 fluorochrome *(1,2)*.

Drug resistance due to reduced drug influx and/or enhanced efflux may be a major cause for failure of chemotherapy in refractory cancer patients. Starting with the pioneering work of Ling, Biedler, Dano, Kessel, and their colleagues *(3–6)* on cell lines made resistant in vitro by exposure to increasing concentrations of colchicine, actinomycin-D, or adriamycin, multiple drug resistance (MDR) was identified as a major target for clinical protocols seeking to overcome the efflux pump and enhance drug retention and sensitivity. The genetic basis and the proteins responsible for drug efflux have been identified *(7)*, and several protocols and drugs were tested to overcome the efflux pump *(8)*. One of the major lessons learned during the previous decade is that drug resistance is multifactorial and the drug-resistant cells use a variety of protective mechanisms to reduce cellular damage.

Several proteins that have the unique ability to act as efflux pumps have been identified. Most of the earlier work focused on MDR gene that codes for the cell membrane-resident P-glycoprotein (P-gp). Subsequent studies have identified two other proteins, MRP and LRP, that reduce cellular drug retention and chemosensitivity *(9,10)*. With the availability of antibodies against the P-glycoproteins, immunocytochemistry was the primary tool for monitoring the expression of these proteins. Subsequently, laser flow cytometry was used to study transport and subcellular distribution of fluorescent drugs *(11,12)*. Because cellular retention and distribution is related to cytotoxicity, these "functional studies" have the potential to supplement the immunocytochemical data and report on the functional activity of the efflux proteins *(13–15)*.

To quantitate markers and mechanisms involved in cellular resistance requires knowledge about a variety of sophisticated laboratory techniques involving immunocytochemistry, flow cytometry, and molecular biology. Unlike immunocytochemistry where one can identify cells with positive or negative P-glycoprotein expression, laser flow cytometry can rapidly determine cellular fluorescent drug retention in the presence or absence of an efflux blocker. However, in spite of its sensitivity, convenience, and rapidity, the use of flow cytometry for functional analysis of drug retention and the effect of efflux blockers can be fraught with the danger that artifacts may lead to erroneous conclusions. We have used a panel of well-characterized cell lines, fluorochromes, and efflux blockers to identify some of the problems in the use of flow cytometry for drug resistance-related marker expression and functional assays *(11–16)*.

Laser flow cytometry can be used for the monitoring of the following parameters related to drug transport and resistance: (1) cellular transport of fluorescent drugs (e.g., anthracyclins, rhodamine 123, Indo-1 AM, Calcein, Hoechst

33342); (2) effect of drugs that either increase drug influx (e.g., amphotericin B) or enhance drug retention by blocking efflux (e.g., verapamil, phenothiazines, cyclosporins, tamoxifen); (3) effect of efflux blocker combinations on drug retention; (4) heterogeneity in drug retention and response to efflux blockers of subpopulations in a tumor; (5) selection of effective efflux blockers and protocols for possible clinical use; (6) rapid identification and sorting of cells (e.g., SP cells) that have efflux as a major phenotypic marker.

## 2. Materials

### 2.1. Indicator Cell Lines

In performing flow cytometric studies on drug transport and efflux, it is important that the procedures used for specimen preparation and analysis are proper to yield the expected results. This makes the use of well-known human or rodent indicator cell lines as controls and calibrators important. Several paired human and mouse parental (drug-sensitive and -resistant) cell lines are available for this purpose. We have used the mouse leukemic P388 cell line and it's cloned adriamycin-resistant P388/R84 cell line for most of our work *(16)*. Another adriamycin (doxorubicin)-resistant cell line, P388/ADR, is widely available from various sources *(6,17)*. These lines are easy to maintain as suspension cultures or in vivo as ascites and have relatively short doubling times (16–18 h). The P388/R84 cell line has multifactorial drug resistance involving drug efflux, detoxification mechanism, and DNA damage/repair *(16)*. It also has relatively stable drug resistance and does not need frequent doxorubicin exposure to maintain the resistant phenotype. Several other well-characterized paired human cell lines useful for the study of drug retention and efflux include human lymphoid cell line, CCRF-CEM, and its vinblastine-resistant subline, CCRF-CEM$_{VLB100}$, developed and studied extensively by Beck and his colleagues *(18)*. Though the parental CCRF-CEM cell line was originally diploid, several tetraploid drug-resistant CCRF-CEM cell lines are available and are easy to maintain in suspension cultures. The human colon carcinoma cell lines, SW620 and its adriamycin-resistant subline, SW620/AD300, are also good paired cell lines to maintain in the lab *(19)*. In the resistant cell line, drug efflux is possibly the major and only mechanism responsible for resistance. The SW620 cell lines grow as monolayers, double in 24 h, and can also be grown as xenografts in athymic mice. However, most of these resistant cell lines need to be continuously grown or frequently rechallenged with drugs to maintain their efflux mechanism.

### 2.2. Fluorochromes

For flow cytometric studies on drug retention and efflux, the dyes chosen must be excitable by a high-pressure mercury arc lamp or emission from a specific laser line. The most commonly used fluorochromes for drug transport studies are doxorubicin (Adriamycin, NSC-123127, Adria Labs, Columbus, OH), daunorubicin, NSC-821151, Calbiochem, San Diego, CA), and rhodamine 123 (Calbiochem). These fluorochromes can be excited from the 488-nm argon laser line. The Hoechst 33342 (Calbiochem) dye is excitable with the mercury arc lamp or the UV laser lines from an argon laser. Bodipy-verapamil (Molecular Probes, Eugene, OR) and the calcium indicator dye Indo-1 AM (Molecular Probes) are two other fluorochromes used for the study of drug transport.

Much of the early drug efflux functional assays relied on the use of important chemotherapeutic antibiotics, Doxorubicin or daunorubicin, for the measurement of drug retention. Daunorubicin is lipophilic and rapidly transported into cells in 15–30 min. The uptake of doxorubicin is much slower and takes 2–3 h to reach maximum. These antibiotics are excited by the standard 488-nm argon laser line and quench their fluorescence on binding to DNA *(11)*. Rhodamine 123 is rapidly transported and its fluorescence, mostly located in the mitochondria, is much brighter than that of daunorubicin or doxorubicin *(21)* (*see* **Note 1**). We have earlier compared the use of two new fluorochromes, SY-38 and SY-3150 *(20)* for monitoring of drug efflux. Different fluorochromes used for transport studies differ in their chemical binding characteristics as well as transport and retention properties. We *(20)* have reported that cellular drug retention data cannot be extrapolated between different fluorochromes, and tumor cells should be tested for their transport characteristics and sensitivity to efflux blockers with drug that will be used for treatment of the patient *(15)*.

The histograms in **Fig. 1** are of normal human peripheral blood lymphocytes, isolated on a Ficoll-Hypaque gradient, incubated with four different fluorochromes: daunorubicin (DNR), rhodamine 123 (RH-123), SY-38 (SY38), and SY-3150 (SY3150). Cells incubated with DNR **(Fig. 1A)** show a single predominant population, while cells incubated with RH-123 **(Fig. 1B)** show a distinct second population (arrow). Similarly, cells incubated with SY38 also showed a second distinct population (arrow). Cells incubated with SY3150 **(Fig. 1D)** did not show any distinct extra populations like those seen in **Fig. 1B** and **Fig. 1C**. The conclusion to be drawn is that the degree of heterogeneity seen depends on the fluorochrome used. In this example, daunorubicin, rhodamine 123, and SY-3150 are not as good as SY-38 for measuring drug transport and efflux.

Other fluorochromes that can be used for study of drug transport are discussed in the Molecular Probes Handbook of Fluorescent Probes and Research Chemicals section on Probes for Cell Adhesion, Chemotaxis, Multidrug Resistance and Glutathione, which the reader may find at www.probes.com/handbook/sections/1506.html.

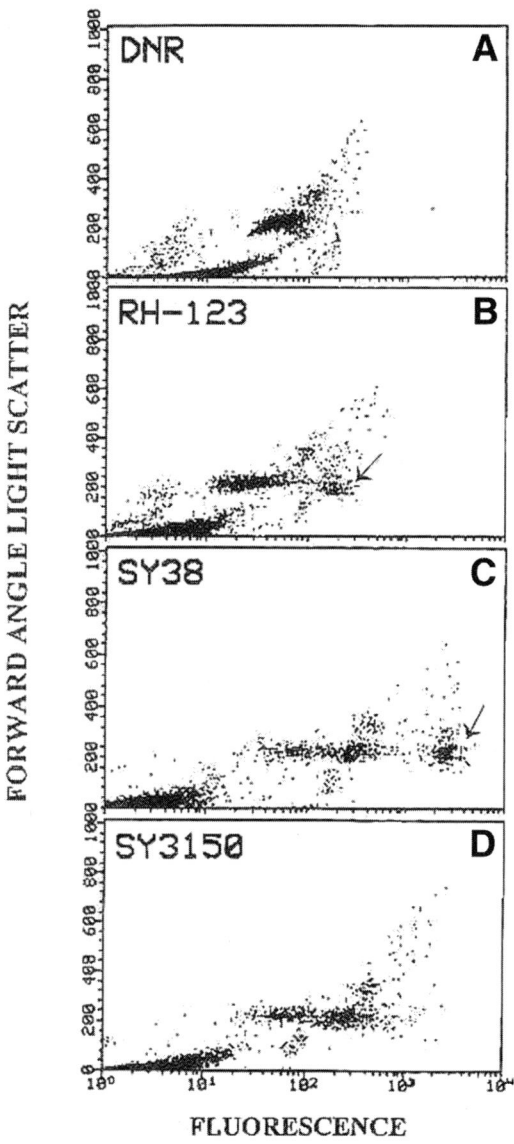

Fig. 1. Dot plots of forward scatter vs drug fluorescence of human peripheral blood lymphocytes incubated with four different fluorochromes (**A–D**). The difference in heterogeneity displayed shows the importance of choosing the best fluorochrome for the cells being studied. (Adapted from **ref. 20**.)

## 2.3. Drug Efflux Blockers

Several well-known drugs with a wide variety of clinical uses have been shown to modulate drug retention. Well-known efflux blockers include calcium channel blockers (e.g., verapamil), immunosuppressive drugs (e.g., cyclosporins), platelet-active agents (e.g., dipyridamole), psychosomatic drugs (e.g., phenothiazines), antimalarials (e.g., quinine), and antiestrogens (e.g., tamoxifen) *(22–24)*. Stein et al. *(25)* have shown that a combination of efflux blockers may have synergistic effect on blocking the pump mechanism (*see* **Note 2**).

## 3. Methods

Protocols for monitoring of drug retention and efflux need to have a control sample, preferably paired cell lines of drug-sensitive and -resistant phenotype; a fluorochrome of interest; a known efflux blocker that will enhance retention of the fluorochrome; and a data acquisition protocol for the flow cytometer.

### 3.1. Control Cell Lines

For calibration and controls, we routinely use log-phase suspension cultures of doxorubicin-resistant P388/R84 cells *(16)*, grown in RPMI 1640 medium supplemented with 10% heat-inactivated fetal bovine serum (FBS), penicillin, and streptomycin. The ID50 for the parental P388 and P388/R84 cells in soft agar assays are 0.0875 and 8.4 µ$M$ of doxorubicin, respectively. Cells ($10^6$/mL) are incubated with doxorubicin (1 µ$M$, 1 h), daunorubicin (0.1 µ$M$, 30 min), or rhodamine 123 (0.1 µ$M$, 15 min) at 37°C. A second aliquot of cells is incubated with the fluorochrome and efflux blocker (verapamil, 10 µ$M$), prochlorperazine (15 µ$M$), or dipyridamole (10 µ$M$). Cells incubated in the presence of the efflux blocker are analyzed for their fluorescence and the laser power and gain/amplification adjusted to record the peak of fluorescence distribution in the second log of a four-log histogram. In resistant cells incubated without the efflux blocker, there is approx one log less fluorescence. Once the laser power, photomultiplier high voltage, and other gains have been optimized (using the resistant cells with and without the efflux blocker), the settings are not changed for running the experimental samples.

#### 3.1.1. Experimental Sample

Cells are recovered by centrifugation of human body fluids (pleural fluid, bone marrow, peripheral blood, ascites fluid) or of solid tumor homogenates dissociated by enzymatic or mechanical means. The supernatant fluid is aspirated and the cell pellet is resuspended and washed in $Ca^{2+}$- and $Mg^{2+}$-free phosphate-buffered saline (PBS). After centrifugation, the pelleted cells are resuspended in fresh tissue culture medium supplemented with 10% heat-inactivated FBS and filtered through a 40-µ$M$ nylon mesh.

*Drug Transport and Efflux* 155

Bone marrow aspirates, peripheral blood, and some body fluid samples may contain large numbers of red blood cells, which need to be removed. These cell pellets are diluted with $Ca^{2+}$- and $Mg^{2+}$-free PBS, layered over Ficoll-Hypaque (Pharmacia Biotech, Uppsala, Sweden) and centrifuged. The mononuclear cell layer is carefully aspirated, washed with $Ca^{2+}$- and $Mg^{2+}$-free PBS, and resuspended in fresh tissue culture medium supplemented with 10% heat-inactivated FBS.

### 3.2. Fluorochromes

Stock solutions of doxorubicin, daunorubicin, or rhodamine 123 are prepared in $Ca^{2+}$- and $Mg^{2+}$-free Hanks' balanced salt solution (HBSS), and fresh working solutions are prepared before each experiment. The final drug concentrations normally used is 1–3 $\mu M$ doxorubicin or daunorubicin or 0.1 $\mu M$ rhodamine 123, and cells may be incubated for 15–60 min at 37°C before flow analysis (*see* **Note 3**).

### 3.3. Efflux Blockers

The blockers we normally use are prochlorperazine, verapamil, or dipyridamole. The stock solutions are prepared in $Ca^{2+}$- and $Mg^{2+}$-free HBSS, and fresh working solutions are prepared before each experiment (*see* **Note 3**). For efflux-blocking experiments, cells incubated with a fluorochrome are incubated with and without the addition of prochlorperazine (20 $\mu M$), verapamil (10 $\mu M$), or dipyridamole (15 $\mu M$) (*see* **Note 4**).

#### 3.3.1. Data Acquisition Protocols

Although our published work on drug retention and efflux has been carried out on a Beckman Coulter XL (Beckman Coulter, Miami, FL) or a Becton Dickinson FACScan (San Jose, CA) equipped with an argon-ion laser, most of the currently available flow cytometers including those with high-pressure mercury illumination have enough excitation power for performing the drug uptake and efflux experiments (*see* **Note 5**). In most studies, forward angle (FS), 90° light scatter (SS), and fluorescence >530 nm (FL1) are measured and the same flow cytometer data acquisition protocol can be used for measuring drug uptake/efflux, efflux blocking, and the separation of live/dead cells with propidium iodide (PI). The flow cytometer desktop is arranged to collect three sets of histograms/scatter plots:

1. A two-parameter FS Y-axis vs SS X-axis histogram for setting the FS gain and visualizing live/dead/debris. Set the gain so that the populations are about midscale and high enough to visually separate cells from debris.

2. A one-parameter log FL1 histogram with the high voltage (HV) set to record fluorescence of the resistant cells incubated with the fluorochrome and the efflux blocker in the second log of a four-log-scale X axis.
3. A two-parameter FS Y-axis vs FL1 X-axis histogram for visualizing drug-sensitive/resistant cells, the effect of blocked/nonblocked cells, or live/dead shift with PI.

Minimums of 10,000 cells are usually analyzed to generate list-mode data files (*see* **Note 6**). In kinetic studies of drug uptake, "time" is used as a parameter along with drug fluorescence. The data acquisition software on most of the commercial flow cytometers has "time" as a parameter. The data acquisition protocol for kinetic drug uptake studies has an additional two-parameter histogram of FL1 Y axis vs time X axis. As time is used as the stopping parameter for data acquisition, more than 10,000 cells may be analyzed in a typical kinetic study, depending on the event rate and cell concentration.

*3.3.2. Types of Assays*

1. For drug uptake/efflux studies, cells are incubated with the fluorochrome with or without the efflux blocker for a given length of time and then analyzed on the flow cytometer. The appearance of subpopulations, which increase their fluorochrome retention in the presence of the efflux blockers, suggests the presence of an active drug efflux pump.

    The multiparameter histograms in **Fig. 2** are of P388 doxorubicin-sensitive (**2A**) and -resistant (**2C**) cells, respectively, incubated for 30 min with 2 µmol of daunorubicin. **Figures 2B** and **2D** are with daunorubicin and 10 µmol of verapamil. The drug fluorescence (X axis) in log scale shows that the resistant cells (**2C**) have a four- to sixfold reduced drug retention vs the drug-sensitive cells. That this reduced retention is due to rapid drug efflux is shown by comparison of **Fig. 2C** and **2D**, where verapamil has blocked the drug efflux pump in the resistant cells, resulting in similar drug retention of the sensitive and the resistant cells.

2. For drug-uptake kinetic studies, the fluorochrome and either PBS or the efflux blocker is added to the cells at time zero ($T_0$) and data acquisition started. The shift in fluorescence intensity vs time is a measure of drug retention, which in resistant cells incubated in the presence of the efflux blockers is significantly enhanced. For these studies it is suggested that the event rate of approx 100 events/s be maintained. As drug uptake is influenced by temperature, it is important to keep the sample tube at 37°C during the entire data acquisition run. This can be achieved by use of a temperature-controlled heated air curtain. Scale the time X axis to suit the known drug uptake characteristics of the fluorochrome. For example, rhodamine 123 and daunorubicin can be studied using a 600-s (10 min) scale, whereas doxorubicin needs 30–60 min to study its transport.

    The contour plots in **Fig. 3** show log fluorescence vs time of P388/R84 cells incubated for 10 min with rhodamine 123 with or without verapamil (top plot). In less than a minute, the drug efflux pump was blocked; and after 10 min of incu-

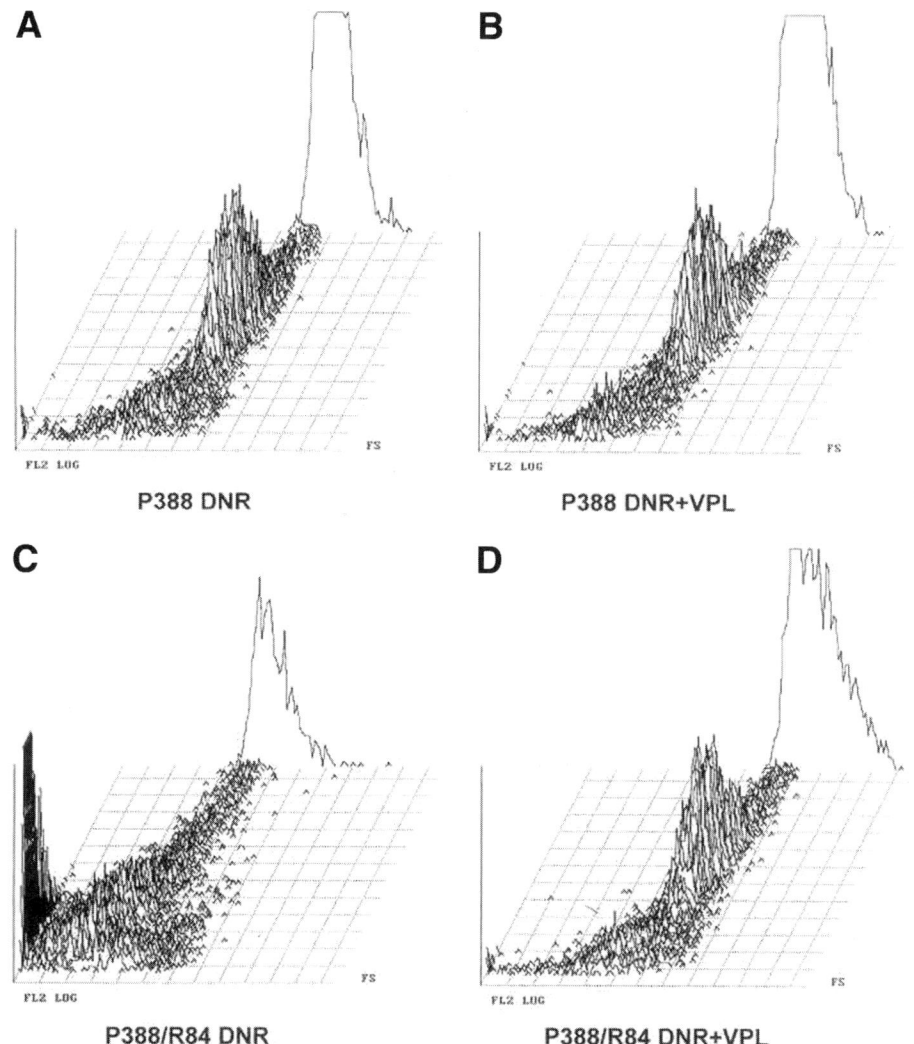

Fig. 2. Uptake and rentention of Daunorubicin in P388 parental drug-sensitive and P388/R84 drug-resistant cells. In P388 cells (**A,B**) and in P388/R84 cells incubated with the efflux blocker verapamil (**D**) a prominent population with high drug retention is seen. In P388/R84 cells incubated with daunorubicin alone, retention is low due to drug efflux (**C**). Adapted from **ref. *30***.

bation, these cells had approximately log higher fluorescence intensity than the control cells.
3. For identification of dead or membrane-permeable cells, it is essential to discriminate between the high fluorescence of these cells and that of the cells that

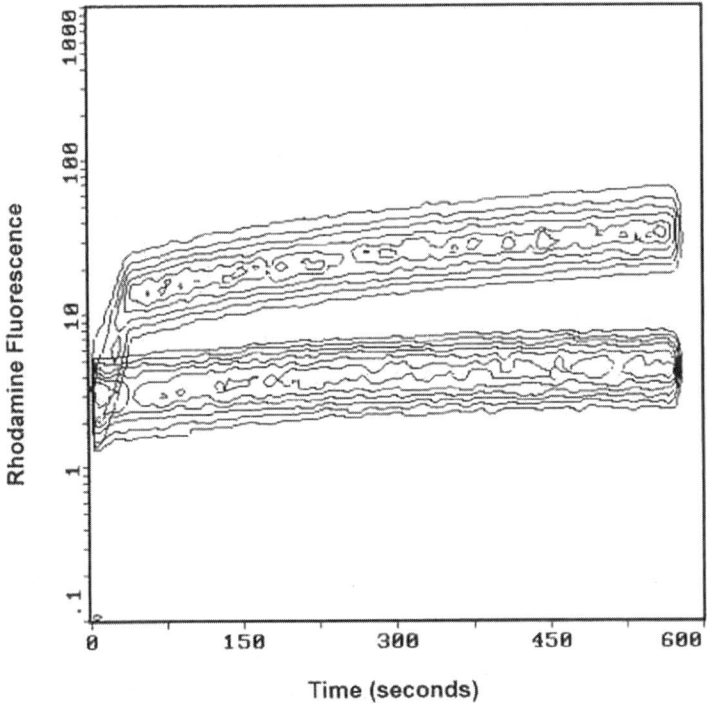

Fig. 3. Time vs fluorescence of rhodamine 123 in P388/R84 cells incubated with drug alone (lower contour plot) or in the presence of the efflux blocker verapamil (upper contour plot). (Adapted from **ref. 30**.)

lack the drug efflux pump. We have described the inclusion of isotonic propidium iodide for staining of dead or membrane-damaged cells in drug kinetic and efflux studies *(20)*. We recommend addition of 25 µg/mL of propidium iodide dissolved in isotonic phosphate buffered saline for this purpose. **Figures 4A** and **4E** are dot plots of murine leukemic P388 and drug-resistant P388/R84 cells incubated with daunorubicin. Based on the forward scatter-vs-log fluorescence dot plots **(Fig. 4E)**, the P388/R84 culture had at least five distinct subpopulations. The single-parameter histograms of drug fluorescence **(Figs. 4B** and **4F)**, do not demonstrate heterogeneity present in the sample. To discriminate among the cells with low drug retention (resistant cells), cells with high retention (sensitive cells), and cells with damaged cell membranes (which cannot efflux the drug), isotonic propidium iodide was added to the cultures to label the membrane permeable cells. The dot plot **(Fig. 4C)** and single-parameter histogram **(Fig. 4D)** show how the procedure can enhance the separation of the subpopulations by dramatically increasing the fluorescence of the membrane-permeable cells. This separation is even more pronounced in the P388/R84 cells, as the live resistant cells efflux the fluorochrome while the membrane-permeable cells **(Figs. 4G** and **4H)** stain brightly with PI

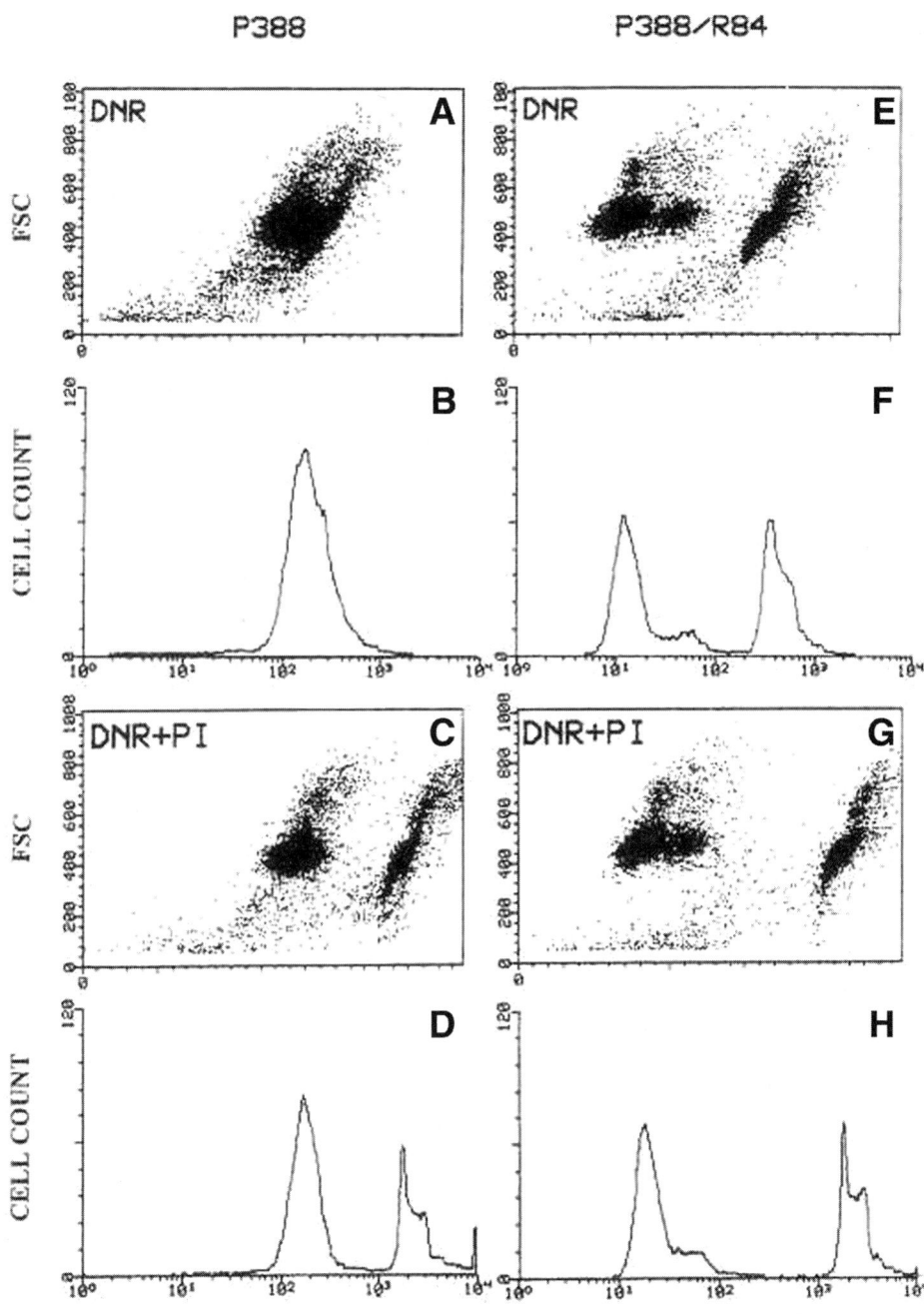

Fig. 4. Use of isotonic propidium iodide for identification of cells with permeable cell membranes or dead cells. (Adapted from **ref. 20**.)

and stand out as distinct populations. This experiment shows that by using PI, one can distinguish between the real heterogeneity of drug retention in a tumor specimen and the artifacts created by the presence of dead, dying, and necrotic cells with leaky dye-permeable membranes.

Drug efflux and sensitivity to efflux blockers is not limited to drug-resistant tumor cells, as P-glycoprotein expression and drug efflux has been reported in a variety of normal cells such as capillary endothelial cells of the brain and testes, adrenal, liver, and CD34-positive bone marrow stem cells. Although once reported to have no P-gp mRNA expression, a significant percentage of normal human peripheral lymphocytes have P-gp expression and efflux that can be blocked. The histograms in **Fig. 5** are of normal human peripheral blood lymphocytes, isolated on a Ficoll-Hypaque gradient, incubated with the fluorochrome SY-38 and the efflux blockers verapamil (Vpl) or dipyridamole (Dpd). **Figure 5A** is a forward-scatter-vs-side-scatter dot plot of these isolated mononuclear cells. The R1 gate identifies small lymphocytes. The forward-scatter-vs-log fluorescence of all the mononuclear cells after incubation with SY-38 is shown in **Fig. 5B** and in the presence of SY-38 and verapamil in **Fig. 5C**. In comparing these two images, it appears that cells in **Fig. 5B** (arrows) have increased their drug retention in the presence of verapamil (**Fig. 5C**). **Figures 5D** and **5E** show the data using the R1 gate region for small lymphocytes, after incubation with SY-38 alone (**Fig. 5D**) or in the presence of verapamil (**Fig. 5E**). This data shows that cells in the R1 gate, which had low SY-38 retention, were sensitive to the efflux blocking action of verapamil or other efflux blockers (dipyridamole, data not shown).

**Figure 6** illustrates daunorubicin retention in tumor cells from pleural effusion of a lung cancer patient after incubation with and without the efflux blockers chlorpromazine (CpZ) or verapamil (VpL). **Figure 6A** shows heterogeneity of daunorubicin retention. **Figure 6B** shows that chloropromazine blocked the efflux pumps, producing a single fluorescence peak, while verapamil did not (**Fig. 6C**). Histograms **6G–I** shows similar analysis of cells retrieved from the patient after 1 mo of therapy *(15)*.

4. For flow cytometric identification of SP stem cells in bone marrow, Goodell et al. *(1)* reported that in murine bone marrow cells incubated with Hoechst 33342 for red vs blue emission, a small subpopulation of cells (SP cells) with reduced drug fluorescence could be recognized. These SP cells appear to have active drug efflux that was blocked by incubation with verapamil, resulting in increased fluorescence. The Hoechst staining method based on drug efflux and blocking is described as a simple, easy, and reproducible way for identification of hematopoietic stem cells. In subsequent dual-wavelength analysis of Hoechst dye-stained human, rhesus and miniature swine bone marrow cells, SP-like cells, were identified as a distinct population of cells that efflux the dye in a manner identical to that of the murine SP cells. Like the murine SP cells, both human and rhesus SP cells are primarily CD34-negative and lineage marker-negative. The rhesus SP population contains a large number of long-term culture-initiating cells (LTC-ICs), thus suggesting that they are primitive hematopoietic cells capable of

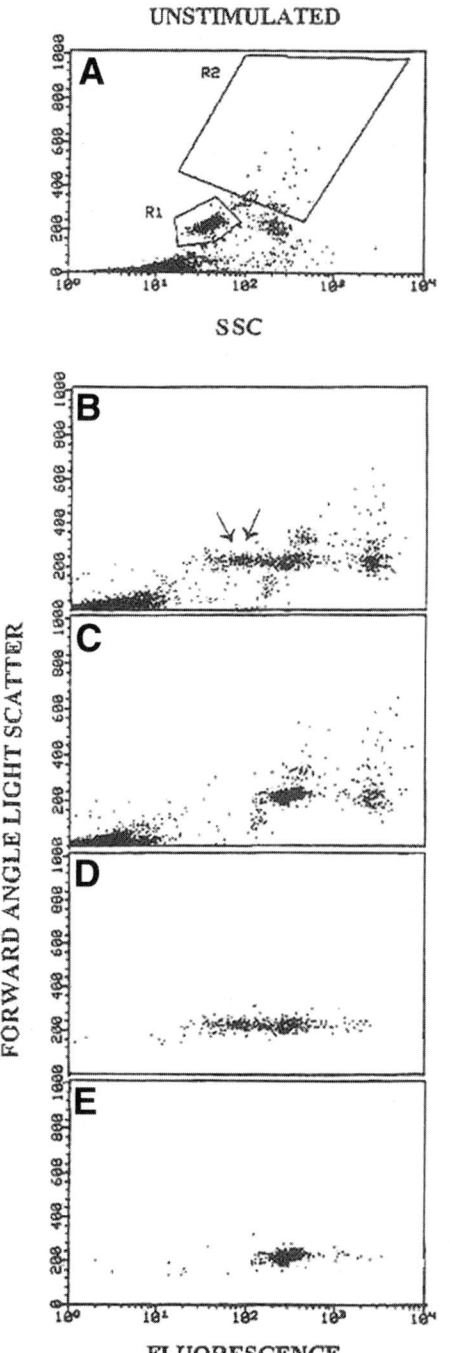

Fig. 5. Dot plots of unstimulated peripheral blood lymphocytes incubated with fluorochrome SY-38. (Adapted from **ref. 20**.)

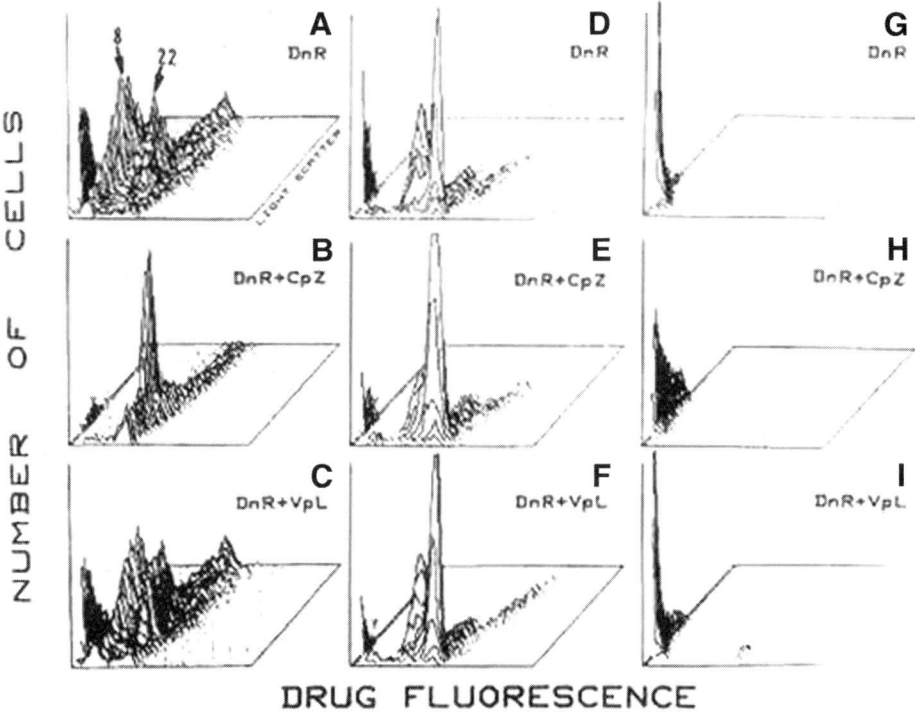

Fig. 6. Daunorubicin retention in tumor cells from the pleural fluid of a lung cancer patient. Note chlorpromazine CpZ (**B**) but not verapamil VpL (**C**) enhanced drug retention, resulting in the emergence of a single population with high drug fluorescence. In samples retrieved after 1 mo of therapy, drug retention was low (**G**), and the efflux blockers did not increase drug retention (**H,I**). (Adapted from **ref. *15*.**)

differentiation into T-cells. In subsequent studies, the Hoechst double-emission method was used to describe the presence of SP cells in a variety of human tissues, including skeletal muscle, heart, brain liver, spleen, umbilical cord, and adult blood. Kim et al. have reported studies suggesting the involvement of the ABCG2 gene of the human ATP-binding cassette superfamily in Hoechst 33342 efflux in transformed MCF cell line *(27)*.

**Figure 7** shows a red-vs-blue dot plot of Hoechst 33342 fluorescence in murine bone marrow cells analyzed on a Quanta™ Analyzer with HBO mercury light excitation (NPE Systems, Pembroke Pines, FL). The arrow in **Fig. 7A** points to the subpopulation (SP) of bone marrow cells with reduced Hoechst retention that are not seen in cells coincubated with the efflux blocker verapamil (**Fig. 7B**).

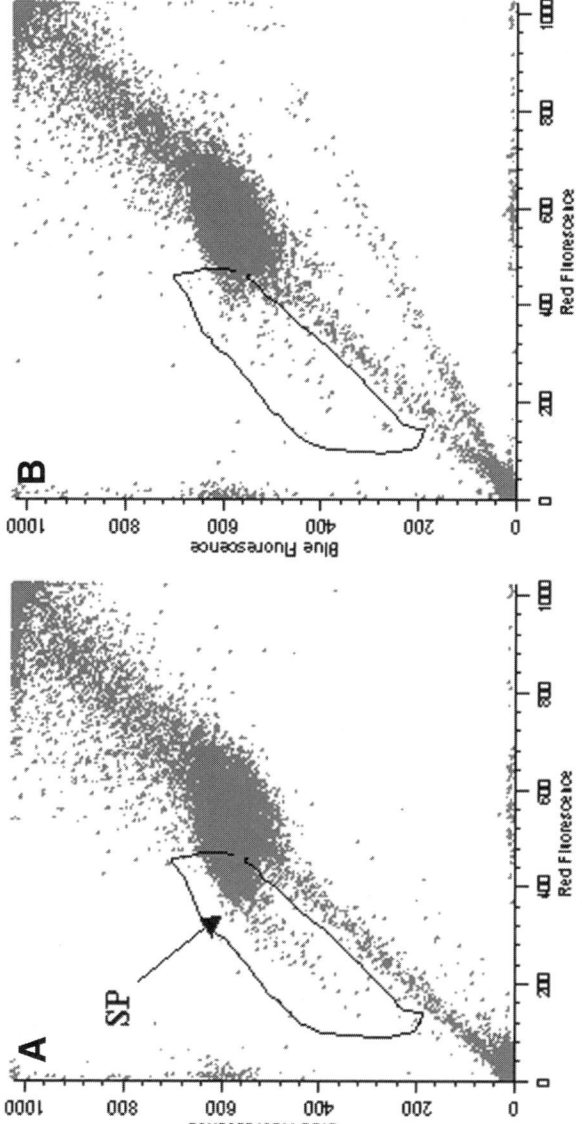

Fig. 7. Two color (red vs blue) emission dot plots of mouse bone marrow cells incubated with Hoechst 33342. In (**A**), the arrow points to the presence of SP cells with low fluorochrome retention. In the presence of the efflux blocker verapamil (**B**), drug retention in most of the SP cells is enhanced. (Data generated by Raquel Cabana on a NPE Quanta Analyzer [NPE Systems, Pembroke Pines, FL].)

## 4. Notes

1. Rhodamine 123 can exhibit a transient increase in binding to mitochondria of dead cells as well as in cells entering the cell cycle from a quiescent state, as reported by Darzynkiewicz et al. *(28)*.
2. Very high concentrations of the fluorochromes or the efflux blockers may be toxic and damage the cell membrane and the efflux pump *(26)*.
3. The pH of the incubating mixture sample is an important factor when considering drug transport and efflux studies, as the excitation maxima of a drug may be shifted or the uptake and efflux rates altered by pH changes *(29)*.
4. Since some of the efflux blockers may bind to glass and rubber or precipitate out of solution under certain experimental conditions, proper precautions should be observed to avoid this artifact.
5. In flow cytometry, one must be sure that pinholes have not developed in aging dichroic filters or that autofluorescence is not generated by high-power excitation of the bandpass filters.
6. Dual-parameter dot plots or scattergrams of forward light scatter vs drug fluorescence are better than single-parameter histograms of cellular fluorescence, because they allow for identification of dead cells and other subpopulations for gating purposes.

## References

1. Goodell, M. A., Brose, K., Paradis, G., Conner, A. S., and Mulligan, R. C. (1996) Isolation and functional properties of murine hematopoietic stem cells that are replicating in vivo. *J. Exp. Med.* **183,** 1797–1806.
2. Storms, R. W., Goodell, M. A., Fisher, A., Mulligan, R. C., and Smith, C. (2000) Hoechst dye efflux reveals a novel CD7(+)CD34(–) lymphoid progenitor in human umbilical cord blood. *Blood* **96,** 2125–2133.
3. Ling, V. (1992) P-glycoprotein and resistance to anticancer drugs. *Cancer* **69,** 2603–2609.
4. Biedler, J. L. (1994) Drug resistance: genotype versus phenotype. *Cancer Res.* **54,** 666–678.
5. Dano, K. (1973) Active outward transport of daunomycin in resistant Ehrlich ascites tumor cells. *Biochim Biophys. Acta* **323,** 466–483.
6. Kessel, D., Botterill, V., and Wodinsky, I. (1968) Uptake and retention of daunomycin by mouse leukemic cells as factors in drug response. *Cancer Res.* **28,** 938–941.
7. Gottesman, M. M. (1993) How cancer cells evade chemotherapy: Sixteenth Richard and Hinda Rosenthal Foundation Award Lecture. *Cancer Res.* **53,** 747–754.
8. Gottesman, M. M. and Pastan, I. (1989) Clinical trials of agents that reverse multidrug-resistance. *J. Clin. Oncol.* **7,** 409–411.
9. Cole, S. P., Bhardwaj, G., Gerlach, J. H., et al. (1992) Overexpression of a transporter gene in a multidrug-resistant human lung cancer cell line. *Science* **258,** 1650–1654.

10. Izquierdo, M. A., Scheffer, G. L., Flens, M. J., et al. (1996) Broad distribution of the multidrug resistance-related vault lung resistance protein in normal human tissues and tumors. *Am. J. Pathol.* **148,** 877–887.
11. Krishan, A. and Ganapathi, R. (1980) Laser flow cytometric studies on the intracellular fluorescence of anthracyclines. Cancer Res. 40, 3895–3900.
12. Durand, R. E. and Olive, P. L. (1981) Flow cytometry studies of intracellular adriamycin in single cells in vitro. *Cancer Res.* **41,** 3489–3494.
13. Krishan, A. and Bourguignon, L.Y. (1984) Cell cycle related phenothiazine effects on adriamycin transport. *Cell. Biol. Int. Rep.* **8,** 449–456.
14. Krishan, A., Sauerteig, A., and Wellham, L. L. (1985) Flow cytometric studies on modulation of cellular adriamycin retention by phenothiazines. *Cancer Res.* **45,** 1046–1051.
15. Krishan, A., Sridhar, K. S., Davila, E., Vogel, C., and Sternheim, W. (1987) Patterns of anthracycline retention modulation in human tumor cells. *Cytometry* **8,** 306–314.
16. Nair, S., Singh, S. V., Samy, T. S., and Krishan, A. (1990) Anthracycline resistance in murine leukemic P388 cells. Role of drug efflux and glutathione related enzymes. *Biochem. Pharmacol.* **39,** 723–728.
17. Inaba, M., Kobayashi, H., Sakurai, Y., and Johnson, R. K. (1979) Active efflux of daunorubicin and adriamycin in sensitive and resistant sublines of P388 leukemia. *Cancer Res.* **39,** 2200–2203.
18. Beck, W. T., Mueller, T. J., and Tanzer, L. R. (1979) Altered surface membrane glycoproteins in Vinca alkaloid-resistant human leukemic lymphoblasts. *Cancer Res.* **39,** 2070–2076.
19. Leibovitz, A., Stinson, J. C., McCombs, W. B. III, McCoy, C. E., Mazur, K. C., and Mabry, N. D. (1976) Classification of human colorectal adenocarcinoma cell lines. *Cancer Res.* **36,** 4562–4569.
20. Krishan, A., Sauerteig, A., Andritsch, I., and Wellham, L. (1997) Flow cytometric analysis of the multiple drug resistance phenotype. *Leukemia* **11,** 1138–1146.
21. Lampidis, T. J., Munck, J. N., Krishan, A., and Tapiero, H. (1985) Reversal of resistance to rhodamine 123 in adriamycin-resistant Friend leukemia cells. *Cancer Res.* **45,** 2626–2631.
22. Tsuruo, T., Iida, H., Tsukagoshi, S., and Sakurai, Y. (1981) Overcoming of vincristine resistance in P388 leukemia in vivo and in vitro through enhanced cytotoxicity of vincristine and vinblastine by verapamil. *Cancer Res.* **41,** 1967–1972.
23. Ganapathi, R., Grabowski, D., Rouse, W., and Riegler, F. (1984) Differential effect of the calmodulin inhibitor trifluoperazine on cellular accumulation, retention, and cytotoxicity of anthracyclines in doxorubicin (adriamycin)-resistant P388 mouse leukemia cells. *Cancer Res.* **44,** 5056–5061.
24. Slater, L. M., Sweet, P., Stupecky, M., Wetzel, M. W., and Gupta, S. (1986) Cyclosporin A corrects daunorubicin resistance in Ehrlich ascites carcinoma. *Br. J. Cancer* **54,** 235–238.
25. Stein, W. D. (1997) Kinetics of the multidrug transporter (P-glycoprotein) and its reversal. *Physiol. Rev.* **77,** 545–590.

26. Krishan, A., Sridhar, K. S., Mou, C., et al. (2000) Synergistic effect of prochlorperazine and dipyridamole on the cellular retention and cytotoxicity of doxorubicin. *Clin. Cancer Res.* **6,** 1508–1517.
27. Kim, M., Turnquist, H., Jackson, J., et al. (2002) The multidrug resistance transporter ABCG2 (breast cancer resistance protein 1) effluxes Hoechst 33342 and is overexpressed in hematopoietic stem cells. *Clin. Cancer Res.* **8,** 22–28.
28. Darzynkiewicz, Z., Traganos, F., Staiano-Coico, L., Kapuscinski, J., and Melamed, M. R. (1982) Interaction of rhodamine 123 with living cells studied by flow cytometry. *Cancer Res.* **42,** 799–806.
29. Alabaster, O., Woods, T., Ortiz-Sanchez, V., and Jahangeer, S. (1989) Influence of microenvironmental pH on adriamycin resistance. *Cancer Res.* **49,** 5638–5643.
30. Krishan, A. (2001) Monitoring of cellular resistance to cancer chemotherapy: drug retention and efflux, in *Methods in Cell Biology, Vol 64* (Darzynkiewicz, Z., Crissman, H. A., and Robinson, J. P., eds.), Academic, San Diego, CA, pp. 193–209.

# 12

## Flow Cytometric Measurement of Functional and Phenotypic P-Glycoprotein

### Monica Pallis and Emma Das-Gupta

#### Summary

The measurement of functional and phenotypic P-glycoprotein by flow cytometry is suitable for cells in suspension, and is particularly appropriate for blood and bone marrow cells. We describe a functional assay for P-glycoprotein using rhodamine 123, an assay for daunorubicin accumulation, and an assay to measure P-glycoprotein levels using the MRK16 antibody. Our protocols include the use of an anti-CD45 antibody for the identification of leukemic blasts. The protocols described in this chapter were designed for use in studies accompanying UK Medical Research Council Trials of patients with Acute Myeloid Leukaemia and High Risk Myelodysplastic Syndrome (>10% blasts). These assays are performed in more than one UK Centre, and hence each assay has been subjected to rigorous reproducibility testing (*1*).

#### Key Words

P-glycoprotein; rhodamine 123; MRK 16; daunorubicin; PSC 833; acute myeloid leukemia.

### 1. Introduction

P-glycoprotein is the product of the *MDR1* gene and functions as a cell membrane pump responsible for the efflux of cationic, lipophilic substances including many drugs. In acute myeloid leukemia, as in other malignancies, overexpression of P-glycoprotein has been associated with resistance to remission-induction chemotherapy (*2,3*). Our growing understanding of the role of P-glycoprotein in chemoresistance has created a demand for accurate, quantitative assays that can be used on clinical samples.

P-glycoprotein is often expressed at low levels and therefore its measurement has proved to be a considerable technical challenge. Multicenter studies have demonstrated lack of agreement between laboratories, with nonetheless a consensus opinion that flow cytometry is a promising way forward *(4,5)*. Flow cytometry has distinct advantages: the population of interest can be selected by appropriate labeling and gating even in a sample with mixed cell types. Furthermore, ratiometric or quantitative results can be generated (ratiometric being defined as the ratio of test to control fluorescence). The French Drug Resistance Intergroup network have demonstrated the impact that ratiometric analytical methods can have on the reproducibility of the result generated: they found that in the analysis of P-glycoprotein expression, assessment of the number of positive cells was subjective, because there was no logical cutoff point between positive and negative values and thus the values obtained by different researchers were far more variable than when P-glycoprotein positivity was calculated ratiometrically as mean fluorescence with P-glycoprotein antibody divided by mean fluorescence with control antibody *(6)*. An additional advantage of ratiometric measurements is that variables such as cytometer type and setup, cellular characteristics such as size and autofluorescence, batch-to-batch variations in reagents, and minor variations between assays are controlled for insofar as they affect both parts of the ratio. As well as being used for measuring proteins, ratiometric flow cytometry can be used for measuring functional multidrug resistance *(5,7)*. The functional assay system is based on the fact that organic, cationic probes (e.g., rhodamine 123), and many drugs (e.g., daunorubicin), diffuse freely across the plasma membrane into cells, but in P-glycoprotein-positive, chemoresistant cells the protein effluxes the probe, unless it is blocked by a specific inhibitor. The accumulation of high levels of probe in the presence of P-glycoprotein inhibitor compared to a low level of probe accumulation in the absence of inhibitor can be used to measure P-glycoprotein-mediated efflux in the cells of interest. A daunorubicin accumulation assay can be used to corroborate the functional P-glycoprotein assay. If a sample has high levels of functional P-glycoprotein in the rhodamine assay, that sample will accumulate only low levels of P-glycoprotein substrate drugs *(8)*. The daunorubicin accumulation assay has its technical basis on the principle that flow cytometric measurements may vary (*see* **Note 1**) and that therefore a constant, nonphysiological material, such as polymeric beads, can be used as an internal standard. Because the beads incorporate a carboxylate group, they bind to the cationic fluorescent drug daunorubicin. A ratio is constructed of cell:bead fluorescence in the presence of drug *(9)*.

Several antibodies are available for measuring P-glycoprotein levels. The MRK 16 antibody binds to an extracellular epitope of the protein and is well suited to flow cytometric applications *(6,7)*.

## 2. Materials

### 2.1. Functional Measurement of P-Glycoprotein-Mediated Rhodamine 123 Retention and Daunorubicin Accumulation

1. Rhodamine 123 (Sigma): Dissolve in water to 100 µg/mL stock solution. Dilute stock 1 in 20 in phosphate-buffered saline (PBS) to a 5-µg/mL working solution. Rhodamine 123 loses fluorescence on freeze/thawing, so keep stock and working solutions wrapped in aluminum foil, at 4°C. We have used the same stock for 2 yr.
2. Daunorubicin (Cerubidine, Rhone Polenc Rorer): Dissolve in water to 500 µg/mL (880 µ$M$) stock. Dilute 1 in 20 in PBS to a 44 µ$M$ working solution. Keep stock and working solutions wrapped in aluminum foil, at 4°C. Discard stock after 6 mo (*see* **Note 2**).
3. PSC 833 (Novartis): For stock solution, dissolve 50 mg in 10 mL ethanol (molar concentration 4.1 m$M$). Store stock at 4°C with plenty of stretch wrapping to minimize evaporation. Also to minimize evaporation, make up several aliquots of working solution A at a time (*see* **Note 3**).
4. Working solution A: mix 100 µL ice-cold stock to 300 µL cold ethanol on ice and immediately make up 20-µL aliquots in precooled lidded vials. Store until needed at 4°C.
5. Working solution B: Immediately prior to use, add 30 µL water to a vial of working solution A.
6. Solvent control for PSC 833: 40% ethanol in water.
7. Rest medium: RPMI 1640, 20% fetal calf serum (FCS), 10 m$M$ HEPES buffer, 2 m$M$ L-glutamine.
8. Test medium: RPMI 1640, 10% FCS, 10 m$M$ HEPES buffer, 2 m$M$ L-glutamine (*see* **Note 4**).
9. PBSAA buffer: PBS with 1% bovine serum albumin (BSA; Sigma, Fraction V) and 0.1% sodium azide. Store at 4°C (*see* **Note 5**).
10. Antibodies:
    a. CD45PerCP (Becton Dickinson) (*see* **Note 6**).
    b. Control IgG1[i] PerCP (Becton Dickinson).
    c. CD45FITC (Becton Dickinson)..
    d. Control IgG1 FITC (Becton Dickinson).
11. 10-µm carboxylate beads (Polysciences, cat. no. 18133).
12. Positive control cells (*see* **Note 7**).

### 2.2. Measurement of P-Glycoprotein Using MRK 16 Antibody

1. PBSAA buffer: PBS with 1% BSA and 0.1% sodium azide. Store at 4°C.
2. Antibodies:
    a. MRK 16 anti-P-glycoprotein antibody (Kamiya) at 500 µg/mL. Make a 1-in-5 working solution in PBSAA to 100 µg/mL (*see* **Note 8**).

**Table 1**
**Summary of Conditions for the Functional Assays**

| Tube number | Incubation temperature (°C) | Tube contents |
|---|---|---|
| 1 | 4 | Cells, rhodamine 123 |
| 2 | 4 | Cells, rhodamine 123 |
| 3 | 37 | Cells, PSC 833, rhodamine 123 |
| 4 | 37 | Cells, PSC 833, rhodamine 123 |
| 5 | 37 | Cells, solvent, rhodamine 123 |
| 6 | 37 | Cells, solvent, rhodamine 123 |
| 7 | 4 | Cells, daunorubicin |
| 8 | 4 | Cells, daunorubicin |
| 9 | 37 | Cells, daunorubicin |
| 10 | 37 | Cells, daunorubicin |
| 11 | 37 | Beads, daunorubicin |
| 12 | 37 | Beads, daunorubicin |

    b. Mouse IgG2a isotype control (Dako), 100 µg/mL.
    c. Rabbit antimouse F(ab')$_2$, FITC-conjugated (Dako).
    d. CD45PerCP (Becton Dickinson).
    e. Control IgG1 PerCP (Becton Dickinson).
3. Serum
    a. 20% normal rabbit serum in PBSAA.
    b. Normal mouse serum.
4. Positive control cells (*see* **Note 7**).

## 3. Methods

### 3.1. The Functional Measurement of P-Glycoprotein-Mediated Rhodamine 123 Retention and Daunorubicin Accumulation

1. Preliminary step, if using thawed cells: Before counting cells, incubate for 1–2 h in rest medium to restore metabolism. During this time, dead cells tend to clump, and the clumps can be picked out using a Pasteur pipet. We usually obtain >90% viability using this method (*see* **Note 9**).
2. Count cells. Pellet $1.1 \times 10^7$ cells at 200$g$ for 5 min. Resuspend (at $1 \times 10^6$/mL) in 11 mL test medium.
3. Label 12 FACS tubes (**Table 1**).
4. Add:  Tubes 3 and 4: 5 µL PSC 833 working solution B.
           Tubes 5 and 6: 5 µL 40% ethanol.
5. Add 1 mL of cells to each of tubes 1–10 (*see* **Note 10**).
6. Place tubes 1, 2, 7, and 8 on ice.
7. Pipet 1 mL of PBSAA buffer into tubes 11 and 12 and add 5 µL well-mixed carboxylate beads.

8. Add: 40 µL rhodamine 123 to tubes 1–6.
   45 µL daunorubicin to tubes 7–12.
9. Vortex well.
10. Loosely cover tubes 3–6 and 9–12 and place in a 37°C $CO_2$ incubator (*see* **Note 11**). Cover the remaining tubes in the ice box. Leave for 75 min.
11. Precool a centrifuge and PBSAA buffer to 4°C. It is vital that after the 75-min incubation, cells are kept cold to prevent further efflux.
12. Pellet all tubes (1–12) at 200$g$ for 5 min. Tip off, resuspend in 3 mL PBSAA, and pellet again. Do not blot; approx 80 µL of cells will be left in the bottom of the tube.
13. Add 300 µL PBSAA to tubes 11 and 12 and leave on ice until time to use the cytometer. Add the antibodies, remembering to keep the tubes cold at all times:
    a. Tubes 1, 3, 5: 10 µL CD45PerCP (*see* **Note 12**).
    b. Tubes 2, 4, 6: 10 µL control IgG1PerCP.
    c. Tubes 7, 9: 5 µL CD45FITC.
    d. Tubes 8, 10: µL control IgG1 FITC.
14. Leave on ice for 15 min, pellet at 4°C, and rinse twice in 1 mL PBSAA.
15. Resuspend in 300 µL PBSAA (*see* **Note 13**).
16. FACS (*see* **Note 14**). Allow plenty of time to establish your settings the first time you do this. Using a Becton Dickinson FACScalibur with a 488-nm argon laser and logarithmic amplification, R123 fluorescence can be collected in FL1 (530-nm bandpass filter), daunorubicin fluorescence in FL2 (585-nm bandpass filter). For tubes 1–6 (rhodamine 123), first set up an acquisition document with two dot plots: forward vs side scatter and FL1 vs FL3. Using tube 1, ensure that all voltages are set correctly. It is particularly important to make sure that the 4°C probe fluorescence is placed well into the first log decade of the cytometer (*see* **Note 15**), **Fig. 1**. Collect data for tubes 1 and 2 and then decide whether any compensation needs to be set (*see* **Note 16**). Remember, the perCP antibody fluorescence should not affect the mean rhodamine 123 fluorescence. Collect data for tubes 3 and 4 and again check that you are satisfied with the compensation and adjust if not. You may not need to make any adjustments, but remember, if you do, return to tube 1 so that all data are collected at the same settings. Collect 5000 events per tube. For the daunorubicin assay, set up a second acquisition document, this time using forward vs side scatter and FL2 vs FL1. Again make sure that the daunorubicin voltage is set high enough for tubes 7–8 fluorescence to appear well into the first log decade (**Fig. 1**). You will need considerable compensation between daunorubicin and the FITC-conjugated antibodies. For tubes 11 and 12, you may need to decrease the side scatter settings, as the beads have very little side scatter compared to leukemia cells (*see* **Note 17**).
17. Analyze your results (*see* **Note 18**). **Figures 2** and **3** indicate examples of appropriate plots and gates. Calculate rhodamine 123 modulation with PSC833 using the formula

$$\frac{\text{tube 3 FL1 MFI} - \text{tube 1 FL1 MFI}}{\text{tube 5 FL1 MFI} - \text{tube 1 FL1 MFI}}$$

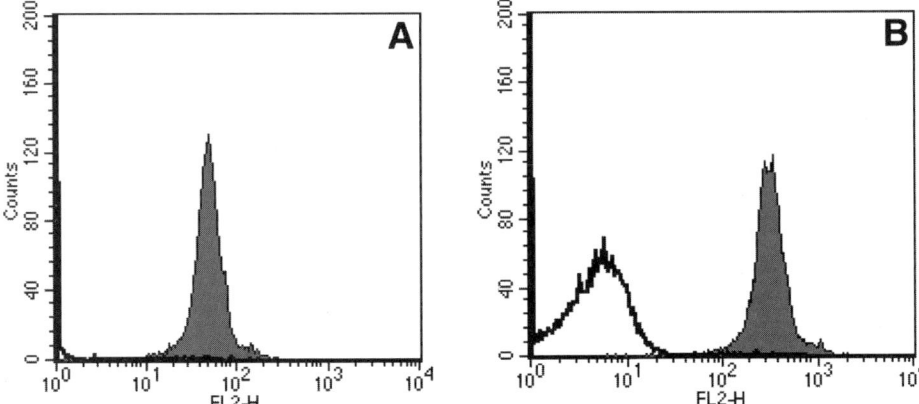

Fig. 1. Illustration of bad (**A**) and good (**B**) voltage settings. Plots **A** and **B** both represent the fluorescence from the same two tubes of cells incubated with daunorubicin at 37°C (shaded histograms) and at 4°C (unshaded histograms). The reason for the difference in the two distributions is that the FL2 voltage in **B** is considerably higher than in **A**. Plot **B** represents data collected with satisfactory fluorescence settings, in which the difference in fluorescence between the two histograms can be measured. Plot **A** represents data collected at such a low voltage that the mean fluorescence of the cells incubated at 4°C is collected in channel 1. This is equivalent to its being "off the scale" and in this case the difference in fluorescence at the two temperatures cannot be measured.

To validate your result, recalculate the modulation ratio on gate 1 cells (i.e., without selecting CD45-low cells) and confirm your calulation using the data from tubes 4, 2, and 6 instead of 3, 1, and 5, respectively.
Calculate the daunorubicin cell:bead ratio using the formula

$$\frac{\text{tube 9 FL2 MFI} - \text{tube 7 FL2 MFI}}{\text{tube 11 FL2 MFI}}$$

Validate your result as for the rhodamine assay, using data from tubes 10, 8, and 12.

### 3.2. Measurement of Surface P-Glycoprotein Using MRK16 Antibody (see *Note 19*)

1. Prepare, rest, and count cells as for the functional assays.
2. Pellet $5 \times 10^5$ cells and resuspend in 200 µL PBSAA.
3. Dispense 80 µL cells per tube into two tubes.
4. Add first layer antibodies:
   Tube 1: 10 µL MRK16 (100-µg/mL working solution) (*see* **Note 20**).
   Tube 2: 10 µL mouse IgG2a isotype control antibody.
5. Vortex well.

6. Incubate for 30 min at room temperature.
7. Wash three times in 1 mL PBSAA.
8. Block both tubes with 80 µL of 20% normal rabbit serum for 30 min.
9. Without removing the rabbit serum, add 5 µL FITC-conjugated rabbit antimouse antibodies. Vortex and incubate on ice for 30 min.
10. Wash twice in 1 mL PBSAA.
11. Add 5 µL normal mouse serum as blocking agent, mix well, and add 5 µL CD45PerCP. Incubate on ice for 15 min.
12. Rinse twice.
13. FACS: As in the functional assay, make sure you have plenty of time and plenty of cells when you do this for the first time. Although there is theoretically no spectral overlap between FITC and PerCP, you will need to confirm that the P-glycoprotein fluorescence is the same in the presence of CD45PerCP and isotype control PerCP. You may wish to add extra tubes omitting either the FITC layer or the CD45PerCP to adjust the compensation settings. Again as in the functional assay (**Fig. 1**), set the voltage to ensure that your isotype control fluorescence appears well into the first log decade.
14. (Optional for most applications, but useful for longitudinal or multicenter studies) Run a set of beads with standardised fluorescence, e.g., Quantum beads (Flow Cytometry Standards) or Fluorospheres (Dako), at the same instrument fluorescence settings as were used for the cells and use these to establish a standard curve and convert the fluorescence results (*see* **Note 21**).
15. Use gating to select leukaemic blasts, and determine the mean FITC intensity of the cells of interest (**Fig. 4**). Unless you are using a standard curve, calculate the ratio of test to control mean fluorescence intensity. Kolmogoroff Smirnoff statistics are available in some flow cytometry software, and these have also been used as a semiquantitative measure of P-glycoprotein expression *(7,8)*.

## 4. Notes

1. In our laboratory we are doing longitudinal studies and therefore we ensure that our instrument is regularly calibrated and that our measurements are standardized. Flow cytometric measurements are often remarkably constant from one day to another, but they can change for no apparent reason (e.g., if the instrument has not been adequately cleaned) and are likely to change when the instrument is serviced. In a longitutinal study, allowances must also be made for the possibility that the analysis will be done on more than one instrument.
2. We have also used a preparation obtained from Sigma that gave very similar results
3. There are several P-glycoprotein inhibitors that can be used in these assays. We are currently using PSC 833 because this agent is being used clinically in a randomized trial and we are planning to compare the results of our in vitro assays with patient outcome. However, preliminary data have shown that the threshold of rhodamine 123 modulation by PSC 833 needs to be set at 1.7 rather than 1.0 on patient cells, i.e., rhodamine retention is modulated to some extent by PSC 833

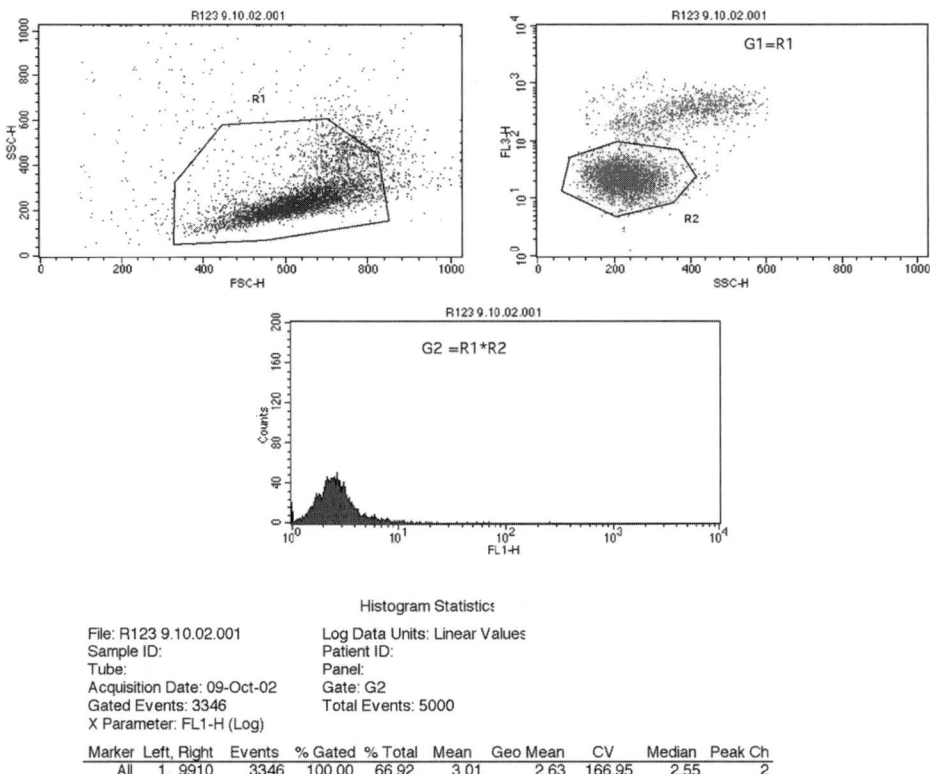

Fig. 2. Example of a rhodamine 123 modulation analysis layout. Illustration of the plots and gates appropriate for the calculation for rhodamine modulation described in **step 17** under **Subheading 3.1.** The last digit on each of the plots is the tube number. Note that the histogram entitled R1239.10.02.003 (tube number 3, cells incubated with PSC833) has much higher rhodamine fluorescence than that of plot R1239.10.02.005 (tube number 5, cells incubated with solvent). This sample has a high rhodamine modulation ratio indicative of functional P-glycoprotein.

even in cells that do not express P-glycoprotein (8). We have also used cyclosporin A extensively with clinical samples, and with the latter agent, the cutoff point for positivity appears to be 1.0. Whichever P-glycoprotein-blocking agent you choose, make sure that you are using a nontoxic dose, e.g., by examining your cells after overnight culture with the agent.
4. It is vital to use a medium with a pH of as near 7.4 as possible. The pH of the medium has a major effect on accumulation of probes. For the same reason, incubation must be in a $CO_2$ incubator—a water bath is not an acceptable substitute.
5. We have found that different brands of albumin alter the results, particularly in the daunorubicin assay.

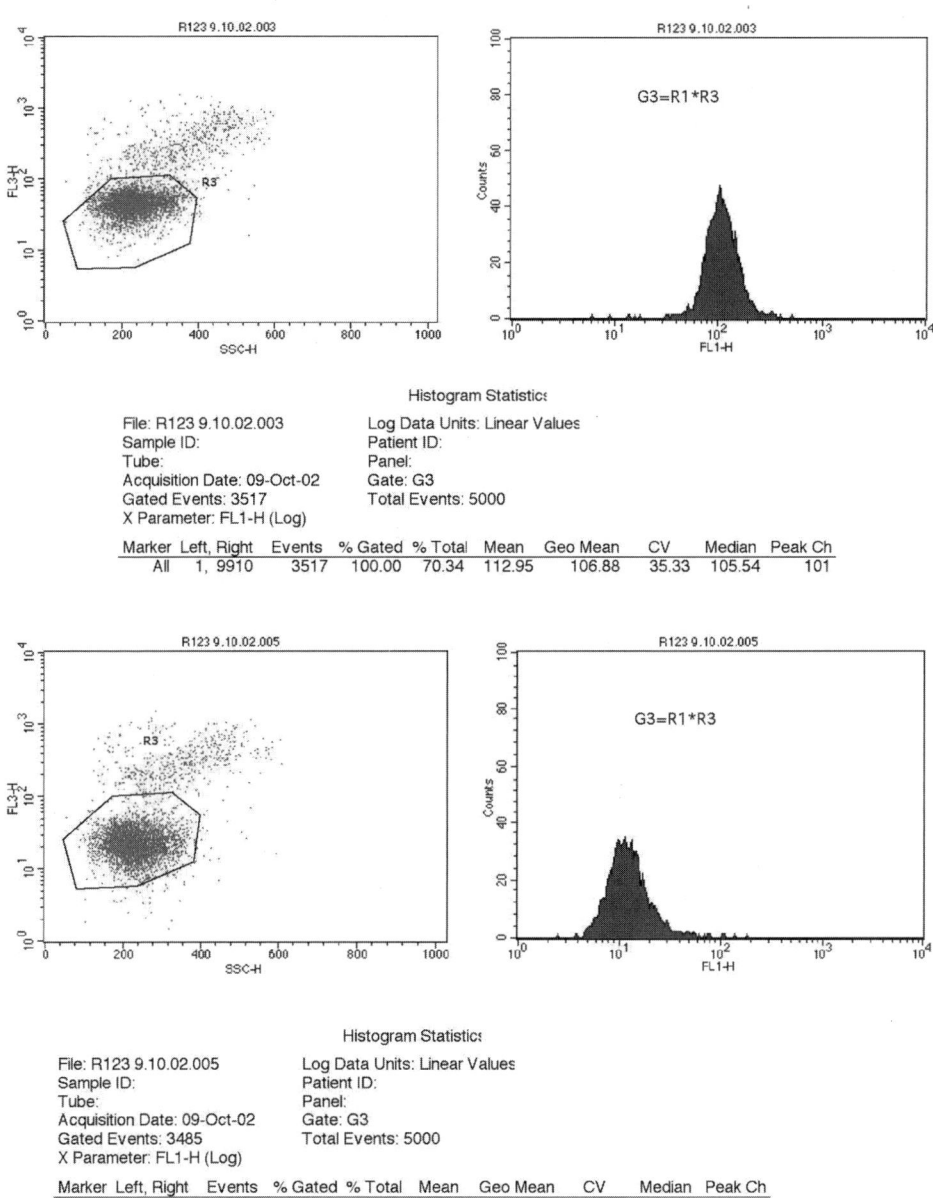

Fig. 2. *(continued)*

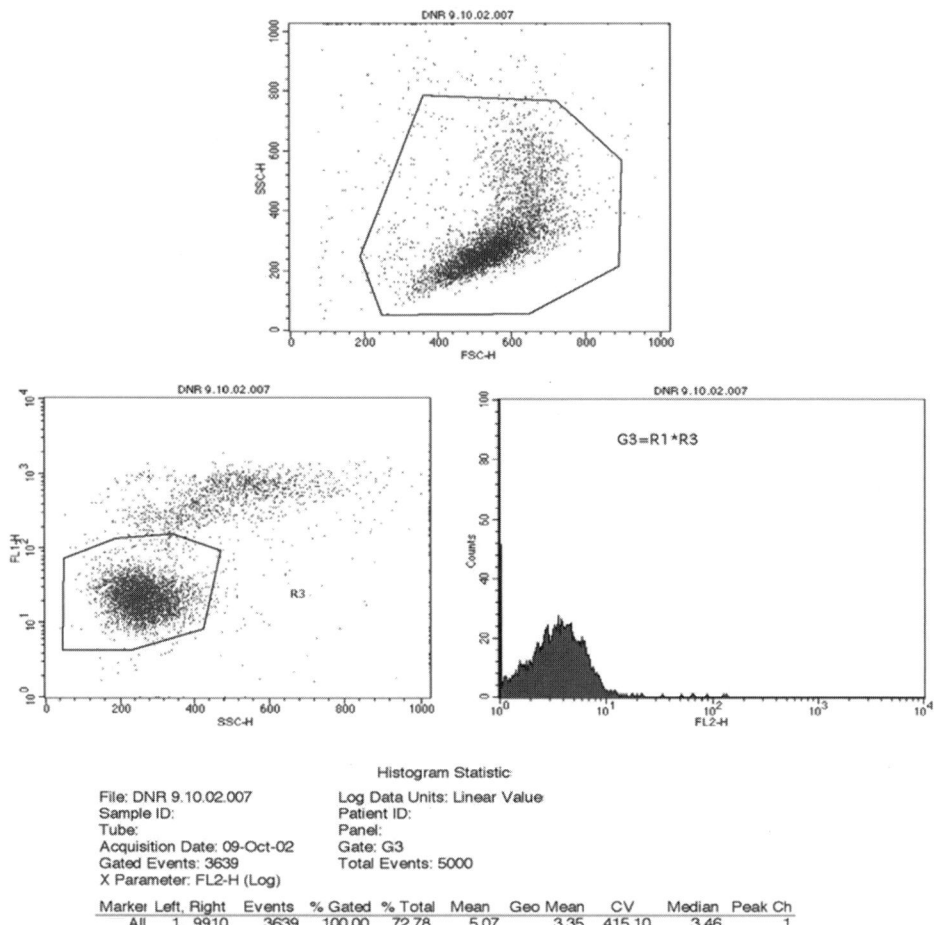

Fig. 3. Example of a daunorubicin uptake analysis layout. Illustration of the plots and gates appropriate to the calculation of the daunorubicin cell:bead ratio described in **step 17** under **Subheading 3.1.** The last digit on each of the plots is the tube number. This is the same sample as in **Fig. 2** and has a low cell:bead fluorescence ratio compared to other samples in our current studies, corroborating the result obtained in the rhodamine assay.

6. It is good practice to use a negative control antibody to CD45 when initially setting up the assays. Even though CD45 is not being measured, an isotype control is necessary to validate the flow cytometric compensation. The fluorescence of rhodamine 123 or of daunorubicin should be the same, whether the cells are counterstained with CD45 or with isotype control antibody. (Compensation should be set by an experienced flow cytometrist, as it is beyond the scope of this chapter.)

Histogram Statistic

| | |
|---|---|
| File: DNR 9.10.02.011 | Log Data Units: Linear Value |
| Sample ID: | Patient ID: |
| Tube: | Panel: |
| Acquisition Date: 09-Oct-02 | Gate: G2 |
| Gated Events: 4405 | Total Events: 5000 |
| X Parameter: FL2-H (Log) | |

| Marker | Left, Right | Events | % Gated | % Total | Mean | Geo Mean | CV | Median | Peak Ch |
|---|---|---|---|---|---|---|---|---|---|
| All | 1, 9910 | 4405 | 100.00 | 88.10 | 89.51 | 82.08 | 61.12 | 74.99 | 71 |

Histogram Statistic

| | |
|---|---|
| File: DNR 9.10.02.009 | Log Data Units: Linear Value |
| Sample ID: | Patient ID: |
| Tube: | Panel: |
| Acquisition Date: 09-Oct-02 | Gate: G3 |
| Gated Events: 3525 | Total Events: 5000 |
| X Parameter: FL2-H (Log) | |

| Marker | Left, Right | Events | % Gated | % Total | Mean | Geo Mean | CV | Median | Peak Ch |
|---|---|---|---|---|---|---|---|---|---|
| All | 1, 9910 | 3525 | 100.00 | 70.50 | 272.16 | 254.41 | 40.91 | 257.13 | 239 |

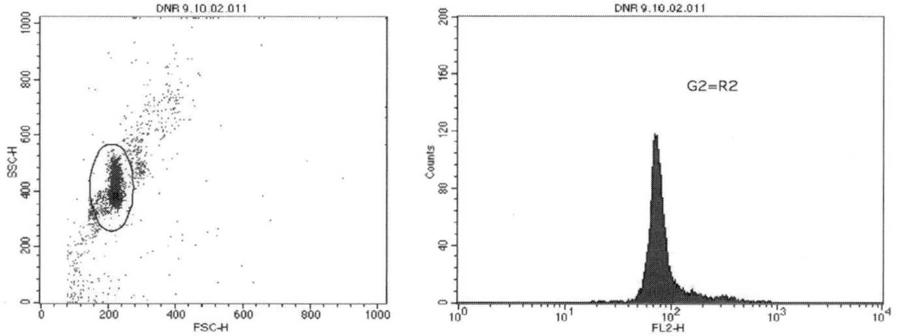

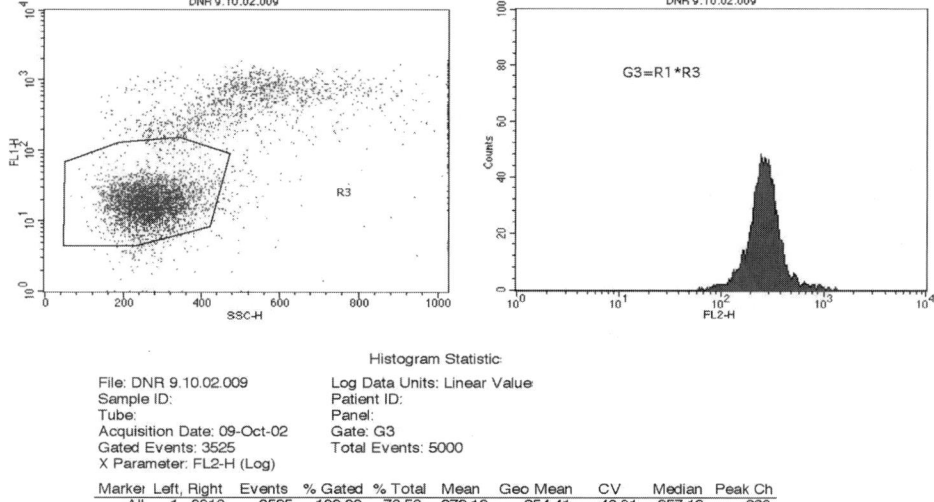

Fig. 3. *(continued)*

7. Choose positive control cells suitable for your application. Try to choose cells that overexpress P-glycoprotein at approximately the same level as your cells of interest. We use TF1 leukemia cells.
8. This dilution is carried out simply in order to obtain the MRK16 at the same concentration as the isotype control antibody, so needs to be adapted if a different isotype control is used.

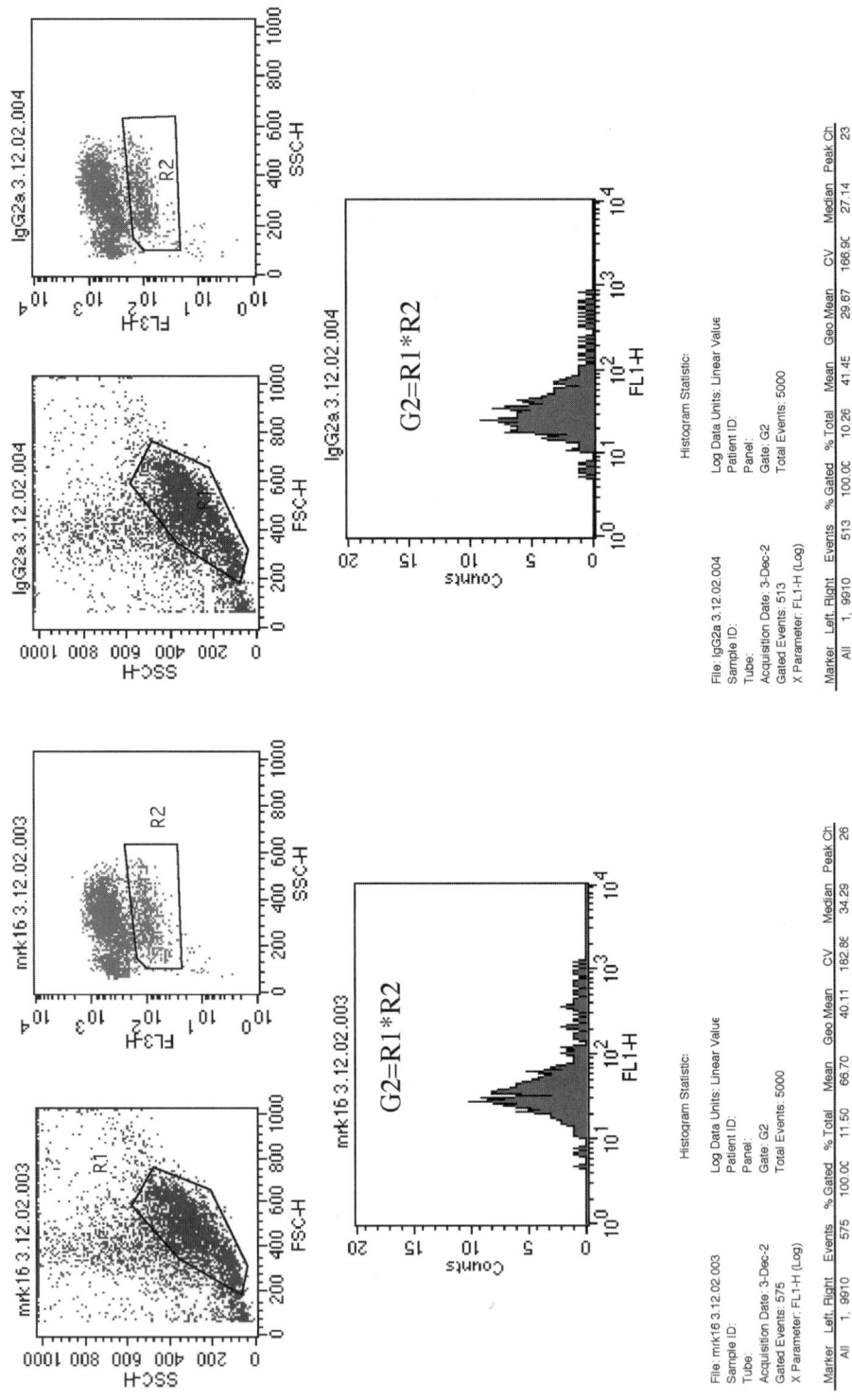

9. After much time wasting, we decided not even to attempt to use or to freeze samples more than 48 h old (e.g., samples that had been in the mail over the weekend). We also discard samples if the post-thaw-and-rest viability is less than 85%
10. The first time you perform this assay, you may wish to set up extra tubes with probes but without antibodies to guide you in setting flow cytometric voltage and compensation.
11. Tubes can be covered in aluminum foil, or two-position lidded FACS tubes can be used. The salient point is to allow the $CO_2$-enriched atmosphere to circulate so that the pH is maintained throughout the incubation.
12. Immature bone marrow cells, including leukaemic blasts, express less CD45 than mature lymphocytes and monocytes *(10)*. We have validated the CD45 gating method of leukaemic blast selection by comparing results obtained in this way with the manual blast count *(11)*.
13. If you are setting up the assay for the first time, resuspend your cells in 1 mL of buffer so that you are less likely to run out of cells while establishing the settings. If you wish to rigorously exclude dead cells, it is possible at this stage to resuspend the cells in a 50-µg/mL solution of propidium iodide, which is only taken up by cells once membrane integrity is lost. Propidium iodide fluoresces very strongly in FL2, such that its fluorescence is easily distinguishable from that of the much more weakly fluorescing daunorubicin in the FL2 channel. However, if you are using antibodies as well, you will now have three fluorochromes on which to check compensation and will need to set up extra tubes with combinations of two fluorochromes to set this correctly.
14. The instrument should be well maintained and calibrated. We calibrate our Becton Dickinson FACscalibur weekly using the Calibrite/Autocomp system.
15. Sensitivity will be completely lost if fluorescence is allowed to accumulate in channel 1. Relative fluorescence intensity numbers generated by a flow cytometer can only be on a linear scale if you, the operator, set the voltages correctly in the first place *(see* **Fig. 1**). This vital point is often not appreciated. It can happen that settings that appear suitable in one assay become inadequate in a subsequent assay, for example, if a new batch of probe is less fluorescent.
16. You may need to ask an experienced flow cytometrist to help you at this stage. Once voltage and compensation settings have been established on your first sample, these settings can be used for subsequent samples, and therefore less flow cytometry expertise is needed.

---

Fig. 4. *(see opposite page)* Example of an MRK 16 analysis layout. Illustration of the plots and gates used to calculate P-glycoprotein levels with MRK 16. (This is not the same sample analyzed in **Figs. 2** and **3**.) The three plots and the statistics on the left are from cells stained with MRK 16, and on the right from cells stained with isotype control. Only a small percentage of cells in this sample fall within the CD45low blast gate (R2). From the two histograms, it would not be logical to decide that some cells are positive and others are negative for P-glycoprotein. However, the mean fluorescence ratio is 40.11/29.67 = 1.35, which represents a positive P-glycoprotein value.

17. A point obvious to the trained but often obscure to novice researchers is that altering scatter settings in the middle of an assay has no effect on fluorescence measurements. However, when comparing fluorescence from two or more tubes, fluorescence settings have to be the same for each tube.
18. In some centers a designated technician will perform the assays for the researcher. Whether or not the flow cytometry is being done for you, make sure that you understand the format of the data. Most modern software is usually set to convert logarithmically generated data into relative fluorescence units. However, sometimes data are displayed as channel numbers on a logarithmic scale.
19. P-glycoprotein can by found within the cell, but be aware that any permeabilization technique used to detect intracellular P-glycoprotein may result in the loss of surface P-glycoprotein. In our hands, MRK 16 is well suited to the measurement of surface protein, but the UIC2 antibody (Immunotech) is better suited to the detection of the intracellular protein.
20. If you are using a different cell type, you will need to perform your own saturation study to determine the optimal dose of antibody.
21. Fluorescent bead standards are used to construct a standard curve of molecules of equivalent (soluble) fluorochrome (mef or mesf). Cellular fluorescence measurements can be converted to mef from the standard curve either manually or with the use of a computer program. This method has the advantage of enabling results from different instruments to be converted to the same scale. We use bead standards in our antibody assays. However, rhodamine 123 fluoresces more brightly than commercially available bead standards, so for our functional assays we rely on ratiometric measurements. We and others have found these to be reproducible in two-center studies *(1,7)*. Note that manufacturers' instructions for the bead standards may recommend that fluorescence voltages be altered in order to fit blank bead fluorescence into the first log decade. However, if the voltages and compensation have been set up with a different system (e.g., Autocomp and Calibrite), remember that the voltages should remain *unchanged* for bead standards as well as for samples.

# References

1. Truran, L., Pallis, M., Fisher J., et al. (2002) Quantitative and comparative flow cytometry for the measurement of multidrug resistance and apoptosis-related variables in acute myeloid leukaemia. A two-centre methodological study. *Hematol. J.* **3 (Suppl. 1),** 308.
2. Krishna, R. and Mayer, L. D. (2000) Multidrug resistance (MDR) in cancer. Mechanisms, reversal using modulators of MDR and the role of MDR modulators in influencing the pharmacokinetics of anticancer drugs. *Eur. J. Pharm. Sci.* **11,** 265–283.
3. Pallis, M., Turzanski, J., Higashi, Y., and Russell, N. (2002) P-glycoprotein in acute myeloid leukemia: therapeutic implications of its association with both a multidrug-resistant and an apoptosis-resistant phenotype. *Leuk. Lymphoma* **43,** 1221–1228.

4. Beck, W. T., Grogan, T. M., Willman, C. L., et al. (1996) Methods to detect P-glycoprotein-associated multidrug-resistance in patients tumors—consensus recommendations. *Cancer Res.* **56,** 3010–3020.
5. Broxterman, H. J., Lankelma, J., and Pinedo, H. M. (1996) How to probe clinical tumor samples for P-glycoprotein and multidrug resistance-associated protein. *Eur. J. Cancer* **32A,** 1024–1033.
6. Marie, J. P., Huet, S., Faussat, A. M., et al. (1997) Multicentric evaluation of the MDR phenotype in leukemia. *Leukemia* **11,** 1086–1094.
7. Broxterman, H. J., Sonneveld, P., Feller, N., et al. (1996) Quality control of multidrug resistance assays in adult acute leukemia: correlation between assays for P-glycoprotein expression and activity. *Blood* **87,** 4809–4816.
8. Pallis, M., Turzanski, J., Langabeer, S., and Russell, N. (1999) Reproducible flow cytometric methodology for measuring multidrug resistance in leaukaemic blasts, in *Recent Advances in Experimental Biology* (Kaspers, G., Pieters, R., and Veerman, A., eds.), Kluwer Academic, NY, pp. 77–88.
9. Pallis, M. and Russell, N. H. (1998) Functional multidrug resistance in acute myeloblastic leukemia: a standardized flow cytometric assay for intracellular daunorubicin accumulation. *Br. J. Haematol.* **100,** 194–197.
10. Borowitz, M. J., Guenther, K. L., Shults, K. E., and Steltzer, G. T. (1993) Immunophenotyping of acute leukemia by flow cytometric analysis: use of CD45 and right angle light scatter to gate on leukemic blasts in three-color analysis. *Am. J. Clin. Pathol.* **100,** 534–540.
11. Das-Gupta, E., Pallis, M., and Russell, N. (1999) Multidrug resistance in CD45/side scatter gated samples from patients with acute myeloblastic leukemia. *Haematologica* **184,** 299a.

# 13

## Measurement of Ceramide and Sphingolipid Metabolism in Tumors

*Potential Modulation of Chemotherapy*

### David E. Modrak

#### Summary

Ceramide is a bioactive lipid involved in the induction of apoptosis and is the precursor to several sphingolipids, including sphingomyelin, the gangliosides, and sphingosine. Ceramide production is increased in response to stress and toxic agents. Because modulation of ceramide levels has been shown to affect sensitivity and/or resistance to therapeutic agents, it will be important to assess the activity of sphingolipid metabolic pathways when investigating the mode of action of antitumor drugs. This chapter summarizes protocols for quantitating the level of apoptosis, the activities of acidic sphingomyelinase, neutral sphingomyelinase, glycosylceramide synthase, sphingomyelin synthase, and ceramidase, and the amount of ceramide in tumor xenografts in nude mice.

#### Key Words

Apoptosis; ceramide; sphingomyelin; acidic sphingomyelinase; neutral sphingomyelinase; glycosylceramide synthase; diacylglycerol kinase; sphingomyelin synthase; ceramidase.

### 1. Introduction

Ceramide has been shown to be a mediator of cellular differentiation and apoptosis in tumor cells *(1–3)* and lies at the center of sphingolipid metabolism (**Fig. 1**). *De novo* synthesis of ceramide results from condensation of serine and palmitoyl-CoA, followed by acylation and desaturation. Desaturation is essential for the apoptosis-inducing activity of ceramide. Ceramide can be glycosylated in the first step on the path to higher-order glycolipids, deacylated to form sphingosine, or sphingomyelin (SM) can be generated through the transfer of choline from phosphatidylcholine. Ceramide can also be generated rapidly through the action of sphingomyelinases *(4,5)*. Furthermore, modulation of sphingolipid metabolism can markedly alter the sensitivity of tumor cells to chemotherapeutics *(6–8)*. Hence, there is a growing interest in the biology of ceramide and sphingolipids as potential modulators of chemosensitivity *(9–11)*.

This chapter describes simple and reproducible assays for ceramide quantitation and the measurement of several key metabolic enzymes leading to and from ceramide. Procedures for measuring additional pathways of sphingolipid metabolism can be found elsewhere *(12,13)*.

## 2. Materials

For the procedures included in this chapter, the following reagents are needed.

### 2.1. Apoptosis Assay

Cy5-conjugated tumor cell specific antibody, Annexin-V-fluorescein, propidium iodide.

### 2.2. Lipid Analysis

The following stock reagents are needed: cardiolipin, diethylenetriaminepentaacetic acid (DETAPAC), octyl-β-D-glycopyranoside, imidazole, ATP, diacylglycerol (DAG) kinase (BioMol), [γ-$^{33}$P]ATP, Mg(NO$_3$)$_2$, and ascorbic acid. In addition, the following solutions must be made in advance.

1. Ammonium molybdate solution: 4.2 mg (NH$_4$)$_6$Mo$_7$O$_{24}$ • 4H$_2$O, 28.6 µL concentrated H$_2$SO$_4$, per mL.
2. BSS buffer: 135 m$M$ NaCl, 4.5 m$M$ KCl, 1.5 m$M$ CaCl$_2$, 0.5 m$M$ MgCl$_2$, 50 m$M$ glucose, 1 m$M$ HEPES, pH 7.2.
3. 2X DAG kinase reaction buffer: 100 m$M$ NaCl, 100 m$M$ imidazole, pH 6.5, 2 m$M$ EDTA, 25 m$M$ MgCl$_2$ (check pH before use).

### 2.3. Enzyme Assays

PMSF (100 m$M$ in isopropanol), antipain, chymostatin, leupeptin, pepstatin A, bovine brain SM (bbSM), phosphatidylserine (PS), [$^3$H-choline]-SM, UDP-glc, UDP-[1-$^3$H]glucose, Na$_2$SO$_4$, *tert*-butylmethylether, NAD$^+$, NBD-hexanoyl-ceramide. In addition, the following solutions must be made in advance.

1. Cell lysis buffer: 0.25 $M$ sucrose, 1 m$M$ EDTA, 1 m$M$ PMSF, 1 m$M$ dithiothreitol (DTT), 1 µg/mL antipain, 1 µg/mL chymostatin, 1 µg/mL leupeptin, and 1 µg/mL pepstatin A.
2. SM sythase reaction buffer: 50 m$M$ Tris-HCl, pH 7.4, 0.25 $M$ sucrose, 150 m$M$ KCl.

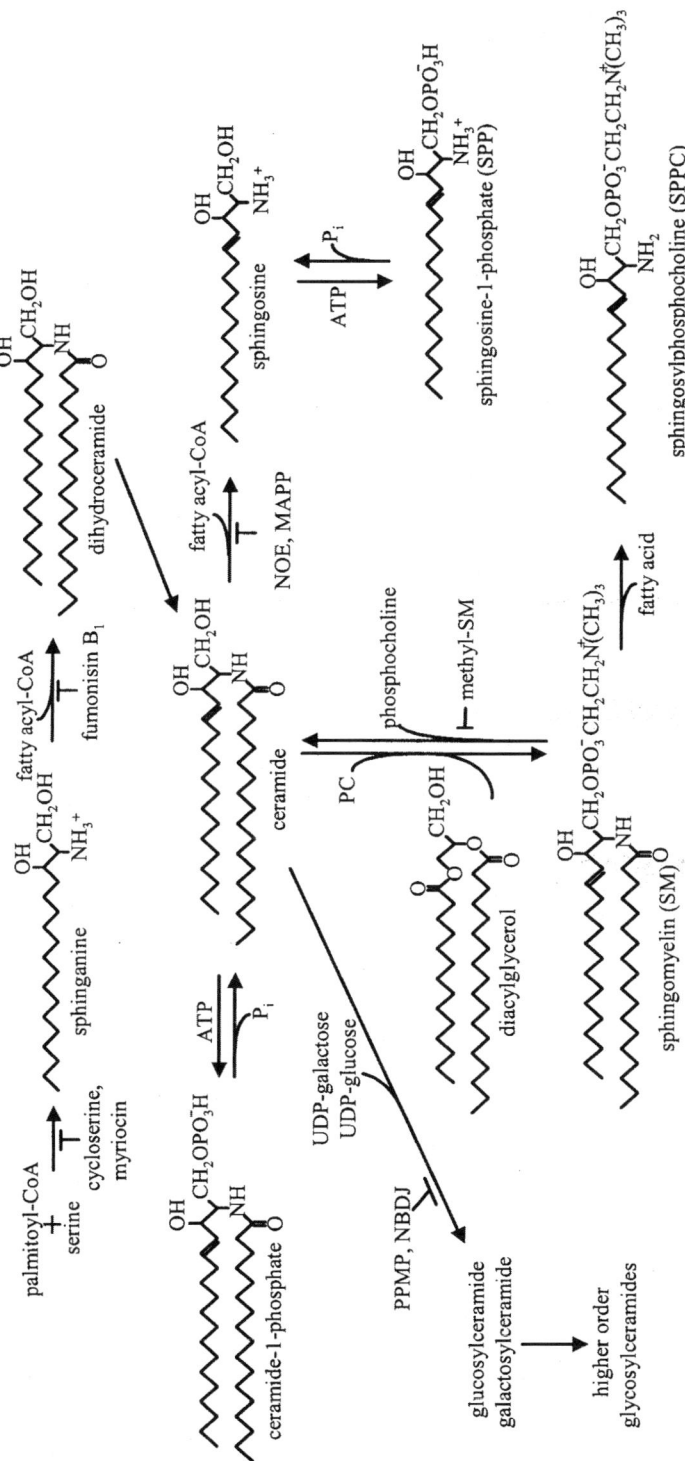

Fig. 1. Sphingolipid metabolism. NOE, N-oleoylethanolamine; MAPP, (1S, 2R)-D-erythro-2-(N-myristolyamino)-1-phenyl-1-propanol; NBDJ, N-butyldeoxynojirimycin; PPMP, DL-threo-1-phenyl-2-palmitoylamino-3-morpholino-1-propanol.

## 3. Methods

Tumor xenografts are grown in nude mice to approximately 0.5 cm$^3$. In our laboratory, we routinely use the human colonic tumor GW-39 as a subcutaneous xenograft. Provided the tumor can be excised cleanly away from normal tissues, any tumor model and any host can be used. On the days of interest, three to five animals from each treatment group are sacrificed; the tumors and other tissues of interest are removed and are kept on ice during processing. The tissues are ground through a large mesh screen with a pestle or plunger from a 5 or 10 mL syringe in 5 vol of cold phosphate-buffered saline (PBS) and returned to ice. At this point, the samples are split into three equal portions for apoptosis and enzyme activity assays and for lipid extraction.

### 3.1. Measurement of Apoptosis

GW-39 human tumor cells express carcinoembryonic antigen (CEA), which can be recognized by the antibody MN-14 *(14)*. Alternatively, any antibody specific for the tumor cells can be used to discriminate between tumor and nontumor stromal cells. The antibody is conjugated to the dye Cy5, available from Amersham Pharmacia. Conjugation of MN-14 using the supplied protocol is straightforward and results in high yields and activity.

1. The tumor suspension is passed through a Pasteur pipet containing a loose glass wool plug about 1–2 cm in length pushed down to the narrow portion of the pipet. The material that flows through contains predominantly single cells as well as some small clusters and cell debris (*see* **Note 1**). The majority of material that could cause clogging of the flow cytometer is trapped in the glass wool.
2. The cells are stained for 10 min on ice with 1 µg MN-14-Cy5 conjugate, 1 µg Annexin-V-fluorescein conjugate (Pharmigen), and 10 µg propidium iodide in 1 mL PBS.
3. Cellular fluorescence of single tumor cells is measured on a FACScaliber flow cytometer (Becton-Dickenson) by gating on the appropriate forward and side scatter regions, using the fluorescence in channel 4 to exclude CEA-negative cells. The percent of cells undergoing apoptosis is the number of cells positive for Annexin-V binding and negative for propidium iodide uptake divided by the total number of CEA-positive cells analyzed (typically approx 95% of cells).

### 3.2. Lipid Analysis

Polypropylene tubes, or other chemically resistant tubes, with tight lids or caps should be used. This procedure is essentially that of Bligh and Dyer *(15)* (*see* **Note 2**).

1. In a 15-mL conical tube, add to the 2 mL sample, 2 mL CHCl$_3$, 4 mL methanol (MeOH) (final vol, 8 mL), and vortex vigorously. The sample can be stored at –20°C overnight if desired.

2. Add 2 mL CHCl₃ and vortex.
3. Add 2 mL water and vortex. Spin sample at 3000 rpm in a Sorvall RT7 centrifuge for 30 min.
4. Transfer the lower organic layer to a clean glass tube and dry under a stream of nitrogen. Warming the tube in a beaker of warm tap water expedites the process. Lipids are stored dried (–20°C) and resuspended in a convenient volume (i.e., 0.5 mL) CHCl₃ : MeOH (2 : 1) prior to use in subsequent assays.

*3.2.1. Total Lipid Phosphate Determination*

This procedure is essentially that of Ames *(16)*. It is effectively linear over the 1 100 nmol phosphate range.

1. Aliquot a portion of the lipids (100 µL or approx one-tenth to one-fifth of the total sample) into a clean (CHCl₃ rinsed) Pyrex tube with a screw cap.
2. Dry lipids under N₂ and resuspend in 100 µL MeOH.
3. Add 30 µL 10% Mg(NO₃)₂ in 95% ethanol and heat gently over a flame with cap off until ethanol evaporates, then heat strongly until brown fumes stop and sample turns white (*see* **Note 3**).
4. After cooling the tubes, add 300 µL 0.5 *M* HCl, cap tightly, and heat in boiling water for 15 min.
5. Cool the tubes to room temperature and add 700 µL freshly made molybdate reaction mix (1 part 100-mg/mL ascorbic acid, 6 parts ammonium molybdate solution). Incubate 1 h at room temperature and read the absorbance at 820 nm (*see* **Note 4**).

*3.2.2. Ceramide Determination*

Several techniques are available for quantitating ceramide levels in cells and tissues *(17–20)*. We prefer the diacylglycerol kinase assay because it is simple and no special equipment beyond thin-layer chromatography (TLC) supplies are needed (*see* **Note 5**). However, it is always advisable to confirm results by other methods, such as liquid chromatography/mass spectrometry (LC-MS), when possible. The following protocol is based on the method supplied with DAG kinase from BioMol (Plymouth Meeting, PA).

1. In a clean 5 mL glass tube, dry the sample lipids (approx one-quarter to one-half of the sample). In separate reactions, $C_{16}$-ceramide is used for generating a standard curve and for comparison with the products of the assay (*see* **Note 5**).
2. Add 100 µL DAGK reaction mix, vortex, incubate at room temperature 30 min. DAGK reaction mix is prepared as follows: For 10 reactions, add the contents of tube #1 (60 µL of 25-mg/mL cardiolipin in CHCl₃, dry down under N₂; add 200 µL of 1 m*M* DETAPAC, bath sonicate 2 min; add 62 µL 825 m*M* octyl-β-D-glycopyranoside, vortex) to tube #2 (500 µL of 2X DAG kinase reaction buffer, 75 µL water, 8 µL of 100 m*M* imidazole, pH 6.5, 80 µL of 1 m*M* DETAPAC, 20 µL of 100 m*M* DTT, 10 µL of 100 m*M* ATP, 35 µL of 1 mg/mL DAG

kinase), vortex the combined solutions, incubate 30 min at room temperature, add 1 µL (10 µCi) [γ-$^{33}$P]ATP and leave on ice until needed.
3. Stop the reaction with 1 mL CHCl$_3$:MeOH:1 N HCl (100:100:1) and 200 µL BSS/EDTA (170 µL BSS plus 30 µL 100 mM EDTA), vortex vigorously, centrifuge 5 min at 1000 rpm in a Sorvall RT7 centrifuge.
4. Transfer the lower organic layer (avoid taking the interface) to a clean glass tube, dry under N$_2$.
5. Resuspend the film in 50 µL of CHCl$_3$:MeOH (1:1) and load the entire sample onto a TLC plate (20 cm long, K6F silica gel 60 A, 250 µm thick; Whatman, Clifton, NJ) spotting 10 µL at a time. Allow the samples to dry completely before continuing. Heating gently with a hair dryer will speed the process.
6. Resolve the lipids using CHCl$_3$:MeOH:acetic acid (glacial) (65:15:5), dry the plate in a chemical hood, cover the plate in plastic wrap, and subject to autoradiography overnight (Kodak XAR film).
7. On the back of the glass TLC plate, mark the positions of the bands corresponding to ceramide-1-PO$_4$ and use a glass cutter to score the glass (*see* **Note 6**). Carefully break the glass into pieces encompassing the ceramide band(s) and count by liquid scintillation (EcoScint, National Diagnostics, Atlanta, GA). The unknown ceramide levels of the samples should be normalized to the total amount of lipid phosphate present in the sample. Alternatively, an internal standard (i.e., C$_6$-ceramide added to the sample before processing) may be used.

### 3.2.3. Total Sphingomyelin Determination

It is possible to determine the total amount of sphingomyelin in the extracted lipids by high-performance liquid chromatography (HPLC) using CH$_3$CN:MeOH:85% H$_3$PO$_4$ (100:10:1) to resolve the lipids on a C$_{18}$ silica column (resuspend the lipids in *n*-hexane:isopropanol [3:1]) before injecting onto column). However, little change is seen in total sphingomyelin content of the tissues as a function of treatment group. More informative would be the total amount of sphingomyelin in separate intracellular compartments, because it is postulated that not all sphingomyelin can be a substrate for activated sphingomyelinase (SMase) *(21)*. A summary of various procedures for measuring the transmembrane distribution of sphingomyelin can be found elsewhere *(22)*.

### 3.3. Enzyme Assays

The third portion of the tissue suspension is centrifuged to collect the cells (3000 rpm Sorvall RT7, 10 min, 4°C) and sonicated as follows to make a crude extract (*see* **Note 7**).

1. Resuspend the cells in fresh, cold lysis buffer. The amount to use is adjusted for the amount of tissue: small tissues, such as brain and kidney, are resuspended in approx 0.5 mL, whereas larger tissues, such as liver and tumor, are resuspended in 1 mL of buffer. Very large tumors may need to be resuspended in 2 mL. In general, approx 1–2 mL of buffer per gram of tissue is used.

## Measurement of Ceramide and Sphingolipid Metabolism

2. Sonicate the samples using a probe sonicator at near-maximum output for five 10-s pulses (model W185, Heat Systems, Ultrasonics, Plainview, NY). Chill the sample on ice for 20 s between pulses.
3. Centrifuge the samples for 5 min at 500g.
4. The supernatant is stored at −80°C.
5. Use 10 µL for a protein determination assay (e.g., Bradford assay).

### 3.3.1. Sphingomyelinases

SMases are responsible for the conversion of sphingomyelin to ceramide and release choline in the process. The differences in water solubility of the substrate and products can be taken advantage of when assaying these enzymes. For both the acidic and neutral SMases, hydrolysis of lipophilic radioactive sphingomyelin, labeled in the choline head group, results in the release of hydrophilic radioactive choline (*see* **Note 8**).

#### 3.3.1.1. ACIDIC SMASE

This assay, and the following one for neutral SMase, were adapted from the work of Liu and Hannun *(23)*.

1. To prepare the reaction mixture, dry under $N_2$ in a glass tube, per reaction, 5 nmol bbSM and 5 nmol PS, from 5 m$M$ stocks in $CHCl_3$:MeOH (9:1). Add 10 µL of 1 $M$ Na-acetate, pH 5.0, 1 µL of 1% Triton X-100, $10^5$ dpm of [$^3$H-choline]-SM, 39 µL of water, and sonicate in a bath sonicator (Fisher FS-14) at approx 37°C. Leave the solution at 37°C until needed, but use within 10 min.
2. Add 50 µL of this mixture to 50 µL tissue extract and incubate 1 h at 37°C in a shaking water bath. The extract should be diluted in 20 m$M$ Na-acetate, pH 5.0, if needed. Typically, 10–200 µg of protein is assayed; however, the amount of protein used will depend on the level of activity present in the tissue.
3. Stop the reaction with 1.5 mL $CHCl_3$:MeOH (2:1) and 200 µL water, vortex and centrifuge 5 min at 500g.
4. Remove 200 µL of the approx 800 µL total aqueous layer, and add 10 mL EcoScint for counting by liquid scintillation.

#### 3.3.1.2. NEUTRAL SMASE

This reaction is similar to that for acidic SMase except for the changes in reaction buffer conditions.

1. For each reaction, 5 nmol each of bbSM and PS are dried and resuspended in 10 µL of 1% Triton X-100, 10 µL of 1 $M$ Tris-HCl, pH 7.4, 0.5 µL of 1 $M$ DTT, 0.5 µL of 1 $M$ $MgCl_2$, 29 µL water, $10^5$ dpm [$^3$H-choline]-SM. The mixture is sonicated in a bath sonicator at approx 37°C. Leave the solution at 37°C until needed, but use within 10 min.
2. Add 50 µL of this mixture to 50 µL tissue extract and incubate 1 h at 37°C in a shaking water bath. The extract should be diluted in 20 m$M$ Tris-HCl, pH 7.4, if

needed. Typically, 10–200 µg of protein is assayed; however, the amount of protein used will depend on the level of activity present in the tissue.
3. Stop the reaction with 1.5 mL $CHCl_3$:MeOH (2:1) and 200 µL water, vortex, and centrifuge 5 min at 500g.
4. Remove 200 µL of the 800 µL total aqueous layer, and add 10 mL EcoScint for counting by liquid scintillation.

3.3.1.3. BASIC SMASE

A SMase with an alkaline pH optimum has been identified in the intestinal lumen of several vertebrates, including humans and rats, and is dependent on the presence of bile salts for activity. It has not been identified in tissues other than the colon mucosa, where it is postulated to aid in the prevention of colon carcinogenesis. A procedure for assaying this enzyme can be found in the paper by Hertervig et al. *(24)*.

*3.3.2. Glycosylceramide Synthase*

Glycosylceramide is the root of over 200 different glycosphingolipids. Glycosylceramide synthase (GCS) has been shown to impart drug resistance when overexpressed *(8)*. As with the SMase assays, this assay also uses differential solubilities to separate the $^3$H-glucose substrate from the $^3$H-glc-cer product and was adapted from the assay described by Shayman and Abe *(25)*.

1. For 10 reactions, dry under $N_2$, 6 µmol of lipids PC:octanoylsphingosine (C8-ceramide):sulfatide (7:2:1 molar ratio), resuspend in 712 µL water, and sonicate in an ice water bath for 10 min. Add 200 µL of 1 *M* Tris-Cl, pH 7.4, 20 µL of 10 m*M* UDP-glc, 20 µL of 1 *M* $MgCl_2$, 2 µL of 1 *M* DTT, 2 µL of 1 *M* EGTA, 40 µL of 100 m*M* $NAD^+$, 4 µL of 1 mCi/mL UDP-[1-$^3$H]-glucose, and vortex (*see* **Note 9**).
2. Add 100 µL of the reaction mixture to 100 µL extract (diluted in 10 m*M* Tris-HCl, pH 7.4) in a glass tube, incubate 1 h at 37°C in a shaking water bath. Occasional brief sonications in a 37°C bath may be necessary if extract particles are seen to be clinging to the sides of the tube.
3. Stop the reaction with 0.8 mL of 5% $Na_2SO_4$ and 5 mL *tert*-butylmethylether, vortex vigorously, and centrifuge for 5 min at 800g.
4. Transfer the upper organic layer to a clean scintillation vial, dry, add 5 mL of scintillation fluid, and count.

*3.3.3. Sphingomyelin Synthase*

At the present time, only dipalmitoyl-[$^3$H-methyl-choline]-phosphatidylcholine (PC) is commercially available and this can be used for assaying SM synthase, although SM synthase prefers unsaturated PC substrates. Alternatively, [$^3$H-methyl-choline]PC may be produced by incubating cells, or injecting rats, with radiolabeled choline and subsequent preparative-scale TLC or

HPLC. The use of fluorescent NBD-ceramide as the substrate for measuring SM synthase activity *(26)* obviates the need for producing radiolabeled PC, but this method does have the drawback that a fluorescence detector attached to the HPLC is needed. To use NBD-ceramide as the substrate, resuspend 6 nmol NBD-ceramide (dried from an ethanol stock) in 40 µL of 1% fatty acid-free bovine serum albumin (BSA). Add 60 µL SM synthase reaction buffer and incubate at 37°C for 30 min before use.

1. To initiate the assay, mix 100 µL NBD-ceramide solution with 100 µL protein (0.5–1 mg) and incubate at 37°C for 1–4 h, as determined from preliminary trials (*see* **Note 10**).
2. Stop the reaction by the addition of 1 mL of mobile phase (850:150:1.5, MeOH:$H_2O$:85% $H_3PO_4$) and incubate 1 h at 37°C. Microfuge the samples at maximum speed at 4°C for 15 min.
3. The products are resolved by HPLC on a $C_{18}$-silica column with the column connected to a fluorescence detector (excitation 455 nm, emission 530 nm) and with the mobile phase described above.

*3.3.4. Ceramidases*

The use of NBD-ceramide as the substrate significantly reduces the cost of this assay. This procedure is essentially that of Nikolova-Karakashian and Merrill *(27)*.

3.3.4.1. ACIDIC CERAMIDASE

1. For 10 reactions, 100 nmol of NBD-hexanoyl-ceramide is dried in a glass tube and resuspended in 10 µL ethanol. Then 90 µL of 1% Triton X-100 is added and 10 µL aliquots are placed in numbered microfuge tubes with tight-fitting caps suitable for organic solvents (*see* **Note 11**).
2. Approximately 0.25–1 mg of protein is added and the volume is adjusted to 50 µL with 250 m*M* Na-acetate, pH 4.5. The tubes are incubated on ice for 10 min to allow the substrate to equilibrate into the membranes.
3. Na-acetate (250 µL, 250 m*M*) is added and the tubes are transferred to a 37°C water bath for 1 h.
4. The reaction is terminated with 1 mL of mobile phase (MeOH:$H_2O$:85% $H_3PO_4$, 850:150:1.5), incubated 1 h at 37°C, and microfuged for 15 min at maximum speed and 4°C.
5. The products are resolved by HPLC on a $C_{18}$-silica column with the column connected to a fluorescence detector (excitation 455 nm, emission 530 nm) and with the mobile phase described above.

3.3.4.2. NEUTRAL CERAMIDASE

This reaction is the same as for acidic ceramidase except that 10 m*M* Tris-HCl, pH 7.4 is substituted for the Na-acetate.

3.3.4.3. BASIC CERAMIDASE

This reaction is the same as for acidic ceramidase except that 10 m$M$ Tris-HCl, pH 9.0, is substituted for the Na-acetate.

## 4. Notes

1. It is important to pack the glass wool tight enough to prevent large particles from flowing through but loose enough to allow the cells to come through. Generally, the former is more problematic than the latter. Microscopic examination of the cell suspension to confirm the absence of large cell clusters is advisable.
2. While the absolute volume of solvents is adjusted according to the amount of starting tissue, the ratios must be maintained at 0.5:1.0:0.4 ($CHCl_3$:MeOH:$H_2O$) before dilution and 1.0:1.0:0.9 after dilution and take into account the amount of water in the sample.
3. If possible, do this step in a chemical fume hood. Also, note that the use of an open flame can be hazardous, to say the least, if volatile organic solvents are nearby. Therefore, use caution and inspect the work area for potentially flammable objects and solutions before starting this procedure.
4. The color continues to develop and reliable data can be obtained up to 24 h after adding the molybdate reaction mix.
5. $C_{16}$-ceramide should be used for generating a standard curve, because small-chain ceramides (i.e., $C_2$) are poor substrates for DAG kinase. The lower limit of detection is approx 10 pmol of ceramide, while the upper limit of usefulness is approximation 600 pmol. Perry and Hannun have recently reviewed several important considerations for using DAG kinase to quantitate ceramide, including kinetic issues and the source of enzyme *(28)*. Provided the enzyme is used in excess, >90% conversion of substrate ceramide to ceramide-1-$PO_4$ is expected. In our experience, the changes in tumor ceramide content are small, of the order of two- to threefold in drug-treated groups compared to untreated groups (unpublished).
6. Often, two bands are seen, presumably corresponding to ceramide species containing fatty acids of different acyl chain lengths. Both bands should be counted together. A phosphatidic acid band will often be seen and will run with a higher $R_f$ than ceramides.
7. In general, preliminary assays should always be run to determine the relationship between the linearity of response and incubation time as a function of protein input. When appropriate, the presence of endogenous substrates should also be taken into account when calculating the specific activity of the sample. Substrates and inhibitors of sphingolipid metabolism are available commercially from various suppliers, such as BioMol (Plymouth Meeting, PA), Avanti Polar Lipids (Alabaster, AL), Sigma-Aldrich (St. Louis, MO), Cayman Chemical (Ann Arbor, MI), American Radiolabeled Chemicals (St. Louis, MO), and ICN (Irvine, CA).
8. The stability of SMases are improved by the addition of protease inhibitors and cooling. Neutral SMase activity is enhanced by DTT and PS *(29)*. On the other hand, acidic SMase is inhibited by DTT. The final concentration of Triton X-100 should be 0.1%, inclusive of any present in the protein sample.

9. PC was noted to stimulate glycosylceramide synthase activity in brain and kidney tissue *(30)*. Sulfatide has been reported to stimulate ceramide galactosyltransferase activity *(31)* but in our hands is not essential for the measurement of this enzyme. Both $NAD^+$ and $NADP^+$ are equally effective stimulators of activity, and Tris buffer inhibits activity at higher concentrations (i.e., >0.1 $M$).
10. In some instances, the activity of endogenous ceramidases may be too great to obtain reliable data on SM synthase. In such cases, it may be necessary to include the ceramidase inhibitors N-oleoylethanolamine at high micromolar concentrations or MAPP [(1S, 2R)-D-erythro-2-(N-myristolyamino)-1-phenyl-1-propanol)] at low micromolar concentrations.
11. Tyrosine phosphorylation may play a role in activating ceramidase and inhibitors of phosphatases added to tissue extracts may maintain ceramidase activity.

## References

1. Jarvis, W. D. and Grant, S. (1998) The role of ceramide in the cellular response to cytotoxic agents. *Curr. Opin. Oncol.* **10,** 552–559.
2. Liu, G., Kleine, L., and Hebert, R. L. (1999) Advances in the signal transduction of ceramide and related sphingolipids. *Crit. Rev. Clin. Lab. Sci.* **36,** 511–573.
3. Pena, L. A., Fuks, Z., and Kolesnick, R. (1997) Stress-induced apoptosis and the sphingomyelin pathway. *Biochem. Pharmacol.* **53,** 615–621.
4. Levade, T. and Jaffrezou, J. P. (1999) Signalling sphingomyelinases: which, where, how and why? *Biochim. Biophys. Acta* **1438,** 1–17.
5. Liu, B., Obeid, L. M., and Hannun, Y. A. (1997) Sphingomyelinases in cell regulation. *Semin. Cell Dev. Biol.* **8,** 311–322.
6. Cabot, M. C., Giuliano, A. E., Han, T. Y., and Liu, Y. Y. (1999) SDZ PSC 833, the cyclosporine A analogue and multidrug resistance modulator, activates ceramide synthesis and increases vinblastine sensitivity in drug-sensitive and drug-resistant cancer cells. *Cancer Res.* **59,** 880–885.
7. Bose, R., Verheij, M., Haimovitz-Friedman, A., Scotto, K., Fuks, Z., and Kolesnick, R. (1995) Ceramide synthase mediates daunorubicin-induced apoptosis: an alternative mechanism for generating death signals. *Cell* **82,** 405–414.
8. Liu, Y. Y., Han, T. Y., Giuliano, A. E., and Cabot, M. C. (1999) Expression of glucosylceramide synthase, converting ceramide to glucosylceramide, confers adriamycin resistance in human breast cancer cells. *J. Biol. Chem.* **274,** 1140–1146.
9. Senchenkov, A., Litvak, D. A., and Cabot, M. C. (2001) Targeting ceramide metabolism—a strategy for overcoming drug resistance. *J. Natl. Cancer Inst.* **93,** 347–357.
10. Kolesnick, R. (2002) The therapeutic potential of modulating the ceramide/sphingomyelin pathway. *J. Clin. Invest.* **110,** 3–8.
11. Modrak, D. E., Rodriguez, M. D., Goldenberg, D. M., Lew, W., and Blumenthal, R. D. (2002) Sphingomyelin enhances chemotherapy efficacy and increases apoptosis in human colonic tumor xenografts. *Int. J. Oncol.* **20,** 379–384.
12. Merrill, A. and Hannun, Y. (eds.) (2000) *Sphingolipid Metabolism and Cell Signalling, Part A, Vol. 311*. Academic, London.

13. Merrill, A. and Hannun, Y. (eds.) (2000) *Sphingolipid Metabolism and Cell Signalling, Part B, Vol. 312.* Academic, London.
14. Hansen, H. J., Goldenberg, D. M., Newman, E. S., Grebenau, R., and Sharkey, R. M. (1993) Characterization of second-generation monoclonal antibodies against carcinoembryonic antigen. *Cancer* **71**, 3478–3485.
15. Bligh, E. G. and Dyer, W. J. (1959) A rapid method of total lipid extraction and purification. *Can. J. Biochem. Physiol.* **37**, 911–917.
16. Ames, B. N. (1966) Assay of inorganic phosphate, total phosphate and phosphatases. *Meth. Enzymol.* **8**, 115–118.
17. Bodennec, J., Brichon, G., Koul, O., El Babili, M., and Zwingelstein, G. (1997) A two-dimensional thin-layer chromatography procedure for simultaneous separation of ceramide and diacylglycerol species. *J. Lipid Res.* **38**, 1702–1706.
18. Morgan, E. T., Nikolova-Karakashian, M., Chen, J. Q., and Merrill, A. H. Jr. (1996) Sphingolipid-dependent signaling in regulation of cytochrome P450 expression. *Meth. Enzymol.* **272**, 381–388.
19. Watts, J. D., Gu, M., Polverino, A. J., Patterson, S. D., and Aebersold, R. (1997) Fas-induced apoptosis of T cells occurs independently of ceramide generation. *Proc. Natl. Acad. Sci. USA* **94**, 7292–7296.
20. Tepper, A. D. and Van Blitterswijk, W. J. (2000) Ceramide mass analysis by normal-phase high-performance liquid chromatography. *Meth. Enzymol.* **312**, 16–22.
21. Liu, P. and Anderson, R. G. (1995) Compartmentalized production of ceramide at the cell surface. *J. Biol. Chem.* **270**, 27,179–27,185.
22. Sillence, D. J., Raggers, R. J., and van Meer, G. (2000) Assays for transmembrane movement of sphingolipids. *Meth. Enzymol.* **312**, 562–579.
23. Liu, B. and Hannun, Y. A. (2000) Sphingomyelinase assay using radiolabeled substrate. *Meth. Enzymol.* **311**, 164–167.
24. Hertervig, E., Nilsson, A., Nyberg, L., and Duan, R. D. (1997) Alkaline sphingomyelinase activity is decreased in human colorectal carcinoma. *Cancer* **79**, 448–453.
25. Shayman, J. A. and Abe, A. (2000) Glucosylceramide synthase: assay and properties. *Meth. Enzymol.* **311**, 42–49.
26. Nikolova-Karakashian, M. (2000) Assays for the biosynthesis of sphingomyelin and ceramide phosphoethanolamine. *Meth. Enzymol.* **311**, 31–42.
27. Nikolova-Karakashian, M. and Merrill, A. H. Jr. (2000) Ceramidases. *Meth. Enzymol.* **311**, 194–201.
28. Perry, D. K. and Hannun, Y. A. (1999) The use of diglyceride kinase for quantifying ceramide. *Trends Biochem. Sci.* **24**, 226–227.
29. Liu, B. and Hannun, Y. A. (1997) Inhibition of the neutral magnesium-dependent sphingomyelinase by glutathione. *J. Biol. Chem.* **272**, 16,281–16,287.
30. Brenkert, A. and Radin, N. S. (1972) Synthesis of galactosyl ceramide and glucosyl ceramide by rat brain: assay procedures and changes with age. *Brain Res.* **36**, 183–193.
31. Shukla, G. S. and Radin, N. S. (1990) Glucosyceramide synthase of mouse kidney: further characterization with an improved assay method. *Arch. Biochem. Biophys.* **283**, 372–378.

# II

# GENOMICS, PROTEOMICS, AND CHEMOSENSITIVITY

# 14

## Gene Expression Profiling to Characterize Anticancer Drug Sensitivity

### James K. Breaux and Gerrit Los

#### Summary

This chapter presents a protocol for using cDNA microarrays to acquire gene expression profiles that characterize anticancer drug sensitivity. The protocol includes steps for drug exposure, RNA isolation, preparation of fluorescently labeled samples, microarray hybridization, data processing, and data analysis. In addition to the detailed protocol, important experimental design issues are discussed, and some preliminary experiments are recommended.

#### Key Words

Cancer; cDNA microarray; chemotherapy; drug sensitivity; drug resistance; gene expression profile.

## 1. Introduction

Resistance to chemotherapy remains a major obstacle in the treatment of cancer patients. A better understanding of the differences between sensitive cells and resistant cells at the molecular level will lead to the development of more efficacious therapies. One molecular aspect that can be studied is mRNA expression, and there is a great deal of evidence that cells that are sensitive to a particular treatment display different transcriptional profiles than cells that are resistant *(1–6)*. A recently developed tool that is extremely useful for acquiring such transcriptional profiles is the DNA microarray, which allows simultaneous detection of the expression levels of thousands of genes. The protocol presented in this chapter is an example of how DNA microarrays can be used to obtain expression profiles that characterize cells that are sensitive or resistant to a particular drug treatment.

Differences in gene expression that confer sensitivity or resistance to a drug might be evident prior to any drug exposure. For example, cells that have high steady-state levels of metallothionein are often resistant to cisplatin (reviewed in **ref. 7**). Alternatively, the altered expression leading to increased sensitivity or resistance may not be apparent until the drug response occurs. For example, it was recently observed that relative mRNA levels of the apoptosis inhibitor survivin *(8)* were similar in two cell lines (one of which was relatively sensitive to cisplatin while the other was relatively resistant) prior to treatment with cisplatin *(9)*. However, at the 24-h time point following drug treatment, survivin mRNA had significantly increased in the resistant cell line, while no significant change was observed in the sensitive cell line. While it remains to be shown whether the increase in survivin mRNA played a direct role in the resistant phenotype, this potentially important difference between the sensitive and resistant cell lines would have been missed if only steady-state expression levels had been studied. Thus, to fully characterize differences in mRNA expression that are associated with sensitive/resistant cells, one should consider obtaining both steady-state expression profiles as well as profiles following drug exposure.

The expression profiles yielded by studies performed as described in this chapter are useful for at least three purposes. First, they will lead to a better understanding of the mechanism of action of the drug treatment being studied (*see* **Notes 1** and **2**). Second, comparison of the profiles of sensitive and resistant cell lines will potentially identify new molecules involved in conferring sensitivity or resistance (*see* **Note 3**). Finally, mRNA expression profiles can often be used to classify samples into groups in which the members of each group have a similar phenotype *(10–20)*. Thus, it might be possible to use expression profiles of tumors to classify the tumors as sensitive or resistant to a particular drug treatment. Some studies have already demonstrated encouraging results that indicate that this approach might be feasible *(21–24)*. The ability to screen patients' tumors for drug sensitivity would be extremely advantageous for patients and would afford physicians the ability to select the optimal therapy for each patient.

### 1.1. Overview of the Protocol

As noted above, profiling can be performed on cells at steady state or following drug treatment. The protocol presented in this chapter is an example of the latter; however, steady-state profiles could be obtained using the same general protocol (*see* **Notes 4** and **5**). An overview of the protocol is displayed in **Figs. 1** and **2**, and the steps are summarized below.

---

Fig. 1. *(see facing page)* Schematic overview of microarray hybridization protocol for gene expression profiling following drug treatment. See **Subheading 1.1.** for details.

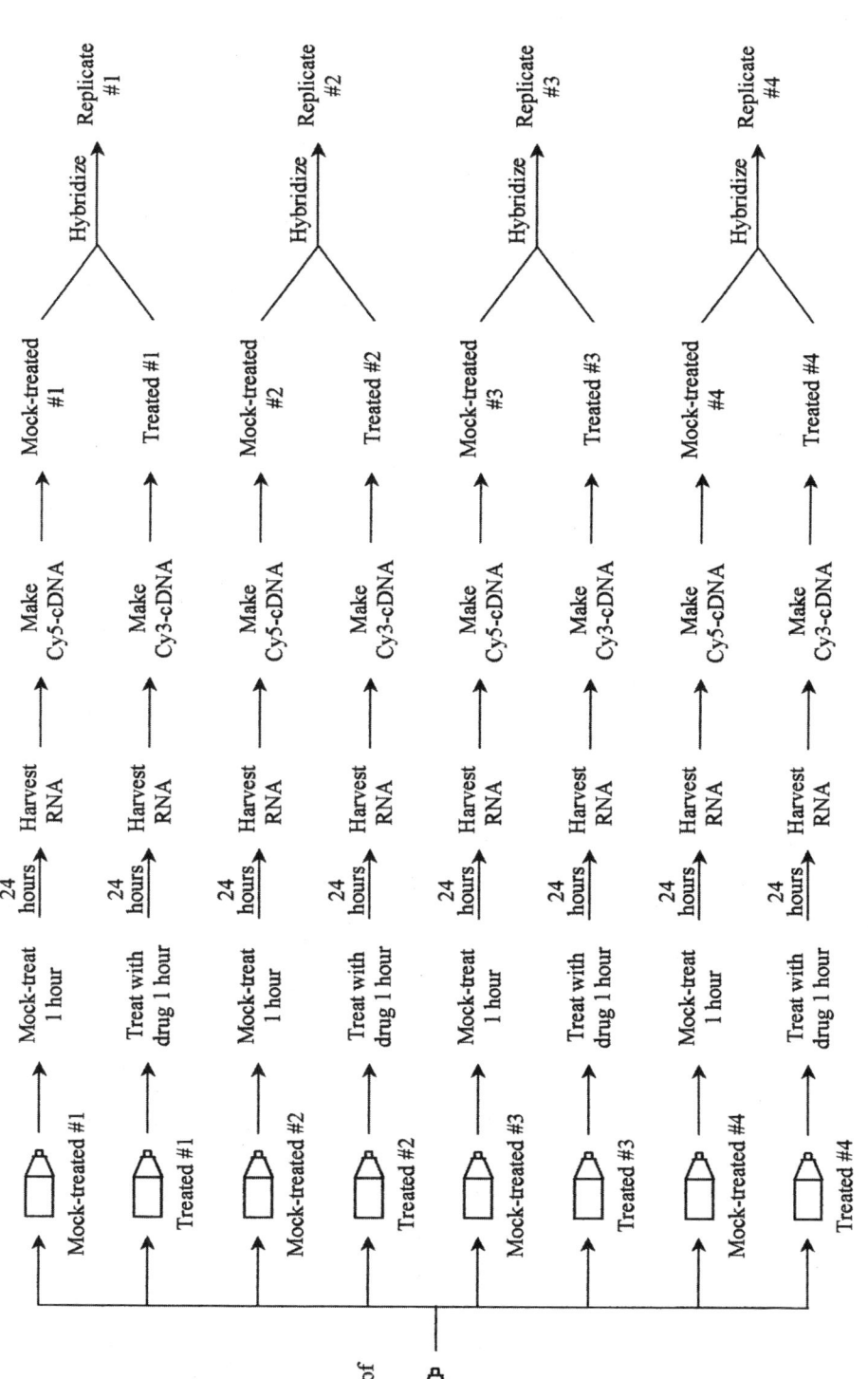

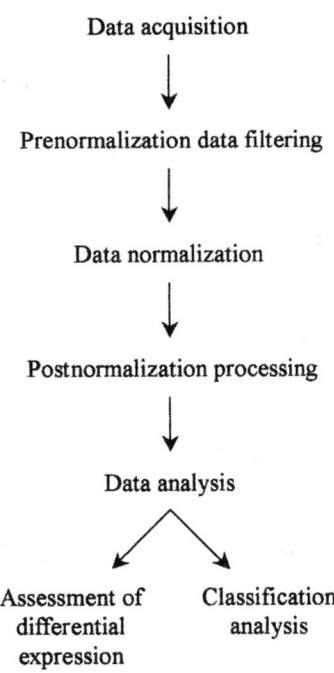

Fig. 2. Overview of acquisition, processing and analysis of microarray data. Displayed are the major steps involved in the acquisition, processing, and analysis of microarray data. The first three steps are performed independently for each microarray. **Data acquisition** entails scanning the microarray, aligning a grid to the resulting image of the microarray, visually inspecting the grid, flagging problematic spots, and extracting data for each spot. The extracted data include the Cy3 intensity and Cy5 intensity for each spot as well as information that is used during the subsequent step: **Prenormalization data filtering.** This step involves removing the data for spots that were flagged during grid alignment or that do not meet certain quality control criteria. In addition, local background intensity can be subtracted from the spots during this step. **Data normalization** refers to a procedure that is used to remove systematic bias in the expression data. During **postnormalization processing**, the data are prepared for the specific type of data analysis that is to ensue. In some cases this involves processing of data from individual arrays (e.g., taking the median intensity for replicate spots on an array, or removing genes for which a minimum number of replicate measurements are not obtained on a given array). In other cases it entails processing of data for multiple arrays (e.g., removing genes for which a minimum number of replicate measurements are not obtained among the arrays to be analyzed). Two general types of data analysis are discussed in the protocol presented in this chapter: **assessment of differential expression** (used to select genes that are differentially expressed with some degree of statistical significance) and **classification analysis** (used to select genes whose expression levels allow the samples being studied to be classified into two or more groups).

# Gene Expression Profiling

The following steps are performed for each cell line to be characterized:

1. Cells are seeded into a tissue culture flask.
2. After the cells become approx 80% confluent, the cells are collected and split into eight flasks. Four of the flasks are designated for treatment and the other four are designated for mock treatment.
3. The cells are allowed to reach a certain level of confluence and then they are mock-treated or treated with drug for an hour.
4. After a 24-h incubation, RNA is harvested from all samples.
5. Cy3-labeled cDNA is generated from the treated samples and Cy5-labeled cDNA is generated from the mock-treated samples.
6. Each Cy3-treated sample is mixed with a Cy5-mock-treated sample, and each mixed sample is allowed to hybridize to a microarray (four microarrays total).
7. The microarrays are scanned, and Cy3 and Cy5 intensity data are acquired.
8. The data are processed and then analyzed to identify differentially expressed genes.

Once differentially expressed genes are identified for each cell line, the lists of differentially expressed genes can be compared to identify changes in expression that are common to multiple sensitive cell lines and those that are common to multiple resistant cell lines. In addition, if expression profiles are obtained for a large enough panel of cell lines, classification analysis can be performed to determine if the expression profiles can be used to classify the cell lines as being sensitive or resistant.

## 1.2. Experimental Design

There are many experimental design issues that are pertinent to the gene expression profiling protocol presented in this chapter. The essential issues are discussed below.

### 1.2.1. Choice of Microarray

DNA microarrays come in two major varieties: (1) the cDNA microarray, in which polymerase chain reaction (PCR)-amplified cDNA molecules are spotted in an array on a glass slide (i.e., each spot in the array contains a single species of cDNA); (2) the oligonucleotide microarray, in which oligonucleotides are spotted on a glass slide or synthesized directly on a quartz wafer (i.e., each spot in the array contains a single species of oligonucleotide representing a specific gene). Most of our experience has involved working with cDNA microarrays, so the protocol presented in this chapter employs that variety. Similar studies could be performed using oligonucleotide microarrays, but significant changes would have to be made to the protocol as it is presented below.

Our protocol assumes that you already have a cDNA microarray that you are planning to use (i.e., we do not explain how to fabricate your own microarray). If you are interested in fabricating a custom microarray, *see* **ref. 25**. If you are looking for a commercially available cDNA microarray, we have had good success using microarrays purchased from Stanford (*see* www.microarray.org/sfgf/) and University Health Network (*see* www.microarrays.ca/).

### 1.2.2. Samples to Be Profiled

Expression profiles for characterizing sensitivity can be derived from tumor cell lines or from tumor biopsies. Our experience has involved working with cell lines, so that is what is described in the following protocol (*see* **Note 6**). The protocol assumes that you have at least two cell lines for which you want to generate expression profiles: one cell line that is sensitive to the drug treatment in question and one that is resistant. For example, you might have a sensitive cell line and a resistant variant that was derived from the sensitive cell line (e.g., through repeated drug exposure—*see* **refs. *26*** and ***27***). Alternatively, you might have a panel of cell lines, some representing sensitive cells and some representing resistant cells. Whatever the case, it is useful to establish the relative level of sensitivity/resistance for each cell line being studied (e.g., by performing colony-forming assays with each cell line—*see* **refs. *26*** and ***27***).

### 1.2.3. Drug Treatment Parameters

Two important experimental design issues related to the drug treatment are the concentration of drug and the length of exposure to be employed. We feel that when performing studies on cells in culture, one should try to simulate the conditions that would be encountered by a tumor in vivo. Thus, if a drug tends to be administered to patients via an iv bolus injection or a 30-min infusion, a 1-h exposure in vitro is more like the clinical situation than a continuous exposure. Similarly, the concentration of drug administered to cells in culture should be within the range of plasma concentrations of the drug that are attainable in patients.

### 1.2.4. Time Point(s) to Be Studied

For a more complete characterization of the changes in expression associated with drug sensitivity/resistance, multiple time points should be studied. However, limiting resources very often preclude the ability to examine multiple time points. If one wants to use the profiles for classification analysis, one time point might be sufficient. For simplicity, the protocol presented in this chapter describes the examination of a single time point (the protocol could easily be adapted to look at more time points). When the objective is to study a single time point, it might be worthwhile to perform a pilot study (with minimal replication, and possibly with only one cell line) in which multiple time points are examined in order to determine if one of them is optimal for the detection of

# Gene Expression Profiling

differentially expressed genes. If none of the time points is found to be optimal, other criteria can be used to select a time point (e.g., you might select the time point that is most clinically relevant or the time point that affords the most convenient experimental setup).

## 1.2.5. Hybridization Format

Because two-color hybridizations allow you to hybridize two samples at the same time to the microarray, you have to make a choice as to what those two samples should be. In the current protocol, we describe how to co-hybridize a mock-treated sample (labeled with Cy5) and a treated sample (labeled with Cy3). An alternative format would be to employ a common reference sample for each hybridization (*see* **Note 7**). For example, you might hybridize mock-treated Cy5 with reference Cy3 on one microarray, and then treated Cy5 with reference Cy3 on another microarray. The obvious disadvantage of employing a reference sample is that you have to perform twice as many hybridizations. However, one important advantage is that you can perform more analyses with the data. For example, if you wanted to compare the expression level of a gene in the treated samples from one cell line to the treated samples in another cell line, you could do such a comparison if you were to co-hybridize all samples with a common reference sample, but you could not do this if you were to co-hybridize mock-treated and treated samples (*see* **Note 8**).

## 1.2.6. Number of Replicates

We feel that it is important to have at least three or four replicates per condition (preferably more) *(28)*. In addition, these replicates should be biological replicates (e.g., independent harvests of RNA, rather than taking multiple aliquots of the same RNA and performing replicated fluorescent cDNA preparation or taking multiple aliquots of the same fluorescent cDNA samples and hybridizing to multiple microarrays). Having at least three biological replicates will ensure that you can assess the statistical significance of the observed changes in gene expression.

Another type of replicate that might be important to do is a dye-switch replicate, in which the dyes used to label the two co-hybridized samples are switched (e.g., for the current protocol, the treated sample would be labeled with Cy5 and the mock-treated sample with Cy3). Some researchers have reported seeing dye-specific effects in which a gene will display higher intensity for one of the dyes regardless of which of the two samples is labeled with that dye. Performing dye-switch hybridizations will help you identify such genes. However, if you are limited as to the number of hybridizations that you can perform, we recommend that you not carry out any dye-switch hybridizations (just realize that you might have a higher number of false positives and negatives than if you had been able to perform the dye-switch hybridizations). Note that dye switching is not necessary if you employ a common reference sample in all hybridizations.

### 1.3. Suggested Preliminary Experiments

If you are performing cDNA microarray experiments for the first time, we highly suggest that you perform some preliminary experiments to validate your technique. The following are two examples of preliminary validation experiments that could be performed:

1. Many microarrays have control spots that contain genes from a different species than the organism being studied. You can generate cRNA for these genes through in vitro transcription, and then spike known amounts of the cRNA into two samples to be labeled (i.e., in **step 1** under **Subheading 3.3.1.**) *(29)*. By spiking different amounts of a gene into the sample to be labeled with Cy3 and the sample to be labeled with Cy5, you can assess your ability to detect differential abundance of that gene. In addition, different genes can be spiked at different ratios so that you can assess your limit of detection.
2. If control spots are not available, an alternative experiment that you can do is simply to perform a hybridization comparing two extremely different cell types (for example, a T-cell vs a fibroblast). The differences in gene expression between such divergent cell types should be large in number (and many of the differences should be large in magnitude as well), so this is a good test of your technique.

## 2. Materials
### 2.1. Cell Culture and Drug Exposure

1. 150-$cm^2$ tissue culture flasks (Fisher; cat. no. 10-126-34).
2. Cell culture medium and supplements appropriate for the particular cell lines being studied.
3. Drug(s) to be studied (*see* **Note 9**).
4. PBS (Invitrogen, cat. no. 14190144).

### 2.2. RNA Isolation

Required materials will depend on which RNA isolation procedure you utilize.

### 2.3. Preparation of Fluorescently Labeled Samples

*2.3.1. Preparation of Aminoallyl-Labeled cDNA (aa-cDNA)*

1. DEPC-treated water, certified nuclease-free (Ambion, cat. no. 9920).
2. 1 $M$ Tris-HCl, pH 8.0 (Ambion, cat. no. 9855G): Dilute to 10 m$M$ Tris-HCl, pH 8.0, with DEPC-treated water.

## Gene Expression Profiling

3. Oligo(dT)$_{20}$-VN (custom order from QIAGEN, http://oligos.qiagen.com): Dilute oligo(dT)$_{20}$-VN to 4 µg/µL with 10 mM Tris, pH 8.0.
4. 50 mM 5-(3-aminoallyl)-dUTP (aa-dUTP; Ambion, cat. no. 8439).
5. Sequencing Grade Solution dNTP Set, 100 mM Solutions (Amersham Biosciences, cat. no. 27-2035-01).
6. Prepare a 25X aa-dUTP/dNTP solution by mixing the following:
   a. 7.5 µL 100 mM dATP (500 µM in final 1X solution).
   b. 7.5 µL 100 mM dCTP (500 µM in final 1X solution).
   c. 7.5 µL 100 mM dGTP (500 µM in final 1X solution).
   d. 2.5 µL 100 mM dTTP (167 µM in final 1X solution).
   e. 10 µL 50 mM aa-dUTP (333 µM in final 1X solution).
   f. 25 µL DEPC-treated water.
7. SuperScript II RNase H⁻ Reverse Transcriptase, including 5X First-Strand Buffer and 0.1 M dithiothreitol (DTT) (Invitrogen, cat. no. 18064014).
8. RNaseOUT Recombinant Ribonuclease Inhibitor (Invitrogen, cat. no. 10777019).
9. 1 M NaOH.
10. 1 M HCl.
11. 1 M Tris-HCl, pH 7.0: Dilute to 10 mM Tris-HCl, with DEPC-treated water.

### 2.3.2. Purification of aa-cDNA

1. 3 M sodium acetate, pH 5.5 (Ambion, cat. no. 9740).
2. QIAquick PCR purification kit (QIAGEN, cat. no.28104).
3. 100% ethanol (AAPER; see www.aaper.com/). Dilute to 75% with DEPC-treated water.

### 2.3.3. Coupling Cy Dye to aa-cDNA

1. DMSO (anhydrous; Sigma-Aldrich, cat. no. 27,685-5).
2. Cy3 Mono-Reactive Dye Pack (Amersham Biosciences, cat. no. PA23001) and Cy5 Mono-Reactive Dye Pack (Amersham Biosciences, cat. no. PA25001). When the tubes are first received, store them unopened at 4°C.
3. Make working aliquots of the Cy dyes as follows:
   a. Resuspend one tube with 33 µL dimethyl sulfoxide (DMSO). Mix well with pipettor.
   b. Aliquot 2 µL to each of 16 0.5-mL PCR tubes.
   c. Dry the samples in a vacuum concentrator (*see* **Note 10**).
   d. Store at 4°C in the dark in a jar containing desiccant (*see* **Note 11**).
4. Prepare NaHCO$_3$ labeling buffer as follows:
   a. Weigh approx 25 mg NaHCO$_3$ in a 1.5-mL microcentrifuge tube.
   b. Add DEPC-treated water so that the final concentration of NaHCO$_3$ is 25 mg/mL.
   c. Vortex until solid is completely dissolved.
   d. Store in 100-µL aliquots at –20°C (should be stable for at least 6 mo) (*see* **Note 12**).

## 2.4. Hybridization

### 2.4.1. Final Sample Preparation

1. Oligo(dA)$_{20}$ (custom ordered from Proligo; see www.proligo.com/).
2. Human Cot-1 DNA (Invitrogen, cat. no. 15279011).
3. Prepare hyb-block as follows:
    a. Mix 100 µg of Oligo(dA)$_{20}$ and 100 µg of Cot-1 DNA in a 1.5-mL microcentrifuge tube.
    b. Add 1/10 vol of 3 $M$ sodium acetate, pH 5.5, and mix well.
    c. Add 2.5 vol 100% ethanol and mix well.
    d. Put at –80°C for at least 1 h (you can do –20°C overnight, too).
    e. Spin at full speed in a microcentrifuge at 4°C for 15 min.
    f. Carefully aspirate (and discard) most of the supernatant using a 1000-µL pipettor. Then aspirate the rest of the supernatant using a 100-µL or 200-µL pipettor.
    g. Add 500 µL of 75% ethanol to wash the pellet. Vortex to mix.
    h. Spin at full speed in a microcentrifuge at 4°C for 15 min.
    i. Carefully aspirate the supernatant with a 1000-µL pipettor until the level is just above the pellet. Flash-spin the sample and then carefully aspirate the rest of the supernatant using a 20-µL pipettor.
    j. Let the pellet air-dry for about 10 min and then resuspend with 10 µL DEPC-treated water. Shake the sample at room temperature for 15 min to ensure complete resuspension. Flash-spin the sample to collect.
4. Formamide (Fisher, cat. no. BP227-500).
5. 20X SSC: Mix 175.3 g NaCl (3 $M$ final) and 88.2 g sodium citrate dihydrate (0.3 $M$ final) in 800 mL NANOpure water. Adjust pH to 7.0. Adjust total volume to 1 L with NANOpure water.
6. 10% sodium dodecyl sulfate (SDS): 50 g SDS: in 500 mL NANOpure water; autoclave or filter before use.
7. 0.1 $M$ DTT (use the tube that comes with SuperScript II RT; *see* **Subheading 2.3.1.**).
8. Osmonics Cameo 3N 0.22-µm syringe filters (Fisher, cat. no. DDR0200300).
9. Prepare hyb-buffer as follows in a 1.5-mL microcentrifuge tube:
    a. Mix 500 µL formamide (50% final) with 239 µL NANOpure water.
    b. Add 250 µL 20X SSC (5X final) and mix.
    c. Add 10 µL 10% SDS (0.1% final) and mix.
    d. Add 1 µL 0.1 $M$ DTT (0.1 m$M$ final) and mix.
    e. Filter into a new 1.5-mL microcentrifuge tube using a syringe filter.
    f. Store at 4°C (*see* **Notes 13** and **14**).

### 2.4.2. Microarray Preparation

1. LifterSlips (Erie Scientific; www.eriesci.com/) (*see* **Note 15**).
2. Slide forceps.
3. BSA (Fisher, cat. no. BP1600-100).

# Gene Expression Profiling

4. Wheaton Coplin jar (Fisher, cat. no. 08-813E).
5. Prepare prehyb-buffer in a 50-mL conical tube as follows (*see* **Note 16**):
   a. Put 0.5 g bovine serum albumin (BSA) (1% final) into the conical tube and dissolve in 37 mL NANOpure water (stir with a small magnetic stir bar).
   b. Add 12.5 mL 20X SSC (5X final) and stir to mix.
   c. Add 500 µL of 10% SDS (0.1% final) and stir to mix.
   d. Filter and pour into a Coplin jar.
   e. Place the Coplin jar containing the prehyb-buffer into a hybridization oven. Preheat the prehyb-buffer to 42°C.
6. Isopropanol (Fisher, cat. no. BP2632-4).

### 2.4.3. Posthybridization Washing (see **Note 17**)

1. Six 24-oz plastic storage containers (can purchase from local grocery store). Label these "Wash container #1" through "Wash container #6."
2. Four 50-mL conical tubes.
3. Two Wheaton slide racks (Fisher, cat. no. 08-812-1B and 08-812-1C).
4. Wash solution #1: 1X SSC, 0.1% SDS (100 mL 20X SSC, 20 mL 10% SDS, 1880 mL NANOpure water).
5. Wash solution #2: 1X SSC (45 mL 20X SSC, 855 mL NANOpure water).
6. Wash solution #3: 0.2X SSC (4.5 mL 20X SSC, 445.5 mL NANOpure water).

## 2.5. Data Processing

1. Microarray scanner (e.g., GenePix 4000A from Axon Instruments; www.axon.com/).
2. Software for image processing and data acquisition (e.g., GenePix Pro; also from Axon Instruments).
3. Software for processing data, e.g.,
   a. Microsoft Excel (Microsoft; www.microsoft.com/).
   b. R statistical computing environment (*see* http://cran.us.r-project.org/).

## 2.6. Data Analysis

1. Software for assessment of differential expression (e.g., Significance Analysis of Microarrays; *see* www-stat.stanford.edu/~tibs/SAM/).
2. Database software (e.g., Microsoft Access; www.microsoft.com/).
3. Software for classification analysis (e.g., Prediction Analysis for Microarrays; *see* www-stat.stanford.edu/~tibs/PAM/).

# 3. Methods
## 3.1. Cell Culture and Drug Exposure (see Note 18)

**Subheadings 3.1.** and **3.2.** are written for the processing of one cell line. The procedure as described below should be performed on all cell lines that are to be profiled.

### 3.1.1. Preparation of Cells for Drug Treatment

1. Expand cells until they are approx 80% confluent in a 150-cm² flask.
2. Collect cells and split into eight separate flasks. Four of these flasks will be for mock treatment and the other four will be for treatment (*see* **Fig. 1**).
3. Monitor the cells and perform the drug treatment when the cells are approx 40–70% confluent (*see* **Note 19**).

### 3.1.2. Drug Treatment

1. Prepare 100 mL cell culture medium with the desired concentration of drug.
2. Remove flasks from the incubator (*see* **Note 20**).
3. For each flask, aspirate the cell growth medium and add 24 mL fresh medium (to the mock-treated flasks) or fresh medium + drug (for the treated flasks).
4. Return the flasks to the incubator for 1 h.
5. After the 1-h incubation, aspirate the medium and wash the cells in each flask with 25 mL PBS (*see* **Note 9**).
6. Aspirate the wash and add fresh cell culture medium.
7. Return flasks to incubator.

## 3.2. RNA Isolation

1. Remove flasks from incubator (*see* **Note 20**). Examine cells under microscope and make a note of their condition (*see* **Note 21**).
2. Aspirate medium. Wash cells with 25 mL PBS.
3. Isolate total RNA from all eight flasks using the standard method employed by your laboratory (*see* **Note 22**).
4. Quantitate the RNA as follows (*see* **Note 23**):
   a. Measure the $A_{230}$, $A_{260}$, and $A_{280}$ using a spectrophotometer.
   b. Calculate [RNA] (*see* **Note 24**):

   $1\ A_{260}$ = 40 ng/µL for RNA when the path length of the cuvet is 1 cm

   [RNA] (µg/µL) = ($A_{260}$ × 40 × df) / 1000 where df is the dilution factor

   c. Calculate the $A_{260} / A_{230}$ and $A_{260} / A_{280}$ ratios. The former should be above 2.0 and the latter should be above 1.9; otherwise, the RNA may not be of high enough quality.

## 3.3. Preparation of Fluorescently Labeled Samples (see Note 25)

The steps in this section explain how fluorescently labeled cDNA is generated from the mRNA in a total RNA sample (*see* **Note 26**). First the mRNA is reverse-transcribed into cDNA using anchored oligo(dT) primers. During this step, a modified nucleotide (aminoallyl-dUTP) is incorporated into the cDNA. After purifying the aminoallyl-labeled cDNA, fluorescent Cy dyes (either Cy3 or Cy5) are coupled to the cDNA molecules via reaction with the aminoallyl groups. Finally, the fluorescently labeled cDNA is purified from any free Cy dye that remains.

The protocol below is written for a single sample. If you are following the experimental design proposed under **Subheading 1.1.**, there will actually be eight samples (four mock-treated samples and four treated samples) for each cell line. In order to minimize potential variability that might occur if samples are prepared on different days, we recommend processing all eight samples simultaneously.

### 3.3.1. Preparation of Aminoallyl-Labeled cDNA (aa-cDNA)

1. Put 25–50 µg of total RNA into a 0.5-mL PCR tube.
2. Add 1 µL (4 µg) oligo(dT)$_{20}$-VN (*see* **Note 27**).
3. Add DEPC-treated water to 16.8 µL total volume, and then mix well with a pipettor set at 10 µL.
4. Incubate at 70°C for 10 min in a thermal cycler; then chill on ice for 10 min. Flash-spin to collect the sample.
5. Finish preparing the reverse-transcription reaction as follows (*see* **Note 28**):
   a. To the RNA sample, add 6 µL 5X Superscript II First-Strand Buffer and vortex to mix.
   b. Add 3 µL 0.1 $M$ DTT (10 m$M$ final) and vortex to mix.
   c. Add 1.2 µL 25X aa-dUTP/dNTP solution and vortex to mix.
   d. Add 1 µL RNaseOUT (1.33 U/µL final) and 2 µL SuperScript II RT (13.3 U/µL final), and then vortex to mix.
   e. Flash-spin the sample to collect.
6. Incubate the sample at 42°C for 2 h in a thermal cycler (*see* **Note 29**).
7. Incubate the sample at 95°C for 5 min in a thermal cycler (*see* **Notes 30** and **31**). Snap-cool by immediately placing the sample on ice. Incubate for at least 2 min and then flash spin.
8. Add 12.9 µL of 1 $M$ NaOH (0.3 $M$ final). Quickly mix 3–4 times with pipettor and then vortex. Flash-spin and then incubate at 65°C in thermal cycler for 30 min (*see* **Note 32**).
9. Flash-spin the sample to collect it, and then neutralize the reaction by adding 12.9 µL of 1 $M$ HCl. Quickly mix 3–4 times with pipettor and then vortex.
10. Add 6.2 µL of 1 $M$ Tris, pH 7.0 (0.1 $M$ final). Vortex to mix.
11. Add 38 µL DEPC-treated water to bring the final volume to 100 µL (*see* **Note 33**). Vortex to mix.

### 3.3.2. Purification of aa-cDNA

QIAquick purification columns are used to purify the aa-cDNA (to remove unincorporated aa-dUTP and the hydrolyzed RNA). The following steps are based on the original protocol from QIAGEN, but several essential modifications are included. These modifications are necessary because the QIAGEN protocol employs Tris buffers, and Tris cannot be present during the coupling step (described under **Subheading 3.3.3.**).

1. Insert a QIAquick column into a collection tube (both are provided with the kit).
2. Add 550 µL Buffer PB (provided with the kit) to the cDNA sample and mix with a pipettor.
3. Add 10 µL of 3 $M$ sodium acetate, pH 5.5, and mix with a pipettor (*see* **Notes 34 and 35**).
4. Transfer the sample to the column and spin the column for 1 min at 11,750$g$.
5. Carefully discard the flow-through (we prefer to aspirate with a pipettor).
6. Add 725 µL 75% ethanol to the QIAquick column to wash. Spin for 1 min at 11,750$g$.
7. Pour out the flow-through and repeat the wash.
8. Pour out the flow-through and then spin the column at 11,750$g$ for an additional minute to remove any residual ethanol.
9. Transfer the column to a clean 1.5-mL microcentrifuge tube.
10. Add 52 µL DEPC-treated water and incubate for 5 min.
11. Elute the cDNA by spinning the column at 11,750$g$ for 1 min.
12. Repeat **steps 10** and **11** (elute into the same microcentrifuge tube). After the second elution, the total volume should be approx 100 µL (*see* **Note 36**).

### 3.3.3. Coupling Cy Dye to aa-cDNA (see Note 37)

1. Concentrate the aa-cDNA sample using a vacuum concentrator. The sample does not need to be completely dry (just less than or equal to 7 µL). Do not overdry the sample.
2. Resuspend the aa-cDNA in 7 µL DEPC-treated water (if the sample is not completely dry, just add DEPC-treated water up to 7 µL). Rinse the walls of the tube as you mix with a pipettor.
3. Flash-spin to collect the sample.
4. Add 3 µL of the $NaHCO_3$ labeling buffer and quickly mix with pipettor.
5. Incubate with shaking for at least 15 min (*see* **Note 38**).
6. Resuspend a prealiquotted tube of Cy dye with 1 µL DMSO.
7. Add the Cy dye to the aa-cDNA and quickly vortex to mix. Flash-spin to collect the sample.
8. Incubate the sample for 1 h in the dark at room temperature.
9. Add 90 µL DEPC-treated water to bring the final volume to 100 µL. Vortex to mix.

### 3.3.4. Purification of Cy Dye-Labeled cDNA

The Cy-labeled cDNA must be purified to remove any uncoupled Cy dye. As with the previous purification, we recommend using QIAquick PCR purification columns. Use the same protocol as described above under **Subheading 3.3.2.** with the following modifications:

# Gene Expression Profiling

1. In **steps 6** and **7**, wash with 725 μL Buffer PE (provided with the kit) (*see* **Note 39**).
2. For **steps 10–12**, dilute Buffer EB (provided with the kit) 1:5 with NANOpure water, and use the resulting buffer for elution (*see* **Note 40**).

## *3.4. Hybridization (see Note 41)*

The hybridization protocol presented below describes the steps involved in setting up a hybridization for a single microarray (e.g., co-hybridizing a Cy3-treated sample and a Cy5-mock-treated sample to a microarray). If you are following the experimental design suggested under **Subheading 1.1.**, there will be four microarrays for each cell line being studied. To minimize variability, all four hybridizations for a given cell line should be set up simultaneously; however, pay special attention to the note at the beginning of **Subheading 3.4.3.**

### *3.4.1. Final Sample Preparation*

1. Quantitate each Cy-labeled sample as follows (*see* **Note 42**):
   a. Remove 20 μL of the sample and mix with 40 μL of 10 m$M$ Tris, pH 7.0.
   b. Prepare a blank by mixing 20 μL elution buffer (i.e., the 1:5 dilution of Buffer EB) with 40 μL of 10 m$M$ Tris, pH 7.0.
   c. Blank the spectrophotometer and then perform a wavelength scan to measure absorbances from 200 to 800 nm.
   d. Calculate [cDNA]:

   $1\ A_{260} = 37$ ng/μL   for cDNA when the path length of the cuvet is 1 cm

   [cDNA] (ng/μL) = ($A_{260} \times 37 \times 3$)   where 3 is the dilution factor

   e. Calculate total yield of cDNA assuming the total volume of the sample is 100 μL (*see* **Note 43**):

   Total yield cDNA (ng) = [cDNA] × 100 μL

   f. Calculate total yield of dNTPs in the cDNA (pmol):

   The average molecular weight of a dNTP is 0.3245 ng/pmol.

   Total yield of dNTPs (pmol) = total yield cDNA/0.3245

   g. Calculate the [Cy dye]:

   The extinction coefficient for Cy3 at 550 nm is 0.15 μ$M^{-1}$cm$^{-1}$.
   The extinction coefficient for Cy5 at 649 nm is 0.25 μ$M^{-1}$cm$^{-1}$.

   [Cy3] (μ$M$) = ($A_{550} \times 3$) / (0.15 × 1 cm)
   [Cy5] (μ$M$) = ($A_{649} \times 3$) / (0.25 × 1 cm)

h. Calculate the total pmol of incorporated dye assuming the total volume of the sample is 100 µL:

$$\mu M = \mu mol/L = pmol/\mu L$$

$$pmol\ dye = [Cy\ dye]\ (pmol/\mu L) \times 100\ \mu L$$

i. Calculate the frequency of incorporation (FOI) expressed as the number of Cy-dUTPs per 1000 dNTPs (*see* **Note 44**):

$$FOI = 1000 \times (pmol\ dye/pmol\ dNTPs)$$

2. Based on the quantitation of the samples, mix the desired amount of the Cy3-labeled sample and the Cy5-labeled sample in a 1.5-mL microcentrifuge tube (*see* **Note 45**).
3. Add 2 µL hyb-block and mix well with a 200-µL pipettor.
4. Dry the sample in a vacuum concentrator. Do not overdry (it is probably better to allow 1 or 2 µL of liquid to remain than to let the sample overdry).
5. Resuspend the sample with 40 µL hyb-buffer (*see* **Note 46**). Incubate with shaking for 10–15 min to facilitate resuspension (*see* **Note 47**).
6. Flash-spin the sample to collect, and then transfer to a 0.5-mL microcentrifuge tube.

### 3.4.2. Microarray Preparation

1. Wash a LifterSlip by dipping in NANOpure water followed by dipping in 100% ethanol. Allow the LifterSlip to air-dry.
2. Add 40 µL NANOpure water to a 50-mL conical tube. This tube will serve as the hyb-chamber for **Subheading 3.4.3., step 6** (*see* **Note 48**).
3. Place a microarray slide in the Coplin jar containing prehyb-buffer (which has been preheated to 42°C). Incubate at 42°C in a hybridization oven for at least 45 min.
4. Wash the slide by dipping approximately 20 times in NANOpure water (*see* **Note 49**).
5. Dip the slide approx 20 times in isopropanol.
6. Dry the slide immediately by spinning at 40*g* for 3 min (*see* **Note 50**).
7. Add the sample to the microarray slide as soon as possible (it was recommended to us not to wait more than 1 h after the prehybridization step is finished).

### 3.4.3. Initiation of Hybridization (see **Note 51**)

1. Denature the sample by incubating at 95°C for 3 min in a thermal cycler.
2. While the sample is denaturing, prepare the microarray slide as follows:
   a. Set the slide array-side-up on a heating block preheated to 42°C.
   b. Take the LifterSlip (cleaned as described under **Subheading 3.4.2.**) and spray with compressed air to remove any dust that might be present.
   c. Carefully set the LifterSlip on top of the slide so that it covers the array.
3. After the 3-min incubation at 95°C, spin the sample at full speed in a microcentrifuge for 2 min.

# Gene Expression Profiling

4. Transfer the sample to a new 0.5-mL microcentrifuge tube (if there is an insoluble pellet, take care not to transfer it).
5. Gently mix the sample in the new tube using the pipettor (do not introduce bubbles), and then immediately apply the sample to the microarray slide (*see* **Note 52**).
6. Carefully place the microarray slide into a hyb-chamber, and seal the hyb-chamber tightly.
7. Place the hyb-chamber into a hyb-oven preheated to 42°C. Incubate for 18 h (*see* **Note 53**).

## 3.4.4. Posthybridization Washing

The wash procedure described below is sufficient for simultaneously washing four microarrays that have been hybridized with similar fluorescent samples (e.g., replicates). It is recommended that microarrays hybridized with fluorescent samples derived from different test conditions (e.g., in the case of this protocol, samples derived from different cell lines) should not be washed together in the same wash containers (i.e., if you want to simultaneously wash microarrays hybridized with fluorescent samples derived from different test conditions, increase the amount of the wash solutions and the number of slide racks and wash containers accordingly). If you are washing only one or two microarray slides, 50-mL conical tubes can be used (one set of conical tubes per slide) instead of the large storage containers, and the amount of the wash solutions can be scaled down.

1. Make sure that all slide racks and wash containers are clean.
2. Prepare wash solutions as described under **Subheading 2.4.3.**
3. Pour wash solutions into wash containers as follows:
   a. Pour 45 mL wash solution #1 into four 50-mL conical tubes.
   b. Pour 450 mL wash solution #1 into Wash containers #1, #2, and #3. Place a slide rack in Wash container #2.
   c. Pour 450 mL wash solution #2 into Wash containers #4 and #5. Place a slide rack in Wash container #5.
   d. Pour 450 mL wash solution #3 into Wash container #6. Place this wash container next to the centrifuge that will be used to dry the slides.
4. Remove the four hyb-chambers from the hyb-oven. Using slide forceps, quickly transfer each slide to a separate 50-mL conical tube containing wash solution #1 (*see* **Notes 54** and **55**).
5. Do the following with each slide (complete all steps for one slide before proceeding with the next one):
   a. Gently dip the slide up and down until the LifterSlip becomes loose.
   b. Slowly remove the slide from the conical tube (make sure that the LifterSlip does not scratch the slide).
   c. Immediately dip and swirl the slide in Wash container #1 for 5 s (*see* **Note 56**).
   d. Transfer the slide to the slide rack sitting in Wash container #2 (*see* **Note 57**).

6. After all slides are in the slide rack in Wash container #2, dip the slide rack up and down in the wash solution for 1 min.
7. Blot the rack on a paper towel and quickly transfer to Wash container #3. Dip the slide rack up and down in the wash for 1 min.
8. Set the slide rack on a paper towel. Pour out the wash in Wash container #3 and add 450 mL fresh wash solution #1. Place the slide-rack back in the wash solution and dip up and down for 1 min.
9. Do the following with each slide (*see* **Note 58**):
   a. Remove the slide from the slide rack.
   b. Immediately dip and swirl the slide in Wash container #4 for 5 s.
   c. Transfer the slide to a slide rack sitting in Wash container #5.
10. Once all slides are in the slide rack in Wash container #5, dip the slide rack up and down in the wash solution for 1 min.
11. Quickly take Wash container #5 (with the slide rack still inside) to the centrifuge that will be used for drying the slides.
12. Blot the slide rack on a paper towel and then transfer to Wash container #6. Dip the slide rack up and down for 1 min.
13. Dry the slides as follows:
    a. Blot the slide rack on a paper towel and then quickly and carefully remove the slide rack handle.
    b. Place the slide rack in a plate holder that is lined with a folded paper towel.
    c. Place the plate holder into the centrifuge (do not forget to balance properly), and spin at 40*g* for 3 min.
    d. Carefully remove the slide rack from the plate holder and place on a paper towel.
    e. Remove each slide and place array-side-up on a paper towel.
    f. Make sure that each slide is dry. If not, quickly dry them with compressed air. Also, if the edges of a slide are wet, blot the edges on a paper towel.
14. Store the slides in the dark.

### 3.4.5. Troubleshooting

Microarray experiments are not trivial, and we have found that unexpected problems can arise at any time. In the event that you have difficulties, we highly recommend that you consult the vast amount of practical information available from the Yahoo! Microarray Group (*see* http://groups.yahoo.com/group/microarray/). Following are some of the major problems that we have encountered, along with some suggested ways to attempt to resolve each problem.

1. If the yield of cDNA is low (*see* **Subheading 3.4.1.**), make sure that your RNA is of high quality and that it is not getting degraded prior to the reverse transcription reaction. In addition to examining the $A_{260}/A_{230}$ and $A_{260}/A_{280}$ ratios (**step 4** under **Subheading 3.2.**), you can also run a small aliquot of the RNA on a 1% agarose gel to determine of the RNA is degraded. (If the 28S rRNA band is not

approximately twice as intense as the 18S rRNA band, the RNA has experienced degradation).

2. If the sample FOI is too low (*see* **Subheading 3.4.1.**):
   a. The 25X aa-dUTP/dNTP solution presented in this protocol yields a 2:1 ratio of aa-dUTP to dTTP. This ratio has worked well for us; however, if incorporation efficiencies are found to be too low (or too high) in your hands, this ratio of dUTP to dTTP might need to be optimized.
   b. It is possible that the prealiquotted Cy dyes (*see* **step 3** under **Subheading 2.3.3.**) have degraded substantially. A potential quick-fix is to resuspend multiple tubes of dye with the same aliquot of DMSO (**step 6** under **Subheading 3.3.3.**). This will increase the concentration of nondegraded Cy dye used in the coupling reaction. A better solution is to make fresh aliquots of the Cy dyes. If you find that this does not solve the problem, you might want to purchase a fresh batch of the Cy dyes from the supplier.
3. If the FOI for Cy3 is very different than the FOI for Cy5, perform **step 2b** for the dye with the lower FOI.
4. If there is substantial nonspecific fluorescence on the microarray (after scanning below):
   a. Scan a slide before prehybridizing to see if there is a problem with the slides.
   b. You might need to optimize the prehybridization of the slides.
   c. This is sometimes caused by the fluorescent sample drying out during the hybridization incubation. If this appears to be occurring, add more NANOpure water to the hyb-chamber and/or make sure that the hyb-chamber is sealed tightly prior to the incubation.
   d. You might need to optimize the washing of the slides.
5. If the median Cy5 intensity is much lower than the median Cy3 intensity (after scanning below): Cy5 is apparently very sensitive to ozone *(30)*; thus, a sudden increase in laboratory ozone levels might cause a severe decrease in Cy5 intensity on your microarrays (in some cases, the decrease in Cy5 intensity is so severe that the data are rendered useless). For suggestions of ways to prevent this effect of ozone, *see* **ref. 30** and www.genisphere.com/. We have also been told that adding DTT to the wash solutions (**steps 4–6** under **Subheading 2.4.3.**) might help as well.

## *3.5. Data Processing* (see *Notes 59 and 60*)

### *3.5.1. Data Acquisition*

1. After the microarray has been hybridized and washed, a scanner is used to measure the Cy3 and Cy5 fluorescence intensities at each spot (*see* **Note 61**). We scan our microarrays with a GenePix 4000A scanner, but there are many other commercially available scanners that can be employed. The Axon scanner is controlled by a software package called GenePix Pro.
2. Scanning of the microarray results in the production of an image for each fluorochrome. GenePix Pro displays a composite of these two images in which each

of the images has been assigned a pseudo-color (a common choice is to display the Cy3 image as green and the Cy5 image as red, although other options are available). The composite image should be examined immediately to determine if a second scan is required. If any of the following scenarios occurs, the scanner PMT settings should be adjusted accordingly, and the microarray should be rescanned (*see* **Note 62**).
    a. The intensities of a large number of spots are saturated (i.e., above the limit of detection of the scanner) in one or both channels.
    b. The intensities of a large number of spots are too low in one or both channels.
    c. The average spot intensity in the Cy3 channel is much higher/lower than the average spot intensity in the Cy5 channel.
3. After the image is successfully acquired, the GenePix software is used to overlay a grid onto the image where each feature in the grid defines the exact location of a spot in the microarray.
    a. Initially, a template grid is manually aligned so that each feature in the grid roughly encircles its corresponding spot on the array.
    b. Then the GenePix Pro automatic alignment functionality is used to more accurately select each spot (i.e., ideally, each feature will be centered at the corresponding spot and it will accurately encircle the spot).
    c. During the automatic alignment, the software flags any features in the grid for which it cannot find a corresponding spot.
4. Next, the grid is visually inspected, and features that do not accurately encircle spots are either adjusted or flagged. In addition, a feature is flagged if the underlying spot is obviously of poor quality (e.g., if it is covered by nonspecific fluorescence).
5. Once the grid alignment is deemed satisfactory, the GenePix software is used to extract data for each spot (*see* **Note 63**), and these data are stored in a tab-delimited text file.

## *3.5.2. Prenormalization Data Processing* (see **Note 64**)

1. Import the tab-delimited text file produced by GenePix into Microsoft Excel (or alternative spreadsheet software).
2. Within Excel, flag spots that do not meet certain quality control criteria. Examples of criteria include:
    a. Flag spot if the spot diameter is <50 μm.
    b. Flag spot if ≥50% of the pixels in both channels are saturated (*see* **Note 65**).
    c. Flag spot if a certain percentage of pixels (e.g., 55 %) in one or both channels are not greater than some minimum intensity value (e.g., the local background +2 standard deviations) (*see* **Note 66**).
3. Remove data for any spots that were flagged during gridding or that were flagged in **step 2**.
4. If desired, subtract local background from the median Cy3 and median Cy5 intensity at each spot (*see* **Note 67**).

## 3.5.3 Data Normalization (see **Note 68**)

The final value that we want to obtain for each gene is a ratio of Cy3 intensity/Cy5 intensity. The ratios that are initially obtained after scanning the microarray are influenced by several factors. One factor is the different abundances of the corresponding genes in the two samples being compared. This is generally the only factor that the researcher wants to measure. Unfortunately, the ratios are also influenced by several sources of systematic variation, including (but not limited to): (1) different incorporation efficiencies of the dyes in the two samples being compared; (2) nonuniform distribution of the Cy3- and Cy5-labeled components of the hybridization sample across the microarray (or some other circumstance that results in nonuniform hybridization of the cDNA molecules labeled with the two dyes); (3) different amounts of degradation of the dyes occurring prior to the time that the microarray is scanned; (4) different intensities of fluorescent light detected from the two dyes as a result of the particular laser power and PMT settings used when the microarray is scanned. Normalization is a process that attempts to remove bias in the ratios that results from these (and any other) nonbiological sources of variation. Normalization is also used to allow a more fair comparison of ratios measured on different microarrays.

The normalization procedure that we employ is a modification of a previously described method *(31,32)*, and our approach was recently proposed by another group *(33)*. The procedure, which is applied independently to the data from each microarray, can be summarized as follows:

1. For each spot that was not filtered out in **Subheading 3.5.2., step 3**, calculate the mean log intensity ($A$) and log ratio of the intensities ($M$) as follows (*see* **Note 69**):
   a. $A = \frac{1}{2}(\log_2 \text{Cy3} + \log_2 \text{Cy5})$, where "Cy3" or "Cy5" is the median intensity (of all pixels within the spot) in the corresponding channel.
   b. $M = \log_2 (\text{Cy3}/\text{Cy5})$.
2. Save these data, along with the $x$ position ($X$) and $y$ position ($Y$) of each spot on the microarray in a text file, and then import the data into the R statistical computing environment.
3. In order to simultaneously remove intensity-dependent bias and position-dependent bias in the log ratios, use the *loess* and *predict.loess* functions (in the *modreg* library) to generate a normalization factor $C(X, Y, A)$ for the log ratio measured at each spot.
4. Subtract the $C(X, Y, A)$ values returned by *predict.loess* from the original $M$ values to yield the final normalized log ratios.
5. Generate scatterplots of $M$ vs $X$, $M$ vs $Y$, and $M$ vs $A$ before and after the normalization. The normalized log ratios should be centered at $M = 0$ (*see* **Notes 70 and 71**).
6. Export the normalized log ratios to a text file, and then import into Excel.

*3.5.4. Postnormalization Data Processing*

1. If the cDNA samples were spotted multiple times on the particular microarray that you are using:
   a. If desired, you can employ additional quality control filtering at this point, such as removing genes for which a minimum number of replicate measurements were not obtained on a given microarray, or removing genes that exhibit excessive variability among the replicate spots (e.g., CV > 0.4).
   b. Calculate the median of the replicate log ratios for a given gene. This is the final log ratio that will be used in subsequent analyses.
2. Prepare the data from multiple microarrays for subsequent data analyses:
   a. If you follow the experimental design suggested under **Subheading 1.1.**, you will have four replicate microarrays for a given cell line. Organize the final log ratios from the four microarrays in a new Excel workbook (i.e., you should end up with a table in which each row contains data for a single gene and each of four columns contains the final log ratios from a single microarray).
   b. Remove genes if they have more than one missing value across the four replicates (i.e., there need to be at least three replicate measurements for a given gene for it to be considered in subsequent analyses).

## *3.6. Data Analysis (see Notes 1–3)*

*3.6.1. Assessment of Differential Expression*

The next step is to perform statistical analysis to select differentially expressed genes for each cell line that was profiled. There are many ways of accomplishing this, but one approach that we have found to be particularly useful is implemented in a software application called Significance Analysis of Microarrays (SAM) (*see* **Note 72**). SAM is implemented as an Excel add-in (*see* www-stat.stanford.edu/~tibs/SAM/). The algorithm employed by SAM has been discussed in detail elsewhere *(34,35)*. The following is a brief description of how SAM can be used to analyze data obtained via the protocol presented in this chapter (for more information, refer to the SAM manual that accompanies the software):

1. Starting with the Excel worksheet prepared under **Subheading 3.5.4., step 2**, format the data according to the directions for a "One class response" in the SAM manual (this should simply amount to inserting a blank row above the first row of data, and inserting a "1" above each of the four columns of log ratios).
2. Select the entire table of data, and then click on the "SAM" button (this button should be on the Excel toolbar after you install SAM).
3. Select the following parameters, and then click on the "OK" button:
   a. Response Type = "One class Response."
   b. Number of Permutations = 100.
   c. Imputation Engine = K-Nearest Neighbors Imputer.

d. Random Number Seed = 1234567 (or click on the button labeled "Generate Random Seed").
4. SAM will generate an observed-vs-expected plot (*see* **ref. 35**). Above the plot on the left, SAM reports the number of significant genes and an estimate of the corresponding number of false significant genes associated with that group of significant genes.
   a. Adjust the significant genes and the number of false significant genes by moving the "Delta Slider" in the "SAM Plot Controller" window (*see* **Note 73**).
   b. Once the number of significant genes and the number of false significant genes are at acceptable levels (*see* **Note 74**), click on the "List Significant Genes" button in the "SAM Plot Controller" window.
5. Repeat **steps 1–4** for all cell lines being profiled. When finished, you will have the following for each cell line:
   a. A list of genes displaying increased abundance (in treated cells relative to mock-treated cells) at the 24-h time point following treatment with the drug in question.
   b. A list of genes displaying decreased abundance (in treated cells relative to mock-treated cells) at the 24-h time point following treatment with the drug in question.
6. Import the lists into a database (e.g., Microsoft Access).
   a. Compare the lists to identify changes in expression that are unique to one or more sensitive cell lines that were profiled.
   b. Compare the lists to identify changes in expression that are unique to one or more resistant cell lines that were profiled.

*3.6.2. Classification Analysis*

If expression profiles are acquired for a panel of cell lines, you can perform classification analysis in order to identify subsets of genes whose expression levels allow the cell lines to be classified as sensitive or resistant. As with the assessment of differential expression, there are many ways to perform classification analysis. A recently proposed method that appears to outperform many of its predecessors is called Prediction Analysis for Microarrays (PAM) (*see* **Note 75**) *(18,36)*. Like SAM, PAM has been implemented as an add-in for Excel (*see* www-stat.stanford.edu/~tibs/PAM/). Following is an example of how PAM could be used to identify a subset of genes that allows discrimination between sensitive and resistant cell lines. For a detailed description of how PAM works, *see* **refs. 18** and **36**.

1. Acquire expression profiles for a large panel of cell lines. For this example, we will say that 50 profiles have been acquired (from 25 sensitive cell lines and 25 resistant cell lines) (*see* **Note 76**).
2. Randomly select five samples from each class. These 10 samples will be used to test the classifier that is discovered. The remaining 40 samples will be used to

train the classifier and identify a subset of genes that allows proper classification of the samples.
3. Format the data for the 40 training samples in an Excel worksheet according to the directions in the PAM manual (supplied with the software). Similarly, format the data for the remaining 10 samples in a second worksheet (in the same workbook).
4. Select the entire table containing the data for the 40 training samples, and then click on the "PAM" button (this button should be on the Excel toolbar after you install PAM).
5. Enter the required information in the opening window (see the PAM manual for details), and then click on the "OK" button.
6. The PAM Controller window will appear. Click on the "Train" button to train the classifier.
7. To view a plot of the training error, click on the "Plot Training Error" button.
8. Click on the "Cross Validate" button to perform cross-validation.
9. Click on the "Plot CV Curves" button to view plots displaying how the misclassification error (determined through cross-validation) varies according to the adjustable parameter called the "threshold." Two plots are displayed: a plot of the combined misclassification error for all classes and a plot of the misclassification error for the individual classes.
10. By looking at the misclassification error plots, select a threshold value at which the misclassification error is sufficiently low (preferably zero). Enter this number in the "Threshold" box.
11. Click on the "Plot CV Probabilities" button to view a plot of the class probabilities associated with the selected threshold value. Repeat this step for multiple threshold values (i.e., change the threshold value in the "Threshold" window and click on the "Plot CV Probabilities" button). Identify the class probability plot that displays optimal class probabilities (ideally, the class probability would be "1" for each sample in its respective class, but this will most likely not happen for all samples).
12. Once an optimal cross-validated class probability plot (and hence, an optimal threshold value) has been selected, enter the optimal threshold value in the "Threshold" window and then click the "List Genes" button. This will generate a list of genes that are in the subset of genes that allows discrimination between the sensitive and resistant classes.
13. To test the classifier with the 10-sample test set:
    a. Make sure that the optimal threshold value is in the "Threshold" window.
    b. Click on the "Predict Test Set" button. Enter the required information in the window that pops up, and then click the "OK" button.
    c. Click on the "Show Prediction" button to see which samples were predicted correctly by the classifier.

## 4. Notes

1. Note the following regarding genes that are found to be differentially expressed in a microarray experiment:

a. To provide additional evidence that a gene is truly differentially expressed under the condition being studied (e.g., in this case, during the response to a drug treatment), the differential expression should be confirmed using an alternative technique that is generally accepted to be more reliable (e.g., quantitative real-time PCR).
   b. Unless proper controls are employed, one does not generally know if a gene displaying altered abundance is doing so because the gene is being transcriptionally regulated or because the stability of the corresponding mRNA is being affected.
   c. Even if the differential expression of a gene is confirmed at the mRNA level, additional studies are required to determine if the gene is affected at the protein level (changes in mRNA abundance do not always correlate with changes in protein level). Furthermore, it should be determined if the condition being studied has any effect on the activity of the protein.
2. A gene that displays differential abundance following drug treatment may be directly involved in the response to the drug. On the other hand, the change in abundance may be due to an indirect effect. Additional studies are required to distinguish between these possibilities.
3. It is important to emphasize that the expression profiles obtained as described in the protocol presented in this chapter are only *correlated* with sensitivity or resistance. Additional studies are required to establish whether the genes that display altered abundance that is a unique characteristic of sensitive/resistant cells are directly involved in conferring sensitivity/resistance to the drug being studied (or if the altered abundance of those genes is merely an indirect effect associated with the sensitive/resistant phenotype).
4. To analyze steady-state differences in gene expression between a sensitive and resistant pair of cell lines, you could do the following:
   a. Omit the drug treatment, and harvest RNA from the cells when they are ≤80–85% confluent).
   b. Generate Cy3-labeled cDNA from the resistant cells and Cy5-labeled cDNA from the sensitive cells.
   c. Co-hybridize the two samples to a microarray (do at least four replicates if possible).
   d. Use SAM (*see* **Subheading 3.6.1.**) to identify genes that are significantly differentially expressed between the sensitive and resistant cell lines.
5. If you wish to generate steady-state expression profiles for a panel of cell lines which range in their level of sensitivity/resistance (i.e., you are not analyzing sensitive/resistant pairs as described in **Note 4**), you might consider co-hybridizing all cell lines with a common reference sample (*see* **Subheading 1.2.5.**).
6. Note the following if you intend to work with tumor biopsies:
   a. To perform an experiment analogous to that described in this chapter, a biopsy could be obtained from a patient before treatment and then at a specific time point after initiation of treatment (e.g., 24 h). These samples would be analogous to the mock-treated and treated samples in the current protocol.

b. If possible, to generate replicate expression profiles you should either take multiple biopsies or acquire multiple samples from each biopsy. The latter could be accomplished by using laser-capture microdissection (e.g., *see* **ref. 37**).

c. When working with tumor specimens, you will most likely have to amplify the RNA (also exemplified in **ref. 37**).

7. The reference sample might be pooled RNA derived from multiple cell lines, or possibly a commercially available reference sample such as the Stratagene Universal Human Reference RNA—*see* www.stratagene.com/). It should be noted that the pooling does not have to occur at the RNA stage. In fact, the variability in the reference sample (between microarrays) would presumably be reduced if the pooling were done after the cDNA is produced.

8. Once you perform the normalization as described under **Subheading 3.5.3.**, there is no accurate way to extract the numerator and the denominator of the ratio corresponding to a given gene. This is because the normalization is applied to the log ratios and not to the Cy3 or Cy5 intensities themselves (i.e., if a particular log ratio is adjusted by a correction factor, $C$, it is not clear how much of $C$ should be applied to the Cy3 intensity and how much should be applied to the Cy5 intensity). This is why if you do co-hybridizations with mock-treated and treated samples, you cannot compare the expression level of a gene in the treated samples from one cell line to the treated samples from another cell line. You can only compare the *ratio* of expression observed for each cell line (i.e., treated cell line 1/mock-treated cell line 1 compared to treated cell line 2/mock-treated cell line 2).

9. Cancer chemotherapeutics are generally toxic. As such, great care needs to be employed when handling them, and they should be properly disposed of according to the environment, health, and safety regulations of your particular institution.

10. These samples should be completely dry, but take care not to overdry.

11. Do not store these aliquots too long. Try to use them within a few weeks.

12. When you thaw an aliquot of $NaHCO_3$ labeling buffer, thaw the solution completely and allow it to reach room temperature. Then vortex to make sure the $NaHCO_3$ is completely in solution.

13. We have not tested how long the hyb-buffer can be stored. It is probably best to make it fresh at least every 2–3 mo.

14. Warm the hyb-buffer to room temperature and mix well before use. Make sure there is no precipitate.

15. We have found these specialized cover slips to be much better for microarray hybridization than any other cover slips that we have tried.

16. We prepare this fresh on the day of hybridization.

17. All wash solutions should be filtered prior to use. We use a single 500-mL, 0.22-µm bottle-top filter (Millipore, cat. no. SCGPS05RE) to filter all wash solutions prepared for a given wash session (the wash solutions are filtered in reverse order so that SDS is not introduced into wash solutions #2 and #3). All wash solutions should be mixed well (e.g., using a magnetic stir bar) before and after filtering.

18. When working with cells, make sure that any solutions that will be added to the cells are at least at room temperature and preferably at 37°C. This is imperative

during the drug treatment and subsequent cell washing (i.e., you do not want to confound the results by subjecting the cells to cold shock as well as treating them with drug).
19. The desired level of confluence at the time of treatment depends on the doubling time of the cells. Generally, you want to have a large number of cells at the time of RNA isolation (to maximize the amount of RNA that can be obtained); however, the cells in the flasks should not be allowed to reach confluence, as this will cause undesirable changes in gene expression. Thus, if the cells will double by the time point at which RNA will be harvested, the cells should be treated when they are approx 40% confluent. If the cells double more slowly, treatment can be initiated at higher levels of confluence.
20. When performing expression analysis, one needs to make a concerted effort not to introduce variability as a result of the way that the samples are processed. Thus, if you cannot work quickly enough during the drug treatment and RNA isolation steps, you might consider doing one or both of the following:
    a. Number and pair the flasks of cells (e.g., mock-treated #1 would be paired with treated #1, etc.). During drug treatment and RNA isolation, always process the samples in the same order and always process paired flasks simultaneously or consecutively (e.g., the order could be mock-treated #1, treated #1, . . . mock-treated #4, treated #4).
    b. During the drug treatment and RNA isolation, do not remove all eight flasks from the incubator at the same time (i.e., work with only two or four flasks at a time).
21. At the time of RNA isolation, cells should be at most approx 80–85% confluent. As cells approach 100% confluence, it is likely that changes in gene expression will occur, and you do not want these changes in expression to confound the results.
22. There are several effective methods available for RNA isolation. Our lab has had good success with the GITC method *(38)*. Other methods include purification using TRIzol LS reagent (Invitrogen, cat. no. 10296010) or purification kits such as those provided by QIAGEN (*see* www1.qiagen.com/). If desired, you can also purify mRNA rather than working with total RNA (in which case the reverse transcription reaction under **Subheading 3.3.1.** should be carried out with 2–4 µg mRNA).
23. If your RNA purification protocol involves ethanol precipitation just prior to the final resuspension in DEPC-treated water (e.g., the GITC method), we recommend storing your RNA at –20°C as an ethanol precipitate (i.e., add the sodium acetate and ethanol to precipitate the RNA and then store at –20°C). Then finish processing the RNA (i.e., spin the pellet down, wash the pellet, resuspend the pellet in DEPC-treated water, and quantitate) immediately prior to doing the RT reaction. Store any leftover RNA in single-use aliquots at –80°C. If your RNA purification protocol does not require ethanol precipitation (e.g., if the RNA is eluted from a column in DEPC-treated water and the RNA does not need to be concentrated), we recommend that you quantitate the RNA immediately after elution and then store it in single-use aliquots at –80°C).

24. The total yield per flask depends on the cell type and the number of cells present. Ideally, you would like to have at least 50 µg per flask. Also, the [RNA] needs to be at least 3.16 µg/µL if you want to start with 50 µg in **Subheading 3.3.1.**
25. Our protocol for preparation of fluorescently labeled samples was derived from multiple publicly available protocols (most notably, those from TIGR (*see* **ref. 25**) and Molecular Probes (*see* www.probes.com/media/pis/mp21664.pdf), as well as from personal experience.
26. Although the "two-step" labeling process (described under **Subheading 3.3.**) takes more time than the alternative "direct incorporation" approach (in which a Cy-dye conjugated nucleotide is incorporated into the cDNA during reverse transcription), we feel that it is superior for the following reasons:
    a. The two-step method is less expensive.
    b. Researchers have found that Cy5-conjugated nucleotides are sometimes incorporated into cDNA at lower frequency than Cy3-conjugated nucleotides. Since the same modified nucleotide (the aminoallyl-dUTP) is incorporated into all samples in the two-step method, such differential incorporation is avoided.
    c. When processing a large number of samples, we find that it is convenient to store the samples (either overnight or longer) after generating cDNA. This is fine for aa-cDNA, but possibly not for Cy-labeled cDNA (due to the notorious instability of the Cy-dyes, it is advisable to use the Cy-labeled cDNA as soon as possible after it is generated).
27. The "anchored" oligo(dT) controls the length of the poly(dT) tails in the cDNA molecules. If the anchor (the nucleotides VN at the 3' end of the oligo, where N represents any nucleotide, and V represents any nucleotide except T) were not included, the poly(dT) tails could be random lengths, and some might be quite long. As a result of the anchor, all poly(dT) tails should have 20 nucleotides.
28. When working with three or more RNA samples, we recommend that you make a premix of the reagents that are added in **step 5**. Make enough of the premix for $n + 1$ samples (where $n$ is the number of RNA samples being processed).
29. If necessary, this incubation can be longer (including overnight); however, you should probably try to be consistent with any samples that you will be comparing.
30. In this step, the Superscript II RT is inactivated, and the RNA:cDNA hybrids are denatured.
31. We have noticed that the caps on the PCR tubes can sometimes pop open soon after the thermal cycler lid is opened. Sometimes a cap can pop open so forcefully that the PCR tube jumps out of the PCR block (potentially spilling some of its contents). To prevent this from occurring, we always make sure to quickly cover the tubes with one hand as soon as the lid is opened (we generally hold a paper towel on top of the tubes because they are quite hot), and then remove the tubes from the PCR block and place them on ice with the other hand.
32. This step results in hydrolysis of the RNA.
33. For **steps 10** and **11**, if you are processing multiple samples simultaneously you can make a premix of 1 $M$ Tris, pH 7.0, and DEPC-treated water so that they can be added in a single step.

34. This step ensures that the pH of the solution is optimal for the binding of DNA to the column; see the QIAquick Spin Handbook (provided with the kit) for more details.
35. For **steps 2** and **3**, if you are processing multiple samples simultaneously you can make a premix of Buffer PB and 3 $M$ sodium acetate, pH 5.5, so that they can be added in a single step.
36. If you are not immediately proceeding with the coupling reaction, the aa-cDNA can be stored at this point (samples should be stored at –20°C because DNA can degrade in the absence of a buffering agent).
37. During all processing involving the Cy dyes, minimize exposure of the samples to light (to prevent photobleaching).
38. This step increases the probability that all of the cDNA has been resuspended and ensures that the sample is well mixed.
39. Follow the instructions in the QIAquick Spin Handbook (provided with the kit) regarding the addition of ethanol to Buffer PE prior to use.
40. Dilution of Buffer EB serves to decrease the amount of extra salt that ends up in the final sample that will be applied to the microarray.
41. Our hybridization protocol was derived from several publicly available protocols (but mainly the protocol from TIGR—*see* **ref. 25**), as well as from personal experience.
42. If you are planning to do a lot of microarray experiments, we suggest that you obtain access to a low-volume spectrophotometer (e.g., the NanoDrop; *see* www.nanodrop.com/). Such a spectrophotometer will allow you to use a much smaller volume when quantitating (i.e., much less of the sample is wasted). Furthermore, the samples can be quantitated without having to dilute them. The protocol described here assumes the reader has access to a spectrophotometer that utilizes 50-μL cuvets, because these spectrophotometers tend to be more common.
43. In our hands, the average yield of cDNA when starting with 50 μg total RNA is approximately 1000 ng.
44. We prefer that the FOI be between 20 and 50. If the FOI falls much below 20, the sample may still yield acceptable signal, but it might be advisable to perform the cDNA preparation again.
45. We prefer to mix equal amounts of the Cy3-cDNA and Cy5-cDNA. After **step 5**, the concentration of cDNA should be 12.5–25 ng/μL for each Cy-cDNA. Since the resuspension volume in **step 5** is 40 μL, this means you should add between 500 and 1000 ng each of the Cy3-cDNA and the Cy5-cDNA. Although we suggest adding equal amounts of cDNA, you would ideally also be mixing similar picomoles of dye. While the picomoles of dye added do not have to be equal, we recommend that you do not let them differ by more than threefold. If you are processing multiple samples (e.g., four treated Cy3 and four mock-treated Cy5 samples), you can match treated Cy3 and mock-treated Cy5 replicates that have similar FOI values (unless the samples were processed in such a way that each mock-treated replicate was paired with a specific treated replicate—*see* **Note 20**).
46. The final volume depends on the size of the LifterSlip required to cover the array. We use a 25 × 60 mm LifterSlip, for which, 40 μL is sufficient volume.

47. From this point on, keep samples at room temperature or above to prevent precipitation of SDS.
48. Specialized hyb-chambers are available from various suppliers, but we have found that the 50-mL conical tubes work well, and they are much less expensive.
49. If you are washing multiple slides simultaneously, you can use slide racks and wash containers similar to **Subheading 3.4.4.** (however, we recommend using a separate slide rack and separate wash containers than the ones used in **Subheading 3.4.4.**).
50. If you are drying only one or two slides, you can simply place each slide in a 50-mL conical tube and spin. Otherwise, the slides will presumably already be in a slide rack, which can be spun in a centrifuge that has plate holders (don't forget to balance properly).
51. If you are setting up multiple hybridizations on the same day, we recommend that you complete the steps under **Subheading 3.4.3.** with one or two samples at a time (i.e., the times at which the microarrays enter the hybridization oven will be slightly staggered).
52. Place the pipet tip right next to the LifterSlip and slowly eject the sample. The sample will be drawn under the LifterSlip.
53. Samples can be allowed to hybridize for longer periods of time (and possibly shorter, too), but you should probably try to be consistent (especially with samples that will be compared).
54. Once the microarrays have been removed from the hybridization oven, do not let them dry until **step 13** (i.e., do not expose them to the air for any substantial length of time).
55. The 50-mL conical tubes used as hyb-chambers can be rinsed and reused for future hybridizations.
56. The purpose of this wash is to quickly get rid of the bulk of the fluorescent sample.
57. We recommend that you always orient the microarray slides a certain way in the slide racks (e.g., put the top of the slide to the right with the array side facing forward). Also, do not use the first slot in the slide rack (the microarray might get damaged by coming into contact with the rack).
58. The purpose of this set of steps is to minimize the transfer of SDS to subsequent washes.
59. There are many commercially available software packages that you can use to process and analyze microarray data. We like to have the freedom to utilize any data processing/analysis techniques that we choose, and we have not found a commercial package that allows us to do that. Thus, we do most of our data processing/analysis using Microsoft Excel and the R statistical analysis environment. If you do not have someone in your lab who is comfortable working with R and with using formulas in Excel, we recommend that you find a software package that is an appropriate alternative.
60. There are also several freely available open-source software packages that you might find useful (*see* **ref. *39***).

# Gene Expression Profiling

61. We recommend that microarrays be scanned as soon as possible after they are washed because in some cases we have seen the fluorescence signal decay substantially in a short amount of time.
62. We prefer to scan each microarray only once if possible. Although each successive scan should cause only a minimal decrease in fluorescence intensity (due to photobleaching), we have observed unacceptable decreases in signal upon repeated scanning. We recommend that you perform a pilot experiment with one or two microarrays and use them to get an idea of what the optimal PMT settings should be.
63. GenePix calculates many statistics for each spot (including the median Cy3 intensity, the median Cy5 intensity, the median Cy3 local background, the median Cy5 local background, and many others). Some of these statistics are used in the subsequent data processing steps.
64. **Steps 2–4** can be carried out automatically if you create template worksheets in Excel. For example, we have a worksheet that is setup to perform **step 2** after the raw data (extracted by GenePix) are pasted into the sheet. Then we have a subsequent worksheet (in the same workbook) that performs **step 3** (and that could potentially perform **step 4**).
65. This criterion is used because if 50% or more of the pixels are saturated, you cannot accurately determine the median intensity of all of the pixels within a spot. The criterion could also be set up to flag a spot if ≥50% of the pixels in *either* channel is saturated, but sometimes you might want to keep data for a spot as long as you can accurately determine the median intensity for at least one of the channels.
66. We generally do not employ a criterion based on minimum intensity because we (and others—*see* **ref. 33**) feel that such a criterion might result in the elimination of potentially useful data.
67. We do not subtract background because we (and others—*see* **ref. 33**) feel that it increases the variance for low-intensity spots. Instead, we try to minimize nonspecific fluorescence through utilizing good technique. If nonspecific fluorescence is encountered, and if it is clearly affecting the intensities of some spots, those spots are flagged during the gridding process.
68. There is no generally accepted procedure for normalization. For the normalization of two-dye hybridizations, we currently prefer the approach presented here. For information regarding alternative approaches, we refer the interested reader to **refs. 32** and **33**. For normalizing Affymetrix microarrays, *see* **ref. 40**. In addition to the three aforementioned references, additional useful articles are listed at bioinformatics.upmc.edu/Help/MicroarrayReferences.html.
69. These calculations can be setup in the second worksheet mentioned in **Note 64**.
70. Please contact us if you would like to see an example R script that was written to carry out **steps 3–5**.
71. There are two parameters passed to the *loess* function that are important for controlling the amount of correction applied to the log ratios: *degree* and *span*. If you feel that the scatterplots of the normalized log ratios (generated in **step 5**) indicate that the log ratios have been corrected too much or not enough, you can

adjust these parameters. The *degree* parameter should be set to either 1 or 2, whereas the *span* argument should be set to a value between 0 and 1 (inclusive). We recommend that *span* be set to the largest value that results in adequate correction of the log ratios (note that "adequate correction" is somewhat subjective).
72. For additional approaches to assessing differential expression, see the references listed at bioinformatics.upmc.edu/Help/MicroarrayReferences.html.
73. The parameter "delta" determines which genes are considered "significant" and is also used to determine the estimated number of false significant genes associated with each list of significant genes. The "Delta Slider" is a convenient way to quickly modify the value of delta so that you can see the effect on the number of significant genes and the number of false significant genes. As delta increases, the number of significant genes and the number of false significant genes will decrease.
74. It should be noted that "acceptable levels" are subjective. For instance, you might be willing to allow a 1% false discovery rate. In this case, an example of an "acceptable level" would be if you could adjust delta such that the significant number of genes were 200 and the number of false significant genes were 2. Regardless of your "acceptable level," what is important is that you can report the estimated false discovery rate associated with any list of "significant" genes.
75. For additional methods for classification analysis, see the references listed at bioinformatics.upmc.edu/Help/MicroarrayReferences.html.
76. If your only goal is to perform classification analysis (and if your resources are limited), it is probably acceptable if you do not perform four replicates per cell line as suggested in the experimental design under **Subheading 1.1.** For classification analysis, an increased number of samples is more important than replication of each sample. Just be aware that if you do not perform at least three replicates for each cell line, you will not be able to reliably select genes that are differentially expressed in each cell line. If replicates are performed, average the log ratios from the replicates before proceeding with **step 2**.

## Acknowledgments

We would like to thank Goli Samimi for critically reading this chapter and for providing helpful comments. In addition, we are very grateful to the many researchers who have made their detailed microarray protocols publicly available on the Internet (especially researchers from TIGR and Molecular Probes). Finally, we would like to thank those members of the Los and Howell labs who have performed expression analysis experiments and have thereby contributed to our personal experience.

## References

1. Kudoh, K., Ramanna, M., Ravatn, R., et al. (2000) Monitoring the expression profiles of doxorubicin-induced and doxorubicin-resistant cancer cells by cDNA microarray. *Cancer Res.* **60,** 4161–4166.

2. Watts, G. S., Futscher, B. W., Isett, R., Gleason-Guzman, M., Kunkel, M. W., and Salmon, S. E. (2001) cDNA microarray analysis of multidrug resistance: doxorubicin selection produces multiple defects in apoptosis signaling pathways. *J. Pharmacol. Exp. Ther.* **299,** 434–441.
3. Sakamoto, M., Kondo, A., Kawasaki, K., et al. (2001) Analysis of gene expression profiles associated with cisplatin resistance in human ovarian cancer cell lines and tissues using cDNA microarray. *Hum. Cell* **14,** 305–315.
4. Maxwell, P. J., Longley, D. B., Latif, T., et al. (2003) Identification of 5-fluorouracil-inducible target genes using cDNA microarray profiling. *Cancer Res.* **63,** 4602–4606.
5. Samimi, G., Manorek, G., Castel, R., et al. (2005) cDNA microarray-based identification of genes and pathways associated with oxaliplatin resistance. *Cancer Chemother. Pharmacol.* **55,** 1–11 [Epub 2005 Jan.].
6. Lamendola, D. E., Duan, Z., Yusuf, R. Z., and Seiden, M. V. (2003) Molecular description of evolving paclitaxel resistance in the SKOV-3 human ovarian carcinoma cell line. *Cancer Res.* **63,** 2200–2205.
7. Kartalou, M. and Essigmann, J. M. (2001) Mechanisms of resistance to cisplatin. *Mutat. Res.* **478,** 23–43.
8. Altieri, D. C. (2001) The molecular basis and potential role of survivin in cancer diagnosis and therapy. *Trends Mol. Med.* **7,** 542–547.
9. Ikeguchi, M., Nakamura, S., and Kaibara, N. (2002) Quantitative analysis of expression levels of bax, bcl-2, and survivin in cancer cells during cisplatin treatment. *Oncol. Rep.* **9,** 1121–1126.
10. Golub, T. R., Slonim, D. K., Tamayo, P., et al. (1999) Molecular classification of cancer: class discovery and class prediction by gene expression monitoring. *Science* **286,** 531–537.
11. Alizadeh, A. A., Eisen, M. B., Davis, R. E., et al. (2000) Distinct types of diffuse large B-cell lymphoma identified by gene expression profiling. *Nature* **403,** 503–511.
12. Bittner, M., Meltzer, P., Chen, Y., et al. (2000) Molecular classification of cutaneous malignant melanoma by gene expression profiling. *Nature* **406,** 536–540.
13. Perou, C. M., Sorlie, T., Eisen, M. B., et al. (2000) Molecular portraits of human breast tumours. *Nature* **406,** 747–752.
14. Ross, D. T., Scherf, U., Eisen, M. B., et al. (2000) Systematic variation in gene expression patterns in human cancer cell lines. *Nat. Genet.* **24,** 227–235.
15. Bhattacharjee, A., Richards, W. G., Staunton, J., et al. (2001) Classification of human lung carcinomas by mRNA expression profiling reveals distinct adenocarcinoma subclasses. *Proc. Natl. Acad. Sci. USA* **98,** 13,790–13,795.
16. Khan, J., Wei, J. S., Ringner, M., et al. (2001) Classification and diagnostic prediction of cancers using gene expression profiling and artificial neural networks. *Nat. Med.* **7,** 673–679.
17. Beer, D. G., Kardia, S. L., Huang, C. C., et al. (2002) Gene-expression profiles predict survival of patients with lung adenocarcinoma. *Nat. Med.* **8,** 816–824.
18. Tibshirani, R., Hastie, T., Narasimhan, B., and Chu, G. (2002) Diagnosis of multiple cancer types by shrunken centroids of gene expression. *Proc. Natl. Acad. Sci. USA* **99,** 6567–6572.

19. van 't Veer, L. J., Dai, H., van de Vijver, M. J., et al. (2002) Gene expression profiling predicts clinical outcome of breast cancer. *Nature* **415,** 530–536.
20. Wigle, D. A., Jurisica, I., Radulovich, N., et al. (2002) Molecular profiling of non-small cell lung cancer and correlation with disease-free survival. *Cancer Res.* **62,** 3005–3008.
21. Staunton, J. E., Slonim, D. K., Coller, H. A., et al. (2001) Chemosensitivity prediction by transcriptional profiling. *Proc. Natl. Acad. Sci. USA* **98,** 10,787–10,792.
22. Zembutsu, H., Ohnishi, Y., Tsunoda, T., et al. (2002) Genome-wide cDNA microarray screening to correlate gene expression profiles with sensitivity of 85 human cancer xenografts to anticancer drugs. *Cancer Res.* **62,** 518–527.
23. Kaneta, Y., Kagami, Y., Katagiri, T., et al. (2002) Prediction of sensitivity to STI571 among chronic myeloid leukemia patients by genome-wide cDNA microarray analysis. *Jpn. J. Cancer Res.* **93,** 849–856.
24. Zembutsu, H., Ohnishi, Y., Daigo, Y., et al. (2003) Gene-expression profiles of human tumor xenografts in nude mice treated orally with the EGFR tyrosine kinase inhibitor ZD1839. *Int. J. Oncol.* **23,** 29–39.
25. Hegde, P., Qi, R., Abernathy, K., et al. (2000) A concise guide to cDNA microarray analysis. *Biotechniques* **29,** 548–550, 552–544, 556 [note that an update to this article can be found at http://pga.tigr.org/PDF/BiotechniquesCookbook_II.pdf].
26. Nakata, B., Barton, R. M., Robbins, K. T., Howell, S. B., and Los, G. (1994) Association between hsp60 mRNA levels and cisplatin resistance in human head and neck cancer cell lines. *Int. J. Oncol.* **5,** 1425–1432.
27. Nakata, B., Albright, K. D., Barton, R. M., Howell, S. B., and Los, G. (1995) Synergistic interaction between cisplatin and tamoxifen delays the emergence of cisplatin resistance in head and neck cancer cell lines. *Cancer Chemother. Pharmacol.* **35,** 511–518.
28. Samimi, G., Manorek, G., Castel, R., et al. (2004) Identification of genes whose expression is associated with oxaliplatin resistance. Submitted.
29. Eickhoff, B., Korn, B., Schick, M., Poustka, A., and van der Bosch, J. (1999) Normalization of array hybridization experiments in differential gene expression analysis. *Nucleic Acids Res.* **27,** e33.
30. Fare, T. L., Coffey, E. M., Dai, H., et al. (2003) Effects of atmospheric ozone on microarray data quality. *Anal. Chem.* [available at http://pubs.acs.org/cgi-bin/asap.cgi/ancham/asap/abs/ac034241b.html].
31. Dudoit, S., Yang, Y. H., Callow, M. J., and Speed, T. P. (2002) Statistical methods for identifying differentially expressed genes in replicated cDNA microarray experiments. *Statist. Sinica* **12,** 111–139.
32. Yang, Y. H., Dudoit, S., Luu, P., et al. (2002) Normalization for cDNA microarray data: a robust composite method addressing single and multiple slide systematic variation. *Nucleic Acids Res.* **30,** e15.
33. Cui, X., Kerr, M. K., and Churchill, G. A. (2002) Data Transformations for cDNA microarray data [available at www.jax.org/staff/churchill/labsite/pubs/].

34. Tusher, V. G., Tibshirani, R., and Chu, G. (2001) Significance analysis of microarrays applied to the ionizing radiation response. *Proc. Natl. Acad. Sci. USA* **98,** 5116–5121.
35. Storey, J. D. and Tibshirani, R. (2003) SAM thresholding and false discovery rates for detecting differential gene expression in DNA microarrays, in *Analysis of Gene Expression Data: Methods and Software* (Parmigiani, G., Garrett, E. S., Irizarry, R. A., and Zeger, S. L., eds.), Springer-Verlag, New York.
36. Tibshirani, R., Hastie, T., Narasimhan, B., and Chu, G. (2002) Class prediction by nearest shrunken centroids, with applications to DNA microarrays. Stanford Technical Report, [available at www-stat.stanford.edu/~tibs/research.html].
37. Ma, X. J., Salunga, R., Tuggle, J. T., et al. (2003) Gene expression profiles of human breast cancer progression. *Proc. Natl. Acad. Sci. USA* **100,** 5974–5979.
38. Kingston, R. E. (1995) Guanidinium Methods for Total RNA Preparation, in *Current Protocols in Molecular Biology* (Ausubel, F. M., Brent, R., Kingston, R. E., et al., eds.), Wiley, New York, pp. 4.2.1–4.2.3.
39. Dudoit, S., Gentleman, R. C., and Quackenbush, J. (2003) Open source software for the analysis of microarray data. *Biotechniques* **(Suppl.),** 45–51.
40. Bolstad, B. M., Irizarry, R. A., Astrand, M., and Speed, T. P. (2003) A comparison of normalization methods for high density oligonucleotide array data based on variance and bias. *Bioinformatics* **19,** 185–193.

# 15

## Identifying Genes Related to Chemosensitivity Using Support Vector Machine

### Lei Bao

### Summary

In an effort to identify genes involved in chemosensitivity and to evaluate the functional relationships between genes and anticancer drugs acting by the same mechanism, a supervised machine learning approach called support vector machine (SVM) is used to associate genes with any of five predefined anticancer drug mechanistic categories. The drug activity profiles are used as training examples to train the SVM and then the gene expression profiles are used as test examples to predict their associated mechanistic categories. This method of correlating drugs and genes provides a strategy for finding novel biologically significant relationships for molecular pharmacology.

### Key Words

Chemosensitivity; anticancer mechanism; gene expression; microarray; support vector machine; drug–gene functional relationship.

### 1. Introduction

The identification of genes involved in chemosensitivity is an important issue in molecular pharmacology. Recent advances in gene expression profiling technologies offer a global approach to understanding complex genetic contributions to chemosensitivity. Scherf and coworkers have pioneered the use of microarrays for chemosensitivity profiling *(1,2)*. The researchers assessed gene expression profiles in a set of 60 human cancer cell lines that have been characterized pharmacologically by treatment with more than 70,000 different agents, one at a time. Because the chemosensitivity feature of a cell line is determined by what types of genes it expresses and by how much these genes express, the task of identification of chemosensitivity genes is transformed into how to correlate the gene expression profiles with drug activity profiles *(1,3–5)*. In this chapter, we present a computational method for association of genes with drugs acting by the same mechanism. It is known that drugs acting by the same mechanism tend to have a common activity pattern, whereas drugs acting by different mechanisms are discriminable among each other *(6)*. This finding demonstrated that drug activity profiles were rich in information about mechanism. From a pattern-recognition view, each drug mechanistic category describes a unique probability distribution for the drug activity vectors in the 60-dimensional drug activity space. If we abstract both the gene expression profile and the drug activity profile as random vectors, we may treat them indiscriminatingly. The main assumption we held was that, when a gene expression vector was predicted with a high possibility to be a sample drawn from the unique probability distribution over a mechanistic category, the gene and the drugs from that mechanistic category were probably biologically related. The rationale of the assumption was that if a gene contributed to the cell's response to a class of drugs acting by the same mechanism, the change of its transcript concentration across different cell lines should, in principle, be consistent with the change of chemosensitivity averaged over drugs from that mechanistic category. Based on this assumption, a newly developed machine learning method called support vector machine (SVM) *(7)* is used to locate such drug–gene relationships. The drug activity profiles are used as training examples to train the SVM and then the gene expression profiles were used as test examples to predict the mechanistic categories into which they fell. This provides for further experiments the uncharacterized gene candidates that might potentially be related to cancer chemotherapy efficacies (*see* **Note 1**). Our approach of bringing genes into the context of drug mechanism will give more information on the gene functions than simply correlating drugs and genes.

## 2. Materials

1. Drug mechanistic labels: 127 well-studied drugs were labeled into each of the six mechanistic categories: 34 alkylating agents (Ak), 31 topoisomerase I inhibitors (T1), 16 topoismerase II inhibitors (T2), 17 RNA/DNA antimetabolites (Ri), 16 DNA antimetabolites (Di), and 13 antimitotic agents (Mi) *(6)*.
2. Drug activity dataset: Drug activity value is expressed as the negative logarithm of $GI_{50}$, ($-\log GI_{50}$, *see* **Note 2**), where $GI_{50}$ was the concentration of the compound needed to cause 50% cell growth inhibition *(8)*. About 1400 compounds (including the aforementioned 127 drugs) whose activity data have been well validated are selected from a public database (http://discover.nci.nih.gov) *(1)* and the compound set is further winnowed to eliminate those with more than five missing values. 1217 compounds passed this filter and their activity data across 50 cell lines (*see* **Note 3**) form a $1217 \times 50$ drug matrix.

3. Gene expression dataset: Gene expression was measured by microarrays and recorded as the base 2 logarithm of the ratios of the relative mRNA level of each cell line to a common reference sample pool (*see* **Note 4**). 6357 genes with less than four missing values and with standard deviations larger than 0.5 are selected from the original gene expression database (http://discover.nci.nih.gov) (*1*). After removing chimera clones, repetitive clones, and clones not included by the Unigene database, 4864 genes are reserved and their expression data across 50 cell lines form a 4864 × 50 gene matrix.

## 3 Methods

### 3.1. Data Pretreatment

1. Any missing value of the two matrices is substituted by the median value of the column to which it belonged. Therefore, we use the median of all the measurements in a cell line as a rough estimation for any missing value of that cell line.
2. Because in the biological context, the similarity in the "shape" (relative change tendency for a drug or a gene) is much more significant than the "magnitude," normalization is done so that every row of the two matrices has a zero mean and a standard deviation of 1.

### 3.2. Overview of SVM

SVM is a two-class supervised learning method. In the linear separable case, SVM has a decision function of the form

$$f(\mathbf{x}) = \text{sgn}(\sum_{i=1}^{N} y_i \alpha_i \cdot \mathbf{x} \bullet \mathbf{x}_i + b) \qquad (1)$$

where $\mathbf{x}$ is a test example and $\mathbf{x}_i$ is the $i$th (of $N$) training example with a class label of $y_i$ ($y_i = 1$ or $-1$). The weight $\alpha_i$ and the constant $b$ are chosen to maximize the margin between the decision surface (hyperplane) of positive and negative examples. Training examples with nonzero weights are called support vectors. Typically the number of support vectors is small compared to the total number of training examples. The decision function involves only dot products between the test example and support vectors. In the linear nonseparable case, two important techniques are introduced to extend the linear separable case: soft margin and kernel trick. A soft margin accepts some misclassifications of the training examples and can be implemented by adding a constant factor to the kernel matrix while keeping other formulations unchanged. The kernel trick substitutes the dot product in **Eq. 1** with a suitable kernel function $K(\mathbf{x}_i, \mathbf{x}_j)$. This procedure is equivalent to mapping the original data into a higher-dimensional feature space and locating a hyperplane there. Several typical kernel functions are

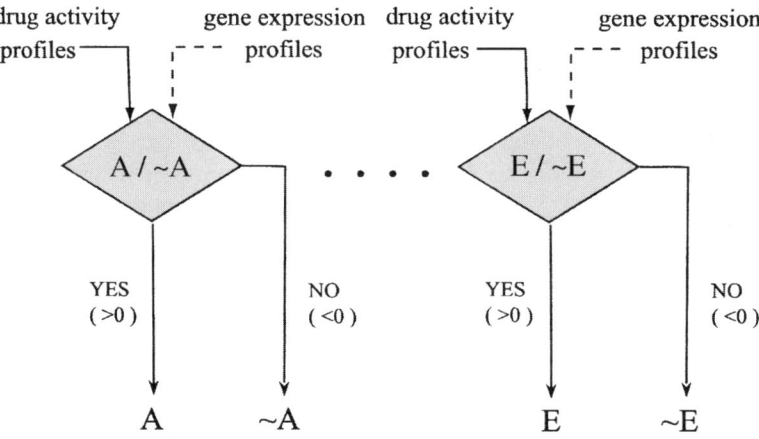

Fig. 1. Illustration of the method. A–E denote the five drug mechanistic categories, Ak, T2, Ri, Di, and Mi. In the training phase, inputs (solid arrows) are the drug activity profiles (drug matrix). Take A/~A classifier as an example, drugs within category A serve as positive training examples, while all the other drugs serve as negative training examples (~A category indicates they do not belong to the category A). In the predicting phase, inputs (dashed arrows) are the gene expression profiles (gene matrix). For each input gene, each of the five trained SVM classifiers gives a discriminant value. If one and only one value is positive, the gene is assigned to the corresponding drug mechanistic category; if all five values are negative, the gene is removed from further study.

$$K(\mathbf{x}_i,\mathbf{x}_j) = (\mathbf{x}_i \bullet \mathbf{x}_j + 1)^d \qquad (2)$$

$$K(\mathbf{x}_i,\mathbf{x}_j) = \exp(-r|\mathbf{x}_i - \mathbf{x}_j|^2) \qquad (3)$$

**Equation 2** is the polynomial kernel function of degree $d$, and **Eq. 3** is the radial basis function.

### 3.3. Optimizing SVM Parameters with Drug Activity Profiles

1. For each mechanistic category, a corresponding SVM classifier is constructed. These classifiers are one-vs-rest classifiers ("one," positive class; "rest," negative class). Taking category Ak as an example, compounds of this category are used as the positive training set, while all the other compounds are used as the negative training set. Because the T1 category is comprised solely of camptothecin derivatives, no SVM classifier is built for this category. Therefore, altogether five SVM classifiers are built and trained (*see* **Fig. 1**). The novelty of our strategy lies in that we train SVM with drug properties, but later we use these classifiers to annotate gene functions (*see* **Note 5**).

2. During the training phase, two parameters need to be specified for a SVM classifier: the penalty magnitude for violating the soft margin and the kernel function. The first parameter is determined in the light of a trade-off between sensitivity and specificity. In this study, the drug mechanistic categories contained very few members relative to the total number of compounds in the data set. Therefore, there is an extreme imbalance between the number of positive and negative training examples. Without any modification, the SVM will misclassify all members of the training set as negative examples in the presence of noise. The problem can be combated by modifying the diagonal of the kernel matrix during the training phase *(9)*. For each positive example, a constant $\lambda(n^+/N)$ is added to the diagonal entity while for each negative example, a constant $\lambda(n^-/N)$ is added, where $N$ is the total number of training examples, and $n^+$, $n^-$ are the number of positive and negative training examples. The scale factor $\lambda$ is set to 0.1. This method assigned a larger penalty to false negatives than to false positives.
3. To determine the optimized kernel function for each SVM classifier (*see* **Note 6**), the training set is randomly split into 10 subsets and a 10-fold cross-validation is carried out. Briefly, for each classifier, one subset is removed, the classifier is trained on the remaining nine subsets and then tested for its ability to classify the withheld subset. This procedure is repeated for each subset in the training set. The cost function to be minimized is defined as $fp + 2fn$, where $fp$ is the number of false positives and $fn$ is the number of false negatives. Again, the false negatives are weighted more heavily because of the imbalance in the number of positive and negative training examples. To eliminate the fortuitous effects introduced by a certain splitting, such splitting/validation procedures are repeated six times and the average cost for the six independent splittings is used to assess the optimal classification. Altogether four typical kernel functions (polynomial kernel functions with powers of 1, 2, 3, and the radial basis kernel) are tested and the one with the best performance is picked up (*see* **Note 7**). After some preliminary computations, we found that as a whole the second-degree polynomial kernel performed better than the first- or third-degree kernel or the radial kernel and is more appropriate in this context. Therefore, the second-degree polynomial kernel is used to build the SVMs.

## *3.4. Predicting Gene Labels Using Gene Expression Profiles*

1. After determination of the optimized parameters, each SVM classifier is trained again. This time all training examples (all 1217 compounds) are used.
2. Every gene from the 4864-gene set is used as a test example and each SVM classifier gave it a scalar discriminant value. The sign of the discriminant value specified whether the gene belonged to the class or not, and its extreme value can be used to rank genes by their memberships. If all the discriminant values are negative, then the gene is labeled as "background class" and removed from further study. If one discriminant value is positive while the other four are negative, the gene is assigned to the corresponding drug mechanistic class (*see* **Note 8**); 19, 13, 18, 22 and 3 genes are assigned to the Ak, T2, Ri, Di, and Mi categories, respectively.

## 3.5. Validating the Method

1. It is known that compounds from the Ak, T2, Ri, and Di categories are able to induce DNA damage and genes involved in the DNA repair process are believed to affect the compound efficacies. The 72 genes assigned to any of these four mechanistic categories are pooled to form a new gene set, which is hereinafter referred as "the 72-gene set" for convenience. If this method is effective, DNA repair-related genes are expected to be more enriched in the 72-gene set than in the original 4864-gene set.
2. To compare the occurrence of DNA repair-related genes in the two sets, annotation record for each gene was retrieved from the SOURCE database (http://source.stanford.edu/) (*see* **Note 9**), the keywords DNA and REPAIR are scanned, and the occurrence is normalized by the number of genes in the two sets, respectively (*see* **Notes 10** and **11**). As expected, the DNA repair-related genes are enriched about eight times more in the 72-gene set than in the 4864-gene set, demonstrating the validity of our method.

## 4. Notes

1. Because only the gene transcript concentrations are taken into account, our method can work only when the drug–gene functional relationships are embodied at the transcriptional level. Given the fact that drug–gene functional relationships may take place at various levels, this method can only identify a subset of all the potential relationships. Another limitation of our method is that *a priori* knowledge of drug mechanistic category is necessary, so drugs with unknown mechanisms are not applicable. However, with more and more drug mechanistic categories identified, this approach would have more use.
2. After this transformation, an increase in the resulting $-\log GI_{50}$ value is consistent with an increase in the cell line's sensitivity to the drug, so $-\log GI_{50}$ is used as the quantitative indicator of drug activity instead of $GI_{50}$ itself.
3. The cell line set used for assessing the gene expression profiles and the cell line set used for assessing the drug activity profiles of the 127 drugs have 50 common members. Only data for these 50 cell lines are used for further calculation.
4. The gene expression profiles are those for untreated cells, therefore the expression data represents sensitivity to therapy rather than the molecular consequences of therapy. cDNA microarray data are fluorescent ratios. Ratio measurements are most naturally processed in log space, because in log space being 2-fold up and 2-fold down has the same magnitude of change in an opposite direction, as we want intuitively.
5. In fact, other machine learning approaches such as neural networks can also be employed in such study. Yet SVM does have several advantages over such machine learning problems. First, SVM avoids overfitting and finding trivial results (a common problem in the machine learning field) by selecting the optimal hyperplane among multiple candidates. Second, SVM condenses the information of the training examples into a small number of support vectors. If all the other

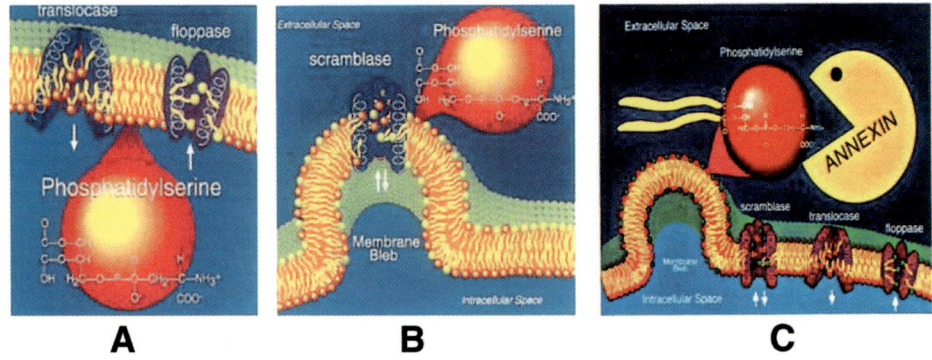

**Color Plate 1, Fig. 1.** (*see* full caption and discussion in Ch. 24 on p. 364.) Molecular basis for Annexin A5 imaging.

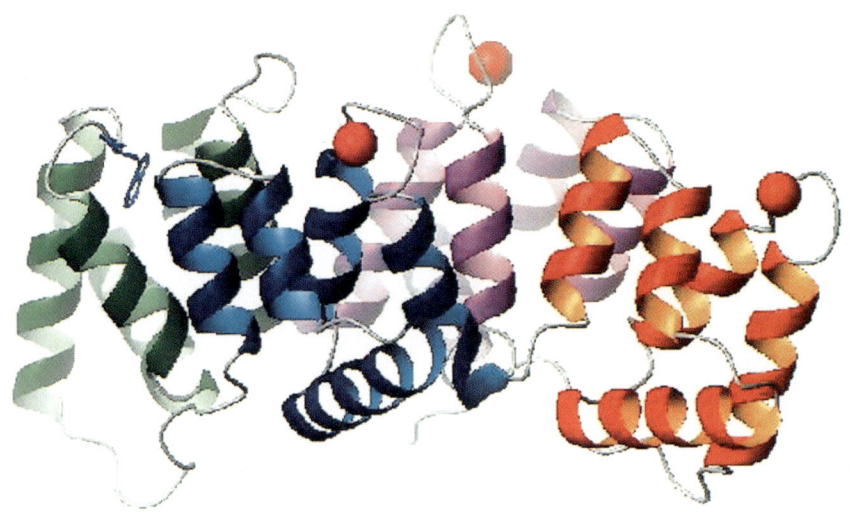

**Color Plate 2, Fig. 2.** (*see* full caption and discussion in Ch. 24 on p. 365.) Molecular structure of human Annexin A5.

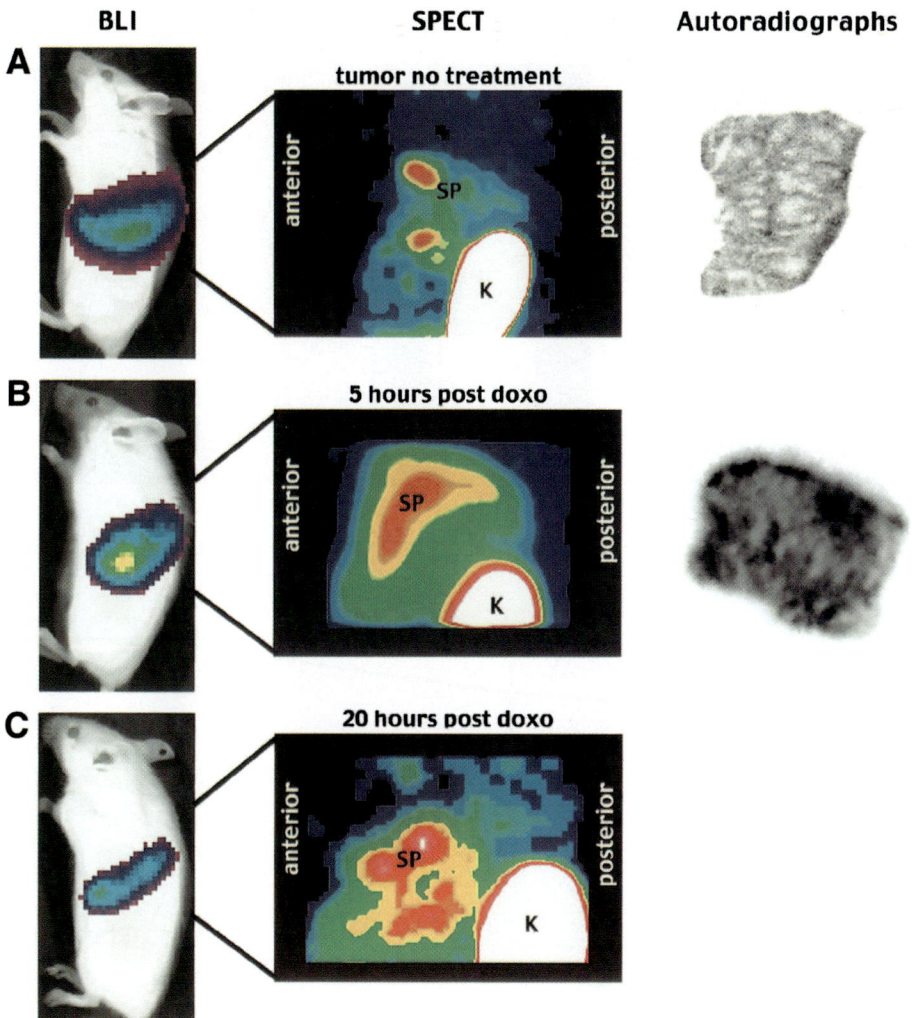

**Color Plate 3, Fig. 5.** (*see* full caption and discussion in Ch. 24 on p. 373.) $^{99m}$Tc-Annexin A5 uptake as seen by SPECT and autoradiography.

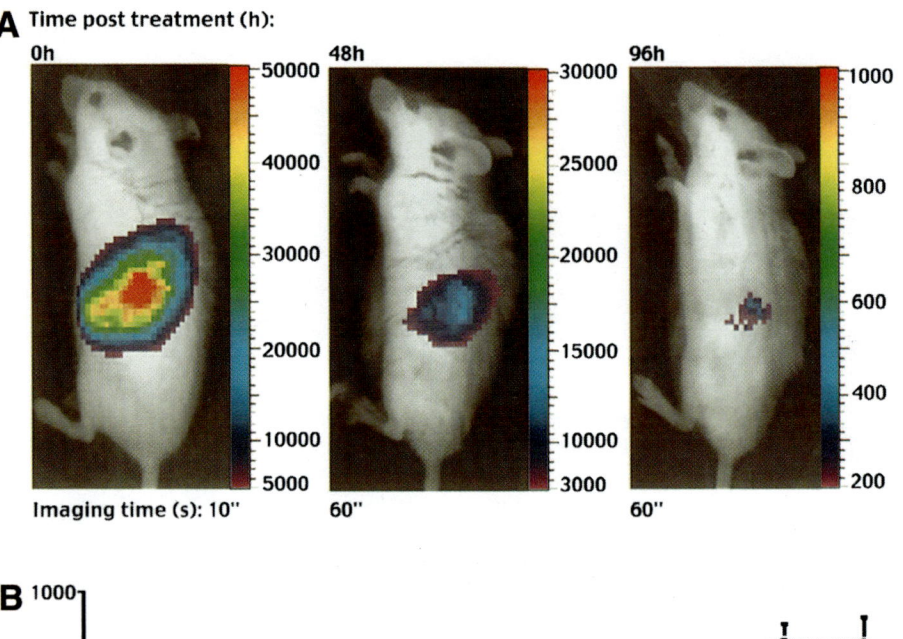
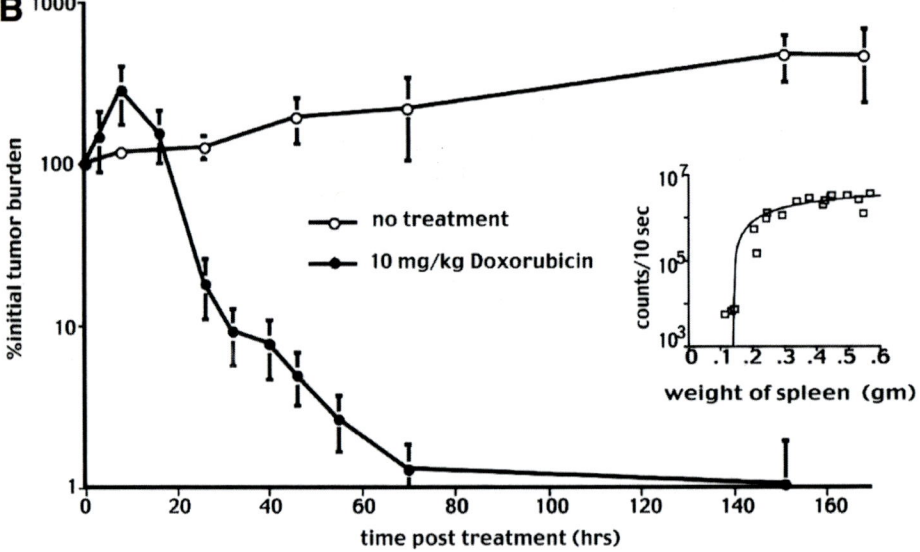

**Color Plate 4, Fig. 6.** (*see* full caption and discussion in Ch. 24 on p. 374.) Evaluation of tumor regression post-doxorubicin treatment.

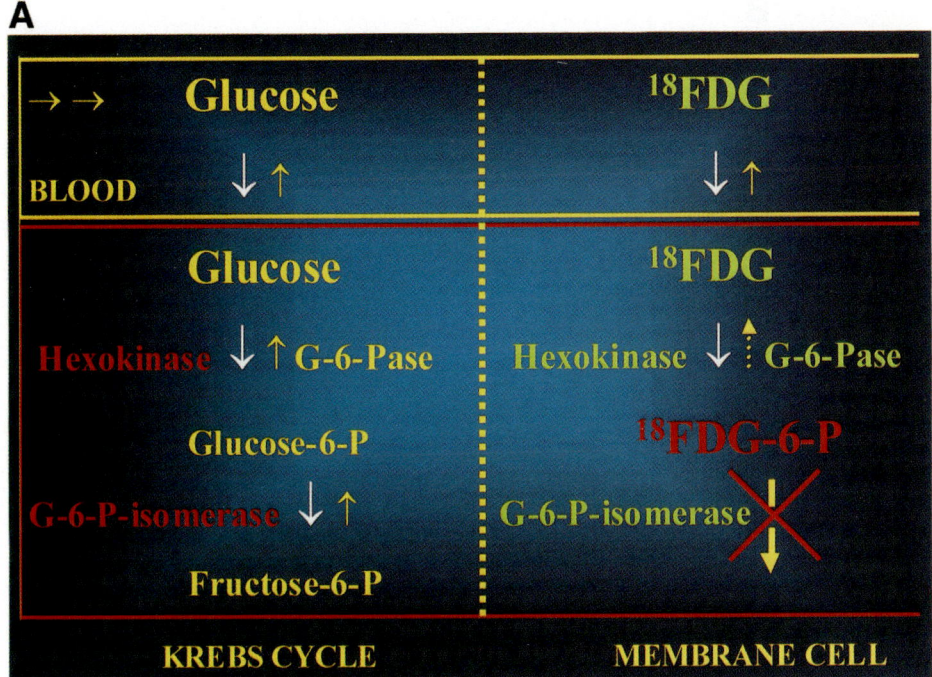

**Color Plate 5, Fig. 1A.** (*see* full caption and discussion in Ch. 26 on p. 418.) Glucose uptake into tumor cells.

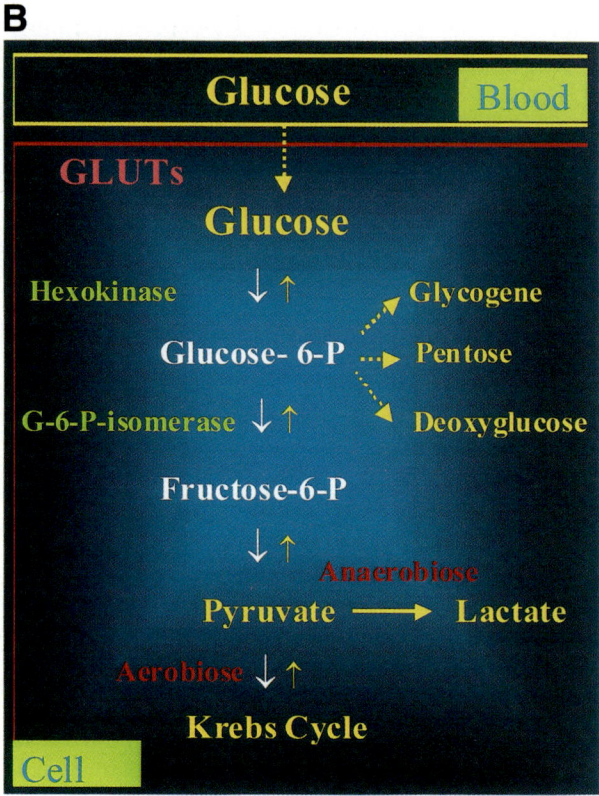

**Color Plate 6, Fig. 1B.** (*see* full caption and discussion in Ch. 26 on p. 419.) $^{18}$FDG uptake into tumor cells.

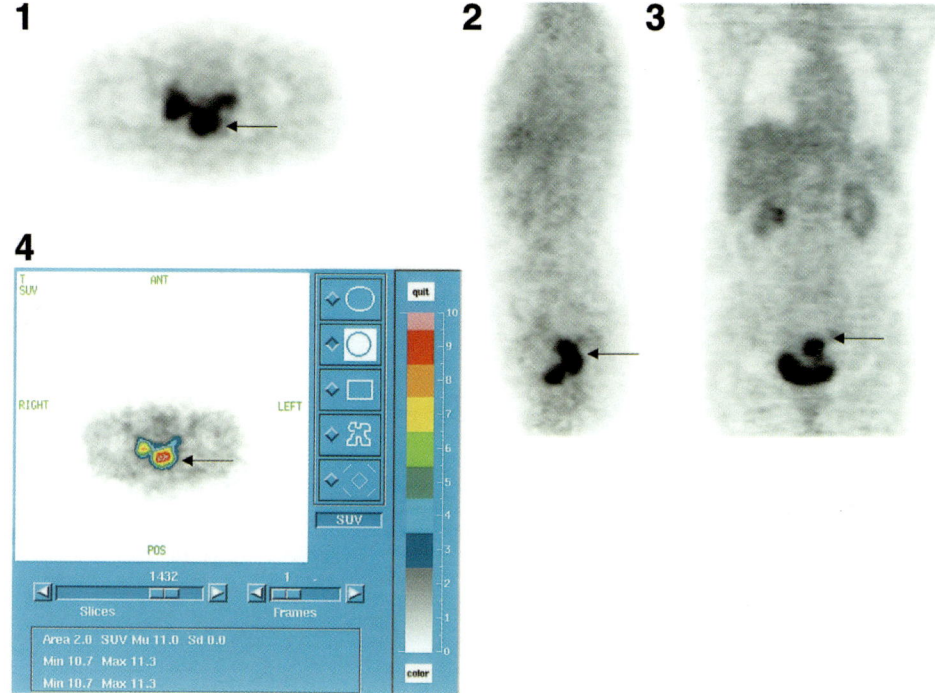

**Color Plate 7, Fig. 3B.** (*see* full caption and discussion in Ch. 26 on p. 427.) Semi-quantitative assessment of $^{18}$FDG uptake with the primary cervical tumor.

training examples are removed and SVM is retrained, the solution would keep unchanged. This allows SVM to classify new examples efficiently, because the majority of the training examples can be safely ignored. Third, the solution of SVM is not affected by the initial conditions. It is worth noting that an emerging machine learning method called the Bayes point machine *(10)*, which takes advantages from both SVM and Bayesian theory, is developing very quickly and is promising to give even better performance than SVM.

6. Given the data set, a proper kernel function and its parameters must be chosen to construct the SVM classifier. This selection is important because the type of kernel function determines the sample distribution in the mapping space. A first-degree kernel is equal to a linear classifier. A second-degree kernel reflects twofold interactions between the measured data, and so on for degree 3. There are no successful theoretical methods for determining the optimal kernel function and its parameters, so we are reduced to trial and error.
7. The SVM software we used was written by William Noble Grundy and can be downloaded at www.cse.ucsc.edu/research/compbio/genex/genex.html. Special attention should be paid to the "-threshold" option during the training phase. Training will halt when the objective function changes by less than this convergence threshold (Default is $10^{-6}$). To get reliable predictions over different runs in the present study, it is vital to set the threshold to $10^{-8}$ or less.
8. We did not encounter the case that a gene has two or more positive discriminant values. If such cases exist, they might be due to the multiple roles of the gene (interesting cases), or they might be due simply to fortuity. We must be more cautious in making inferences in such cases.
9. In the SOURCE database, four fields contained function annotation information. They are the fields of Summary Function, Gene Ontology Annotations, Other Ontology Annotations, and Enzymatic Function. We searched all these four fields for certain key words and compared their frequency in the two gene sets.
10. Using the phrase "DNA repair" could cause some false negatives, so we used DNA and REPAIR as the searching criterion. However, the latter could result in some false positives, therefore, for the 72-gene set, each gene bearing the key words was also manually looked through to make sure that they are indeed involved in the expecting biological process to eliminate false positives. This procedure is not applied to the original 4864-gene set, because bearing the false positives in the 4864-gene set would only lead to a more conservative estimation for the occurrence difference.
11. To eliminate the possibility that the difference in the occurrence of DNA repair-related genes is due simply to more annotated genes in the 72-gene set than in the 4864-gene set, occurrence normalized by the number of annotated genes was also calculated, and the result remained unchanged.

## References

1. Scherf, U., Ross, D. T., Waltham, M., et al. (2000) A gene expression database for the molecular pharmacology of cancer. *Nat. Genet.* **24,** 236–244.

2. Ross, D. T., Scherf, U., Eisen, M. B., et al. (2000) Systematic variation in gene expression patterns in human cancer cell lines. *Nat. Genet.* **24,** 227–235.
3. Butte, A. J., Tamayo, P., Slonim, D., Golub, T. R., and Kohane, I. S. (2000) Discovering functional relationships between RNA expression and chemotherapeutic susceptibility using relevance networks. *Proc. Natl. Acad. Sci. USA* **97,** 12,182–12,186.
4. Musumarra, G., Condorelli, D. F., Scire, S., and Costa, A. S. (2001) Shortcuts in genome-scale cancer pharmacology research from multivariate analysis of the National Cancer Institute gene expression database. *Biochem. Pharmacol.* **62,** 547–553.
5. Bao, L., Guo, T., and Sun, Z. R. (2002) Mining functional relationships in feature subspaces from gene expression profiles and drug activity profiles. *FEBS Lett.* **516,** 113–118.
6. Weinstein, J. N., Kohn, K. W., Grever, M. R., et al. (1992) Neural computing in cancer drug development: predicting mechanism of action. *Science* **258,** 447–451.
7. Cortes, C. and Vapnik, V. (1995) Support-vector networks. *Machine Learning* **20,** 273–293.
8. Boyd, M. R. and Paull, K. D. (1995) Some practical considerations and applications of the National Cancer Institute In Vitro Anticancer Drug Discovery Screen. *Drug Dev. Res.* **34,** 91–109.
9. Brown, M. P., Grundy, W. N., Lin, D., et al. (2000) Knowledge-based analysis of microarray gene expression data by using support vector machines. *Proc. Natl. Acad. Sci. USA* **97,** 262–267.
10. Herbrich, R., Graepel, T., and Campbell, C. (2001) Bayes point machines. *J. Machine Learning Res.* **1,** 245–279.

# 16

## Genetic Manipulation of Yeast to Identify Genes Involved in Regulation of Chemosensitivity

### Giovanni L. Beretta and Paola Perego

#### Summary

Fission and budding yeast have been regarded as valuable tools for studying several cellular processes in eukaryotic cells and have been exploited as model systems for the identification of determinants of chemosensitivity. Indeed, yeast mutants of DNA repair and cell cycle checkpoint pathways exhibit increased sensitivity to selected antitumor drugs, thereby allowing us to establish the role of specific genes in drug response. The basic cellular functions of simple eukaryotic organisms and mammalian cells are conserved. Thus, the features of yeast, such as a small genome, a fast growth rate, and a peculiar life cycle, which allows easy genetic manipulation, can provide advantages in the identification of determinants of chemosensitivity. Here we focus on methods developed in fission yeast with particular reference to gene disruption, transformation, and mutagenesis approaches. These methods could be useful in an attempt to develop target-specific therapeutic strategies.

#### Key Words

Gene disruption; transformation; mutagenesis; fission yeast; chemosensitivity.

## 1. Introduction
### 1.1. Gene Disruption: Knockout Construction

Gene inactivation is a key step in dissecting out gene/protein functions. The possibility of engineering specific DNA sequences into the yeast genome relies on the fact that in yeast nearly all recombination is homologous, so that an incoming DNA molecule is targeted with fidelity to the corresponding genomic location. Homologous recombination was first exploited to modify genes in two steps. With this approach, a circular plasmid carrying the mutant gene can be integrated into the genome, generating transformants with two copies of the

From: *Methods in Molecular Medicine, vol. 111: Chemosensitivity:
Vol. 2: In Vivo Models, Imaging, and Molecular Regulators*
Edited by: R. D. Blumenthal © Humana Press Inc., Totowa, NJ

target gene separated by plasmid sequences. The plasmid sequences can then be removed along with the wild-type copy of the gene, by a second recombination event between the duplicated sequences, leaving the altered copy of the gene *(1,2)*. The one-step gene disruption technique (**Fig. 1A**) allows the insertion of a selectable gene into the target gene, thereby disrupting it *(3)*. A short yeast DNA sequence (fewer than 50 bp) is enough for homologous recombination, and the DNA fragment required for gene disruption can be generated by polymerase chain reaction (PCR). The PCR amplified fragment (gene disruption cassette) provides a selectable phenotype (usually a resistance or prototrophic marker) surrounded by 30–50 bp flanking the sequence to delete. Disruption of multiple genes in a yeast strain can be achieved by (1) sequential deletion through gene disruption cassettes with different selectable phenotypes or (2) removal of the disruption cassette from the genome and further use to disrupt another gene. In this regard, a gene disruption cassette flanked by *loxP* sites works efficiently as expression of Cre recombinase removes the cassette in 80–90% of the cells. Autonomously replicating plasmids carrying Cre recombinase are available with different selectable markers *(4,5)*.

### *1.2. Transformation of Yeast*

A prerequisite for molecular manipulation of any organism is availability of reliable and efficient means for introducing exogenous DNA into the cell. Various techniques can be used for transforming yeast, including electroporation, protoplast, or lithium acetate transformation *(7–10)*. Each technique suffers from limitations such as low efficiency of DNA transfer (lithium acetate transformation) or complexity (protoplast transformation).

### *1.3. Mutagenesis Techniques*

Generating mutants to identify new genes and their properties is the starting point for many molecular studies. Site-specific mutagenesis and other recombinant DNA techniques are increasingly used and are the methods of choice when changes in specific genes or genetic sites are needed.

The best mutagens are those that induce high frequencies of base-pair substitutions and little lethality. The widely used alkylating agents ethylmethane sulfonate (EMS) and nitosoguanidine (NG) fulfil these criteria, but are highly specific in their action as they almost exclusively produce transitions at G–C sites *(13)*. Ultraviolet light (254 nm UV) is also a fairly efficient mutagen, and it has the advantage of producing a greater range of substitutions including transitions and transversions, and frameshift mutations *(14,15)*. Here we focus on EMS and NG. The former is safer to use, but the latter is a more potent mutagen.

**A** ONE-STEP GENE DISRUPTION

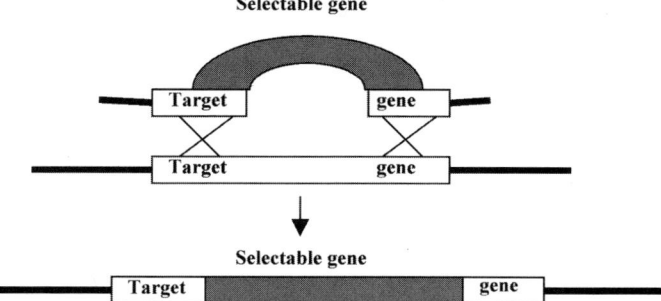

**B**
**Disrupted gene**

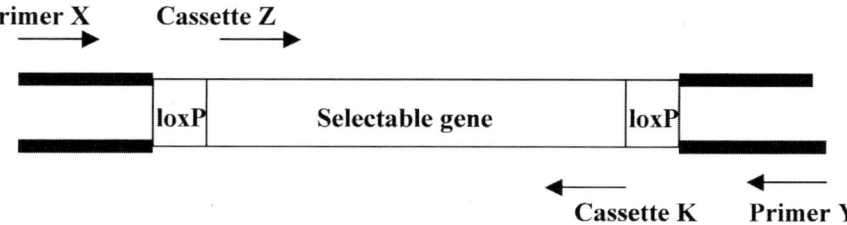

**Undisrupted gene**

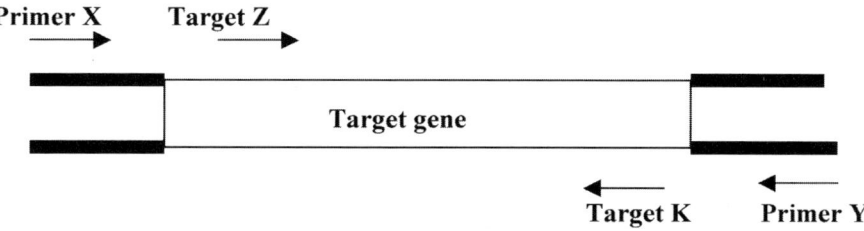

Fig. 1. (**A**) One step-gene disruption. This technique allows the insertion of a selectable gene (usually a resistance or prototrophy marker) into the target gene thereby disrupting it. A short of yeast DNA sequence (fewer than 50 bp) is enough for homologous recombination and the DNA fragment required for gene disruption can be generated by PCR. (**B**) Checking gene disruption. A successful gene disruption is verified by testing for PCR products using the DNA of the disruption mutant as template. Primer pairs: primer X/cassette K and cassette Z/primer Y will yield a PCR product only if the gene is disrupted correctly. The deletion of the target should also be verified by confirming that primer pairs primer X/target K and target Z/primer Y do not yield a PCR product.

### 1.3.1. In Vitro Generalized Mutagenesis: Degenerate PCR Mutagenesis

Degenerate PCR can be easily and reproducibly used to introduce mutations into cloned DNAs. It is based on the fidelity of *Taq* polymerase, which is decreased by adding $Mn^{2+}$ to the buffer and increasing the dCTP and dTTP concentration in the PCR mix *(16)*.

### 1.3.2. Site-Directed Mutagenesis: Oligonucleotide-Directed Mutagenesis

The method has the advantage of limiting the mutations introduced into the gene to the region of the gene corresponding to the oligonucleotide. Any nucleotide can be changed by synthesizing the appropriate mutant oligonucleotide. Oligonucleotide can be used to generate a library of point mutants that can be subsequently screened. Here we focus on the two most used techniques: quick change and cassette mutagenesis.

In the quick-change technique, the mutation present in the synthesized oligonucleotide is introduced into the full-length gene by *Pfu* DNA polymerase-mediated linear amplification. The template in the amplification reaction is the full-length wild-type gene carried on a plasmid. The primers used for linear amplification are precisely complementary to each other, and both include the mutation to be introduced. Because the two primers are complementary, the reaction amplifies the entire plasmid, generating a product corresponding to the entire plasmid. This final product is a circular DNA with nicks at the 5' end of each primer. The parental template DNA, which is naturally methylated, is digested with a methylation-sensitive enzyme (*DpnI*) and the product of the reaction is transformed into *Escherichia coli*. Only the newly synthesized plasmid including the oligonucleotides with the incorporated mutations will be left undigested by the *DnpI* and will be able to transform *E. coli*, resulting in efficient recovery of the mutagenized full-length gene.

Cassette mutagenesis involves construction of a point mutant or libraries of point mutants. The mutations present in the oligonucleotide used for PCR are used to amplify a DNA fragment-containing restriction site also engineered into the PCR primers. These restriction sites are then used to introduce the PCR fragment into the full-length gene (**Fig. 2**).

---

Fig. 2. *(see facing page)* Cloning by gap repair. The cloning vector carrying the gene to be mutated is digested with restriction enzymes 1 and 2, generating a gapped vector. If the PCR fragment generated has usable restriction sites, or if the PCR primers incorporate restriction sites at each end of the PCR fragment, these may be used directly to clone the mutagenized DNA into the gapped vector (cloning using restriction site). An efficient alternative is homologous recombination to repair a gapped plasmid using a cotransformed PCR fragment as template (cloning using recombitional gap repair).

# Genetic Manipulation of Yeast

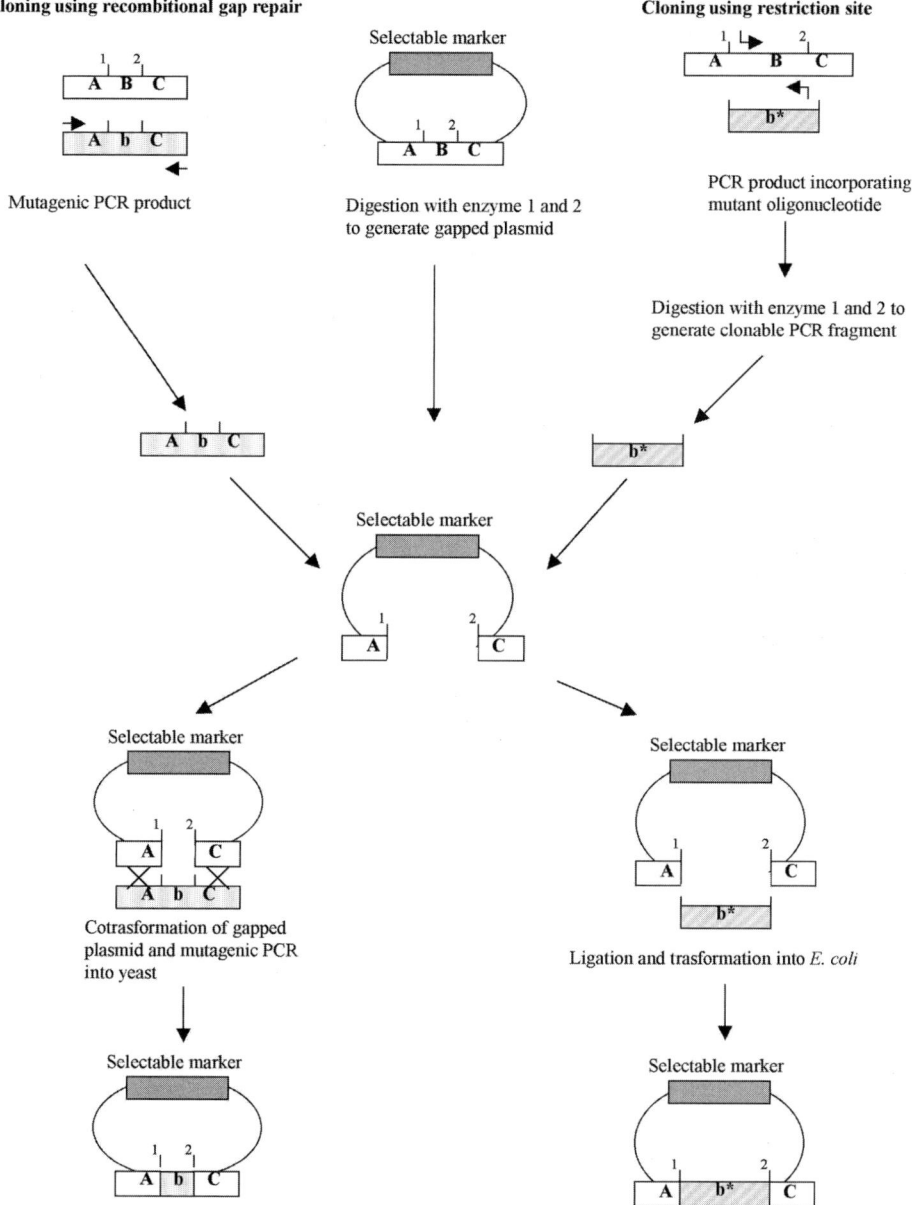

## 2. Materials
### 2.1. One-Step Gene Disruption: PCR-Based Gene Disruption Technique
1. *Taq* DNA polymerase (5 U/µL with 10X buffer): any supplier.
2. dNTP mix (2.5 m$M$ of each dNTP).

### 2.2. Transformation of Yeast
*2.2.1. Electroporation Procedure*

1. Buffer A: 10 m$M$ Tris-HCl, pH 8.0, 1 m$M$ EDTA.
2. 1 $M$ sorbitol.

*2.2.2. Protoplast Procedure*

1. Buffer B: 20 m$M$ citrate/phosphate, pH 5.6, 40 m$M$ EDTA, 30 m$M$ 2-mercaptoethanol (0.2% v/v, added after autoclaving).
2. Buffer C: 50 m$M$ citrate/phospate, pH 5.6, 1.2 $M$ sorbitol. Adjust to pH 5.6 with 5 $M$ NaOH and add 30 m$M$ 2-mercaptoethanol (0.2% v/v, added after autoclaving), 25 mg NovoZym 234.
3. Buffer D: 10 m$M$ Tris-HCl, pH 7.6, 1.2 $M$ sorbitol.
4. Buffer E: 10 m$M$ Tris-HCl, pH 7.6, 10 m$M$ CaCl$_2$, 1.2 $M$ sorbitol.
5. Buffer F: 10 m$M$ Tris-HCl, pH 7.6, 10 m$M$ CaCl$_2$, 20 m$M$ polyethylene glycol (PEG) 4000.
6. Buffer G: 10 m$M$ Tris-HCl, pH 7.6, 10 m$M$ CaCl$_2$, 1.2 $M$ sorbitol, 0.5 mg/mL yeast extract, 5 µg/mL supplements.

*2.2.3. Lithium Acetate Procedure*

1. Buffer H: 0.1 $M$ lithium acetate (adjusted the pH to 4.9 with acetic acid).
2. 50% (w/v) PEG 4000.

### 2.3. Mutagenesis Techniques
1. 4% EMS.
2. Buffer I: 50 m$M$ Tris-malate, pH 6.
3. 1-mg/mL NG in buffer I. Mutagens are powerful carcinogens: they have to be handled in a proper hood, using protective clothing, gloves, and eye protection.

*2.3.1. In Vitro Generalized Mutagenesis: Degenerate PCR Mutagenesis*

1. *Taq* DNA polymerase (5 U/µL with 10X buffer): any supplier.
2. Restriction enzymes (20 U/µL with 10X buffer): any supplier.

*2.3.2. Site-Directed Mutagenesis: Oligonucleotide-Directed Mutagenesis*

1. *Pfu* DNA polymerase (2.5 U/µL) supplied with 10X buffer: any supplier.
2. *Dpn*I (20 U/µL) supplied with 10X buffer: any supplier.

### 2.3.2.1. Cassette Mutagenesis: Construction of a Point Mutant or Libraries of Point Mutants

1. *Pfu* DNA polymerase (2.5 U/µL) supplied with 10X buffer: any supplier.
2. T4 DNA ligase (400 U/µL) supplied with 10X ligase buffer: any supplier.
3. Restriction enzymes: any supplier.

## 3. Methods

### 3.1. One-Step Gene Disruption: PCR-Based Gene Disruption Technique

#### 3.1.1. Primer Design

1. *Disruption cassette primers.* The sequences flanking the target gene are added to the 5′ ends as follows: 30–50 nucleotides of the top/bottom strand immediately upstream/downstream of the sequences to delete (the nucleotides immediately before the ATG/after the stop codon) are added to the 5′-ends of each PCR primer.
2. *Disruption confirmation primers.* The PCR primers flanking the target gene are chosen so that the product formed in conjunction with the PCR primers within the disruption cassette (cassette K and cassette Z primers in **Fig. 1B**) or within the target gene (target K and target Z primers) is 300–1000 nucleotides in length. The primers should be 17–28 nucleotides with the melting temperature around 65°C. As shown in **Fig. 1B**, a successful gene disruption is verified by testing for PCR products using the described primers (X and Y) with DNA of the disruption mutant as template. Primer pairs: primer X/cassette K and cassette Z/primer Y will yield a PCR product only if the gene is disrupted correctly. The deletion of the target should also be verified by confirming that primer pairs (primer X/target K and target Z/primer Y) do not yield a PCR product.

#### 3.1.2. Preparative PCR of Gene Disruption Cassette

##### 3.1.2.1. From Plasmid DNA

1. Prepare a mix (46 µL total volume) containing: 5 µL 10X *Taq* DNA polymerase, 4 µL of 10 m*M* dNTP mix (2.5 m*M* each dNTP), 2 µL of 1 ng/µL template DNA (*see* **Note 1**), 34 µL H$_2$O. Keep the tube on ice and add 1 µL of *Taq* DNA polymerase (5 U/µL).
2. Dispense 46-µL aliquots into PCR tubes.
3. Add 2 µL of 25 µ*M* upstream primer and 2 µL of 25 µ*M* downstream primer.
4. Add H$_2$O instead of DNA to the negative control tube. Keep everything on ice until placing tubes in thermocycler.
5. Thermocycler parameters: Hot start, 94°C, 3 min; denaturation, 94°C, 1.5 min; annealing, 57°C, 2 min; extension, 72°C, 3 min; final extension, 72°C, 3 min. Run 35 cycles. Note that a large number of cycles is crucial.
6. Assay 2 µL on a 1% agarose gel (concentration should be approx 50 ng/µL).

##### 3.1.2.2. From Gene Disruption Cassette Present in Yeast Genome

The gene disruption cassette can be amplified as one product using primers flanking the disrupted gene (primer X and primer Y in **Fig. 1B**).

1. Use as template DNA from yeast cells freshly grown on solid medium. Gently touch the surface of the colony (avoid contact with agar) with a plastic pipet tip attached to the pipettor. Place the tip into a 50-µL PCR reaction mix and pipet up and down once. Too many cells or the presence of agar will inhibit the reaction.
2. Assay 10 µL of the PCR reactions on agarose gel, because less PCR product is available when starting from a colony as compared to preparative PCR where a plasmid is used as template. No purification or precipitation of the PCR product is necessary before transformation.

*3.1.3. Yeast Transformation*

For yeast transformations, *see* **Subheading 3.2.** The amount of the PCR-amplified DNA used for each transformation is about 2–5 µg.

*3.1.4. Checking for Correct Gene Disruption by PCR*

1. Pick up some colonies of transformants grown on selective agar plates (4–10 from each transformant). Use the wild-type strain as a negative control and start from freshly grown yeast cells as a template for the PCR. Gently touch the surface of the colony (avoid contact with agar) with a plastic pipet tip attached to the pipettor. Place the tip into a 50-µL PCR reaction mix and pipet up and down once. Too many cells or the presence of agar will inhibit the reaction.
2. Use the primers designed according to the rules described above.
3. Set up a 50-µL PCR as described above.
4. Add loading dye to each reaction and run 20 µL on agarose gel (*see* **Notes 1–3**).

## *3.2. Transformation of Yeast*

*3.2.1. Electroporation Procedure*

The electroporation technique is extremely simple and efficient, and includes three steps.

1. Preparation of electrocompetent cells. An overnight culture grown with vigorous shaking at 30°C to 1.3–1.5 $OD_{595}$ is diluted the next morning and grown until the yeast enters exponential growth phase. The subsequent step of centrifugation and washing in sterile water achieves the goals of 500–1000-fold concentrating the cells and reducing the culture conductivity.
2. Electroporation. An aliquot of yeast electrocompetent cells is transferred to a sterile tube. Then ≤100 ng of DNA is added to the cell suspension, mixed, and incubated on ice for about 5 min. The DNA should be dissolved in a small volume (e.g., 5 µL) of a low-ionic-strength buffer (A) or water to avoid flashover. Transfer to a 0.2-cm sterile electroporation cuvet. Pulse at 1.5 kV, 25 µF, 200 Ω. Apparatus and cuvets are commercially available. Immediately add 1 mL of cold 1 *M* sorbitol to the cuvet, pipet gently, and mix the contents. Transfer to a culture tube.

3. Plating. Aliquots of transformation reaction are plated spreading on selective medium. No incubation in a shaker is required after resuspension and transfer of the reaction from the cuvette; plate as soon as possible.

### 3.2.2. Protoplast Procedure

1. Grow a 200-mL culture to an $OD_{595}$ of 0.2–0.5 ($4 \times 10^6$–$1 \times 10^7$ cells/mL) in appropriate medium.
2. Harvest cells, decant supernatant, and resuspend the pellet in 10 mL of buffer B.
3. Harvest cells and resuspend the contents in 5 mL of buffer C.
4. Incubate at 37°C for 15–30 min until spheroplasts have formed.
5. Add 35 mL of buffer D.
6. Spin gently at 720g for 5 min and wash twice in 20 mL of buffer D, each time resuspending gently in 1 mL. At the last resuspension, take an aliquot and count the number of protoplasts with a hemacytometer.
7. Resuspend at $2$–$5 \times 10^8$ protoplasts/mL in buffer E (*see* **Note 4**).
8. Using 100 µL protoplast/transformation, add 1–10 µg of transforming DNA. Incubate at room temperature for 15 min (*see* **Notes 5** and **6**).
9. Add 1 mL of buffer F and incubate at room temperature for 15 min.
10. Spin at 720g for 5 min, drain well, and resuspend the protoplast in 0.2–0.5 mL of buffer G. Incubate at 30°C for 30–60 min.
11. Plate out 0.2-mL aliquots onto well-dried minimal sorbitol plates.

### 3.2.3. Lithium Acetate Procedure

1. Grow a 150-mL culture in appropriate medium to an $OD_{595}$ of 0.2–0.5 ($4 \times 10^6$–$1 \times 10^7$ cells/mL).
2. Harvest cells at 1620g for 5 min at room temperature.
3. Wash cells in 40 mL water and spin them down as in **step 2**.
4. Resuspend the cells at $1 \times 10^9$ cells/mL in buffer H and dispense 100 µL aliquots into 2-mL tube. Incubate at 30°C for 60–120 min. Cells will sediment at this stage.
5. Add 1 µg of DNA in 15 µL total volume and mix by gentle vortexing. Completely resuspend cell sedimented during the incubation. Add 290 µL of 50% (w/v) PEG 4000 prewarmed at 30°C. Mix by gentle vortexing and incubate at 30°C for 50 min.
6. Heat-shock at 43°C for 15 min and keep at room temperature for 10 min.
7. Centrifuge at 4500g for 2 min. Carefully remove the supernatant.
8. Resuspend the cells in 1 mL of appropriate medium.
9. Add 9 mL of medium to have a final vol of 10 mL and incubate with shaking at 30°C for 60 min or longer.
10. Plate aliquots of less than 0.3 mL onto appropriate medium. If necessary, centrifuge the cells at this stage and resuspend in 1 mL of medium to spread more cells on a plate.

## 3.3. Mutagenesis Techniques

### 3.3.1. EMS Mutagenesis

1. Grow up 100 mL of yeast cells in appropriate medium to an $OD_{595}$ of 0.2–0.5 ($4 \times 10^6$–$1 \times 10^7$ cells/mL).
2. Harvest cells at 1620g for 5 min and resuspend at $1 \times 10^8$ cells/mL in fresh medium.
3. Take 2 mL, transfer to a 50-mL plastic capped tube and add 2 mL of 4% EMS (2% final concentration) (*see* **Note 7**).
4. Leave the cells at room temperature in the fume hood for 3 h with gentle shaking.
5. Transfer 1 mL to a 1.5-mL tube, harvest the cells, and wash three times with 1 mL of sterile 0.9% NaCl.
6. Dilute the cells as required and plate onto medium. The percentage of survival should be approximately 50% (this percentage is strain dependent) (*see* **Notes 8** and **9**).
7. EMS is inactivated using and excess of 5% sodium thiosulfate.

#### 3.3.1.1. NG Mutagenesis

1. Grow 100 mL of yeast cells in appropriate medium to an $OD_{595}$ of 0.2–0.5 ($4 \times 10^6$–$1 \times 10^7$ cells/mL).
2. Take 10 mL and harvest cells at 1620g for 5 min. Wash once with 10 mL of buffer I.
3. Resuspend cells in buffer I at $1.4 \times 10^8$ cells/mL. Mix 700 µL of cells with 300 µL of 1-mg/mL NG in the same buffer (*see* **Note 7**). Incubate at 30°C for 30, 60, and 90 min with occasional vortexing.
4. Remove 100 µL of cells and dilute with 900 µL of buffer I. Wash twice with 1 mL of buffer I and once with medium.
5. Cells are then resuspended in 1 mL of medium and incubated for 4 h at 25°C and plated. The percentage of survival should be approximately 40, 15, and 3% for 30, 60, and 90 min, respectively (though percentages are strain dependent) (*see* **Notes 8** and **9**).
6. NG is inactivated using overnight bleaching.

#### 3.3.1.2. Introduction of Point Mutation into Cloned Genes

Many techniques are available for introducing sequence changes into cloned yeast genes. Point mutations can be introduced by generalized mutagenesis or oligonucleotide-directed mutagenesis. The latter approach allows the choice of the exact position/nature of the nucleotide or amino acid change to make and can be used for generating a library of point mutants. In the case of limited knowledge of the protein functional domains, a generalized method to obtain mutants across the entire gene is appropriate. With both approaches, the mutations must be introduced into the full-length gene. Three basic approaches are available for generalized mutagenesis: the quick-change method, recombinational gap repair, and cloning by natural restriction site. The following Subheadings focus on in vitro generalized mutagenesis and site-directed mutagenesis.

### 3.3.1.3. IN VITRO GENERALIZED MUTAGENESIS: DEGENERATE PCR MUTAGENESIS

1. *PCR conditions.* The plasmid to be mutagenized, carrying the wild-type gene, is subjected to a PCR reaction. In 50 μL final volume add: 20 fmol template; 0.3 μ*M* each primer; 0.5 m*M* $MnCl_2$; 0.2 m*M* dATP; 0.2 m*M* dGTP; 1 m*M* dCTP; 1 m*M* dTTP; 1X *Taq* polymerase buffer. Keep on ice and add 1 μL *Taq* DNA polymerase.
2. Thermocycler parameters: hot start, 94°C, 3 min; denaturation, 98°C, 5 s; annealing/extension, 62°C, 6 min/cycle; the number of cycles is dependent on the desired mutation rate. Using the given conditions the reported mutation rate was 0.66% per base pair after 10 duplications of the template *(17)*. Assay 2 μL on a 1% agarose gel (concentration should be approx 50 ng/μL).
3. *Plasmid gapping by restriction enzymes.* The plasmid is first gapped by restriction enzymes uniquely present in the gene of interest. Reaction conditions: 5 μg plasmid vector carrying the cloned gene of interest; 20 U restriction enzyme 1; 20 U restriction enzyme 2; 1X buffer (giving optimal activity for both enzymes). If the two enzymes are not compatible, reactions should be performed separately (*see* **Note 10**).
4. Incubate 2–4 h at the appropriate temperature (depending on the enzymes used). After gapping, the plasmid can be gel purified to remove undigested or singly digested vector.
5. *Cloning PCR-mutagenized fragment by gap repair.* Once the mutagenized PCR fragment is generated, it must be introduced into the gapped vector. If the fragment has usable restriction sites, or if the PCR primers incorporate restriction sites at each end of the PCR fragment, these may be used directly to clone the mutagenized DNA into the gapped vector. An efficient alternative is homologous recombination to repair a gapped plasmid using a cotrasformed PCR fragment as template (**Fig. 2**) *(18)*.
6. Transformation mix: 0.1–1 μg of gapped plasmid; 3–5X molar excess of PCR product. Transform these DNAs into an appropriately marked yeast strain deleted, if possible, for the chromosomal locus of the mutated gene (*see* **Note 11**). Plate on media selective for the marker on the gapped plasmid.

### 3.3.2. Site-Directed Mutagenesis: Oligonucleotide-Directed Mutagenesis

1. *Design of primers.* The primers should be synthesized precisely complementary to each other and the $T_m$ must be at least 78°C. The mutation is placed in the middle of the primer with at least 12 bp of wild-type sequence on each side of the mutation site.
2. *Amplification reaction.* In a thermocycler tube, make a 50-μL reaction containing 1 μg template DNA (*see* **Note 12**), 250 μ*M* each dNTP, 1X *Pfu* buffer, 3 m*M* $MgSO_4$ (final), 30 pmol of each mutagenic primer. Heat the tube at 95°C and add 1 μL of *Pfu* DNA polymerase. Cycle for 16 rounds using the following condition: 95°C, 40 s; 53°C, 60 s; 68°C, 2 min per kb of template plasmid length.

3. *Digestion of product with DpnI.* After cycling, check the amplification by running on a agarose gel. If there is product, remove 5 µL, add to a total of 20 µL the digestion buffer and 10 U of *DpnI*. Digest for 1 h at 37°C.
4. *Transformation into E. coli.* Transform 1 µL of the digested product into *E. coli*.

3.3.2.1. CASSETTE MUTAGENESIS: CONSTRUCTION OF A POINT MUTANT OR LIBRARIES OF POINT MUTANTS

1. *Primer design.* The oligonucleotide must have four distinct regions. Region 1, at the 3′ end of the oligonucleotide, is a region of perfect homology with the target gene. When using degenerate oligonucleotides to construct libraries of mutants, this constant region must be 25 nucleotides in length to guarantee that mutation in the degenerate oligonucleotide exactly 5′ to this region are not biased against in the subsequent PCR step. Region 2 incorporates the desired point mutation or, in the case of libraries of mutants, multiple mutations. Region 3 includes the restriction site and can also include a further constant region, depending on the distance between the site to be mutagenized and the restriction site. Region 4, exactly 5′ to the restriction site, is the "clamp" of several nucleotides to allow efficient digestion with the restriction enzyme whose site has been incorporated in region 3 of the oligonucleotide. Many restriction enzymes will not digest restriction sites present at the very end of the DNA fragment, and so, depending on the restriction enzyme, the "clamp" may be necessary to get efficient digestion of the PCR product.
2. *PCR amplification.* This step is identical to that described above.
3. *Enzyme digestion of plasmid vector and amplified fragment DNA.* After amplification, the PCR product and the plasmid vector are digested with the restriction enzymes.
4. *Cloning by ligase enzyme.* The ligase reaction (20 µL final volume) is performed using: 0.1–1 µg of digested plasmid; 3–5X molar excess of digested PCR product; 1 µL ligase; 1X ligase buffer (*see* **Notes 13** and **14**). Incubate at 16°C for 16 h. This step regenerates the full-length gene.
5. *Transformation into E. coli.* Transform this DNA into *E. coli* cell.

## 4. Notes

1. If the template used in the PCR to produce the disruption cassette is a plasmid capable of replicating autonomously in the yeast cells, a significant number of transformants will inherit the plasmid rather than the disruption cassette. This can be minimized by cleaving the plasmid with a restriction enzyme that does not cut into disruption cassette or, even better, by using a plasmid that cannot replicate autonomously as template.
2. In some cases genes are difficult to disrupt. They include: (a) genes lying in a duplicated region for which it is necessary to check the flanking sequences to be sure that they are not repeated elsewhere in the genome; (b) genes flanked by long stretches of simple sequences [e.g., poly(AT)] for which a new deletion oligonucleotide including the unique flanking sequence is required to reach gene disruption. For some genes a few transformants can be obtained using the usual

45 bp of flanking homology, and a gene disruption cassette flanked by 90 bp is required to increase the number of transformants. However, in some cases longer regions of sequence homology can give rise to pseudo-stable transformants, likely due to circularization of the sequence.
3. In many cases, gene deletion is accompanied by duplication of the gene of interest. The duplicated gene appears to be linked to the disrupted gene *(6)*. These events can be due to duplication of the entire chromosome or of a portion of it, which includes the disrupted gene. Thus, the absence of the deleted gene must be confirmed by a PCR assay.
4. Storage of protoplasts. Protoplast can be aliquoted, stored at −70°C in buffer E, and used for at least 2 mo.
5. Transformation efficiency. The transformation efficiency can be determined by calculating the number of transformants in 1 mL of resuspended cells per 1 µg plasmid per $10^8$ cells. For example, if the transformation of $1.0 \times 10^8$ cells with 100 ng plasmid resulted in 500 colonies on a plate spread with 1 µL of suspension:

Transformation efficiency =
$500 \times 1000$(plating factor) $\times 10$(plasmid factor) $\times 1$(cell/transformation $\times 10^8$)

Transformation efficiency = $5 \times 10^6$ trasformants/1.0 µg plasmid/$10^8$ cells. Transformation efficiency declines as plasmid concentration is increased *(8,11)*.
6. Optimization of the protoplast transformation. Transformation frequency can be increased using lipofectin *(12)*. For this purpose, follow the protocol to **step 8** and after the 15-min incubation of the protoplast with DNA add 100 µL of 10 m*M* Tris-HCl, pH 7.6, 10 m*M* CaCl$_2$, 1.2 *M* sorbitol, 66-µg/mL lipofectin and incubate a further 15 min at room temperature. Proceed to **step 9** and follow the rest of the protocol.
7. Mutagen concentration. A balance between high mutation frequency with avoidance of multiple mutations and reasonable high survival is required. The highest proportion of mutants per treated cell is usually found at concentrations giving 10–50% survival. Concentrations that kill more than 95% of cells should be avoided, as they may select multicell clusters or atypically resistant variants spontaneously occurring in all cell populations or multiple mutants.
8. Growth conditions after treatment. After exposure to mutagens, yeast culture should be allowed to grow for several generations under nonselective conditions, to enhance the expression of mutations. With some mutagens, such as EMS, mutations occur mainly during S-phase, and repaired damage can continue to produce mutations in successive generations. Growth is also required to promote dilution and turnover of gene products, or the synthesis of new ones, to allow the full expression of the mutant or revertant phenotype. In addition, cells may require time to recover from mutagen damage, which could transiently prevent some cells from growing. Plating dilutions of treated cells in solid medium, to get colonies for screening, has the advantage that each induced mutation identified is of independent origin.
9. Mutant "cleanup." Since treated strains often contain mutations in several genes, the mutant phenotype initially observed may be a misleading result of several individual genetic alterations. It is usually helpful to "clean up" the strain by placing

the mutation of interest in a nonmutagenized genetic background by repeated backcrossing to an untreated isogenic strain or, if the mutant locus is known, by PCR-cloning the mutant gene and transfer to an untreated strain by gene replacement.
10. Efficiency. The efficiency of the methods depends on (a) the extent of homology between the ends of PCR fragment and the gapped plasmid and (b) the underlying rate of nonhmologous end joining (NHEJ) that results in recircularization of the plasmid without incorporation of the PCR fragment. The two enzymes used to gap the plasmid should be chosen so that the generated ends are not substrates for efficient relegation by NHEJ. The plasmid can be gapped either with enzymes generating blunt ends, or by two different enzymes generating noncompatible ends. Both ends of the PCR product to be cloned must share homology with the ends of the gapped plasmid. Commonly, the PCR fragment carries around 200 bp of homology with the gapped plasmid *(18)*.
11. Maximize the number of transformants. It is recommended that the number of transformants be maximized during transformation, as this will determine the final number of mutants of the library.
12. The template must be prepared from a methylation-competent strain of *E. coli*.
13. Blunt-ended and single-base-pair overhang ligations require about 50 times as much enzyme to achieve the same extent of ligation as cohesive-ended DNA fragments.
14. Blunt-end ligation may be enhanced by addition of PEG or hexamine chloride.

## References

1. Orr-Weaver, T. L., Szostak, J. W., and Rothstein, R. J. (1981) Yeast transformation: a model system for the study of recombination. *Proc. Natl. Acad. Sci. USA* **78**, 6354–6358.
2. Orr-Weaver, T. L., Szostak, J. W., and Rothstein, R. J. (1983) Genetic applications of yeast transformation with linear and gapped plasmids. *Meth. Enzymol.* **101**, 228–245.
3. Rothestein, R. J. (1983) One-step gene disruption in yeast. *Meth. Enzymol.* **101**, 202–211.
4. Guldener, U., Heck, S., Fielder, T., Beinhauer, J., and Hegemann, J. H. (1996) A new efficient gene disruption cassette for repeated use in budding yeast. *Nucleic Acids Res.* **24**, 2519–2524.
5. Delneri, D., Tomlin, G. C., Wixon, J. L., et al. (2000) Exploring redundancy in the yeast genome: an improved strategy for use of the cre-loxP system. *Gene* **252**, 127–135.
6. Hughes, T. R., Roberts, C. J., Dai, H., et al. (2000) Widespread aneuploidy revealed by DNA microarray expression profiling. *Nat. Gen.* **25**, 333–337.
7. Ito, H., Fukada, Y., Murata, K., and Kimura, A. (1983) Transformation of intact yeast cells treated with alkali cations. *J. Bacteriol.* **153**, 163–168.
8. Gietz, R. D. and Woods, R. A. (2002) Transformation of yeast by lithium acetate/single-stranded carrier DNA/polyethylene glycol method. *Meth. Enzymol.* **350**, 87–93.

9. Uno, I., Fukami, K., Kato, H., Takenawa, T., and Ishikawa, T. (1988) Essential role for phosphatidylinositol 4,5-bisphosphate in yeast cell proliferation. *Nature* **333,** 188–190.
10. Prentice, H. L. (1991) High efficiency transformation of *Schizosaccharomyces pombe* by electroporation. *Nucleic Acids Res.* **20,** 621.
11. Becker, D. M. and Guarente, L. (1991) High-efficiency transformation of yeast by electroporation. *Meth. Enzymol.* **194,** 182–187.
12. Allshire, R. C. (1990) Introduction of large linear minichromosomes into *Schizosaccharomyces pombe* by an improved transformation procedure. *Proc. Natl. Acad. Sci. USA* **87,** 4043–4047.
13. Kohalmi, S. E. and Kunz, B. A. (1988) Role of neighbouring bases and assessment of strand specificity in ethylmethanesulphonate and N-methyl-N'-nitro-N-nitrosoguanidine mutagenesis in the SUP4-o gene of *Saccharomyces cerevisiae*. *J. Mol. Biol.* **204,** 561–568
14. Kunz, B. A., Pierce, M. K., Mis, J. R., and Giroux, C. N. (1987) DNA sequence analysis of the mutational specificity of u.v. light in the SUP4-o gene of yeast. *Mutagenesis* **2,** 445–453.
15. Lee, G. S., Savage, E. A., Ritzel, R. G., and von Borstel, R. C. (1988) The base-alteration spectrum of spontaneous and ultraviolet radiation-induced forward mutations in the URA3 locus of *Saccharomyces cerevisiae*. *Mol. Gen. Genet.* **214,** 396–404.
16. Caldwell, R. C. and Joyce, G. F. (1992) Randomization of genes by PCR mutagenesis. *Meth. Appl* **2,** 28–33.
17. Lawrence, C. W. (2002) Classical mutagenesis techniques. *Meth. Enzymol.* **350,** 189–199.
18. Muhlrad, D., Hunter, R., and Parker, R. A. (1992) Rapid method for localized mutagenesis of yeast genes. *Yeast* **8,** 79–82.

# 17

## Real-Time RT-PCR (Taqman®) of Tumor mRNA to Predict Sensitivity of Specimens to 5-Fluorouracil

### Tetsuro Kubota

#### Summary

5-Fluorouracil (5-FU) is still a key drug in the treatment of various kinds of advanced cancer, including breast and gastrointestinal carcinomas. To predict the sensitivity of colorectal cancer to 5-FU, mRNA is extracted from surgically obtained cancer specimens and expression of thymidylate synthetase (TS), dihydropyrimidine dehydrogenase (DPD), thymidine phosphorylase (TP), uridine phosphorylase (UP), es-nucleoside transporter (NT), and E2F1 are detected by real-time reverse transcription polymerase chain reaction (RT-PCR) (TaqMan®). Previous results have shown that the catabolic rate-limiting enzymes DPD and NT, which are important membranous transporter of nucleosides, may regulate the sensitivity to 5-FU.

#### Key Words

mRNA; RT-PCR; dihydropyrimidine dehydrogenase; nucleoside transporter; antitumor activity; 5-fluoruracil.

### 1. Introduction

5-Fluorouracil (5-FU) was first synthesized by Heidelberger et al. in 1957 *(1)*, and it has been used for the treatment of various solid cancers for over 45 yr. In Japan, 5-FU derivatives such as tegafur, doxifluridine (5′-DFUR), and UFT have been developed since the 1970s and used in oral therapy for cancer. Also, in the United States and Europe, development of UFT/leucovorin (LV), capecitabine, eniluracil/5-FU, S-1, etc., began in the 1990s, and oral cancer therapy with fluorinated pyrimidines has attracted attention *(2)*. When a meta-analysis was conducted on nine randomized clinical trials that compared 5-FU with 5-FU plus intravenous LV for the treatment of advanced colorectal cancer, therapy with 5-FU plus LV showed a highly significant benefit over single-agent 5-FU in terms of tumor response rate, although this increase in response did not result in a discernable improvement of overall survival. This result suggested that large numbers of patients in both groups did not respond to treatment *(3)*.

Several genes result in expression of proteins that affect the efficacy of 5-FU. Thymidylate synthetase (TS) is a target enzyme of 5-FU, in which an active metabolite, 5-fluorouridine monophosphate, will combine with TS accompanied by a cofactor, 5,10-methylene tetrahydrofolate, to prevent *de novo* DNA synthesis. Several studies suggest that high TS expression will result in 5-FU resistance *(4–6)*. Dihydropyrimidine dehydrogenase (DPD) is the first and rate-limiting catabolizing enzyme of 5-FU. Thymidine phosphorylase (TP) and uridine phosphorylase (UP) are the initial phosphorylating enzymes of 5-FU, which will be anabolized to 5-fluorouridine monophosphate, and TP is also known as the key enzyme responsible for conversion to the metabolite doxifluridine, which is also a metabolite of newly investigated capecitabine. es-nucleoside transporter (NT) is an equilibrium membranous transporter of pyrimidines, which do not depend on the sodium pump *(7)*. E2F1 codes a representative transcriptional enzyme responsible for regulating transcriptional expression of several important messages, including TS and topoisomerase I, which might be involved in 5-FU resistance.

Salvage of preformed nucleosides requires transport across the plasma membrane by sodium-dependent (concentrative) and sodium-independent (equilibrative) mechanisms. The assessed NT mRNA in the present study codes NBMPR-sensitive equilibrative nucleoside transporter (es or ENT1), which transports nucleoside from higher to lower concentration, of which transportation will be inhibited by nitrobenzylmercaptopurine riboside (NBMPR). For 5-FU resistance, NT may efflux the active metabolites of 5-FU (5-fluorouridine and 5-fluorodeoxyuridine) to the outsides of tumor cells. On the other hand, the elevation of NT might also cause more cellular uptake of thymidine to rescue cells from thymine-less death by TS inhibition. The role of these various enzymes and transport proteins under consideration are shown in **Fig. 1**.

Takechi et al. have investigated an mRNA differential display analysis to compare transcripts from the NUGC-3 human gastric tumor cell line and its 5-FU-resistant subline to identify genes differentially expressed in association with resistance to 5-FU *(7)*. We have previously reported that expression of (DPD) mRNA will predict the sensitivity of human tumor xenografts *(8)* and human gastric cancer specimens *(9)* to 5-FU. In this chapter, we describe the detection methodology to monitor expression of six genes associated with 5-FU sensitivity, TS, DPD, TP, UP, NT, and E2F1 mRNA by real-time reverse transcription polymerase chain reaction (RT-PCR) (TaqMan®). The correlation between the 5-FU sensitivity (results of MTT assays) of the resected speci-

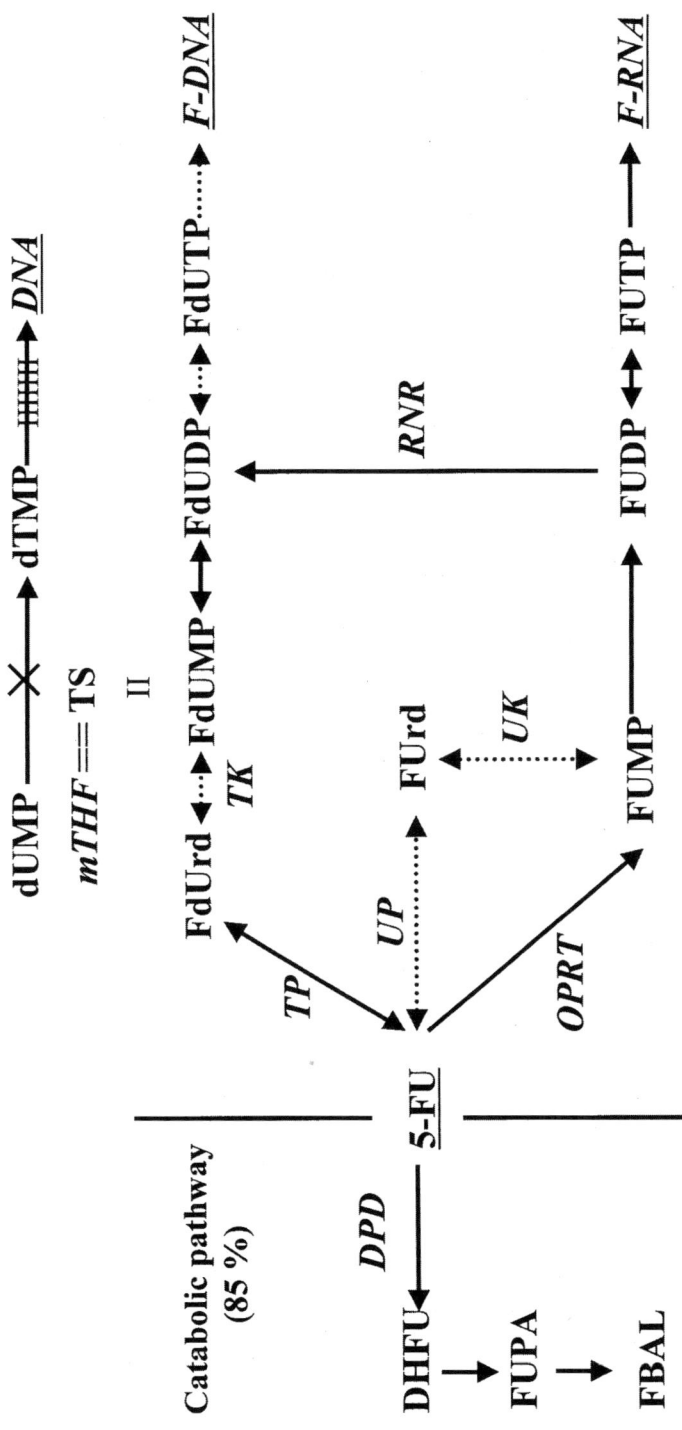

Fig. 1. Metabolic pathway of 5-fluorouracil. Abbreviations: dUMP, deoxyuridine monophosphate; dTMP, deoxyuridine triphosphate; mTHF, methylenetetrahydrofolate; TS, thymidylate synthetase; FdUrd, fluorodeoxyuridine; FdUMP, fluorodeoxyuridine monophosphate; FdUDP, fluorodeoxyuridine diphosphate; FdUTP, fluorodeoxyuridine triphosphate; TK, thymidine kinase; TP, thymidine phosphorylase; UP, uridine phosphorylase; FdUrd, fluorodeoxyuridine; UK, uridine kinase; RNR, ribonucleotide reductase; OPRT, orotate phosphorybosyl transferase; FUMP, fluorouridine monophosphate; FUDP, fluorouridine diphosphate; FUTP, fluorouridine triphosphate; DPD, dihydropyrimidine dehydrogenase; DHFU, dihydrofluorouracil; FUPA, fluoroureidopropionic acid; FBAL, fluoro-β-alanine.

**Table 1**
**Correlation Between Chemosensitivity to 5-FU and Expression of mRNA**

| Factor | Coefficient of correlation | $P$ value |
|---|---|---|
| TS | 0.16 | 0.1363 |
| DPD | 0.244 | 0.0229* |
| NT | 0.257 | 0.0156* |
| TP | 0.222 | 0.0376* |
| E2F1 | 0.246 | 0.0216* |

*Statistically significant.
The gene expression of colorectal carcinoma detected by real time RT-PCR was compared with their sensitivity to 5-fluorouracil detected by MTT assay *(10)*.

mens and mRNA expression is shown in **Table 1** *(10)*. DPD, NT, TP, and E2F1 mRNAs showed statistically significant correlations with 5-FU sensitivity represented as I.R. at $P < 0.05$, while no statistical correlations were observed between TS mRNA expression and 5-FU sensitivity. Therefore, the resistance mechanisms of 5-FU may include several changes in cellular functions, while the catabolic rate-limiting DPD and membranous transporter NT will mainly regulate the clinically relevant resistant mechanism. The ability to monitor expression of these key genes involved in 5-FU sensitivity appear to be a useful tool at predicting response to 5-FU therapy.

## 2. Materials

1. 5-FU: Kyowa Hakko Kogyo, Tokyo, Japan.
2. RNeasy mini kit: Qiagen, Chatsworth, CA.
3. RNase-Free DNase Set: Qiagen, Chatsworth, CA.
4. rRNasin ribonuclease inhibitor: Promega, Madison, WI.
5. Moloney murine leukemia virus reverse transcriptase: GIBCO BRL.
6. 50 m$M$ Tris-HCl (pH 8.3), 75 m$M$ KCl, 3 m$M$ MgCl$_2$, 10 m$M$ dithiothreitol (DTT), and 0.5 m$M$ dNTPs.
7. Primer Express software: PE Biosystems, Foster City, CA.
8. Primers and TaqMan probes for glyceraldehyde-3-phosphate dehydrogenase (GAPDH): PE Biosystems, Foster City, CA.
9. Quencher dye: TAMRA.
10. ABI PRISM 7700 Detection System: PE Biosystems, Foster City, CA.
11. TaqMan universal PCR Master Mix: PE Biosystems, Foster City, CA.
12. MDA-MB-231 human breast tumor cells: American Type Culture Collection, Manassas, VA.

## 3. Methods

### 3.1. RNA Wxtraction and cDNA Synthesis from Patient Tumor Samples (see Note 1)

Total RNA is isolated using RNeasy mini kit, and DNase treatment is performed using RNase-Free DNase Set, following the manufacturer's instructions (*see* **Note 2**).

Reverse transcription with up to 10 µg of total RNA is carried out in a total volume of 100 µL containing 250 pmol oligo $(dT)_{18}$, 80 U rRNasin ribonuclease inhibitor, and 500 U Moloney murine leukemia virus reverse transcriptase (Gibco BRL) in 50 m$M$ Tris-HCl (pH 8.3), 75 m$M$ KCl, 3 m$M$ $MgCl_2$, 10 m$M$ DTT, and 0.5 m$M$ dNTPs. Initially, the total RNA solution mixed with oligo $(dT)_{18}$ is heated at 70°C for 10 min and immediately chilled on ice, then the other reagents are added. First-strand cDNAs are obtained after 15 min at 30°C and after 60 min at 42°C (*see* **Note 3**).

### 3.2. Primers and TaqMan Probes

Primers and TaqMan probes for TS, DPD, TP, UP, and E2F1 are designed using the Primer Express software (*see* **Notes 4** and **5**). Primers and TaqMan probes for glyceraldehyde-3-phosphate dehydrogenase (GAPDH) are purchased from PE Biosystems. The probes are labeled with a reporter dye (FAM) situated at the 5′ end of the oligonucleotide and a quencher dye (TAMRA) located at the 3′ end. The sequences of primers and probes are summarized in **Table 2**.

### 3.3. PCR Procedure

Quantification of target cDNA (TS, DPD, TP, UP, and E2F1) and an internal reference gene (GAPDH) is conducted using a fluorescence-based real-time PCR method (TaqMan PCR using ABI PRISM 7700 Detection System) *(11)*. The PCR is carried out in a final volume of 25 µL mixture containing cDNA equivalent to 1–10 ng of total RNA, 200 n$M$ each primer, 100 n$M$ probe, and 12.5 µL TaqMan universal PCR Master Mix (containing 1X TaqMan buffer, 200 µ$M$ dATP, dCTP, dGTP, and 400 µ$M$ dUTP, 5 m$M$ $MgCl_2$, 1.25 U of AmpliTaqGold, 0.5 U of AmpErase UNG) purchased from PE Biosystems. Thermal cycling conditions are 50°C for 2 min and 95°C for 10 min, followed by 45 cycles at 95°C for 15 s and 60°C for 1 min (*see* **Notes 6–8**).

### 3.4. Relative Quantification of Gene Expression

Relative quantification of gene expression is performed using the relative standard curve method. The standard curve is created automatically by the ABI PRISM 7700 Detection System by plotting the threshold cycle ($C_T$) against

## Table 2
## Sequence of PCR Primers and Sequence-Specific Probes for Target Genes

| Gene (GenBank accession no.) | Primer/probe | Sequence | Corresponding cDNA sequence |
|---|---|---|---|
| TS (X02308) | Forward primer | GAATCACATCGAGCCACTGAAA | 882–1099 |
| | Reverse primer | CAGCCCAACCCCTAAAGACTGA | |
| | Probe | TTCAGCTTCAGCGAGAACCCAGA | |
| DPD (U09178) | Forward primer | AATGATTCGAAGAGCTTTTGAAGC | 1755–1862 |
| | Reverse primer | GTTCCCCGGATGATTCTGG | |
| | Probe | TGCCCTCACCAAAACTTTCTCTCTT GATAAGGA | |
| TP (M63193) | Forward primer | CCTGCGGACGGAATCCT | 700–770 |
| | Reverse primer | GCTGTGATGAGTGGCAGGCT | |
| | Probe | CAGCCAGAGATGTGACAGCCACCGT | |
| UP (X90858) | Forward primer | TGACTGCCCAGGTAGAGACTATCC | 586–792 |
| | Reverse primer | AGACCTATCCCACCAGAAGTGC | |
| | Probe | TGCTCCAACGTCACTACATCCGCAT | |
| E2F1 (M96577) | Forward primer | AGGAGTTCATCAGCCTTTCCC | 1325–1426 |
| | Reverse primer | CCCCAAAGTCACAGTCGAAGAG | |
| | Probe | CCCACGAGGCCCTCGACTACCAC | |
| NT (AF079117) | Forward primer | TCTTCATGGCTGCCTTTGC | 1295–1373 |
| | Reverse primer | GGCTTCACTTTCTTGGGCC | |
| | Probe | TCGCCAGCCTCTGCATGTGCTT | |
| GAPDH (M33197) | Forward primer | GAAGGTGAAGGTCGGAGTC | 66–291 |
| | Reverse primer | GAAGATGGTGATGGGATTTC | |
| | Probe | CAAGCTTCCCGTTCTCAGCC | |

The probes were labeled with a reporter dye (FAM) situated at the 5′-end of the oligonucleotide and a quencher dye (TAMRA) located at the 3′-end.

*Abbreviations:* TS, thymidylate synthetase; DPD, dihydropyrimidine dehydrogenase; TP, thymidine phosphorylase; UP, uridine phosphorylase; NT, es-nucleoside transporter.

each input amount (containing 16, 4, 1, 0.25, 0.063, 0.016, 0.0039 ng) of control total RNA (total starting RNA), prepared from MDA-MB-231 human breast tumor cells (American Type Culture Collection, Manassas, VA). The coefficient of linear regression ($r$) for each standard curve should be more than 0.990. For each unknown sample, the relative amount is calculated using linear regression analysis from their respective standard curves. A relative target gene expression value is obtained by division of the target gene value by the GAPDH value as an internal reference gene (*see* **Notes 9** and **10**).

## 4. Notes

1. *Patient samples.* All patients with advanced cancer must give their written informed consent for gene analysis of their specimens. Surgical specimens are stored at –80°C until gene expression analysis is performed. The protocol should be approved by the Institutional Review Board of each institute.
2. *Specimen preservation and RNA extraction.* It is important to prevent RNA degradation as much as possible. After first trimming surgical specimens into approximately 5-mm pieces, they are promptly frozen in liquid nitrogen (trimming should be performed before freezing, because it is difficult to cut frozen specimens). The specimens are then immersed in liquid nitrogen and stored at –80°C until protein denaturation in the RLT buffer included in the RNeasy kit. Care must be taken when thawing frozen specimens, because the RNA decomposes readily. Total RNA is isolated with the RNeasy kit, according to the manufacturer's instructions.
3. *cDNA preparation.* Although random 6-mer can be substituted for oligo$(dT)_{18}$ for cDNA synthesis, because oligo $(dT)_{18}$ acts specifically on mRNA, the final detection sensitivity is increased.
4. *Location of primers and TaqMan probes.* Since oligo $(dT)_{18}$ is used for cDNA synthesis, primers/probes are located near the 3′ end of mRNA, within 1500 bases from the 3′ end).
5. *Design of primers and TaqMan probes.* The standard conditions for the design of primers/probes with Primer Express software are (a) annealing temperature of 58–60°C for primers and 68–70°C for probes; (b) not choosing G on the 3′ end of probes; (c) choosing probes that include more Cs than Gs in the sequence; (d) choosing primers that contain less than two G(s) and/or C(s) within five bases from the 3′ end.
6. *Protocol for thermal cycling.* Because it is convenient if a thermal-cycle protocol that can be used for all genes is established, the concentration of primers, probes, and TaqMan universal PCR master mix and the conditions of a thermal cycle are standardized.
7. *Formatting of 96-well reaction plate.* In the standard protocol, expression of four genes including GAPDH is measured per plate. Placing the internal standard, GAPDH, in every plate minimizes the measurement error between plates. Twenty-four wells (one-fourth of the 96 wells) are used per gene: 7 wells for a positive control dilution sequence, 1 well for a blank ($H_2O$), and 16 wells to measure a target gene (8 samples × 2 wells). Duplicate samples are sufficient to confirm reproducibility.
8. *Sample preservation and the primer/probe mixture.* Because it is easy to make errors in the dilution process, all the diluted solutions (positive control, measurement sample, and primer/probe) are divided into several aliquots according to the quantity to be necessary for one experiment. Frozen aliquots can be stored for several weeks.
9. *Positive control for relative quantification of gene expression.* Absolute quantification of gene expression requires the preparation of an RNA construct with a

poly A tail for every gene. Preparing many different RNA constructs is very laborious, and preserving intact RNA constructs is not easy. Because RNA prepared from clinical specimens decomposes easily, absolute quantification values are greatly influenced by the degree of degradation. For the above reasons, a relative quantification standardized with a positive control is more suitable for measurements in clinical specimens. cDNA prepared from the human breast cancer cell line MDA-MB-231, which has been found to express comparatively high levels of TS, DPD, TP, UP, E2F1, and NT mRNA in a preliminary test, was used as a positive control in this study, making it unnecessary to prepare another positive control for every gene. In our laboratory, frozen stocks of cDNA solution derived from several human cancer cell lines are always prepared in advance for use as positive controls according to the gene to be measured.

10. *Dilution sequence of the positive control.* cDNA as the positive control is diluted fourfold in seven steps: 16, 4, 1, 0.25, 0.063, 0.016, and 0.0039 ng of reverse-transcribed total RNA. The dynamic range for measurement corresponds to 4096-fold ($4^6$-fold). This seems to provide a sufficient range to quantify gene expression.

## References

1. Heidelberger, C., Chaudhuri, N. K., Danenberg, P., et al. (1957) Fluorinated pyrimidines, a new class of tumor-inhibitory compounds. *Nature* **179**, 663–666.
2. Liu, G., Franssen, E., Fitch, M. I., and Warner, E. (1997) Patient preference for oral versus intravenous palliative chemotherapy. *J. Clin. Oncol.* **15**, 110–115.
3. Advanced colorectal cancer meta-analysis project (1992). Modulation of fluorouracil by leucovorin in patients with advanced colorectal cancer: evidence in terms of response rate. *J. Clin. Oncol.* **10(6)**, 892–903.
4. Johnston, P. G., Lenz, H. J., Leichman, C. G., et al. (1995) Thymidylate synthase gene and protein expression correlate and are associated with response to 5-fluorouracil in human colorectal and gastric tumors. *Cancer Res.* **6**, 1407–1412.
5. Lenz, H. J., Leichman, C. G., Danenberg, K. D., et al. (1996) Thymidylate synthase mRNA level in adenocarcinoma of the stomach: a predictor for primary tumor response and overall survival. *J. Clin. Oncol.* **14**, 176–182.
6. Leichman, C. G., Lenz, H. J., Leichman, L., et al. (1997) Quantitation of intratumoral thymidylate synthase expression predicts for disseminated colorectal cancer response and resistance to protracted-infusion fluorouracil and weekly leucovorin. *J. Clin. Oncol.* **15**, 3223–3229.
7. Takechi, T., Koizumi, K., Tsujimoto, H., and Fukushima, M. (2001) Screening of differentially expressed genes in 5-fluorouracil-resistant human gastrointestinal tumor cells. *Jpn. J. Cancer Res.* **92(6)**, 696–703.
8. Ishikawa, Y., Kubota, T., Otani, Y., et al. (1999) Dihydropyrimidine dehydrogenase activity and messenger RNA level may be related to the antitumor effect of 5-fluorouracil on human tumor xenografts in nude mice. *Clin. Cancer Res.* **5**, 883–889.

9. Ishikawa, Y., Kubota, T., Otani, Y., et al. (2000) Dihydropyrimidine dehydrogenase and messenger RNA levels in gastric cancer: Possible predictor for sensitivity to 5-fluorouracil. *Jpn. J. Cancer Res.* **91,** 105–112.
10. Yoshinare, K., Kubota, T., Watanabe, T., et al. (2003) Gene expression in colorectal cancer and in vitro chemosensitivity to 5-fluorouracil:.a study of 88 surgical specimens. *Cancer Sci.*, **94,** 633–638.
11. Fukushima, M., Okabe, H., Takechi, T., Ichikawa, W., and Hirayama, R. (2002) Induction of thymidine phosphorylase by interferon and taxanes occurs only in human cancer cells with low thymidine phosphorylase activity. *Cancer Lett.* **187,** 103–110.

# 18

## Use of Proteomics to Study Chemosensitivity

### Julia Poland, Silke Wandschneider, Andrea Urbani, Sergio Bernardini, Giorgio Federici, and Pranav Sinha

#### Summary

Chemoresistance remains an unresolved problem in clinical oncology. Therefore it is important to identify molecular factors that lead to an understanding of the mechanisms of drug resistance in cancer cells. On the protein-expression level, this can be done using proteomics, which has become the focus of significant interest and research over the past decade.

We describe an easy and practicable standardized technique that can be used to study global protein expression in chemosensitive and chemoresistant cancer cells to find candidate proteins that are potentially associated with the drug-resistant phenotype. As an example, fractionation of human neuroblastoma cells using two-dimensional polyacrylamide electrophoresis, spot detection, image analysis, and finally protein identification is illustrated.

#### Key Words

Proteomics; proteome analysis; two-dimensional electrophoresis; isoelectric focusing; immobilized pH gradients; mass spectrometry; cancer cell lines; chemosensitivity; chemoresistance.

## 1. Introduction

Chemotherapy is often the only remaining therapeutic option for advanced cancer stages, but its success is limited by the existence of intrinsic, primary drug resistance and particularly the development of secondary, acquired drug resistance. Chemoresistance remains an unresolved problem in clinical oncology. One approach to identify new molecular factors potentially associated with the drug-resistant phenotypes of various types of cancer is the proteomics technique. Proteome analysis is most commonly accomplished by the combination of two-dimensional polyacrylamide gel electrophoresis (2D-PAGE) and mass spectrometry (MS) and allows the identification and quantification of the proteins expressed by cells, tissues, or an organism in a high-throughput manner.

Screening of the global protein expression of chemosensitive and chemoresistant cancer cells using proteomics can be applied as a first step in order to find candidate proteins that may be involved in mechanisms of drug resistance. Subsequently, other studies focusing directly on these proteins can be performed based on the proteomics data, including confirmation studies (e.g., Western blotting) and functional studies (e.g., transfection experiments) to prove the validity of the results.

In the following, fractionation of chemosensitive and chemoresistant cells to find differentially expressed proteins will be exemplified using parental, chemosensitive human neuroblastoma cell lines and their counterparts exhibiting drug resistance toward etoposide.

The methods described for separation and identification of the global proteome of these cells (*see* **Note 1**) include the following steps: sample solubilization and protein determination, two-dimensional electrophoresis with immobilized pH gradients followed by sodium dodecyl sulfate (SDS) polyacrylamide electrophoresis, spot detection using silver staining for analytical gels and coomassie staining for preparative gels, computer-assisted image analysis using sophisticated 2DE analysis software, and finally, protein identification using mass spectrometry. Using these methods, several thousand of proteins can be resolved on a single gel.

## 2. Materials

### 2.1. Chemicals

1. Agarose L, Pharmalyte™ 3–10 for IEF and DryStrip cover fluid from Amersham-Biosciences (Stockholm, Sweden).
2. Acrylamide (99.9% purity) [toxic!], piperazine diacrylamide (PDA), N,N'-methylene-bis-acrylamide (Bis) (electrophoresis purity reagent) [hramful!], sodium diodecyl sulfate (SDS) [harmful!]; N,N,N',N'-tetramethyl-ethylenediamine (TEMED), ammonium persulfate (APS) and Lyphochek assayed chemistry control level 1 and 2 (used to obtain standard curves that were run with each protein determination) were from Bio-Rad Laboratories (Hercules, CA, USA).
3. CHAPS (3-[(Cholamidopropyl)dimethylammonio]-1-propanesulfonate) [irritant!], spermine (N,N'-bis[3-aminopropyl]-1,4-butanediamine), DTT (DL-Dithiothreitol) [harmful!], bromphenol blue and a-cyano-4-hydroxycinnamic acid were from Sigma-Aldrich (Steinheim, Germany), porcine methylated trypsin (sequencing grade) was supplied by Promega (Mannheim, Germany).
4. Urea (ultrapure), EDTA disodium salt [harmful!], Tris-HCl [irritant!] and iodacetamide [toxic!] were from Fluka (Buchs, Switzerland).
5. Denatured ethanol 100% was from Herbeta (Berlin, Germany), coomassie brilliant blue G 250 (pure) from Severa (Heidelberg, Germany) and ammonium bicarbonate from ICN Biomedicals (Eschwege, Germany).

6. From Merck (Darmstadt, Germany), the following reagents were purchased (highest purity grade): hydrochloric acid 37%, trichloroacetic acid (TCA), thiourea [harmful!], tris(hydroxymethyl)-aminomethan (Tris) [irritant!], silver nitrate, sodium thiosulfate pentahydrate [irritant!], sodium bicarbobate, sodium acetate anhydrous, methanol [toxic!], glycerol, glycine, glutardialdehyde solution 25% [toxic!], formaldehyde solution min. 37% [toxic!], 1-Butanol [harmfum!], ammonium sulfate, acetic acid 100%, ortho-phosphoric acid 85%, acetonitrile [toxic!] and thimerosal.

## 2.2. Sample Solubilization and Protein Determination

1. Elisa reader and microtiter plates for protein determination.
2. Solubilization buffer [prepare fresh or store aliquots without dithiothreitol (DTT) at –20°C]: 7 $M$ urea, 2 $M$ thiourea, 4% (w/v) CHAPS, 20 m$M$ spermine, 40 m$M$ DTT.

## 2.3. Two-Dimensional Electrophoresis

1. IPGphor isoelectric focusing unit (Amersham Biosciences), including 18-cm strip holders.
2. Immobiline DryStrips (Amersham Biosciences), pH 3–10 NL, 18 cm for standard fractionation; for zoom gels use narrow pH ranges (*see* **Note 1**).
3. ISO-DALT casting chamber and accessories; ISO-DALT cassettes (20 × 24 cm, 1.5 mm spacer).
4. Rehydration buffer for IEF: 8 $M$ urea, 2% (w/v) CHAPS, 0.5% (v/v) pharmalytes 3-10 (40%), bromphenol blue (a few granules), 20 m$M$ DTT. Prepare aliquots of the buffer (for instance, 1- or 2-mL portions), freeze at –20°C (without DTT); before rehydration, add DTT from a fresh 1 $M$ stock solution.
5. Stock solution "buffer D": 1.5 $M$ Tris, adjust to pH using 6 $M$ HCl (final pH: 8.8).
6. Stock solution "T30 C0.5": 29.85% (w/v) acrylamide, 0.15% (w/v) PDA (*see* **Note 2**).
7. Final gel solution for the second dimension (T15 C0.5): 25% (v/v) buffer D, 0.043% (w/v) sodium thiosulfate pentahydrate, 50% (v/v) T30 C0.5. After degassing, add SDS from a 10% stock solution to a final concentration of 1% (v/v), then 0.02% (v/v) TEMED, and finally 0.5% (v/v) APS of a freshly prepared 10% (w/v) solution.
8. Equilibration solution (prepare 200 mL): 6 $M$ urea, 30% (v/v) glycerol, 2% (w/v) SDS, 50 m$M$ Tris-HCl, pH 8.8. Separate solution in two 100-mL portions, add 1 g DTT to solution 1 and 4 g iodoacetamide to solution 2.
9. Sealing solution: 212 m$M$ glycine, 12 m$M$ Tris, 0.1% (w/v) SDS, 0.5% (w/v) agarose, bromphenol blue (a few granules).
10. Running buffer: 25 m$M$ Tris, 192 m$M$ glycine, 0.1% (w/v) SDS.

## 2.4. Staining

1. Large covered plastic boxes (not less than 30 × 35 cm).
2. Shaker.

### 2.4.1. Silver Staining

1. Fixation: 50% (v/v) ethanol, 10% (v/v) acetic acid.
2. Incubation (I): 0.5 $M$ sodium acetate, 0.2% (w/v) sodium thiosulfate pentahydrate, 30% (v/v) ethanol, 0.5% (v/v) glutardialdehyde.
3. Staining: 0.1% (w/v) silver nitrate, 0.01% (v/v) formaldehyde.
4. Incubation (II): 2.5% (w/v) sodium carbonate.
5. Development: 2.5% (w/v) sodium carbonate, 0.01% (v/v) formalin, 0.05% (w/v) sodium bicarbonate, 0.02% (w/v) thimerosal.
6. Stop solution: 0.05 $M$ EDTA disodium salt.

### 2.4.2. Coomassie Staining for Preparative Runs (see **Note 3**)

1. Fixation: 50% (v/v) methanol, 2% (v/v) phosphoric acid (85%).
2. Incubation: 34% (v/v) methanol, 2% (v/v) phosphoric acid (85%), 17% (w/v) ammonium sulfate.
3. Staining: 34% (v/v) methanol, 2% (v/v) phosphoric acid (85%), 17% (w/v) ammonium sulfate, 0.066% (w/v) coomassie brilliant blue G-250.

### 2.5. Image Analysis

1. Gel scanner (e.g., densitometer 710, Bio-Rad).
2. Image analysis software (e.g., PDQuest, Bio-Rad).

### 2.6. Protein Identification

1. MALDI-TOF-MS equipment (e.g., MALDI-R Micromass-Waters, Reflex IV time-of-flight instrument, Bruker-Daltonik) and accessories.
2. ZipTip C18 (Millipore, Eschborn, Germany).

## 3. Methods

In summary, the methods described below outline (1) sample solubilization and protein determination, (2) two-dimensional electrophoresis, (3) staining, (4) image analysis, and (5) protein identification. **Figure 1** shows a schematic representation of the individual steps.

### 3.1. Sample Solubilization and Protein Determination

Human chemosensitive and etoposide-resistant neuroblastoma cells have been established previously. For details regarding cell culture and establishment of the chemoresistant cells, *see* **ref. 1**.

---

Fig. 1. *(see facing page)* Schematic representation of the individual steps of proteomics: (1) sample solubilization and protein determination, (2) two-dimensional electrophoresis, (3) staining, (4) image analysis, and (5) protein identification.

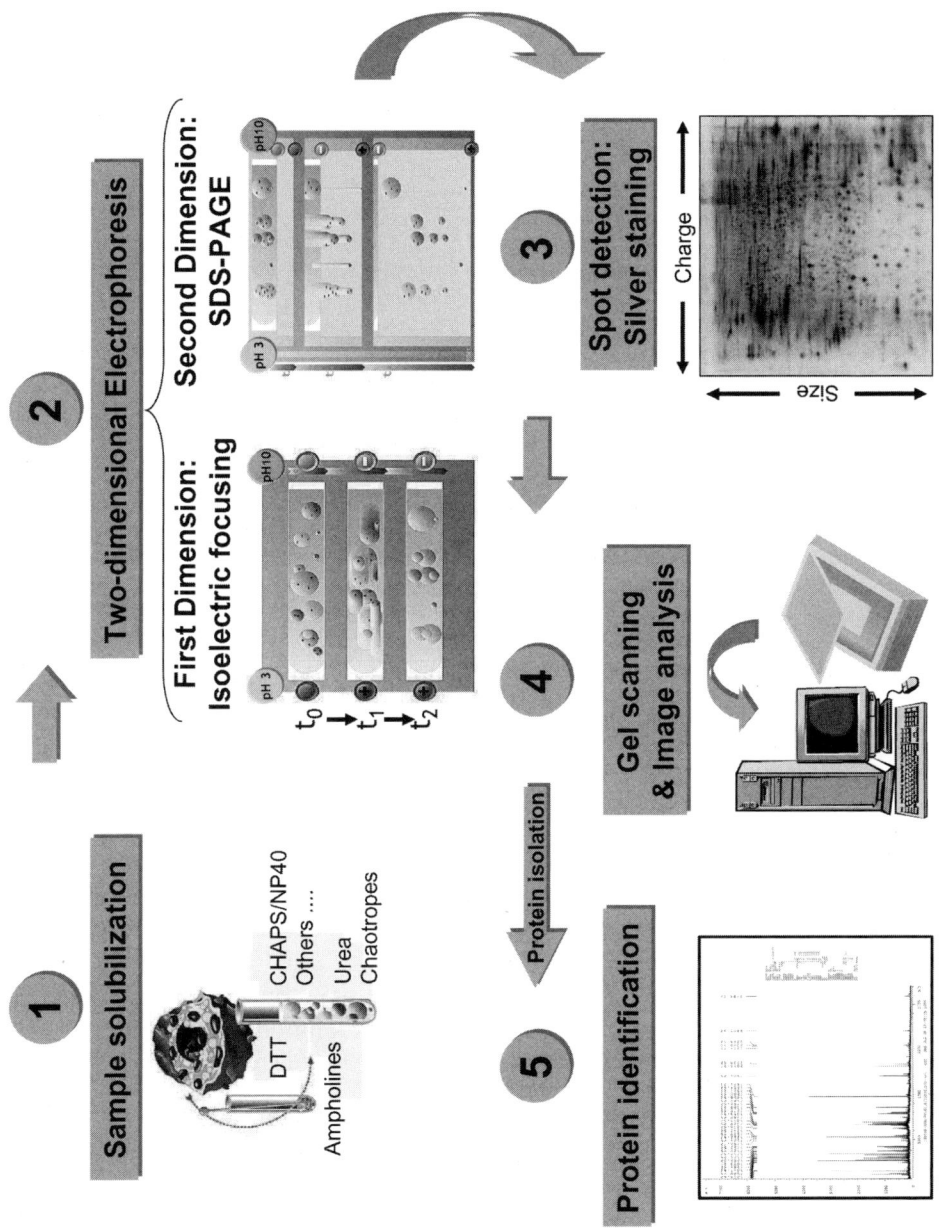

Each cell pellet (at an average 50 million cells) is solubilized according to Rabilloud *(2)*, using the solubilization buffer containing DTT/spermine to precipitate nucleic acids and DTT as a reducing agent.

1. A small volume of buffer is added to the pellet (cell pellet:lysis buffer ratio approx 1:1), followed by incubation for 60 min at room temperature and removal of precipitated nucleic acids using a pipet.
2. After centrifugation for 60 min at 105,000*g* to remove finely dispersed insoluble material, the supernatant is collected and stored in aliquots at –80°C.
3. For protein determination, an aliquot of the protein extract is diluted 1:5/1:10 and the protein concentration in the lysates is measured using an adapted trichloroacetic procedure described in **ref. *3***.
4. 35-µL sample + 100 µL of 0.1 *N* HCl + 25 µL 20% trichloroacetic acid (TCA) are pipetted successively on a microtiter plate.
5. A calibration curve using four different concentrations between 5.35 and 0.135 µg/µL of Validate N as well as a high and a low control (Validate A) is run with each protein determination.
6. Optical density values are supposed to lie in the middle range of the calibration curve. For each sample and control, double measurement is performed.

## *3.2. Two-Dimensional Electrophoresis*

In this section, fractionation of proteins is described using high-resolution two-dimensional electrophoresis under denaturing conditions. The technique was developed by O'Farrell and others in 1975 *(4–6)*. The method is carried out in two independent steps, separating the proteins by two different intrinsic properties (charge/mass). In the first dimension, proteins are separated by their charge in a pH gradient, while the second dimension, carried out orthogonally to the first dimension, is based on the different molecular weights of the proteins. The classical separation technique in the first dimension has been further evolved and optimized with introduction of immobilized pH gradients *(7)*. We illustrate isoelectric focusing with IPGs using a commonly used system (IPGphor isoelectric focusing unit by Amersham Biosciences) that allows electrically assisted rehydration.

### *3.2.1. First Dimension*

1. Prior to isoelectric focusing, individual ready-cast IPG strips (Immobiline DryStrip pH 3-10NL, 18 cm) are placed with the gel side facing down in thermally conductive ceramic holders containing 350 µL total volume of rehydration buffer (*see* **Subheading 2.3.**) including sample (for details, see the user manual, *2-D Electrophoresis using IPGs—Principles and Methods* from Amersham Biosciences).
2. For analytical runs (used to find differentially expressed proteins), a total protein amount of 50 µg is applied; for preparative runs (used to isolate proteins from the

gel for identification with MS), a total protein amount of 1 mg is loaded on each strip (see **Note 3**).
3. 2 mL of DryStrip cover fluid is applied into each strip holder.
4. Electrically assisted rehydration and isoelectric focusing is carried out using the following parameters (50 µA per gel strip, 20°C) with step-by-step increasing voltage: 30 V for 6 h, 60 V for 6 h, 200 V for 1 h, 500 V for 1 h, 1000 V for 1 h, 8000 V (gradient) for 30 min, 8000 V for 3½h.

### 3.2.2. Second Dimension

1. 15% acrylamide, 0.5% cross-linked slab-gels (20 × 24 cm, 1.5-mm spacer) for the second dimension are prepared using the ISO-DALT casting box, allowing casting of 20 gels simultaneously (see **Note 4**).
2. The gels are carefully overlaid with water-saturated butanol.
3. After the first dimension, the individual strips are equilibrated for 10 min in 100 mL equilibration buffer containing 1 g DTT followed by 10 min equilibration in another 100 mL of the same buffer containing 4 g iodoacetamide (see **Note 5**).
4. The strips are then sealed on top of 15% polyacrylamide gels (T15 C0.5) using solution E.
5. Electrophoresis is performed in the ISO-DALT tank designed for 10 gels containing 20 L of the standard Laemmli buffer *(8)* used for SDS-PAGE (solution F).
6. SDS-PAGE is performed at 10 mA per gel constant for 1 h.
7. The rest of the run is completed at 25 mA per gel until the tracking dye reaches the bottom of the gel (see **Note 6**).

## 3.3. Staining

### 3.3.1. Analytical Run: Silver Staining Protocol

Gels are stained according to protocols published by Heukeshoven and Dernick *(9,10)* (see also **Note 7**). The solutions used are listed under **Subheading 2.4.1.** The sequence of the procedure is as follows (use approximately 2.5 L of each solution for simultaneous staining of 10 gels):

1. Fix the gels for at least 2 h or overnight in fixing solution (A).
2. Incubate for 2 h in incubation (I) (B).
3. Rinse 2 × 20 min in distilled water.
4. Stain for 30 min using staining solution (C).
5. Rinse each gel individually in a separate box for a few seconds in distilled water.
6. Incubate each gel individually in a separate box for 1 min in incubation (II) (D).
7. Develop the gels for 5–20 min in developer (E).
8. Stop the reaction with stop solution (F).

### 3.3.2. Preparative Run: Coomassie Staining Protocol

For preparative use, a modified Neuhoff procedure *(11)* is used (see also **Note 3**). The solutions used are listed under **Subheading 2.4.2.** The following steps are performed:

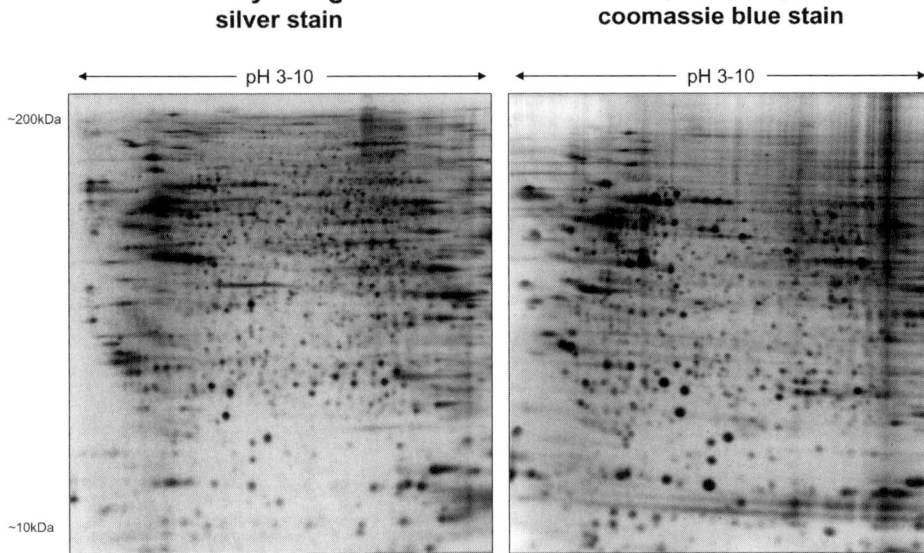

Fig. 2. 2D electropherogrammes of the parental, chemosensitive neuroblastoma cell line SH-SY5Y. *Left side:* analytical, silver-stained gel (50 µg protein). *Right side:* preparative, coomassie-stained gel (1 mg protein).

1. Fix the gels for 6–16 h in fixation solution (A).
2. Rinse 3 × 30 min in distilled water.
3. Incubate for 1 h in incubation solution (B).
4. Stain with solution for 3–5 d (C)—the box should be properly taped up (airtight) to avoid contamination!
5. Destain for 3–6 h using distilled water.

## *3.4. Image Analysis*

After the analytical run, image analysis of the silver-stained gels using sophisticated 2D software is performed. **Figure 2** shows representative electropherogrammes of the parental, chemosensitive human neuroblastoma cell line SH-SY5Y. The 2D gel on the left shows fractionation of 50 µg total protein followed by silver staining of the gel (analytical run), while the image on the right shows a preparative gel of the same sample after coomassie staining. In this case, 1 mg total protein extract was applied. Comparison of the images shows changes between the spot patterns received after coomassie staining and silver staining, respectively (*see also* **Note 3**).

In **Fig. 3** differentially expressed spots are illustrated. Using the 2D image software PDQuest, "differential protein expression" has been defined as a fourfold increase (upregulated proteins) or decrease (downregulated proteins) of optical density. In this range, artefacts caused by sample application, protein determination, or staining differences can most likely be excluded.

**Figure 3a** gives an example of differential overexpression (spot A), while **Fig. 3b** provides an example of differential underexpression (spot B) in the etoposide-resistant clone in comparison to the chemosensitive neuroblastoma cell line. The spots are marked in the original gel scans as well as in the Gaussian image, which is a synthetic image derived from the filtered image (not shown). The filtered image is a copy of the original scan that has been filtered and processed.

1. After scanning of the individual gels, automated spot detection and background subtraction is applied to the gels, followed by creation of matchsets including a normalization step. Triplets of the chemosensitive cells and the chemoresistant cells are matched in two individual lower-level matchsets (level 1 matchset).
2. Subsequently, chemosensitivity vs chemoresistance is compared in a higher-level machtset (level 2 matchset) containing the two lower-level matchsets. This procedure is demonstrated schematically in **Fig. 4**. In **Table 1**, the data of the two differentially expressed spots are presented, including average optical density (OD) and resulting expression factor as well as the name of the protein identified.

## *3.5. Protein Identification*

For identification of differentially expressed protein spots detected by computer-assisted image analysis (*see* **Subheading 3.4.**), preparative gels compatible with MS have been fabricated.

1. Coomassie-stained protein spots are isolated using pipet tips trimmed to the size of the individual spot using a scalpel (*see* **Note 8**).
2. Proteins are digested with porcine methylated trypsin in 40 m$M$ ammonium bicarbonate at 37°C for 6–8 h. The reaction is stopped by freezing.
3. Manually, MALDI mass spectra are recorded in the positive-ion mode with delayed extraction on a Reflex II time-of-flight instrument equipped with a SCOUT multiprobe inlet and a 337-nm nitrogen laser.
4. Mass spectra are obtained by averaging 50–200 individual laser shots.
5. Calibration of the spectra is performed internally by a two-point linear fit using the autolysis products of trypsin at $m/z$ 842.50 and $m/z$ 2211.10.
6. Automatically, MALDI mass spectra are recorded on a M@LDI™ equipped with a 96-well-plate sample target plate and a 337-nm nitrogen laser.
7. Calibration is performed externally by multiple-point polynomial order using a solution of polyethylene glycol in saturated α-cyano-4-hydroxycinnamic acid in acetone.
8. For the mass spectrometric analysis of tryptic digests, MALDI samples are prepared by reverse-phase extraction using ZipTip C18 according to the manufacturer (Millipore).

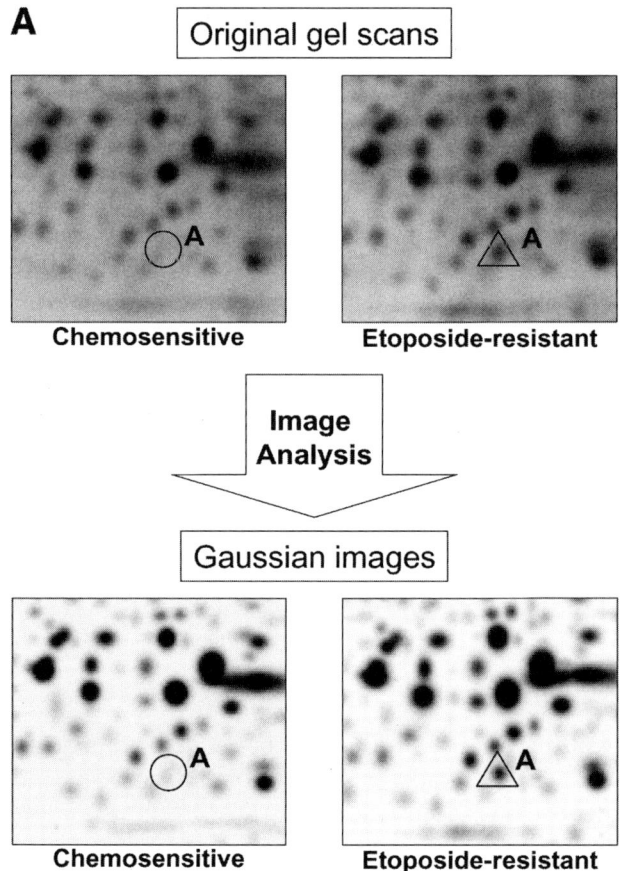

Fig. 3A. Close-up of two regions of the gels showing examples for differentially expressed spots. The spots are marked on the original gel scan as well as on the gaussian images obtained during computer-assisted image analysis. Differentially overexpressed spot (A) in the etoposide-resistant clone in comparison to the chemosensitive neuroblastoma cell line.

9. Elution and spotting is obtained with a 50% acetonitrile/water solution saturated with α-cyano-4-hydroxycinnamic acid, depositing onto individual spots on the target.
10. Database search with the measured monoisotopic peptide masses is performed against the NCBInr database using the peptide search routines MS-Fit (http://prospector.ucsf.edu/ucsfhtml4.0/msfit.htm), ProFound (http://prowl.rockefeller.edu/profound_bin/WebProFound.exe), and MASCOT (www.matrixscience.com).
11. Database searches with fragments generated by PSD experiments are accomplished using the search algorithm MS-Tag (http://prospector.ucsf.edu/ucsfhtml4.0/mstagfd.htm).

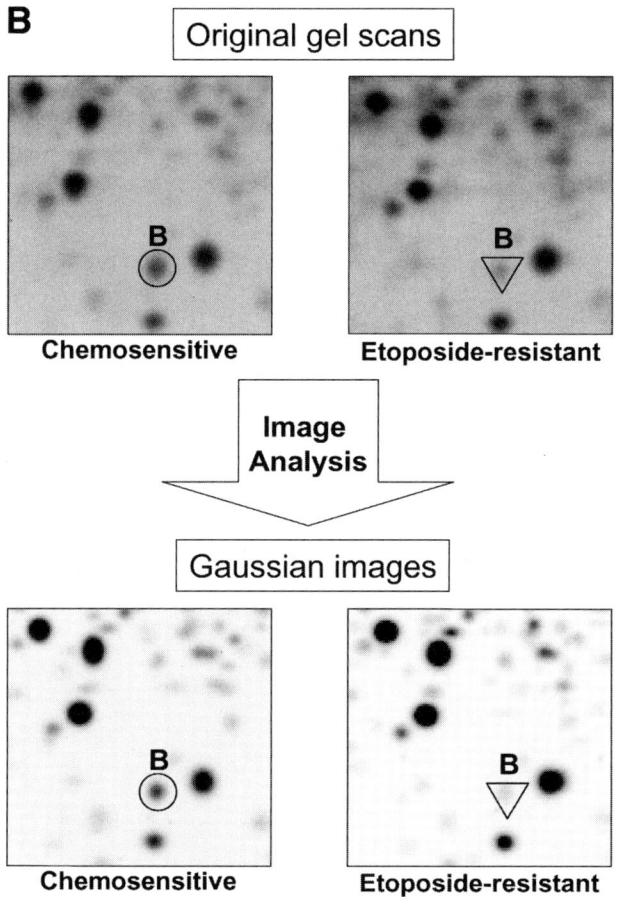

Fig. 3B. Differentially underexpressed spot (B) in the etoposide-resistant clone in comparison to the chemosensitive neuroblastoma cell line.

## 4. Notes

1. In this chapter we describe the basic tools of proteomics to study global protein expression. The gels used here allow resolution of proteins with isoelectric points between 3 and 10 and molecular weights between 8.5 and 230 kDa, resulting in a total of around 1500–4000 protein spots per gel (mainly high-abundance proteins), depending on the sample used. For special problems it may be reasonable to use narrow pH ranges ("zoom gels") to increase resolution of spots in a certain area. Additionally, fractionation of very acidic/basic proteins needs special experimental conditions. The sample solubilization described above is suitable to receive total protein extracts from the cell. Alternatively, protocols for subcellular fractionation (e.g., membrane fraction, nuclear fraction) can be applied to study functional organization of cells and aspects of dynamic changes in the proteome *(12–14)*.

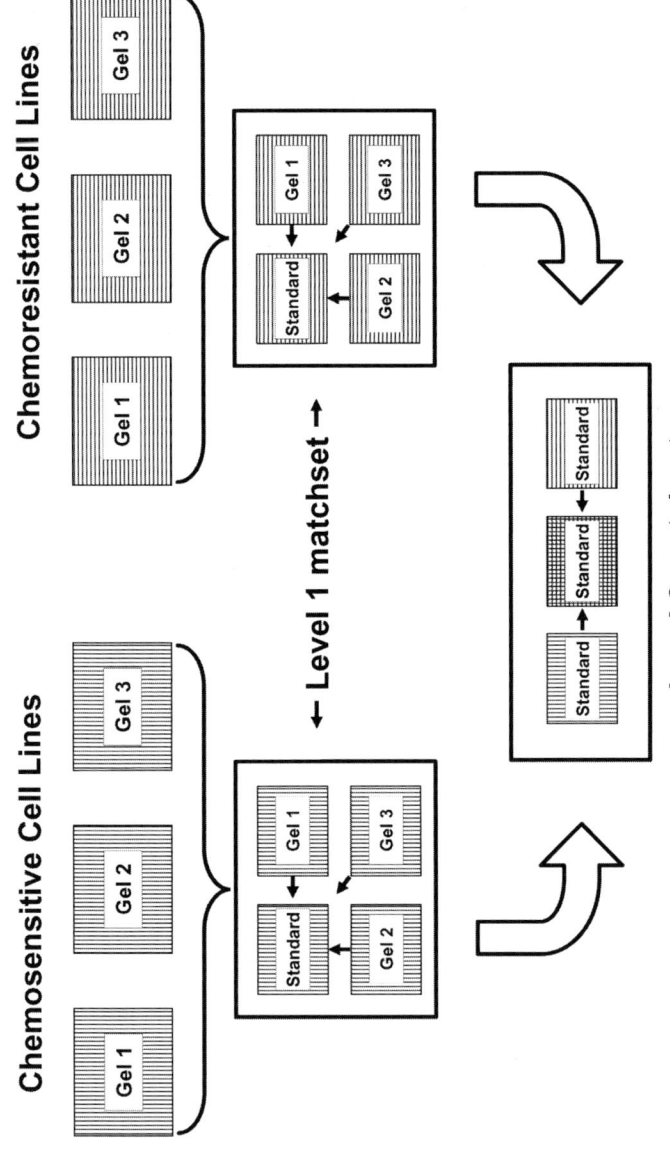

Fig. 4. Schematic representation showing structure of level 1 and level 2 matchsets.

## Table 1
### Data of the Differentially Expressed Spots Obtained from Image Analysis and Mass Spectrometry

| Spot | Average OD in chemosensitive cells | Average OD in chemoresistant cells | Expression in resistant cells | Expression factor | Identified protein |
|---|---|---|---|---|---|
| A | 43.6 | 328.1 | Upregulated | 7.5 | Peroxiredoxin 1 |
| B | 592.7 | 116.2 | Downregulated | 5.1 | dUTP Pyrophosphatase |

2. Alternatively to PDA, N,N'-methylene-bis-acrylamide (Bis) can be used as crosslinker. The advantage of PDA is an increase in gel strength; moreover, it is supposed to cause reduction of silver stain background in SDS-PAGE.
3. Preparative coomassie-stained gels may cause some problems. First, the staining is about 100 times less sensitive than silver staining, thus requiring application of a very high protein amount (at least 1 mg). Second, certain protein spots do not bind coomassie brilliant blue, making spot cutting impossible. Take care that the spot pattern of coomassie-stained gels may be different to the one of silver-stained gels (clearly apparent in **Fig. 2**). In special cases (e.g., availability of very little sample or failing of detection of important spots by coomassie), it might be reasonable to use MALDI-compatible silver staining protocols *(15,16)*. Using the protocol published by us, the amount of sample to be loaded on the gel can be conveniently reduced to about 100 µg total protein. The greatest problem of MALDI-compatible silver staining is contamination with keratins due to the increase of the keratin:protein ratio. Circumventing this problem requires stringent conditions of cleanliness, but complete avoidance is hardly possible.
4. Make sure that the glass cassettes for gel casting are properly cleaned (e.g., use detergent followed by wiping with ethanol and remove dust with air pressure), to avoid artefacts in the gel.
5. Insufficient equilibration (unequal DTT:iodoacetamide ratio) may cause point streaking after silver staining. A possible solution to allow proper shaking of several IPG strips simultaneously without disarrangement of the strips is the use of a multiphor II chamber (Amersham Biosciences) and electrode clamps to fix the gels or individual equilibration in tubes.
6. Recycling of Laemmli buffer can increase separation time and may reduce quality of the gels due to consumption of buffer components. Although it is expensive, we recommend the use of "new" buffer for every run.
7. This silver staining protocol was preferred to ammoniacal silver staining (e.g., the protocol published by Hochstrasser et al.: www.expasy.ch/ch2d/protocols/protocols.fm4.html), although ammoniacal staining procedures are slightly more sensitive. The major advantage of the protocol utilized here is the fact that development can be extended to much longer periods (up to 20 min compared with

max 5 min if the Hochstrasser protocol is used), therefore clearly increasing the reproducibility from gel to gel. Additionally, aldehyde-free ammoniacal silver methods often show "hollow spots" or strong protein-to-protein variation.
8. For a small number of spots, manual spot picking is fine. Use gloves, scissors, and one-way material to avoid contamination. Alternatively (especially if hundreds of spots must be isolated for creation of comprehensive databases or if the equipment is available anyway), spot-picking machines, for instance, available from Bruker Daltonics, Genetix, Bio-Rad, or Amersham Biosciences, can be used.

## References

1. Bernardini, S., Bellincampi, L., Ballerini, S., et al. (2002) Role of GST P1-1 in mediating the effect of etoposide on human neuroblastoma cell line Sh-Sy5y. *J. Cell Biochem.* **86,** 340–347.
2. Rabilloud, T. (1998) Use of thiourea to increase the solubility of membrane proteins in two-dimensional electrophoresis. *Electrophoresis* **19,** 758–760.
3. Cheung, C. K., Mak, Y. T., and Swaminathan, R. (1987) Automated trichloroacetic acid precipitation method for urine total protein. *Ann. Clin. Biochem.* **24,** 140–144.
4. O'Farrell, P. H. (1975) High resolution two-dimensional electrophoresis of proteins. *J. Biol. Chem.* **250,** 4007–4021.
5. Klose, J. (1975) Protein mapping by combined isoelectric focusing and electrophoresis of mouse tissues. A novel approach to testing for induced point mutations in mammals. *Humangenetik* **26,** 231–243.
6. Scheele, G. A. (1975) Two-dimensional gel analysis of soluble proteins. Charaterization of guinea pig exocrine pancreatic proteins. *J. Biol. Chem.* **250,** 5375–5385.
7. Bjellqvist, B., Ek, K., Righetti, P. G., et al. (1982) Isoelectric focusing in immobilized pH gradients: principle, methodology and some applications. *J. Biochem. Biophys. Meth.* **6,** 317–339.
8. Laemmli, U. K. (1970) Cleavage of structural proteins during the assembly of the head of bacteriophage T4. *Nature* **227,** 680–685.
9. Heukeshoven, J. and Dernick, R. (1995) Effective blotting of ultrathin polyacrylamide gels anchored to a solid matrix. *Electrophoresis* **6,** 103–112.
10. Klose, J. and Kobalz, U. (1995) Two-dimensional electrophoresis of proteins: an updated protocol and implications for a functional analysis of the genome. *Electrophoresis* **16,** 1034–1059.
11. Neuhoff, V., Arold, N., Taube, D., and Ehrhardt, W. (1988) Improved staining of proteins in polyacrylamide gels including isoelectric focusing gels with clear background at nanogram sensitivity using Coomassie Brilliant Blue G-250 and R-250. *Electrophoresis* **9,** 255–262.
12. Dreger, M., Bengtsson, L., Schoneberg, T., Otto, H., and Hucho, F. (2001) Nuclear envelope proteomics: novel integral membrane proteins of the inner nuclear membrane. *Proc. Natl. Acad. Sci. USA* **98,** 11,943–11,948.
13. Schirmer, E. C. and Gerace, L. (2002) Organellar proteomics: the prizes and pitfalls of opening the nuclear envelope. *Genome Biol.* **3,** REVIEWS1008.

14. Dreger, M. (2003) Proteome analysis at the level of subcellular structures. *Eur. J. Biochem.* **270,** 589–599.
15. Shevchenko, A., Wilm, M., Vorm, O., and Mann, M. (1996) Mass spectrometric sequencing of proteins silver-stained polyacrylamide gels. *Anal. Chem.* **68,** 850–858.
16. Sinha, P., Poland, J., Schnolzer, M., and Rabilloud, T. (2001) A new silver staining apparatus and procedure for matrix-assisted laser desorption/ionization-time of flight analysis of proteins after two-dimensional electrophoresis. *Proteomics* **1,** 835–840.

# III

## IN VIVO ANIMAL MODELING OF CHEMOSENSITIVITY

# 19

## Clinically Relevant Metastatic Breast Cancer Models to Study Chemosensitivity

### Lee Su Kim and Janet E. Price

#### Summary

Metastatic disease, notably to the lungs, liver, bone, and brain, is the most common cause of death from breast cancer, despite advances in surgical and clinical management. Two basic principles govern the process of metastasis: first, that tumors are heterogeneous populations of cells; and second, that the process of metastasis is a sequence of events that depends on tumor cell properties and interactions with the microenvironment at the sites of metastasis. In theory, inhibitors targeted at any of the steps of metastasis have the potential to inhibit metastatic progression. In vitro assays cannot simulate accurately the complex process of metastasis, and the use of appropriate animal models is necessary to model the process, and for testing the impact of targeted inhibitors on the growth and development of breast cancer metastasis. Animal models of the growth and metastasis of rodent and human breast cancer cells have been developed, including models that target the metastatic growth in key organs sites such as the bone and brain.

#### Key Words

Animal models; metastasis; breast cancer.

### 1. Introduction

Once breast cancer has been diagnosed, the most important question is whether the cancer is confined to the breast or has spread to distant sites. The majority of the deaths of women with breast cancer result from the growth of metastases that are nonresponsive to therapy *(1)*. The development of more effective therapies should be based on a better understanding of the mechanisms responsible for the spread of cells from the breast to distant sites, including lymph nodes, bone, brain, liver, and lungs. A variety of in vitro and in vivo models have been developed to study the biology of metastasis *(2)*. In general, in vitro assays have been designed to model distinct steps in the process, for example, invasion through reconstituted basement membranes *(3)*, or specific binding to endothelial cells isolated from organs where the cancer cells commonly form metastases *(4,5)*. Such in vitro assays have great practical value for evaluating specific tumor cell behaviors, yet their limitations for predicting in vivo malignancy should always be considered. It is probably impossible to simulate accurately all the events of the metastatic process with in vitro models, especially considering the events that involve interactions with components of the microenvironment at the site of metastasis *(6)*. Thus, animal models using transplantable tumors that can grow and metastasize predictably in a suitable host have become standard systems for analyzing the metastatic phenotype and for testing the efficacy of antimetastatic therapies. The most common animal models are rodent tumor models, using transplantable tumors, or spontaneously arising or carcinogen-induced mammary tumors of rats and mice *(7)*. More recently, transgenic mice with various oncogenes targeted to the mammary epithelium have become available, and some are suitable for testing specific forms of therapy, such as those designed for tumors that overexpress *HER2/ neu (8,9)*. Immunodeficient rodents, most commonly athymic (also known as nude) or SCID mice, have been used widely for xenograft studies with human cancers. Not all human cancers or established tumor cell lines will grow successfully in immunodeficient mice, at least from a subcutaneous (sc) route of inoculation, the most common and for practical purposes the easiest technique to use. The approach of injecting human tumor cells into the normal equivalent mouse organ, known as orthotopic injection, has been adopted as a way to improve tumor take and growth, and has also been shown to increase the likelihood of metastasis *(10)*. For breast cancer cells the appropriate site for implantation is the mammary fatpad (mfp) and there is extensive literature describing growth-modulating effects of the mfp on normal, preneoplastic, and malignant mammary epithelial cells *(11,12)*. Injection of human breast cancer cells into the mfp has been shown to result in improved tumor take and growth rates compared with sc injection, and has allowed the selection of more metastatic variants of human breast cancer cells, by isolating cells from the metastatic lesions in the immunodeficient mice *(13,14)*. However, while mfp injection generally improves tumor takes and growth rates, the number of cell lines that reproducibly form spontaneous metastases is disappointingly low, especially because the majority of the commonly used breast cancer cell lines were established from metastases *(2)*. The orthotopic xenotransplantation of histologically intact fragments of human cancers, such as tumor specimens taken directly from the patient, can result in enhanced reproduction of the metastatic potential of the cancer cells *(15)*. An explanation for this may be that stromal elements in the tissue fragments allow for continued expression of genes essential for malignant growth and metastasis. In contrast, when the tumor cells are separated from stroma and grown in tissue culture, the tumor–stroma interactions are lost and metastasis-promoting gene expression may be reduced or silenced. However, while the use of histologically intact tissue xenografts has proven advantages, one disadvantage is that of limited tissue availability compared with the use of established cancer cell lines. These, at least in theory, provide consistent and reproducible models in different laboratories.

Clinical observations suggest that responses of breast cancer metastases to chemotherapy can be influenced by the anatomical location of the lesions, possibly related to differences in microenvironmental stresses *(16)*. Differential chemosensitivity of metastases in different organs may be a function of heterogeneity of the tumor population, with different clones metastasizing to different organs. However, the influence of the organ microenvironment cannot be ignored. Results from experimental tumor models have shown that the same tumor implanted in different organs can have different responses to a chemotherapeutic drug *(17)*. For example, sensitivity of mouse mammary tumor cells to different chemotherapy agents was assessed in vivo, comparing responses in sc tumors with response of the cells in bone marrow, spleen, liver, lungs, and brain. The sc tumors were generally sensitive, while cells in liver and brain were less sensitive to alkylating agents. Cells in bone marrow showed variable sensitivity to different agents, and addition of an antiangiogenic compound markedly increased killing of bone marrow micrometastases by cyclophosphamide *(18)*. Thus the tissue microenvironment may contribute to the sensitivity of metastatic cells to chemotherapy, and modulating the stroma (in this case by inhibiting angiogenesis) can have an impact on the response to treatment.

Experimental models have been developed that can target tumor cells to different organs to simulate metastasis in specific sites, and therefore be used for studying response of tumor cells growing in different organ environments. Intravenous (iv) injection of tumor cells into the tail vein of mice usually results in lung metastasis, and injection into the spleen or into the hepatic portal vein can generate experimental metastases in the liver *(19,20)*. Experimental models of brain metastasis have used direct injection into the brain parenchyma, or introduction of cells into the internal carotid artery *(21)*. Injection of tumor cells into the left heart (intracardiac, ic) leads to widespread distribution of metastases, including bone and bone marrow *(22)*. This model has been used successfully as a model for osteolytic bone metastasis using the MDA-MB-231 human breast cancer cell line *(23)*. Direct injection of breast cancer cells into the bone (e.g., tibia or femur) can result in localized tumors *(24,25)*. Although the direct injection approach cannot be used to investigate events in the initial steps of bone metastasis, it can be used for studies of interactions between tumor cells and the bone microenvironment. Spontaneous bone metastasis by human breast cancer cells is rarely seen *(26)*, but a mouse mammary tumor model, 4T1, syngeneic to BALB/c, is reported form bone metastases from mfp tumors. Clones of the original tumor were isolated and characterized with increased bone-metastasizing ability *(27)*. This, and other studies using human tumor lines, are examples of using an animal model to isolate variants with increased metastatic ability, in some cases for metastasis to a specific site *(14,28)*. Such variants can then be used for further phenotypic characterization, and also for preclinical therapy models.

This chapter describes three techniques for metastasis models using human breast cancer cells: mammary fatpad injection, intracardiac injection, and intracarotid injection.

## 2. Materials

1. Human tumor cell lines, free of *Mycoplasma* and murine pathogenic viruses (reovirus type 3, pneumonia virus, K virus, Theiler's encephalitis virus, Sendai virus, minute virus, mouse adenovirus, mouse hepatitis virus, lymphocytic choriomeningitis virus, ectromelia virus, lactate dehydrogenase virus). Checking the cell lines for these viruses will reduce the risk of introducing pathogens into the animal facility.
2. Nude mice, 6 wk old at start of experiment.
3. Culture medium with serum.
4. Phosphate-buffered saline (PBS) without $Ca^{2+}$ and $Mg^{2+}$.
5. Trypsin-EDTA: 0.25% w/v trypsin and 0.02% w/v EDTA in PBS without $Ca^{2+}$ and $Mg^{2+}$. Prepare a fresh trypsin solution before harvesting cell cultures.
6. Sterile instruments and surgical supplies for necropsy and surgery (forceps, scissors, sutures, and sterile cotton tips [Q-tips] for intracarotid artery injection, and 12-mm wound clips and wound-clip applier).
7. Alcohol wipes and Betadine scrub, or equivalent antiseptic scrub solution.
8. Mouse restraint device for intracarotid artery injections (small board and rubber bands).
9. Sterile 1-mL tuberculin syringes and 27-gage (G) × 1/2-in (13-mm) needles; plastic cannula prepared from a disposable tuberculin syringe for intracarotid artery injections.
10. Anesthesia; either ip injection of 50 mg/kg Nembutal (sodium pentobarbital) in PBS, or an inhalation anesthetic such as Metofane (methoxyflurane).
11. Dissecting microscope.
12. Warming lamp or pad.
13. Calipers for tumor measurements.
14. 10% neutral buffered formalin.

Two critical elements for working with immunodeficient mice are the facility in which they are housed, and the areas used for experimental manipulations. Ideally, the animals should be housed in a Specific-Pathogen-Free (SPF) Barrier Facility, in microisolator cages. All manipulations should be performed in laminar-airflow workstations, or an area that is designated solely for work with immunodeficient animals. Depending on the facility, working with the immunodeficient mice may require changing into surgical scrubs, sterile coveralls, caps, masks, shoe covers, and gloves. Work patterns must be organized such that working with and monitoring immunodeficient animals precedes any work with immunocompetent mice on the same day.

## 3. Methods
### 3.1. Preparation of Cells for Injection

1. Aspirate culture medium from cultures of tumor cells that are between 75% and 90% confluent (plate cells, or add fresh medium the previous day to obtain actively growing cultures) (*see* **Note 1**). Wash with 10 mL of PBS per 75-cm$^2$ flask; add 1–2 mL of the trypsin-EDTA solution. Incubate for 30 s to 1 min, then agitate, shake, or tap the flask in the palm of one hand to detach the cells.
2. Resuspend the cells in 10 mL of culture medium and transfer to a centrifuge tube. Spin at 200$g$ for 10 min, and resuspend the pellet in PBS.
3. Determine cell number, and adjust the concentration for the appropriate inoculum volume, by centrifugation and resuspension in a smaller volume of PBS.
4. Place the suspension in ice and proceed immediately to inject the cells.

### 3.2. Mammary Fatpad Injection

1. Anesthetize a female mouse, lay it on one side, and clean the skin of the opposite side in preparation for surgery. Make a 5-mm incision in the skin over the lower lateral thorax. Open a pocket under the skin in a cranial direction with the blades of the scissors, so that the mammary fatpad can be seen.
2. Vortex the cell suspension and draw it up into a 1-mL syringe. Place a 27-G needle on the syringe and expel any air bubbles.
3. Insert the needle into the fatty tissue of the mammary fatpad, and inject 0.1 mL with $2 \times 10^6$ cells for the MDA-MB-435 human breast cancer cell line (*see* **Note 2**). The inoculum should form a bubble inside the fatpad, and not leak into the sc space. Close the incision with wound clips, and monitor the mouse until recovered from the anesthesia. Return the mouse to a clean cage.
4. Monitor mice daily for overall condition, and measure tumor growth once or twice weekly (*see* **Note 3**). Hold the mouse by grasping it firmly in one hand. Secure the scruff of the mouse neck between thumb and forefinger with the tail between the third and fourth fingers and the palm of the hand and use calipers to measure two diameters of the tumor. Calculate the mean diameter to graph out tumor growth over time. The diameter measurements can also be used to estimate tumor volume, using the formula

$$\text{Tumor volume} = \frac{x^2 y}{2}$$

where $x$ is the smaller diameter of the tumor and $y$ is the larger.

5. When the tumor reaches a maximum size of 1.5 cm, either kill the mouse or remove the tumor. The MDA-MB-435 cell line can form tumors of this size in 10–12 wk. If the tumors are removed, kill mice 4–6 wk later.
6. Euthanize mice and examine for metastases, principally in lungs and lymph nodes, but examine the abdomen also. Fix organs or tissues in formalin and prepare sections for histology if required. If a mouse had been showing abnormal balance or movements, remove the brain for histology (*see* **Note 4**).

### 3.3. Intracardiac Injection

1. Anesthetize a mouse, place on its back on a clean work surface, and clean the skin over the chest.
2. Vortex the cell suspension and draw 0.1–0.2 mL into a tuberculin syringe with a 27-G needle, leaving a small bubble of air on below the syringe plunger. Insert the needle into the second intercostal space 3 mm to the left of the sternum, directing the tip into the center of the chest, to a depth of 6 mm. Pulsatile flow of red blood into the hub of the needle will indicate correct placement of the needle in the left ventricle, and gentle aspiration may be needed if red blood does not appear immediately.
3. Slowly inject 0.05–0.1 mL of suspension over 20–30 s. Do not inject the air bubble.
4. Withdraw the needle, place the mouse on its side, and allow it to recover from the procedure, with supplemental heat if necessary. Return the mouse to a clean cage after it has completely recovered from the anesthetic.
5. Observe the mice daily for signs of tumor burden, including paralysis, hunched posture, or weight loss. Euthanize when moribund or at predetermined time points, and necropsy and preserve tissue for histology if required. Examination of the skeleton by radiography can detect skeletal lesions. The incidence and distribution of metastases may vary for different tumor cell lines (*see* **Note 5**).

### 3.4. Intracarotid Artery Injection

1. Prepare a plastic cannula by melting and stretching the hub of a 1-mL disposable syringe, to create a <30-G cannula.
2. Anesthetize a mouse with ip injection of sodium pentobarbital (50 mg/kg) and restrain on its back on a clean board. Stabilize the head by placing a rubber band under the upper incisors and around the board.
3. Clean the neck of the mouse with alcohol and Betadine.
4. Cut the skin of the neck with a midline incision, and place the mouse under a dissecting microscope. With blunt dissection, expose the trachea and muscles to expose the right common carotid artery (*see* **Note 6**).
5. Prepare the artery distal to the point of division of the internal and external carotid arteries.
6. Place and tie a ligature of 5-0 black silk suture in the common carotid artery, proximal to the point of injection.

7. Place and loosely tie a second ligature at the point of division of the internal and external carotid arteries. Place a sterile cotton tip under the artery just distal to the injection site.
8. Vortex the prepared cell suspension at the required concentration ($1 \times 10^5$ cells in 0.1 mL) and fill the syringe.
9. Nick the common carotid artery with microscissors between the ligatures. Lifting the cotton tip can control back-flow bleeding from distal vessels. Insert the plastic cannula through the hole into the vessel lumen and thread forward into the internal carotid artery. Slowly inject the cell suspension, withdraw the cannula, and tighten the second ligature.
10. Close the skin incision with clips or sutures. Allow the mouse to recover, using a heat lamp if necessary, and when it is fully mobile, place it in a clean cage.
11. Inspect the mice daily, watching for signs of tumor growth, including the development of paralysis, abnormal movements, swelling of the skull, and weight loss. Typically, the survival time of mice injected with $1 \times 10^5$ MDA-MB-231 human breast cancer cells was 50–60 d, killing mice that displayed these signs and not using death as the end point *(29)*.

## 4. Notes

1. Preparation of cell suspensions: Some of the variability in repeat experiments with a particular cell line, or from published results from other laboratories, may arise from inconsistencies in techniques or poor-quality preparation of the cells for injections. To optimize the results and consistency between experiments, thaw a vial from frozen stocks of the cell line and expand the cells in tissue culture to obtain the required cell number. The cells should be in subconfluent, actively growing cultures. The cells from confluent cultures are more likely to form clumps or aggregates, depending on the cell type. In addition, the degree of confluence in vitro has been reported to regulate gene expression, which might affect the in vivo behavior. The important point is to be consistent in using good cell preparation techniques. High viability is essential. The method described generally yields cell suspensions with high viability (98–100%, by trypan blue dye exclusion). If a suspension has less than 90% viability, or if the cells are in clumps, it is best to discard these cells and start with a fresh culture. For experimental metastasis assays using iv injection, clumps of cells, or dead cells mixed with live tumor cells might artificially increase the number of tumor colonies formed. Using $Ca^{2+}$- and $Mg^{2+}$-free buffer will retard formation of clumps, and gentle vortexing may help to break up loose clusters, but if cells come off the tissue culture flask in clumps, it is best to start with fresh, less confluent cultures. Too vigorous pipetting or mixing may be more likely to damage the cells than break up the clumps. As stated above, once the suspension has been prepared, proceed to inject as soon as possible. Keeping the suspension on ice will reduce the formation of cell aggregates.
2. Breast cancer models: The method described uses an estrogen receptor (ER)-negative breast cancer cell line. Cell lines that express ER may not grow unless

the nude mice are supplemented with estrogen. One commonly used method is the implantation of slow-release pellets of 17β-estradiol (from Innovative Research of America, Sarasota, FL). A 60-d-release 0.72-mg pellet will support the growth of the ER-positive MCF-7 breast cancer cell line (from injection of $5 \times 10^6$ cells into the mammary fatpad).

3. All of the animal procedures (housing conditions, experimentation, surgical procedures, euthanasia and anesthesia, etc.) will probably be regulated by an institutional body such as an Institutional Animal Care and Use Committee. In the United States this committee is charged with ensuring compliance with guidelines and requirements established by the Public Health Service (PHS) *Policy on Humane Care and Use of Laboratory Animals*, the U.S. Department of Health and Human Services *Guide for the Care and Use of Laboratory Animals*, and the Animal Welfare Act of 1966 as amended. Experimental design should take into account the well-being of the mice and use appropriate procedures to reduce pain and suffering. In the context of this chapter this means careful monitoring of mice for development of tumor burden, appropriate animal handling and surgical procedures, and the humane use of euthanasia. Using a moribund end point, rather than a death end point for a study, is more practical if the point of the study is to assess the extent of tumor spread. Recognizing the signs of tumor development comes with experience, and regular monitoring of the condition of the animals. Autolysis of mouse tissues starts rapidly, and it is easier to monitor, measure, and recover metastases from freshly killed mice than from those dead for more than an hour or two. Furthermore, if tissues are needed for analyses, such as nucleic acid extraction or immunohistochemistry, these should be harvested immediately after killing the mouse. If a veterinary medicine department is administering the animal facility, this is a source for advice on small animal surgery, anesthesia, euthanasia, and necropsy techniques. Inhalation of Metofane is a rapid and easy means of anesthesia, and is ideal for short procedures, as the mice will recover rapidly. Metofane is a hazardous agent, and should therefore be used only in a suitable fume hood or with appropriate ventilation. It is also not currently manufactured in the United States. Alternative inhalant anesthetics, such as isoflurane and halothane, require specialized vaporizer apparatus. Injectable anesthetics such as Nembutal (sodium pentobarbital, 50 mg/kg injected ip) have longer induction and recovery times. When using anesthesia on nude mice, take precautions to prevent hypothermia, and do not be too liberal with alcohol and surgical scrub fluids. Use a warming pad or lamp during the recovery phase, but do not let the mouse overheat either.

4. Scoring the metastases: The simplest method is to count the numbers of metastases visible on the surface of the target organs. An alternative to aid detection of metastases is to fix the organs in Bouin's fixative. The metastases will be white lesions against the yellow-stained normal tissue. Counting surface lesions does not include microscopic disease, which can be detected in histological sections, although quantitation of metastases in multiple organ sections is labor-intensive. Depending on the model used and site of metastasis, the weights or volumes of organs may be used to estimate the tumor burden (discussed in **ref. *20***). The use

of fluorescent markers, notably green fluorescent protein (GFP) *(30)* can facilitate the detection of cells and micrometastases. Another technique that requires transfection of the tumor cells is introduction of a luciferase gene. When animals with luciferase-expressing tumors are injected with the substrate luciferin, the resulting chemoluminescence can be measured noninvasively, and is proportional to the tumor burden *(26,31)*. Both techniques require specialized equipment for detecting and measuring the fluorescence or luminescence. How the metastatic burden is measured will dictate the choice of test used for statistical analysis. For comparisons of numbers of metastases estimated by surface counting, use a nonparametric test such as the Mann-Whitney rank sum test. Consider the analysis to be used when planning the study, to ensure that there are enough animals per experimental group to achieve statistical significance. If possible, allow for the loss of one or two mice (from early morbidity, or reasons unrelated to the experiment) and still have enough data points for valid statistical analyses.
5. The distribution pattern and the length of time before metastases develop may differ for each cell line, and may also differ from what has been published for a particular cell line. In the first experiment with a cell line, monitor the mice closely and, if necessary, wait longer than expected for the mice to show signs of metastatic tumor burden. Killing mice at different time points can also be done to monitor and establish the time course of growth of metastases (assessed macroscopically or in histological sections). No or fewer metastases than expected could be the result of a number of factors, including the health and housing conditions of the mice, and the cell preparation techniques. Variants of some human tumor cell lines have arisen, possibly resulting from different tissue culture techniques, which vary considerably in their tumorigenic and metastatic phenotypes. To save time and resources, it may be prudent to obtain a particular cell line from an investigator who is currently using the cells for in vivo studies.
6. Intracarotid artery injection is a challenging technique. Previous experience with microsurgery is an advantage, and taking time to practice the technique is probably essential. An assistant who can monitor the level of anesthesia in the mice, and hand supplies or instruments to the operator, will also be helpful. Close postprocedure monitoring of the injected mice is recommended. If there is high mortality in the first few days after injection, the dose or volume of the inoculum may need to be reduced in subsequent experiments.

## References

1. Hortobagyi, G. N. (2000) Developments in chemotherapy of breast cancer. *Cancer* **88,** 3073–3079.
2. Price, J. E. (1996) Metastasis from human breast cancer cell lines. *Breast Cancer Res. Treat.* **39,** 93–102.
3. Albini, A. P., Iwamoto, Y., Kleinman, H. K., et al. (1987) A rapid in vitro assay for quantitating the invasive potential of tumor cells. *Cancer Res.* **47,** 3239–3245.
4. Cheng, H. C., Abdel-Ghany, M., Elble, R. C., and Pauli, B. U. (1998) Lung endothelial dipeptidyl peptidaseIV promotes adhesion and metastasis of rat breast

cancer cells via tumor surface associated fibronectin. *J. Biol. Chem.* **273**, 24,207–24,215.
5. Lehr, J. E. and Pienta, K. J. (1998) Preferential adhesion of prostate cancer cells to a human bone marrow endothelial cell line. *J. Natl. Cancer Inst.* **90**, 118–123.
6. Liotta, L. A. and Kohn, E. A. (2001) The microenvironment of the tumour–host interface. *Nature* **411**, 375–379.
7. Heppner, G. H., Miller, F. R., and Shekhar, P. V. M. (2000) Non-transgenic models of breast cancer. *Breast Cancer Res.* **2**, 331–334.
8. Hutchinson, J. N. and Muller, W. J. (2000) Transgenic mouse models of human breast cancer. *Oncogene* **19**, 6130–6137.
9. Lachman, L. B., Ozpolat, B., Rao, X. M., Kiriakova, G., and Price, J. E. (2001) DNA vaccination against HER2/*neu* reduces breast cancer incidence and metastasis. *Cancer Gene Ther.* **8**, 259–268.
10. Fidler, I. J. (1990) Critical factors in the biology of human cancer metastasis: Twenty-eighth G. H. A. Clowes Memorial Award Lecture. *Cancer Res.* **50**, 6130–6138.
11. Lochter, A. and Bissell, M. J. (1995) Involvement of extracellular matrix constituents in breast cancer. *Semin. Cancer Biol.* **6**, 165–173.
12. Simian, M. Hirai, Y., Navre, M., Werb, Z., Lochter, A., and Bissell, M. J. (2001) The interplay of matrix metalloproteinases, morphogens and growth factors is necessary for branching of mammary epithelial cells. *Development* **128**, 3117–3131.
13. Price, J. E., Polyzos, A., Zhang, R. D., and Daniels, L. M. (1990) Tumorigenicity and metastasis of human breast carcinoma cell lines in nude mice. *Cancer Res.* **50**, 717–721.
14. Lev, D. C., Kiriakova, G., and Price, J. E. (2003) Selection of more aggressive variants of the GI101A human breast cancer cell line: a model for analyzing the metastatic phenotype of breast cancer. *Clin. Exp. Metastasis* **20**, 515–523.
15. Hoffman, R. M. (1999) Orthotopic metastatic mouse models for anticancer drug discovery and evaluation: a bridge to the clinic. *Invest. New Drugs* **17**, 343–359.
16. Kamby, C., Ejlertsen, B., Andersen, J., et al. (1988) The pattern of metastases in human breast cancer. Influence of systemic adjuvant therapy and impact on survival. *Acta Oncol.* **27**, 715–719.
17. Wilmanns, C., Fan, D., O'Brian, C. A., et al. (1993) Modulation of doxorubicin sensitivity and level of p-glycoprotein expression in human colon carcinoma cells by ectopic and orthotopic environments in nude mice. *Int. J. Oncol.* **3**, 413–418.
18. Holden, S. A., Emi, Y., Kakeji, Y., Northey, D., and Teicher, B. A. (1997) Host distribution and response to antitumor alkylating agents of EMT-6 tumor cells from subcutaneous tumor implants. *Cancer Chemother. Pharmacol.* **40**, 87–93.
19. Tarin, D. and Price, J. E. (1981) Influence of microenvironment and vascular anatomy on "metastatic" colonization potential of mammary tumors. *Cancer Res.* **41**, 3604–3609.
20. Welch, D. R. (1997) Technical considerations for studying cancer metastasis *in vivo*. *Clin. Exp. Metastasis* **15**, 272–306.

21. Zhang, R. D., Fidler, I. J., and Price, J. E. (1991) Relative malignant potential of human breast carcinoma cell lines established from pleural effusions and a brain metastasis. *Invasion Metastasis* **11,** 204–215.
22. Arguello, F., Baggs, R. B., and Frantz, C. N. (1988) A murine model of experimental metastases to bone and bone marrow. *Cancer Res.* **48,** 6879–6881.
23. Guise, T. A.,Yin, J. J., Taylor, S. D., et al. (1996) Evidence for a causal role of parathyroid hormone-related protein in the pathogenesis of human breast cancer-mediated osteolysis. *J. Clin. Invest.* **98,** 1544–1549.
24. Kjonniksen, I., Winderen, M., and Fodstad, O. (1994) Validity and usefulness of human tumor models established by intratibial inoculation in nude rats. *Cancer Res.* **54,** 1715–1719.
25. Wang, C. Y. and Chang, Y. W. (1997) A model for osseous metastasis of human breast cancer established by intrafemur injection of the MDA-MB-435 cells in nude mice. *Anticancer Res.* **17,** 2471–2474.
26. Rosol, T. J., Tannehill-Gregg, S. H., LeRoy, B. E., Mandl, S., and Contag, C. H. (2003) Animal models of bone metastasis. *Cancer* **97,** 748–757.
27. Lelekakis, M., Moseley, J. M., Martin, T. J., et al. (1999) A novel orthotopic model of breast cancer metastasis to bone. *Clin. Exp. Metastasis* **17,** 163–170.
28. Yoneda, T., Williams, P. J., Hiraga, T., Niewolna, M., and Nishimura, R. (2001) A bone-seeking clone exhibits different biological properties from the MDA-MB-231 parental human breast cancer cells and a brain-seeking clone in vivo and in vitro. *J. Bone. Miner. Res.* **16,** 1486–1495.
29. Kim, L. S., Huang, S., Lu, W., and Price, J. E. (2004) Vascular endothelial growth factor expression promotes the growth of breast cancer brain metastases in nude mice. *Clin. Exp. Metastasis* **21,** 107–118.
30. Hoffman, R. M. (1998) Orthotopic tranplant mouse models with green fluorescent protein-expressing cancer cells to visualize metastasis and angiogenesis. *Cancer Metastasis Rev.* **17,** 271–277.
31. El Hilali, N., Rubio, N., Martinez-Villacampa, M., and Blanco, J. (2002) Combined noninvasive imaging and luminometric quantification of luciferase-labeled human prostate tumors and metastases. *Lab. Invest.* **82,** 1563–1571.

# 20

## Orthotopic Metastatic (MetaMouse®) Models for Discovery and Development of Novel Chemotherapy

**Robert M. Hoffman**

### Summary

Currently-used rodent tumor models, including transgenic tumor models, or subcutaneously growing human tumors in immunodeficient mice, do not sufficiently represent clinical-cancer, especially with regard to metastasis and drug sensitivity. In order to obtain clinically-accurate models, we have developed the technique of surgical orthotopic implantation (SOI) to transplant histologically intact fragments of human cancer, including tumors taken directly from the patient, to the corresponding organ of immunodeficient rodents. It has been demonstrated in approx 100 publications describing 10 tumor types that SOI allows the growth and metastatic potential of the transplanted tumors to be expressed and reflect clinical cancer. These clinically-accurate and relevant SOI models of human cancer have enabled discovery and evaluation of novel antitumor and antimetastatic agents including antiangiogenic drugs. The green fluorescent protein (GFP) and red fluorescent protein (RFP) genes, cloned from bioluminescent organisms, have now been introduced into a series of human and rodent cancer cell lines in vitro to stably express GFP and RFP in vivo in SOI mouse models. With these fluorescent tools, tumors and metastasis in host organs can be externally imaged down to the single-cell level. The combination of fluorescent protein-based imaging in SOI models enables real-time antitumor, antimetastatic, and antiangiogenic drug evaluation including high-throughput in vivo screening. These SOI models are uniquely useful for innovative drug discovery and mechanism studies and serve as a bridge linking preclinical and clinical drug development.

### Key Words

Surgical orthotopic implantation; metastasis; fluorescent proteins; imaging.

From: *Methods in Molecular Medicine, vol. 111: Chemosensitivity: Vol. 2: In Vivo Models, Imaging, and Molecular Regulators*
Edited by: R. D. Blumenthal © Humana Press Inc., Totowa, NJ

# 1. Introduction

## 1.1. Background of Surgical Orthotopic Implantation (SOI) Mouse Models of Human Cancer

Over the past 16 years, we have presented a new approach to the development of clinically accurate rodent models for human cancer based on our invention of surgical orthotopic implantation. The SOI models have been described in approx 100 publications *(1–101)* and in four patents.* SOI allows human tumors of all the major types of human cancer to reproduce clinical-like tumor growth and metastasis in the transplanted rodents *(1–101)*. The use of the SOI models are reviewed for discovery and development of novel chemotherapy agents.

## 1.2. Surgical Orthotopic Implantation of Tumor Fragments

The SOI models circumvent the cell disaggregation step used in previous orthotopic models. Instead of injecting cell suspensions into the orthotopic site, we have developed microsurgical technology to transplant tumor fragments orthotopically *(1–101)*. The development of SOI technology led to a profound improvement in the results achieved in that the metastatic rates and sites in the transplanted mice reflect the clinical pattern. The advantages of SOI appear quite general, having been seen in comparison to orthotopic implantation of cell suspensions for bladder *(2,3)*, lung *(4,9,10,24,26,27)*, stomach *(5,14,18)*, kidney *(72)*, and colon cancers *(1,6,8,16,32,66–70)* (*see* **Note 1**).

In an example of head-to-head comparison of SOI with orthotopic transplantation of cell suspensions, SOI of stomach cancer tissue fragments resulted in metastases in 100% of the nude mice with extensive primary growth. Metastases were found in the regional lymph nodes, liver, and lung, as is characteristic of this cancer *(5)*. In contrast, orthotopic injection of suspensions of stomach cancer cells to the nude mouse stomach resulted in lymph-node metastases in only 6.7% of those mice bearing tumors and no distant metastases.

We also compared the metastatic rate of human renal cell carcinoma SN12C in two orthotopic nude mouse models *(72)*, SOI of tumor tissue and orthotopic injection of cell suspensions were compared in the kidney. The primary tumors resulting from SOI were larger and much more locally invasive than primary tumors resulting from orthotopic transplantation of cell suspension. SOI generated higher metastatic rates than orthotopic transplantation of cell suspensions. The differences in metastatic rates in the involved organs (lung,

---

*U.S. Patents 5,569,812 and 5,491,284; European Patent 0437488; Japanese Patent 2664261.

liver, and mediastinal lymph nodes) were two- to threefold higher in SOI compared to orthotopic transplantation of cell suspensions ($p < 0.05$). Median survival time in the SOI model was 40 d, which was significantly shorter than that of orthotopic transplantation of cell suspensions (68 d) ($p < 0.001$). Histological observation of the primary tumors from the SOI model demonstrated a much richer vascular network than the orthotopic transplantation of cell suspension model. Lymph node and lung metastases were larger and more cellular in the SOI model compared to the orthotopic transplantation of cell suspensions.

We conclude that the tissue architecture of the implanted tumor tissue in the SOI model plays an important role in the initiation of primary tumor growth, invasion, and distant metastasis. These studies demonstrate directly that the implantation of histologically intact tumor tissue orthotopically allows accurate expression of the clinical features of human renal cancer in nude mice. Experiments showed that distant tumor growth in the SOI models were true time-dependent metastases resulting from clinical-like routes and not due to cells shed in transplantation *(17)*. Thus, the SOI models are a significant improvement, allowing the full metastatic potential of human tumors to be expressed in a rodent model.

## 1.3. Discovery of Basic Aspects of Metastasis and Possible New Therapeutic Targets

It was shown with the SOI colon cancer models that liver colonization is the governing process of colon cancer liver metastasis *(32)*. This study further confirmed Paget's seed and soil hypothesis and demonstrated that the liver colonization event is a potential therapeutic target to prevent metastasis.

We have developed a new antimetastatic chemotherapeutic strategy for combination with hepatic resection for liver metastasis in nude mice. The procedure involves ip administration of 5-fluorouracil (5-FU) 2 h before hepatic resection. Therapy was then continued for 4 consecutive d. We termed this strategy neo-neoadjuvant chemotherapy. The regime significantly prolonged animal survival compared to 5-FU adjuvant chemotherapy, surgery alone, 5-FU without surgery, or the untreated control. The 5-FU neo-neoadjuvant chemotherapy had a 50% survival of 68 d, compared to 41 d for 5-FU neoadjuvant treatment, 32 d for 5-FU adjuvant therapy, 30 d for surgery only, 28 d for 5-FU without surgery, and 26 d for control. Two animals in the neo-neoadjuvant group were free of tumor when sacrificed at d 165 postsurgically. The results in this study indicate that new treatment strategies for resecting liver metastasis should be further explored and that the novel regimes introduced in the study of the model could be of great value for designing further clinical trials *(73–75)*.

## 1.4. Development of Patient-Tumor SOI Models

The first model developed with SOI was for human patient colon cancer *(1)*. The human patient and human xenograft colon tumors transplanted by SOI resulted in clinically-relevant natural history such as liver metastasis, lymph node metastasis and peritoneal carcinomatosis *(1)*. The initial "take" rates for human patient colon tumors transplanted by SOI were greater than 80%. Banks of patient tumors that are established in the SOI models are being developed for all the major tumor types.

## 1.5. Drug Discovery with SOI Mouse Models of Cancer

### 1.5.1. Angiogenesis Inhibitors

Tanaka et al. *(80)* used a human primary-tumor resection model *(17)* in which the transplanted tumor was resected after an SOI of a human colorectal cancer line to estimate the efficacy of an angiogenesis inhibitor on metastasis. The angiogenesis inhibitor evaluated was FR-118487, a member of the fumagillin family. One milligram per kilogram per day of FR-118487 was administered subcutaneously to nude mice for 1, 2, or 4 wk through osmotic pumps. Liver metastasis developed in seven of nine control mice, two of six mice that underwent the tumor resection 2 wk after transplantation (early resection), and in all seven of the mice that underwent tumor resection 4 wk after transplantation (late resection). In short-time treatment protocols, FR-118487 administration immediately after early resection completely inhibited both hepatic and peritoneal metastases. However, short-time treatment administration after late resection had no effect on liver metastasis. Prolonged treatment of FR-118487 inhibited both hepatic and peritoneal metastases after late resection.

The efficacy of the combination of vascular endothelial growth factor-neutralizing antibody (VEGFab) and mitomycin C (MMC) was evaluated in an SOI model of human gastric cancer *(81)*. The MT-2 gastric carcinoma line was transplanted by SOI into 62 nude mice. Liver metastasis developed 6 wk after transplantation. The VEGFab (100 µg/mouse) was administered ip in the VEGFab-alone group ($n = 14$) and the combination VEGFab-MMC group ($n = 16$) twice a week beginning on d 10 after transplantation. MMC (2 mg/kg) was administered in the MMC-alone group ($n = 16$) and the combination VEGFab-MMC group ($n = 16$) on d 10, 17, and 24 after transplantation. Compared with the control group, in which saline solution was administered ip, all three treatments significantly inhibited primary tumor growth. Liver metastasis developed in 9 mice of the control group, 3 of 14 in the VEGFab group, and 4 of 10 in the MMC group. In contrast, no mice had liver metastasis in the combination-therapy group. However, a significant body weight loss and a decrease in spleen weight were observed in the MMC and combination groups, with no significant difference between the two groups.

The therapeutic effect of the VEGFAb on liver metastasis of an endocrine neoplasm was also evaluated in an SOI model *(82)*. EN-1, a xenotransplanted human intestinal endocrine neoplasm, was transplanted by SOI on the cecum of nude mice, which resulted in liver metastasis. The treated group ($n = 19$) received 100 µg/mouse of VEGFAb ip on alternate days from d 10 after SOI. The control group ($n = 19$) received saline. Liver metastasis developed in 16 of 17 control mice and in 2 of 19 treated mice ($p < 0.01$). VEGFAb did not cause any body-weight loss.

To evaluate VEGFAb further, two human colon carcinoma cell lines (TK4 and TK 13) and two gastric carcinoma cell lines (MT2 and MT5) were transplanted by SOI into nude mice *(83)*. VEGFab (100 µg/mouse) or the same volume of saline was administered ip on alternative days from d 10 after transplantation. With each of the four xenografts, VEGFab significantly inhibited both primary tumor growth and macroscopic liver metastasis. Body-weight loss was not observed.

The effect of the angiogenesis inhibitor, TNP-470, on primary tumor growth, liver metastasis, and peritoneal dissemination was evaluated in SOI models of human gastric cancers *(84)*, MT-2 and MT-5. TNP-470 showed a significant inhibitory effect on the growth of the primary tumor when given at a dose of 30 mg/kg on alternate days from d 7 after SOI (early treatment). However, growth of the MT-2 primary tumor was not inhibited by administration beginning on d 14 after transplantation (late treatment). Liver metastasis was inhibited by early treatment of TNP-470 and was significantly more effective than late treatment. Peritoneal dissemination also was inhibited.

Colon tumor xenograft TK-4 was transplanted by SOI and treated with TNP-470 (30 mg/kg) on alternate days beginning on d 10 after SOI. TNP-470 significantly inhibited hepatic metastasis formation *(85)*.

The antimetastatic effect of TNP-470 was further investigated in SOI models of human colon cancer cell lines TK-3, TK-4, and TK-9 *(86)*. TNP-470 (20 or 30 mg/kg) was given sc every other day beginning on d 10 after implantation. There was no difference in the weight of the primary tumors in the control and treated groups. In the mice given 20 mg/kg TNP-470, liver metastasis developed in 3 of 10 cases. In the 30-mg/kg group, metastasis developed in only 1 of 17 mice. In contrast, metastases developed in 22 of 32 mice of the control group. The number of metastatic foci was also significantly less in the treated groups. Although TNP-470 effectively prevented liver metastasis, it had no effect on the growth of the primary tumor.

The antitumor and antimetastatic efficacy of TNP-470 and MMC were investigated in the TK-4 SOI model of human colon cancer *(87)*. TNP-470 was given sc on alternate days for 5 wk beginning on d 10 after SOI. MMC was administered ip once a week beginning on d 10 after SOI. In the control group, liver metastases developed in 9 of 10 mice, including 3 with more than 20 metastatic foci. Liver metastasis also developed in 8 of 10 mice receiving MMC. In contrast, liver metastasis developed in only 2 of 8 mice in the TNP-470 group, and neither of these animals had numerous metastases.

### 1.5.2. Metalloproteinase Inhibitors

Matrix metalloproteinases have been implicated in the growth and spread of metastatic tumors. This role was investigated in an SOI model of human colon cancer in nude mice using the matrix metalloproteinase inhibitor BB-94 (batimastat). Administration of BB-94 or vehicle (phosphate-buffered saline, pH 7.4, containing 0.01% Tween-80) commenced 7 d after tumor implantation (20 animals/group). Animals received 30 mg/kg BB-94 ip once daily for the first 60 d and then three times weekly. Treatment with BB-94 caused a reduction in the median weight of the primary tumor from 293 mg in the control group to 144 mg in the BB-94 treated group ($p < 0.001$). BB-94 treatment also reduced the incidence of local and regional invasion, from 12 of 18 mice in the control group (67%) to 7 of 20 mice in the treated group (35%). Six mice in the control group were also found to have metastases in the liver, lung, peritoneum, abdominal wall, or local lymph nodes. Only two mice in the BB-94 group had evidence of metastatic disease, in both cases confined to the abdominal wall. The reduction in tumor progression observed in the BB-94-treated group translated into an improvement in the survival of this group, from a median survival time of 110 d in the control group to a median survival time of 140 d in the treated group ($p < 0.01$). Treatment with BB-94 was not associated with any obvious toxic effect, and these results suggest that such agents may be effective as adjunctive cancer therapies *(28)*.

CT1746 is an orally active synthetic MMP inhibitor that has a greater specificity for gelatinase A, gelatinase B, and stromelysin than for interstitial collagenase and matrilysin. CT1746 was evaluated in a SOI model of the metastatic human colon tumor cell line Co-3. Animals were gavaged with CT1746 twice a day at 100 mg/kg for 5 d after the SOI of Co-3 for 43 d. In this model, CT1746 significantly prolonged the median survival time of the tumor-bearing animals, from 51 to 78 d. Significant efficacy of CT1746 was observed on primary tumor growth, with 32% reduction in mean tumor area at d 36. Six of 20 treated animals had no detectable spread and metastasis at autopsy, compared to 100% incidence of secondaries in control groups. Efficacy of CT1746 could also be seen on reducing tumor spread and metastasis to individual organ sites such as the abdominal wall, cecum, and lymph nodes compared to vehicle and untreated controls. Chronic administration of a peptidomimetic MMP inhibitor via the oral route thus inhibited primary tumor growth, spread, and metastasis with increase in survival, thereby converting aggressive cancer to a more controlled indolent disease *(47)*.

The efficacy of the MMP inhibitor MMI-166 was evaluated on tumor growth, angiogenesis, and metastasis in an SOI model of the liver metastatic TK-4 human colon cancer line. The synergistic effects of MMI-166 and MMC were evaluated in this model. MMI-166 was administered orally (po) at a dose of 200 mg/kg, 6 d/wk for 5 wk. MMC was administered ip at a dose of 2 mg/kg/wk for 5 wk. The combination group was treated with MMI-166 and MMC. MMI-166 alone did not inhibit primary tumor growth, but significantly inhibited liver metastasis compared with the control group and MMC group. Significant antitumor and antimetastatic effects of the combination therapy were also demonstrated *(78,79)*.

### 1.5.3. Cytosine Analogs

The cytosine analog gemcitabine was evaluated on the human pancreatic cancer cell BxPC-3 using SOI in mice. GFP expression in the tumor enabled high-resolution fluorescent visualization of primary and metastatic growth. Five weeks after SOI, the mice were randomized into three groups: Group I received exploratory laparotomy only. Group II underwent surgical resection of the pancreatic tumor without further treatment. Group III underwent tumor resection followed by adjuvant treatment with gemcitabine, 100 mg/kg every 3 d for four doses, starting 2 d after resection. The mice were sacrificed at 13 wk following implantation, and the presence and location of recurrent tumor was recorded. Gemcitabine reduced the recurrence rate to 28.6%, compared to 70.6% with resection only. Gemcitabine reduced metastatic events 58% in the adjuvant group compared to resection only. This study, demonstrating that gemcitabine is effective as adjuvant chemotherapy postpancreatectomy, suggests adjuvant treatment of pancreatic cancer with this drug clinically *(91)*.

A red fluorescent protein (RFP)-expressing MIA-PaCa-2 human pancreatic cancer line was evaluated for CPT-11 and gemcitabine efficacy in an SOI model *(101)*. Rapid tumor growth and widespread metastases developed in untreated mice within 2 wk, leading to a median survival of 21 d. In contrast, significant tumor growth suppression and consequent increase in survival (32.5 d) were achieved with CPT-11. Gemcitabine highly improved survival (72 d) by inducing transient tumor regression over the first 3 wk. However, at this time, growth and dissemination occurred despite continued treatment, suggesting the development of tumor resistance. The antimetastatic efficacy of each drug was followed noninvasively in real time by imaging the RFP-expressing tumor and metastases, and was confirmed by fluorescent open imaging of autopsy specimens.

We have demonstrated the ability of a novel, p.o.-administered cytosine analog, CS-682, to effectively prolong survival and inhibit metastatic growth in an imageable SOI mouse model of MIA-PaCa-2 pancreatic cancer expressing RFP *(92)*. Mice were treated with various p.o. doses of CS-682 on a five-times-per-week schedule until death. At a dose of 40 mg/kg, CS-682 prolonged survival compared with untreated animals (median survival 35 d vs 17 d). At nontoxic doses, CS-682 effectively suppressed the rate of primary tumor growth. CS-682 also decreased the development of malignant ascites and the formation of metastases, which were reduced significantly in number in the diaphragm, lymph nodes, liver, and kidney. RFP tumor fluorescence enabled noninvasive real-time comparison between groups during treatment and facilitated identification of micrometastases in solid organs at autopsy. The antimetastatic efficacy of CS-682 and its p.o. availability confer significant advantages and clinical potential to this agent for pancreatic cancer.

We subsequently showed that adjuvant treatment with the cytosine analog CS-682 results in a highly significant increase in survival in the SOI MIA-PaCa-2 human pancreatic cancer mouse model *(93)*. Seven days after implantation, mice were randomized into eight groups, depending on whether they were to be treated by tumor resection, 5 wk of CS-682 chemotherapy at 40–60 mg/kg qd, or both. Throughout the course of treatment, noninvasive optical whole-body imaging based on brilliant RFP expression of the tumor permitted visualization and quantification of primary, metastatic, and recurrent disease. Total tumor burden correlated negatively with survival. Untreated mice died of disseminated disease with a median survival of 26 d. Surgical resection alone conferred a small but significant survival advantage (median survival 28 d). Primary CS-682 treatment at all doses also significantly prolonged survival compared to untreated animals, and was more effective than surgery alone at doses of 50 and 60 mg/kg (median survival 34 d and 38.5 d, respectively). Maximal survival (median 48 d, with 30% of animals surviving longer than 60 d) was achieved by adjuvant CS-682, 50 mg/kg, given after surgical resection of the primary pancreatic tumor (compared to surgery alone). The results demonstrate that adjuvant oral administration of CS-682 for pancreatic cancer is highly effective and with acceptable toxicity, suggesting its potential for cure of this disease in appropriate combinations *(93)*.

High-resolution magnetic resonance (MR) imaging techniques in a liver metastatic mouse model were also employed to assess CS-682 (94). Efficacy of CS-682 was visualized in real time by MR imaging on initial seeding and subsequent growth of liver metastases. The relative efficacies of CS-682 and two agents used clinically, gemcitabine and 5-FU, were compared in this model. CS-682 was found to demonstrate superior efficacy by delaying onset and inhibiting growth of liver metastasis compared to gemcitabine, 5-FU, and control. The overall occurrence of metastases was decreased by 62% by CS-682, 18% by gemcitabine, and 35% by 5-FU. CS-682 increased the lifespan of the treated animals significantly, by 28 d above the 29-d median survival without treatment, compared to 11 d by gemcitabine and 14 d by 5-FU. The increased survival in CS-682-treated animals correlated with the antimetastatic activity of this compound. These preclinical findings support the potential clinical utility of CS-682 in the treatment of liver metastasis.

*1.5.4. Camptothecins*

We determined the antitumor and antimetastatic efficacy of the camptothecin analog DX-8951f in SOI metastatic mouse models of pancreatic cancer *(77)*. DX-8951f showed efficacy against two human pancreatic tumor cell lines in this model. These cell lines were transduced with GFP, enabling high-resolution visualization of tumor and metastatic growth. The DX-8951f studies included both an early and advanced-cancer model. In the early model, utilizing the human pancreatic cancer lines MIA-PaCa-2 and BxPC-3, treatment began when the orthotopic primary tumor was approx 7 mm in diameter. DX-8951f was significantly effective against both MIA-PaCa-2 and BxPC-3. In contrast, gemcitabine did not have significant efficacy against MIA-PaCa-2. Although gemcitabine showed significant activity against BxPC-3 primary tumor growth, it was not effective on metastasis. In the model of advanced disease, utilizing BxPC-3, treatment started when the orthotopic primary tumor was 13 mm in diameter. DX-8951f was significantly effective in a dose-response manner on the BxPC-3 primary tumor. DX-8951f also demonstrated antimetastatic activity in the late-stage model, significantly reducing the incidence of lymph node metastasis while eliminating lung metastasis. In contrast, gemcitabine was only moderately effective against the primary tumor and ineffective against metastasis at both sites in the late-stage model. Therefore, DX-8951f showed significantly higher efficacy than gemcitabine, the standard treatment for pancreatic cancer.

*1.5.5. 5-FU-Based Treatments*

The antitumor activities of 5-FU and MMC against the PANC-4 human pancreatic cancer cell line were determined in an SOI model. Slight local tumor growth inhibition with equivalent incidence of metastases to the liver and the peritoneum as the control were observed in the mice treated with 5-FU. In contrast, mice treated with MMC had considerably reduced local tumor growth without liver and peritoneal metastases *(19)*.

S-1 (tegafur [FT], 0.4 5-chloro-2,4-dihydroxypyridine [CDHP], potassium oxonate [Oxo]), resulted in biochemical modulation of 5-FU. The therapeutic effect of S-1 on the SOI models of human colon cancer TK-13 with high metastatic potential to the liver was evaluated. The animals were randomly divided into three groups (control [n = 17], UFT [combination of FT and uracil] [n = 18], and S-1 [n = 17]). S-1 or UFT was administered orally at an equitoxic dose (S-1, 7.5 mg/kg; UFT, 17.5 mg/kg as FT) for 37 consecutive days beginning 10 d after the transplantation. S-1 showed higher tumor growth inhibition than UFT and also showed significant efficacy on liver metastasis, while UFT did not. Liver metastasis developed in only 2 of the 17 mice in the S-1 group, whereas it developed in 9 of the 17 and 7 of the 18 in the control and UFT groups, respectively *(89)*.

The effectiveness of oral 5-FU in suppressing liver metastasis was assessed in a highly metastatic SOI mouse model targeting the liver *(90)*. Doses of 20 and 25 mg/kg of oral 5-FU significantly suppressed primary tumor growth and liver metastasis. The efficacy of 5-FU was visualized by whole-body fluorescence imaging of the GFP-expressing tumor and its subsequent metastases. Toxicity was observed only in the 30-mg/kg dose. Furthermore, the nontoxic doses of 5-FU significantly prolonged survival in these animals.

### 1.5.6. Interferons

The efficacy of recombinant human γ-interferon (IFN-γ) was evaluated for the treatment of human pleural adenocarcinoma in an SOI model of the human non-small-cell lung cancer cell line H-460 *(45)*. IFN-γ was tested in three different dosages (25,000, 50,000, and 100,000 U) vs an untreated control through ip injection twice a day for 5 d, which was started 48 h after SOI. The results showed that IFN-γ can prolong the survival time of the tumor-bearing animals. The symptoms and signs of hypoxia, such as restricted physical activity and cyanosis due to primary tumor growth in the thoracic cavity, as well as cachexia, developed much earlier in the control than in the IFN-γ-treated mice. The mice in the control group had succumbed by d 23 after tumor implantation. However, at that time 67% of the mice in the 100,000 U-treated group, 15% of the mice in the 50,000 U-treated group, and 16% of the mice in the 25,000 U-treated group were still alive. The orthotopically-transplanted tumor grew rapidly and metastasized to the lung and liver in the untreated control. In the IFN-γ-treated groups, both primary tumor growth and metastasis were reduced, probably accounting for the increased survival rate. The results demonstrated dose-dependent efficacy of IFN-γ in suppressing symptomology, primary tumor growth, invasiveness, and metastasis of the human lung cancer cell line H-460, and increased survival of the tumor-bearing animals.

### 1.5.7. Cisplatin Analogs

An SOI model of the human colon cancer cell line Co-3 in nude mice was treated with two doses of platinum analogs {Pt(cis-dach)(DPPE)•(2NO$_3$)} and

{Pt(trans-dach)(DPPE)•(2NO$_3$)} *(76)*. The analogs were evaluated for antimetastatic efficacy in comparison to two doses of cisplatin. Unlike the untreated control group, there were no mesenteric lymph node metastases in the groups treated with the high or low doses of both forms of the DPPE platinum analogs as well as the cisplatin-treated group. However, much more body-weight loss occurred in the cisplatin-treated group than the DPPE-treated groups. The results obtained with SOI animal model of colon cancer demonstrated both cis- and trans-forms of DPPE had as strong an inhibitory effect on metastasis as that of cisplatin, but with much less toxicity.

An SOI model of the human RT-4 bladder tumor in nude mice resulted in local growth, invasion, regional extension, and metastases as well as distant metastases to other organ sites and lymph nodes, thus mimicking the bladder cancer patient *(56)*. This metastatic bladder tumor animal model was treated with two doses of the platinum analog {Pt(cis-dach)(DPPE)•(2NO$_3$)} compared to two doses of cisplatin. Unlike the untreated control group or the group treated with the low dose of cisplatin, there were no metastases in either the high- or low-dose platinum-analog-treated groups and the high-dose cisplatin-treated group.

### 1.5.8. Liposomes

Adriamycin (ADM) was encapsulated in a galactose-conjugated hepatotropic liposome (hLip-ADM). Its ability to enhance the antitumor effect while reducing toxicity was compared with that of free ADM and a control Lip-ADM (cLip-ADM) *(88)*. An SOI model of human colon cancer xenograft TK-4 was used to induce liver metastases in mice. Liver metastasis in animals treated with hLip-ADM was inhibited (0/11), whereas liver metastases developed in 10 of 12 mice in the control group and in 5 of 12 mice given cLip-ADM. hLip-ADM did not have a significant inhibitory effect on primary tumor growth assessed 6 wk after transplantation. These findings indicate that hLip-ADM may be an effective strategy for inhibiting liver metastases from human colon cancer.

### 1.5.9. Antisense Oligonucleotides

The efficacy of a phosphorothioate antisense oligonucleotide (ASO) for KDR/Flk-1 (KDR/Flk-1-ASO), an endothelial cell-specific vascular endothelial growth factor (VEGF) receptor, was investigated on peritoneal dissemination and angiogenesis of a human gastric cancer cell line in nude mice. GFP-transduced NUGC-4 (NUGC-4-GFP) human gastric cancer was implanted into the peritoneal cavity of nude mice. KDR/Flk-1-ASO, KDR/Flk-1-SO, or phosphate-buffered saline (PBS) were administrated from d 7 to 14, 200 µg/mouse, once a day. The mice were sacrificed on d 28. Disseminated peritoneal tumor nodules expressing GFP were visualized by fluorescence microscopy. KDR/Flk-1-ASO significantly decreased the extent of peritoneal dissemination of the tumors. The number of cells undergoing apoptosis was significantly increased in the KDR/Flk-1-ASO-treated tumors. Microvessel density was significantly reduced in the KDR/Flk-1-ASO-treated tumor nodules. The KDR/Flk-1 antisense strategy, therefore, decreases tumor dissemination, apparently by inhibiting angiogenesis *(46)*.

### 1.5.10. Immunotherapy

The efficacy of immunochemotherapy using OK-432 along with 5-FU or MMC on an SOI model of Col-2-JCK, a human colon cancer, was evaluated. When combined with OK-432, both 5-FU and MMC reduced liver metastases, with synergistic reduction of primary tumor growth, demonstrating the potential of combining immunotherapy with chemotherapy against metastases *(16)*.

An SOI model of human gastric cancer model was also used to evaluate the efficacy of immunochemotherapy using OK-432 along with 5-FU or MMC *(18)*. SC-I-NU, a human stomach cancer line, was used in these studies. One-quarter- or one-half-maximum tolerated doses (MTDs) of 5-FU or MMC resulted in a significant reduction of stomach tumor growth, while liver metastases were not reduced, possibly due to suppression of natural killer (NK)-cell activity by both drugs. In contrast, when combined with OK-432, half-MTDs of 5-FU or MMC significantly reduced liver metastases, with synergistic reduction of stomach tumor growth, possibly reflecting a rescue of NK-cell activity by treatment with OK-432.

### *1.6. New Directions*

We have developed novel imaging technology to externally visualize primary and tumor growth and metastasis in mice by use of tumor cells expressing GFP and RFP.* This fluorescence imaging technology presents many new possibilities, including real-time visualization of tumor progression, metastasis, and drug response. With these fluorescent tools, single cells from tumors and metastases can be externally imaged. GFP- and RFP-expressing tumors of the colon, prostate, breast, brain, liver, lymph nodes, lung, pancreas, bone, and other organs have also been visualized externally (*see* **Note 2**).

We used GFP-labeled or RFP-labeled HT-1080 human fibrosarcoma cells to determine clonality of metastasis by simple fluorescence visualization of metastatic colonies after mixed implantation of the red and green fluorescent cells. Resulting pure red or pure green colonies were scored as clonal, whereas mixed yellow colonies were scored as nonclonal. In a spontaneous metastasis model originating from footpad injection in severe combined immunodeficient

---

*U.S. Patents 6,232,523, 6,235,968, 6,251,384, 6,649,159, 6,759,038 and Australia Patent 749,338.

mice, 95% of the resulting lung colonies were either pure green or pure red, indicating monoclonal origin, whereas 5% were of mixed color, indicating polyclonal origin. In an experimental lung metastasis model established by tail vein injection in severe combined immunodeficient mice, clonality of lung metastasis was dependent on cell number. With a minimum cell number injected, almost all (96%) colonies were pure red or green and therefore monoclonal. When a large number of cells were injected, almost all (87%) colonies were mixed color and therefore heteroclonal. Spontaneous metastasis may be clonal because they are rare events, thereby supporting the rare-cell clonal origin of metastasis hypothesis. The clonality of the experimental metastasis model depended on the number of input cells. The simple fluorescence method of determining clonality of metastases can allow large-scale clonal analysis in numerous types of metastatic models *(96)*.

A simple yet powerful technique for delineating the morphological events of tumor-induced angiogenesis and other tumor-induced host processes has been developed with dual-color fluorescence. The method clearly images implanted tumors and adjacent stroma, distinguishing unambiguously the host and tumor-specific components of the malignancy. The dual-color fluorescence imaging is effected by using RFP-expressing tumors growing in GFP-expressing transgenic mice. This model shows with great clarity the details of the tumor–stroma interaction, especially tumor-induced angiogenesis and tumor-infiltrating lymphocytes. The GFP-expressing tumor vasculature, both nascent and mature, could be readily distinguished interacting with the RFP-expressing tumor cells. GFP-expressing dendritic cells were observed contacting RFP-expressing tumor cells with their dendrites. GFP-expressing macrophages were observed engulfing RFP-expressing cancer cells. GFP lymphocytes were seen surrounding cells of the RFP tumor, which eventually regressed. Dual-color fluorescence imaging visualizes the tumor–host interaction by whole-body imaging and at the cellular level in fresh tissues, dramatically expanding previous studies in fixed and stained preparations *(97)*.

## 2. Materials

1. 8-0 and 7-0 surgical sutures (Suture Express, Mission, KS).
2. 6-0 back silk sutures (Suture Express, Mission, KS).
3. RPMI 1640 containing 10% fetal bovine serum (FBS) (Fisher Scientific, Pittsburgh, PA, cat. no. 10-040-CV).
4. Geneticin (Life Technologies, Grand Island, NY, cat. no. G418).
5. Cloning cylinders (Bel-Art Products, Pequannock, NJ).
6. RetroXpress vector pLEIN (Clontech Laboratories, Palo Alto, CA).
7. DsRed-2 vector (Clontech Laboratories, Palo Alto, CA).
8. Fluorescence microscope equipped with a mercury 100-W lamp power supply (Olympus Optical, Tokyo, Japan, cat. no. BH 2-RFCA).

9. Leica fluorescence stereo microscope (Leica, Deerfield, IL, cat. no. LZ12).
10. Long-pass filter GG475 (Chroma Technology, Brattleboro, VT, cat. no. GG475).
11. C5810 3-chip cooled color CCD camera (Hamamatsu Photonics Systems, Bridgewater, NJ, cat. no. C5810).
12. High-resolution Sony VCR (Sony, Tokyo, Japan, model no. SLV-R1000).
13. Image Pro Plus 3.1 software (Media Cybernetics, Silver Spring, MD).
14. pLNCX2 vector (Clontech Laboratories, Palo Alto, CA).
15. Transgenic C57/B6-GFP mice, obtained from Dr. M. Okabe, Research Institute for Microbial Diseases, Osaka University, Osaka, Japan.
16. pLEIN retroviral vector (Clontech Laboratories, Palo Alto, CA).
17. Isoflurane (Iso-thesia) (Burns Veterinary Supply, Vancouver, WA).
18. 50 mg ketamine (Burns Veterinary Supply, Vancouver, WA, cat. no. Ketaset).

## 3. Methods
### *3.1. General Construction of Models* (100)
#### *3.1.1. Mice*

1. Four-to-six-week-old outbred *nu/nu* mice of both sexes are used for the orthotopic transplantation.
2. All the mice are maintained in a pathogen-free environment.
3. Cages, bedding, food, and water are autoclaved and changed regularly.
4. All the mice are maintained in a daily cycle of 12-h period of light and darkness.
5. Bethaprim Pediatric Suspension (containing sulfamethoxazole and trimethoprim) is added to the drinking water.
6. Mice are periodically sent to the University of Missouri to test for pathogens.
7. All animal studies are conducted in accordance with the principles and procedures outlined in the *National Institutes of Health Guide for the Care and Use of Laboratory Animals* under assurance number A3873-1.

#### *3.1.2. Specimens*

1. Fresh surgical specimens are kept in Earle's minimum essential medium (MEM) at 4°C and obtained as soon as possible from hospitals.
2. Transplantation should take place within 24 h of surgical excision.
3. Before transplantation, each specimen is inspected, and all necrotic and suspected necrotic tumor tissue is removed.
4. To take into account tumor heterogeneity, each specimen is equally divided into five parts, separated, and each part is subsequently cut into small pieces of about 1 mm$^3$ size.
5. Tumor pieces for each transplantation are taken from five parts of each specimen equally. In our experience, a typical colon tumor specimen of 1–2 g provides sufficient material for initial surgical orthotopic implantation of more than 20 mice. Additional SOI models of this same tumor can subsequently be generated by a single passage using SOI.

6. It should be noted that patient tumors are routinely passaged orthotopically to produce large cohorts. One hundred mice or more can be readily transplanted in the first passage, which are more than sufficient for treatment studies.

### 3.2. Examples of Surgical Orthotopic Implantation (100)

#### 3.2.1. Colon Cancer

##### 3.2.1.1. Colonic Transplantation (100)

1. Nude mice are anesthetized, and the abdomen is sterilized with iodine and alcohol swabs.
2. A small mid-line incision is made and the colocecal part of the intestine is exteriorized.
3. Serosa of the site where tumor pieces are to be implanted is removed.
4. Eight pieces of 1-mm$^3$-size tumor are implanted on the top of the animal intestine.
5. An 8-0 surgical suture is used to penetrate these small tumor pieces and attach them on the wall of the intestine.
6. The intestine is returned to the abdominal cavity, and the abdominal wall is closed with 7-0 surgical sutures.
7. Animals are kept in a sterile environment. Tumors of all stages and grades can be utilized (1).

##### 3.2.1.2. Intrahepatic Transplantation

1. Nude mice are anesthetized with isoflurane (Forane) inhalation.
2. An incision is made through the left upper abdominal pararectal line and peritoneum.
3. The left lobe of the liver is carefully exposed and the liver is cut about 3 mm with scissors.
4. Two to three pieces of 1–2-mm$^3$ size are put on the nude mouse liver and attached immediately with double sutures using 8-0 nylon with an atramatic needle.
5. After confirmation that no bleeding is occurring, the liver is then returned to the peritoneal cavity.
6. The abdomen and skin are then closed with 6-0 back silk sutures (30).

#### 3.2.2. Prostate Cancer

Two tumor fragments (1 mm$^3$) from a subcutaneous tumor are implanted by SOI in the dorsolateral lobe of the prostate in each of five nude mice.

1. After proper exposure of the bladder and prostate following a lower mid-line abdominal incision, the capsule of the prostate is opened and the two tumor fragments are inserted into the capsule.
2. The capsule is then closed with an 8-0 surgical suture.
3. The incision in the abdominal wall is closed with a 6-0 surgical suture in one layer (11,65).
4. The animals are kept under isoflurane anesthesia during surgery (64).

### 3.2.3. Lung Cancer

1. The mice are anesthetized by isoflurane inhalation.
2. The animals are put in a position of right lateral decubitus, with four limbs restrained.
3. A 0.8-cm transverse incision of skin is made in the left chest wall.
4. Chest muscles are separated by sharp dissection and costal and intercostal muscles are exposed.
5. A 0.4–0.5-cm intercostal incision between the third and fourth ribs on the chest wall is made and the chest wall is opened.
6. The left lung is taken up by a forceps and tumor fragments are sewn promptly into the upper lung with one suture.
7. The lung is then returned into the chest cavity.
8. The incision in the chest wall is closed by a 6-0 surgical suture.
9. The closed condition of the chest wall is examined immediately and, if a leak exists, it is closed by additional sutures.
10. After closing the chest wall, an intrathoracic puncture is made by using a 3-mL syringe and 25G 1/2 needle to withdraw the remaining air in the chest cavity.
11. After the withdrawal of air, a completely inflated lung can be seen through the thin chest wall of the mouse.
12. Then the skin and chest muscle are closed with a 6-0 surgical suture in one layer *(61)*.

### 3.2.4. Pancreatic Cancer (92)

1. Pancreatic tumors in the exponential growth phase, grown subcutaneously in nude mice, are resected aseptically.
2. Necrotic tissues are cut away, and the remaining healthy tumor tissues are cut with scissors and minced into 1-mm$^3$ pieces in RPMI 1640 medium.
3. Mice are then anesthetized and their abdomens are sterilized with alcohol.
4. An incision is then created through the left upper abdominal pararectal line and peritoneum.
5. The pancreas is carefully exposed and two tumor pieces are transplanted onto the middle of the gland using a single 8-0 surgical suture.
6. The pancreas is then returned into the peritoneal cavity, and the abdominal wall and the skin are closed in two layers using 6-0 surgical sutures.
7. All procedures are performed with a 7× microscope (Olympus) or standard surgical loupes.

## 3.3. Evaluation of Growth and Metastasis of Orthotopically Transplanted Tumors

1. The mice are autopsied and analyzed histologically for the presence of local growth and metastases upon sacrifice after they become moribund.
2. Mice are killed if they develop signs of distress. For example, for the colon tumor models, distress symptoms include a decline in performance status and weight loss due to cachexia or drug treatment.

### Orthotopic Metastatic (MetaMouse®) Models

3. At autopsy, the colon and all peritoneal organs, lymph nodes, liver, and lungs are resected and processed for routine histological examination for tumors after careful microscopic examination.
4. Metastases are considered to have occurred if at least one microscopic metastatic lesion is found in any of the animals.
5. The growth of locally-growing tumors is determined by caliper measurement. This is possible for colon tumors because the body wall is so thin.
6. Caliper measurements of the primary tumor can also allow determination of tumor regression.
7. The primary tumor is weighed at autopsy.

#### *3.4. Fluorescence Imaging of Tumors and Metastases with GFP and RFP*

*3.4.1. Isolation of Stable High-Expression GFP Tumor Cells* **(95,98,99)**

1. The GFP expression vector RetroXpress vector pLEIN is purchased from Clontech Laboratories (Palo Alto, CA). The pLEIN vector expresses GFP and the neomycin resistance gene on the same bicistronic message which contains an IRES site.
2. For GFP gene transduction, 20%-confluent cancer cells are incubated with a 1:1 precipitated mixture of retroviral supernatants of PT67 packaging cells and RPMI 1640 (Gibco) containing 10% fetal bovine serum (FBS) (Gemini Bio-products, Calabasas, CA) for 72 h.
3. Fresh medium is replenished at this time.
4. Cells are harvested by trypsin/EDTA 72 h postinfection and subcultured at a ratio of 1:15 into selective medium which contains 200 µg/mL of geneticin (G418) (Life Technologies, Grand Island, NY).
5. The level of G418 is increased to 800–1000 µg/mL gradually.
6. Clones expressing GFP are isolated with cloning cylinders (Bel-Art Products, Pequannock, NJ) by trypsin/EDTA and are amplified and transferred by conventional culture methods.

*3.4.2. Isolation of Stable High-Expression RFP Tumor Cells* **(92)**

1. The pDsRed-2 vector (Clontech Laboratories, Palo Alto, CA) is used to engineer MIA-PaCa-2 clones stably expressing RFP. This vector expresses RFP and the neomycin resistance gene on the same bicistronic message and has been demonstrated to exhibit low toxicity in mammalian cell lines.
2. pDsRed-2 is produced in PT67 packaging cells.
3. RFP transduction is initiated by incubating 20%-confluent MIA-PaCa-2 cells with retroviral supernatants of the packaging cells and DMEM for 24 h.
4. Fresh medium is replenished at this time and cells are allowed to grow in the absence of retrovirus for 12 h.
5. This procedure is repeated until high levels of RFP expression, as determined using fluorescence microscopy, are achieved.
6. Cells are then harvested by trypsin/EDTA and subcultured into selective medium that contains 200 µg/mL G418.

7. The level of G418 is increased to 2000 μg/mL stepwise.
8. Clones expressing high levels of RFP are isolated with cloning cylinders as needed and are amplified and transferred using conventional culture methods.
9. High-RFP-expression clones are isolated in the absence of G418 for 10 passages to select for stable expression of RFP in vivo.

### 3.5. Fluorescence Microscopy

#### 3.5.1. Fluorescence Slide Microscopy (97)

1. An Olympus BH 2-RFCA fluorescence microscope equipped with a mercury 100-W lamp power supply is used.
2. To visualize both GFP and RFP fluorescence at the same time, excitation light is produced through the D425/60 bandpass filter and 470 DCXR dichroic mirror.
3. Emitted fluorescence light is collected through the long-pass filter GG475 (Chroma Technology).

#### 3.5.2. Fluorescence Animal Microscopy (98)

1. A Leica fluorescence stereo microscope, model LZ12, equipped with a mercury lamp and a 50-W power supply, is used.
2. Selective excitation of GFP is produced through a D425/60 bandpass filter and a 470 DCXR dichroic mirror.
3. Emitted fluorescence is collected through a long-pass filter (GG475).
4. A Hamamatsu C5810 3-chip cooled color charge-coupled device camera (Hamamatsu Photonics, Bridgewater, NJ) is used to acquire images.
5. Images that are processed for contrast and brightness and then analyzed with the use of Image Pro Plus 3.1 software (Media Cybernetics, Silver Spring, MD).
6. High-resolution images of 1024 × 724 pixels are captured directly on an IBM PC or continuously through video output on a high-resolution Sony VCR (model SLVR1000; Sony, Tokyo).

### 3.6. External, In Vivo Whole-Body Imaging

1. External, in vivo imaging was performed in a fluorescent light box illuminated by fiberoptic lighting at 470 nm (Lightools Research, Encinitas, CA).
2. Emitted fluorescence is collected through a long-pass filter GG475 on a Hamamatsu C5810 three-chip cooled color CCD camera.
3. High-resolution images of 1024 × 724 pixels are captured directly on an IBM PC or continuously through video output on a high-resolution Sony VCR model SLV-R1000.
4. Images are processed for contrast and brightness and analyzed with the use of Image Pro Plus 3.1 software.
5. Real-time determination of tumor burden is performed by quantifying fluorescent surface area.

## 3.7. GFP Transgenic Animals (97)

1. Transgenic C57/B6-GFP mice are obtained from the Research Institute for Microbial Diseases (Osaka University, Osaka, Japan).
2. The C57/B6-GFP mice expressed the *Aequorea victoria* GFP under the control of the chicken β-actin promoter and cytomegalovirus enhancer. All of the tissues from this transgenic line, with the exception of erythrocytes and hair, fluoresced green under excitation light.
3. The GFP gene, regulated as described above, is crossed into nude mice on the C57/B6 background.
4. Both immunocompetent and nude GFP transgenic mice are used as host for RFP-expressing tumors.

## 4. Notes

1. SOI using intact tumor tissue was an important breakthrough that achieved metastatic rates in the models that reflect clinical cancer. Although orthotopic implantation of tumors was developed before SOI, cell suspensions were injected in contrast to intact tissue, which severely limited the metastatic potential of the tumor. Thus SOI demonstrates the need for intact tissue for successful orthotopic implantation.
2. The use of tumor genetically engineered to express GFP or RFP was a second important breakthrough that allowed whole-body fluorescence imaging of tumor growth, metastasis, and angiogenesis in the SOI models. Imaging enables real-time visualization of drug response on primary and metastatic growth as well as angiogenesis without perturbing the animal, using only illumination by blue light. Prior to development of GFP and RFP imaging, orthotopic tumor growth and metastasis could be observed only upon sacrifice of the mouse.

## References

1. Fu, X., Besterman, J. M., Monosov, A., and Hoffman, R. M. (1991) Models of human metastatic colon cancer in nude mice orthotopically constructed by using histologically-intact patient specimens. *Proc. Natl. Acad. Sci. USA* **88,** 9345–9349.
2. Fu, X., Theodorescu, D., Kerbel, R. S., and Hoffman, R. M. (1991) Extensive multi-organ metastasis following orthotopic onplantation of histologically-intact human bladder carcinoma tissue in nude mice. *Int. J. Cancer* **49,** 938–939.
3. Fu, X. and Hoffman, R.M. (1992) Human RT-4 bladder carcinoma is highly metastatic in nude mice and comparable to ras-H-transformed RT-4 when orthotopically onplanted as histologically-intact tissue. *Int. J. Cancer* **51,** 989–991.
4. Wang, X., Fu, X., and Hoffman, R. M. (1992) A new patient-like metastatic model of human lung cancer constructed orthotopically with intact tissue via thoracotomy in immunodeficient mice. *Int. J. Cancer* **51,** 992–995.
5. Fu, X., Guadagni, F., and Hoffman, R. M. (1992) A metastatic nude-mouse model of human pancreatic cancer constructed orthotopically from histologically-intact patient specimens. *Proc. Natl. Acad. Sci. USA* **89,** 5645–5649.

6. Hoffman, R. M. (1992) Patient-like models of human cancer in mice. *Curr. Perspect. Mol. Cell. Oncol.* **1(B)** 311–326.
7. Kuo, T.-H., Kubota, T., Watanabe, M., et al. (1992) Orthotopic reconstitution of human small-cell lung carcinoma after intravenous transplantation in SCID mice. *Anticancer Res.* **12,** 1407–1410.
8. Fu, X., Herrera, H., Kubota, T., and Hoffman, R. M. (1992) Extensive liver metastasis from human colon cancer in nude and scid mice after orthotopic onplantation of histologically-intact human colon carcinoma tissue. *Anticancer Res.* **12,** 1395–1398.
9. Wang, X., Fu, X., and Hoffman, R. M. (1992) A patient-like metastasizing model of human lung adenocarcinoma constructed via thoracotomy in nude mice. *Anticancer Res.* **12,** 1399–1402.
10. Wang, X., Fu, X., Kubota, T., and Hoffman, R. M. (1992) A new patient-like metastatic model of human small-cell lung cancer constructed orthotopically with intact tissue via thoracotomy in immunodeficient mice. *Anticancer Res.* **12,** 1403–1406.
11. Fu, X., Herrera, H., and Hoffman, R. M. (1992) Orthotopic growth and metastasis of human prostate carcinoma in nude mice after transplantation of histologically intact tissue. *Int. J. Cancer* **52,** 987–990.
12. Hoffman, R. M. (1992) Histoculture and the immunodeficient mouse come to the cancer clinic: rational approaches to individualizing cancer therapy and new drug evaluation (Review). *Int. J. Oncol.* **1,** 467–474.
13. Furukawa, T., Fu, X., Kubota, T., Watanabe, M., Kitajima, M., and Hoffman, R. M. (1993) Nude mouse metastatic models of human stomach cancer constructed using orthotopic implantation of histologically-intact tissue. *Cancer Res.* **53,** 1204–1208.
14. Furukawa, T., Kubota, T., Watanabe, M., Kitajima, M., Fu, X., and Hoffman, R. M. (1993) Orthotopic transplantation of histologically intact clinical specimens of stomach cancer to nude mice: correlation of metastatic sites in mouse and individual patient donors. *Int. J. Cancer* **53,** 608–612.
15. Fu, X. and Hoffman, R. M. (1993) Human ovarian carcinoma metastatic models constructed in nude mice by orthotopic transplantation of histologically-intact patient specimens. *Anticancer Res.* **13,** 283–286.
16. Furukawa, T., Kubota, T., Watanabe, M., et al. (1993) Immunochemotherapy prevents human colon cancer metastasis after orthotopic onplantation of histologically-intact tumor tissue in nude mice. *Anticancer Res.* **13,** 287–291.
17. Kuo, T.-H., Kubota, T., Watanabe, M., et al. (1993) Early resection of primary orthotopically-growing human colon tumor in nude mouse prevents liver metastasis: further evidence for patient-like hematogenous metastatic route. *Anticancer Res.* **13,** 293–297.
18. Furukawa, T., Kubota, T., Watanabe, M., Kuo, T. H., Kitajima, M., and Hoffman, R. M. (1993) Differential chemosensitivity of local and metastatic human gastric cancer after orthotopic transplantation of histologically-intact tumor tissue in nude mice. *Int. J. Cancer* **54,** 397–401.
19. Furukawa, T., Kubota, T., Watanabe, M., Kitajima, M., and Hoffman, R. M. (1993) A novel "patient-like" treatment model of human pancreatic cancer constructed

using orthotopic transplantation of histologically-intact human tumor-tissue in nude mice. *Cancer Res.* **53,** 3070–3072.
20. Kuo, T.-H., Kubota, T., Watanabe, M., et al. (1993) Site-specific chemosensitivity of human small-cell lung carcinoma growing orthotopically compared to subcutaneously in SCID mice: the importance of orthotopic models to obtain relevant drug evaluation data. *Anticancer Res.* **13,** 627–630.
21. Furukawa, T., Kubota, T., Watanabe, M., et al. (1993) A metastatic model of human colon cancer constructed using cecal implantation of cancer tissue in nude mice. *Jpn. J. Surg.* **23,** 420–423.
22. Fu, X., Le, P., and Hoffman, R. M. (1993) A metastatic orthotopic transplant nude-mouse model of human patient breast cancer. *Anticancer Res.* **13,** 901–904.
23. Astoul, P., Colt, H. G., Wang, X., and Hoffman, R. M. (1993) Metastatic human pleural ovarian cancer model constructed by orthotopic implantation of fresh histologically-intact patient carcinoma in nude mice. *Anticancer Res.* **13,** 1999–2002.
24. Astoul, P., Wang, X., and Hoffman, R. M. (1993) "Patient-like" nude and SCID-mouse models of human lung and pleural cancer (Review). *Int. J. Oncol.* **3,** 713–718.
25. Kubota, T., Inoue, S., Furukawa, T., et al. (1993) Similarity of serum-tumor pharmacokinetics of antitumor agents in man and nude mice. *Anticancer Res.* **13,** 1481–1484.
26. Astoul, P., Colt, H. G., Wang, X., and Hoffman, R. M. (1994) A "patient-like" nude mouse model of parietal pleural human lung adenocarcinoma. *Anticancer Res.* **14,** 85–92.
27. Astoul, P., Colt, H. G., Wang, X., et al. (1994) A "patient-like" nude mouse metastatic model of advanced human pleural cancer. *J. Cell Bichem.* **56,** 9–15.
28. Wang, X., Fu, X., Brown, P.D., Crimmin, M. J., and Hoffman, R. M. (1994) Matrix metalloproteinase inhibitor BB-95 (Batimastat) inhibits human colon tumor growth and spread in a patient-like orthotopic model in nude mice. *Cancer Res* **54,** 4726–4728.
29. Hoffman, R. M. (1994) Orthotopic is orthodox: why are orthotopic-transplant metastatic models different from all other models? *J. Cell Biochem.* **56,** 1–3.
30. Togo, S., Shimada, H., Kubota, T., Moossa, A. R., and Hoffman, R. M. (1995) Seed to soil is a return trip in metastasis. *Anticancer Res.* **15,** 791–794.
31. Togo, S., Shimada, H., Kubota, T., Moossa, A. R., and Hoffman, R. M. (1995) Host organ specifically determines cancer progression. *Cancer Res.* **55,** 681–684.
32. Kuo, T.-H., Kubota, T., Watanabe, M., et al. (1995) Liver colonization competence governs colon cancer metastasis. *Proc. Natl. Acad. Sci. USA* **92,** 12,085–12,089.
33. Togo, S., Wang, X., Shimada, H., Moossa, A. R., and Hoffman, R. M. (1995) Cancer seed and soil can be highly selective: human-patient colon tumor lung metastasis grows in nude mouse lung but not colon or subcutis. *Anticancer Res.* **15,** 795–798.
34. Dutton, G. (1996) AntiCancer Inc. scientists identify a key governing step in the metastasis of cancer. *Genet. Eng. News* **16,** 1, January 15.
35. Holzman, D. (1996) Of mice and metastasis: a new for-profit model emerges. *J. Natl. Cancer Inst.* **88,** 396–397.

36. Leff, D. N. (1996) MetaMouse models colon cancer metastasis with clinical potential. *BioWorld Today* **7,** 1, January 8.
37. Sun, F. X., Tang, Z. Y., Liu, K. D., et al. (1996) Establishment of a metastatic model of human hepatocellular carcinoma in nude mice via orthotopic implantation of histologically intact tissues. *Int. J. Cancer* **66,** 239–243.
38. An, Z., Wang, X., Kubota, T., Moossa, A. R., and Hoffman, R. M. (1996) A clinical nude mouse metastatic model for highly malignant human pancreatic cancer. *Anticancer Res.* **16,** 627–631.
39. Riordan, T. (1996) A technique is said to ease attachment of tumors to mice, making them little cancer patients. *The New York Times*, Patents Column, March 4.
40. Murray, G., Duncan, M., O'Neil, P., Melvin, W., Fothergill, J. (1996) Matrix metalloproteinase-1 is associated with poor prognosis in colorectal cancer. *Nat. Med.* **2,** 461–462.
41. Hoffman, R. M. (1996) Fertile seed and rich soil: development of patient-like models of human cancer by surgical orthotopic implantation of intact tissue, in *Update Series: Comprehensive Textbook of Oncology* (Schimpff, S. C., et al., eds.), Williams & Wilkins, Baltimore, vol. 3, pp. 1–10.
42. Sun, F.-X., Tang, Z.-Y., Liu, K.-D., et al. (1996) Metastatic models of human liver cancer in nude mice orthotopically constructed by using histologically intact patient specimens. *J. Cancer Res. Clin. Oncol.* **122,** 397–402.
43. Astoul, P., Wang, X., Colt, H. G., Boutin, C., and Hoffman, R. M. (1996) A patient-like human malignant pleural mesothelioma nude-mouse model. *Oncol. Rep.* **3,** 483–487.
44. Colt, H. G., Astoul, P., Wang, X., Yi, E. S., Boutin, C., and Hoffman, R. M. (1996) Clinical course of human epithelial-type malignant pleural mesothelioma replicated in an orthotopic-transplant nude mouse model. *Anticancer Res.* **16,** 633–639.
45. An, Z., Wang, X., Astoul, P., Danays, T., and Hoffman, R. M. (1996) Interferon gamma is highly effective against orthotopically-implanted human pleural adenocarcinoma in nude mice. *Anticancer Res.* **16,** 2545–2551.
46. Kamiyama, M., Ichikawa, Y., Ishikawa, T., et al. (2002) VEGF receptor antisense therapy inhibits angiogenesis and peritoneal dissemination of human gastric cancer in nude mice. *Cancer Gene Ther.* **9,** 197–201.
47. An, Z., Wang, X., Willmott, N., et al. (1997) Conversion of highly malignant colon cancer from an aggesssive to a controlled disease by oral administration of a metalloproteinase inhibitor. *Clin. Exp. Metastasis* **15,** 184–195.
48. Hoffman, R. M. (1997) Fertile seed and rich soil: the development of clinically relevant models of human cancer by surgical orthotopic implantation of intact tissue, in *Anticancer Drug Development Guide: Preclinical Screening, Clinical Trials, and Approval* (Teicher, B., ed.), Humana, Totowa, NJ, pp. 127–144.
49. Chishima, T., Miyagi, Y., Wang, X., et al. (1997) Cancer invasion and micrometastasis visualized in live tissue by green fluorescent protein expression. *Cancer Res.* **57,** 2042–2047.

50. Inada, T., Ichikawa, A., Kubota, T., Ogata, Y., Moossa, A. R., and Hoffman, R. M. (1997) 5-FU-induced apoptosis correlates with efficacy against human gastric and colon cancer xenografts in nude mice. *Anticancer Res.* **17,** 1965–1972.
51. Chishima, T., Miyagi, Y., Wang, X., et al. (1997) Metastatic patterns of lung cancer visualized live and in process by green fluorescent protein expression. *Clin. Exp. Metastasis* **15,** 547–552.
52. Chishima, T., Miyagi, Y., Wang, X., et al. (1997) Visualization of the metastatic process by green fluorescent protein expression. *Anticancer Res.* **17,** 2377–2384.
53. Chishima, T., Yang, M., Miyagi, Y., et al. (1997) Governing step of metastasis visualized *in vitro. Proc. Natl. Acad. Sci. USA* **94,** 11,573–11,576.
54. Tomikawa, M., Kubota, T., Matsuzaki, S. W., et al. (1997) Mitomycin C and cisplatin increase survival in a human pancreatic cancer metastatic model. *Anticancer Res.* **17,** 3623–3626.
55. Chishima, T., Miyagi, Y., Li, L., et al. (1997) The use of histoculture and green fluorescent protein to visualize tumor cell host interaction. *In Vitro Cell. Dev. Biol.* **33,** 745–747.
56. Chang, S.-G., Kim, J. I., Jung, J.-C., et al. (1997) Antimetastatic activity of the new platinum analog {Pt(cis-dach)(DPPE). (2NO$_3$} in a metastatic model of human bladder cancer. *Anticancer Res.* **17,** 3239–3242.
57. Dev, S. B., Nanda, G. S., An, Z., Wang, X., Hoffman, R. M, and Hofmann, G. A. (1997) Effective electroporation therapy of human pancreatic tumors implanted in nude mice. *Drug Delivery* **4,** 293–299.
58. An, Z., Wang, X., Geller, J., Moossa, A. R., and Hoffman, R. M. (1998) Surgical orthotopic implantation allows high lung and lymph node metastatic expression of human prostate carcinoma cell line PC-3 in nude mice. *Prostate* **34,** 169–174.
59. Nanda, G. S., Sun, F. X., Hofmann, G. A., Hoffman, R. M., and Dev, S. B. (1998) Electroporation therapy of human larynx tumors HEp-2 implanted in nude mice. *Anticancer Res.* **18,** 999–1004.
60. Nanda, G. S., Sun, F. X., Hofmann, G. A., Hoffman, R. M., and Dev, S. B. (1998) Electroporation enhances therapeutic efficacy of anticancer drugs: treatment of human pancreatic tumor in animal model. *Anticancer Res.* **18,** 1361–1366.
61. Yang, M., Hasegawa, S., Jiang, P., et al. (1998) Widespread skeletal metastatic potential of human lung cancer revealed by green fluorescent protein expression. *Cancer Res.* **58,** 4217–221.
62. Sun, F.-X., Sasson, A. R., Jiang, P., An, Z., Gamagami, R., Li, L., Moossa, A. R., and Hoffman, R. H. (1999) An ultra-metastatic model of human colon cancer in nude mice. *Clin. Exp. Metastasis* **17(1),** 41–48.
63. Kiguchi, K., Kubota, T., Aoki, D., et al. (1998) A patient-like orthotopic implantation nude mouse model of highly metastatic human ovarian cancer. *Clin. Exp. Metastasis* **16,** 751–756.
64. Yang, M., Jiang, P., Sun, F. X., et al. (1999) A fluorescent orthotopic bone metastasis model of human prostate cancer. *Cancer Res.* **59,** 781–786.

65. Wang, X., An, Z., Geller, J., and Hoffman, R. M. (1999) A high malignancy orthotopic nude mouse model of the human prostate cancer LNCaP. *Prostate* **39**, 182–186.
66. Kanai, T., Konno, H., Tanaka, T., et al. (1997) Effect of angiogenesis inhibitor TNP-470 on the progression of human gastric cancer xenotransplanted into nude mice. *Int. J. Cancer* **71**, 838–841.
67. Konno, H., Tanaka, T., Kanai, T., Maruyama, K., Nakamura, S., and Baba, S.(1996) Efficacy of an angiogenesis inhibitor, TNP-470, in xenotransplanted human colorectal cancer with high metastatic potential. *Cancer* **77(8),** 1736–1740.
68. Konno, H., Tanaka, T., Matsuda, I., et al. (1995) Comparison of the inhibitory effect of the angiogenesis inhibitor, TNP-470 and mitomycin C on the growth and liver metastasis of human colon cancer. *Int. J. Cancer* **61,** 268–271.
69. Konno, H., Tanaka, T., Baba, M., et al. (1997) Antitumor effect of angiogenesis inhibitors on colon cancer. *Biotherapy* **11,** 993–996.
70. Tanaka, T., Konno, H., Matsuda, I., Nakamura, S., and Baba, S. (1995) Prevention of hepatic metastasis of human colon cancer by angiogenesis inhibitor TNP-470. *Cancer Res.* **55,** 836–839.
71. Konno, H., Arai, T., Tanaka, T., et al. (1998) Antitumor effect of neutralizing antibody to vascular endothelial growth factor on liver metastasis of endocrine neoplasm. *Jpn. J. Cancer Res.* **89,** 933–939.
72. An, Z., Jiang, P., Wang, X., Moossa, A. R., and Hoffman, R. M. (1999) Development of a high metastatic orthotopic model of human renal cell carcinoma in nude mice: benefits of fragment implantation compared to cell-suspension injection. *Clin. Exp. Metastasis* **17,** 265–270.
73. Rashidi, B., An, Z., Sun, F.-X., et al. (1999) Minimal liver resection strongly stimulates the growth of human colon cancer in the liver of nude mice. *Clin. Exp. Metastasis* **17,** 497–500.
74. Rashidi, B., Gamagami, R., Sasson, A., et al. (2000) An orthotopic mouse model of remetastasis of human colon cancer liver metastasis. *Clin. Cancer Res.* **6,** 2556–2561.
75. Rashidi, B., An, Z., Sun, F.-X., Moossa, A. R., and Hoffman, R. M. (2000) Antimetastatic intraoperative chemotherapy of human colon tumors in the livers of nude mice. *Clin. Cancer Res.* **6,** 2464–2468.
76. Rho, Y.-S., Lee, K.-T., Jung, J.-C., et al. (1999) Efficacy of new platinum analog DPPE in an orthotopic nude mouse model of human colon cancer. *Anticancer Res.* **19,** 157–162.
77. Sun, F.-X., Tohgo, A., Bouvet, M., et al. (2003) Efficacy of camptothecin analog DX-8951f (Exatecan Mesylate) on human pancreatic cancer in an orthotopic metastatic model. *Cancer Res.* **63,** 80–85.
78. Ohta, M., Konno, H., Tanaka, T., et al. (2001) Effect of combination therapy with matrix metalloproteinase inhibitor MMI-166 and mitomycin C on the growth and liver metastasis of human colon cancer. *Jpn. J. Cancer Res.* **92,** 688–695.

79. Oba, K., Konno, H., Tanaka, T., et al. (2002) Prevention of liver metastasis of human colon cancer by selective matrix metalloproteinase inhibitor MMI-166. *Cancer Lett.* **175,** 45–51.
80. Tanaka, T., Konno, H., Baba, S., et al. (2001) Prevention of hepatic and peritoneal metastases by the angiogenesis inhibitor fr-118487 after removal of growing tumor in mice. *Jpn. J. Cancer Res.* **92,** 88–94.
81. Matsumoto, K., Konno, H., Tanaka, T., et al. (2000) Combination therapy with vascular endothelial growth factor neutralizing antibody and mitomycin C on human gastric cancer xenograft. *Jpn. J. Cancer Res.* **91,** 748–752.
82. Konno, H., Arai, T., Tanaka, T., et al. (1998) Antitumor effect of a neutralizing antibody to vascular endothelial growth factor on liver metastasis of endocrine neoplasm. *Jpn. J. Cancer Res.* **89,** 933–939.
83. Kanai, T., Konno, H., Tanaka, T., et al. (1998) Anti-tumor and anti-metastatic effects of human-vascular-endothelial-growth-factor-neutralizing antibody on human colon and gastric carcinoma xenotransplanted orthotopically into nude mice. *Int. J. Cancer* **77,** 933–936.
84. Kanai, T., Konno, H., Tanaka, T., et al. (1997) Effect of angiogenesis inhibitor TNP-470 on the progression of human gastric cancer xenotransplanted into nude mice. *Int. J. Cancer* **71,** 838–841.
85. Konno, H., Tanaka, T., Kanai, T., Maruyama, K., Nakamura, S., and Baba, S. (1996) Efficacy of an angiogenesis inhibitor, TNP-470, in xenotransplanted human colorectal cancer with high metastatic potential. *Cancer* **77,** 1736–1740.
86. Tanaka, T., Konno, H., Matsuda, I., Nakamura, S., and Baba, S. (1995) Prevention of hepatic metastasis of human colon cancer by angiogenesis inhibitor TNP-470. *Cancer Res.* **55,** 836–839.
87. Konno, H., Tanaka, T., Matsuda, I., et al. (1995) Comparison of the inhibitory effect of the angiogenesis inhibitor, TNP-470, and mitomycin C on the growth and liver metastasis of human colon cancer. *Int. J. Cancer* **61,** 268–271.
88. Matsuda, I., Konno, H., Tanaka, T., and Nakamura, S. (2001) Antimetastatic effect of hepatotropic liposomal adriamycin on human metastatic liver tumors. *Surg. Today* **31,** 414–420.
89. Konno, H., Tanaka, T., Baba, M., et al. (1999) Therapeutic effect of 1 M tegafur-0.4 M 5-chloro-2,4-dihydroxypyridine-1 M potassium oxonate (S-1) on liver metastasis of xenotransplanted human colon carcinoma. *Jpn. J. Cancer Res.* **90,** 448–453.
90. Wang, J.-W., Yang, M., Wang, X., et al. (2003) Antimetastatic efficacy of oral 5-FU imaged by green fluorescent protein in real time. *Anticancer Res.* **23,** 1–6.
91. Lee, N. C., Bouvet, M., Nardin, S., et al. (2001) Antimetastatic efficacy of adjuvant gemcitabine in a pancreatic cancer orthotopic model. *Clin. Exp. Metastasis* **18,** 379–384.
92. Katz, M. H., Bouvet, M., Takimoto, S., Spivac, D., Moossa, A. R., and Hoffman, R. M. (2003) Selective antimetastatic activity of cytosine analog CS-682 in a red fluorescent protein orthotopic model of pancreatic cancer. *Cancer Res.* **63,** 5521–5525.

93. Katz, M. H., Bouvet, M., Takimoto, S., Spivack, D., Moossa, A. R., and Hoffman, R. M. (2004) Survival efficacy of adjuvant cytosine-analog CS-682 in a fluorescent orthotopic model of human pancreatic cancer. *Cancer Res.* **64,** 1828–1833.
94. Wu, M., Mazurchuk, R., Chaudhary, N. D., et al. (2003) High-resolution magnetic resonance imaging of the efficacy of the cytosine analog 1-[2-C-Cyano-2-deoxy-β-D-arabino-pentofuranosyl]-$N^4$-palmitoyl cytosine (CS-682) in a liver-metastasis athymic nude mouse model. *Cancer Res.* **63,** 2477–2482.
95. Hoffman, R. (2002) Green fluorescent protein imaging of tumour growth, metastasis, and angiogenesis in mouse models. *Lancet Oncol.* **3,** 546–556.
96. Yamamoto, N., Yang, M., Jiang, P., et al. (2003) Determination of clonality of metastasis by cell-specific color-coded fluorescent-protein imaging. *Cancer Res.* **63,** 7785–790.
97. Yang, M., Li, L., Jiang, P., Moossa, A. R., Penman, S., and Hoffman, R. M. (2003) Dual-color fluorescence imaging distinguishes tumor cells from induced host angiogenic vessels and stromal cells. *Proc. Natl. Acad. Sci. USA* **100,** 14,259–14,262.
98. Yang, M., Baranov, E., Li, X.-M., et al. (2001) Whole-body and intravital optical imaging of angiogenesis in orthotopically implanted tumors. *Proc. Natl. Acad. Sci. USA* **98,** 2616–621.
99. Yang, M., Baranov, E., Wang, J.-W., et al. (2002) Direct external imaging of nascent cancer, tumor progression, angiogenesis, and metastasis on internal organs in the fluorescent orthotopic model. *Proc. Natl. Acad. Sci. USA* **99,** 3824–3829.
100. Hoffman, R. M. (1999) Orthotopic metastatic mouse models for anticancer drug discovery and evaluation: a bridge to the clinic. *Invest. New Drugs* **17,** 343–359.
101. Katz, M., Takimoto, S., Spivac, D., Moossa, A. R., Hoffman, R. M., and Bouvet, M. (2003) A novel red fluorescent protein orthotopic pancreatic cancer model for the preclinical evaluation of chemotherapeutics. *J. Surg. Res.* **113,** 151–160.

# 21

## Preclinical Testing of Antileukemic Drugs Using an In Vivo Model of Systemic Disease

### Richard B. Lock, Natalia L. Liem, and Rachael A. Papa

#### Summary

Acute lymphoblastic leukemia (ALL) is predominantly a disease of the bone marrow that disseminates to multiple organ sites throughout the body and, without aggressive treatment, eventually results in multiorgan failure and death. Experimental models that mimic the dissemination of ALL have been difficult to establish, principally due to the poor engraftment efficiency of normal and malignant human hematopoietic cells in various strains of immune-deficient mice. The recent availability of mouse strains that are even more immunocompromised than established strains such as the nude (*nu/nu*) or severe combined immunodeficient (SCID) mouse has presented opportunities to establish improved experimental models of human leukemia. In this chapter we outline the methodology to (1) establish continuous xenografts from primary childhood ALL biopsies in nonobese diabetic/SCID (NOD/SCID) mice and (2) utilize these xenograft models of systemic disease to test established and experimental drugs while monitoring leukemia progression in "real time" by serial monitoring of murine peripheral blood. These experimental models will be useful for the preclinical evaluation of novel therapies.

#### Key Words

Xenograft; NOD/SCID; acute lymphoblastic leukemia; chemotherapy; preclinical testing.

## 1. Introduction

The development of multiagent chemotherapy to treat childhood acute lymphoblastic leukemia (ALL) represents one of the most significant success stories in cancer research of the past 40 years *(1)*. Children diagnosed with this disease now have greater than a 70% likelihood of long-term survival, although the survival rates for adults and infants with this disease are considerably lower *(1–3)*. Despite this relative success, ALL remains one of the most common causes of death from disease in children, and treatment options for those patients who undergo early bone marrow relapse are limited, with allogeneic bone marrow transplantation the best option for long-term survival *(4)*. Furthermore, as significant numbers of children now survive their disease and move into adulthood, the delayed consequences of their treatments are becoming apparent. Such long-term effects include growth retardation, impaired intellectual function, neuroendocrine disorders, cardiac toxicity, impaired reproductive ability, and increased incidence of secondary malignancies *(2,5)*.

Therefore, although the majority of children are cured, it is necessary to identify novel therapeutic approaches that more effectively target leukemia cells and spare normal cell toxicity, as well as those that can eradicate disease that has become resistant to conventional agents. The number of new agents available for testing in patients far exceeds the availability of children who are eligible for clinical trials. Consequently, it is likely that significant improvements in the treatment of childhood ALL will rely on the use of experimental models that are highly reflective of the clinical disease state. The evaluation of novel therapies in these preclinical models will facilitate their prioritization for future clinical trials.

Historically, the use of immunodeficient murine strains, such as the severe combined immunodeficient (SCID) mouse, for the engraftment of ALL cells has led to disappointing results *(6,7)*. For example, in a single study of 681 bone marrow biopsy samples, only 104 (15.3%) successfully engrafted in SCID mice, and the ability to engraft did not predict treatment outcome *(6)*. The nonobese diabetic/SCID (NOD/SCID, NOD/LtSz-scid/scid) mouse strain, which is less immunocompetent than SCID mice due to defects in natural killer cell, complement, and macrophage function *(8)*, has recently been shown to be more receptive to engraftment of normal and malignant human hematopoietic cells *(9–17)*. We have also reported the engraftment of 20 childhood ALL biopsy samples in NOD/SCID mice *(18)*. Importantly, childhood ALL cells established as xenografts in NOD/SCID mice appear to retain the phenotypic and genotypic characteristics of the original patient sample *(13,18)*. Moreover, the in vivo responses to the *Vinca* alkaloid, vincristine, of a subset of xenografts tested correlated with the length of the respective patients first remission *(18)*, providing additional evidence of the clinical relevance of the model.

The objectives of this chapter are to describe the methodology to (1) establish continuous xenografts in NOD/SCID mice using primary childhood ALL biopsy specimens and (2) utilize these experimental models for the preclinical evaluation of established and novel chemotherapeutics. Both methods allow monitoring of leukemia progression in "real time" by the serial sampling of the murine peripheral blood, and will thereby minimize the number of experimental animals required to generate statistically valid data.

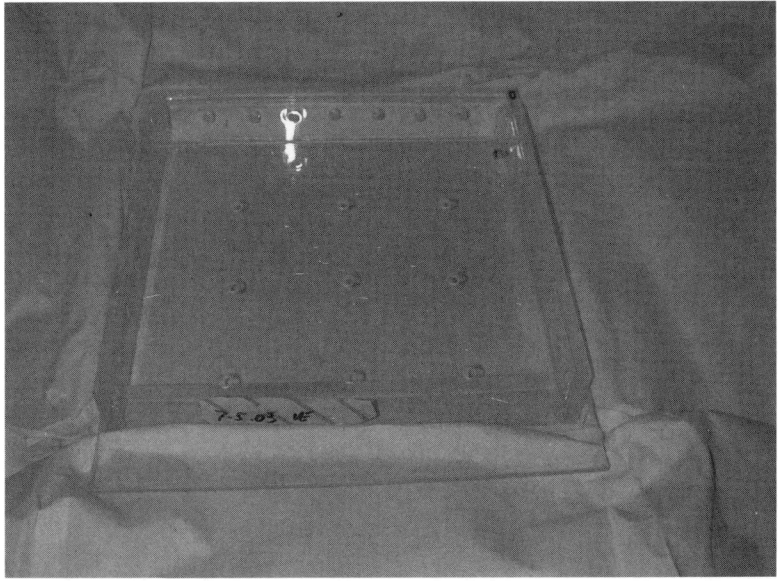

Fig. 1. Ventilated Perspex container, used for irradiating mice, positioned on sterile drapes.

## 2. Materials

1. Six- to 8-wk-old NOD/SCID mice housed in a Specific-Pathogen-Free environment for at least 1 wk prior to experimentation.
2. Sterilized cages, food, and water.
3. Perspex box, gas-sterilized (ethylene oxide), to contain mice while being irradiated **(Fig. 1)**.
4. Sterile drapes.
5. Autoclaved mouse transporter.
6. Sterile plastic 25-g "phantom" mice.
7. Fresh or cryopreserved mononuclear cell preparations from bone marrow biopsies of acute lymphoblastic leukemia patients.
8. Complete medium: RPMI1640 medium containing 10% fetal bovine serum (FBS).
9. Trypan blue.
10. Hemocytometer.
11. Calcium- and magnesium-free phosphate-buffered saline (PBS).
12. High-wattage infrared heat lamp.
13. Perspex mouse restrainer **(Fig. 2)**.
14. 23-gauge × 1¼-in syringe needles; 1-mL syringes.
15. Sterile 0.5-mL microcentrifuge tubes containing 15 µL of heparin solution (1000 IU/mL).

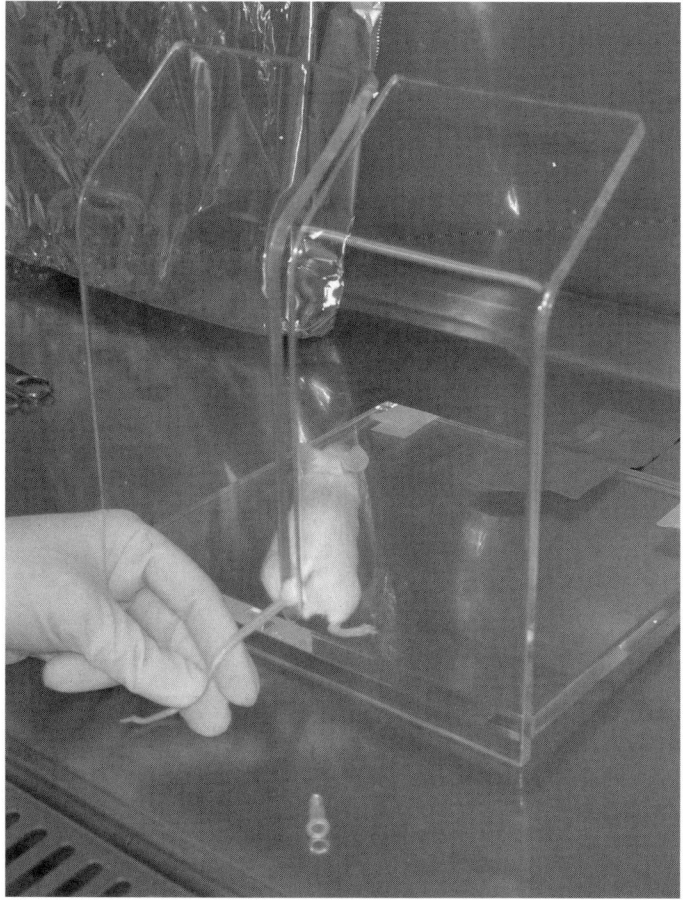

Fig. 2. Mouse positioned in Perspex restrainer inside biological safety cabinet for tail-vein injection or bleeding.

16. Antibodies: fluorescein isothiocyanate (FITC)-conjugated antimurine and allophycocyanin (APC)-conjugated antihuman CD45 (leukocyte common antigen, Ly-5), and FITC- and APC-conjugated antimurine IgG isotype control antibodies (BD Biosciences) (store at 4°C in the dark).
17. Ammonium chloride solution: 8.3% ammonium chloride, 1.0% sodium bicarbonate, 0.4% disodium EDTA in distilled water, pH 7.3.
18. Flow cytometry buffer: 1% FBS and 0.1% sodium azide in PBS. *Note:* sodium azide is toxic and should be handled with caution.
19. Flow cytometry tubes.
20. Multiparameter flow cytometer, FACSCalibur flow cytometer (BD Immunocytometry Systems), or equivalent.

21. Terumo U-100 1.0-mL insulin syringes with 27-gauge × ½-in needle.
22. 1.5-mL microcentrifuge tubes containing 0.5 mL sterile PBS.
23. Complete medium: RPMI1640 medium containing 10% FBS.
24. Autoclaved tea strainer.
25. 5-mL syringes.
26. 70-µm cell strainers (BD Labware, Franklin Lakes, NJ).
27. Normal mouse serum.
28. Sterilized surgical instruments for mouse surgery and bone dissociation.
29. Lymphoprep (Nycomed, Sydney, Australia).
30. 1 mL cryostorage vials.
31. Freezing-down apparatus or Cryo 1°C Freezing Containers (Mr Frosty, Nalgene).
32. Terumo U-100 1.0-mL insulin syringes with 29-gauge × ½-in needle.
33. Chemotherapeutic drugs: cytosine arabinoside; water-soluble dexamethasone (Sigma, cat. no. D2915); methotrexate (Pharmacia & Upjohn); vincristine (Sigma); daunorubicin (Pharmacia & Upjohn). Store all drugs protected from light and dilute in PBS immediately prior to use.

## 3. Methods

### 3.1. Establishing Continuous Xenografts from Childhood ALL Biopsies in NOD/SCID Mice

Historically, the engraftment efficiency of normal and malignant human hematopoietic cells in strains of immune-deficient mice, such as SCID (severe combined immunodeficient) mice, has been low *(6,7)*. More recently, the NOD/SCID mouse strain was shown to be receptive to engraftment of normal and malignant human hematopoietic cells *(9–17)*. We have previously described the engraftment in NOD/SCID mice of 20 childhood ALL biopsies obtained at diagnosis or relapse from patients who encompassed a broad range of disease subtypes and treatment outcomes *(18)*. The following describes a method for establishing continuous ALL xenografts as models of systemic disease in NOD/SCID mice, in which engraftment is monitored by estimating the proportion of human leukemia cells in the mouse peripheral blood.

1. On the morning of transplantation, place a maximum number of eight mice into a sterile Perspex mouse box, and wrap in sterile drapes to prevent contamination from the surrounding air (**Fig. 1**). Expose the mice to 250 cGy of total-body irradiation at a dose rate of 325 cGy/min (or equivalent), by parallel-opposed 4-MV rays (*see* **Note 1**).
2. Retrieve leukemia biopsy samples from cryostorage (*see* **Note 2**), and thaw the vials rapidly by placing in a 37°C water bath. Using a 1-mL pipet, transfer the cell suspension into a 15-mL centrifuge tube. Add 10 mL of prewarmed complete medium, dropwise for the first 5 mL (*see* **Note 3**). Centrifuge the cells at 200*g* for 5 min, discard the supernatant, and resuspend the cells in 10 mL complete medium. Estimate the concentration of viable cells and allocate between 2 and 10 million

cells per mouse (*see* **Note 4**). Recentrifuge the cell suspension and resuspend the cells in ice-cold sterile PBS such that each mouse will receive the appropriate number of cells in a volume of 100 µL. Transfer the cell suspension to 1.5-mL microcentrifuge tubes and place on ice until transplantation.

3. Set up the mouse holder in a biological safety cabinet as depicted in **Fig. 2**. Warm each mouse by placing it near the heat lamp for 20 s, or until the tail veins appear dilated. Using a 23-gauge × 1¼-in needle attached to a 1-mL syringe, draw up the cell suspension and carefully eliminate any air bubbles from the syringe. Place the mouse in the restrainer and, holding the tail with the lateral vein exposed, gently insert the needle to a depth of approximately 1 cm, being careful not to extrude through the opposite side of the vein. Slowly inject 100 µL of cell suspension into the tail vein and remove the needle (*see* **Note 5**). Compress the puncture site using a sterile tissue until bleeding has ceased (usually 20–40 s). Return the mouse to its box and examine daily for general well-being.

4. Begin to monitor for engraftment during the second week after transplantation. Warm each mouse by placing it near the heat lamp for approximately 20 s. While holding the mouse in the restrainer (**Fig. 2**), pierce the lateral tail vein using a 23-gauge × 1¼-in needle. Collect 3–4 drops (50–75 µL) of blood into a 0.5-mL microcentrifuge tube containing 15 µL of heparin. Stop the bleeding as described in **step 3** (*see* **Notes 6–8**).

5. Transfer 50–75 µL of blood from each tube into a flow cytometry tube. To each tube add 94 µL of flow cytometry buffer, 5 µL of APC-conjugated antihuman CD45, and 1 µL of FITC-conjugated antimouse CD45. Incubate at room temperature in the dark for 30 min (*see* **Notes 9** and **10**). To each tube then add ammonium chloride solution to the equivalent of 8 vol of the original blood volume (400–600 µL) and incubate the tubes at 37°C for 5 min in the dark to lyse the red blood cells. Add 3 mL of flow cytometry buffer to each tube to neutralize the ammonium chloride and centrifuge at 200*g* for 5 min at room temperature. Discard the supernatant and resuspend the pellet in 150 µL of flow cytometry buffer. Analyze samples by dual-color flow cytometry with appropriate compensation settings for FITC (FL1, 530 nm) and APC (FL4, 670 nm), acquiring 10,000 events per sample. Calculate the proportion of human versus murine $CD45^+$ cells to determine the extent of dissemination of leukemia into the peripheral blood. This method is able to reliably detect 0.1% human $CD45^+$ cells in murine peripheral blood.

6. When the proportion of human $CD45^+$ cells in the peripheral blood exceeds 50%, or at the first indication of morbidity (>20% weight loss, lethargy, ruffled fur), sacrifice the mice by cervical dislocation (*see* **Note 11**). To determine the extent of leukemic infiltration of mouse organs, collect the blood (by cardiac puncture, transfer to a 0.5-mL microcentrifuge tube containing 15 µL of heparin), spleen, liver, lungs, kidney, and brain (*see* **Note 12**). In addition, collect the bone marrow by flushing the femurs with 10 mL of complete medium using a 27-gauge × ½-in needle. Prepare cell suspensions of spleen (and additional organs that you wish to cryopreserve) by placing individual organs into a sterile tea strainer and homog-

enizing with complete medium using the plunger of a 5-mL syringe to mince the tissues. Subsequently prepare single-cell suspensions by filtering the homogenates through 70-μm cell strainers into 50-mL tubes. For tissues for which complete organs are not required, place a tissue segment into a 1.5-mL microcentrifuge tube containing 0.5 mL of PBS and macerate with the plunger of a 1-mL syringe. For flow cytometric estimation of leukemic infiltration, transfer 50–100 μL of cell suspension to a flow cytometry tube, add 50-μL of mouse serum, and incubate for 5 min at room temperature. To each tube add 94 μL of flow cytometry buffer, 5 μL of APC-conjugated antihuman CD45, and 1 μL of FITC-conjugated antimouse CD45. Carry out the remainder of the procedure as described in **step 5** (*see* **Note 13**).
7. For use in secondary transplantations, immunophenotype analysis *(18)*, or other laboratory investigations, purify mononuclear cells from spleens and bone marrow by Ficoll density gradient centrifugation, as follows: underlay 35 mL of cell suspension in complete medium with 15 mL of Lymphoprep in a 50-mL screw-cap tube; centrifuge at 800*g* for 30 min at 20°C; collect the interphase (mononuclear cell) layer and transfer to a clean tube; dilute up to 50 mL with complete medium and centrifuge at 200*g* for 10 min at room temperature; discard the supernatant and wash the cells again with complete medium. Calculate the total number of viable cells using 0.2% trypan blue and cryopreserve in 20–40-million-cell aliquots in FBS containing 10% dimethyl sulfoxide (DMSO) (*see* **Note 14**). For use in secondary and tertiary transplantations to establish continuous xenografts, thaw cryopreserved cells and process exactly as described for primary cells in **step 2**. Inoculate and monitor mice exactly as described above (*see* **Note 15**).

## 3.2. Preclinical Drug Testing Using Childhood ALL Xenograft Models of Systemic Disease

Because of the ethical implications of testing new drugs/compounds on humans, and the increasing disparity between the number of patients eligible for clinical trials and the availability of new agents, it is likely that significant improvements in the therapy of leukemia will depend on the use of relevant preclinical experimental models to prioritize novel therapies for future clinical trials. We have developed an experimental model of systemic disease from childhood ALL biopsy specimens, which uses serial sampling of peripheral blood to assess antileukemic effects of established or novel compounds in "real time" *(18)*.

1. Based on the growth characteristics of your xenograft models, determine the appropriate number of mice required in control and drug-treated groups to achieve sufficient statistical power for the planned experiments *(19)*.
2. Determine the optimal dose, dosing schedule, and route of administration for the drug to be tested in NOD/SCID mice. This is best achieved by treating groups of three mice with a range of drug doses and carefully monitoring for signs of

morbidity (weight loss, ruffled fur, lethargy). The highest dose of drug that does not cause significant levels of toxicity should be chosen for subsequent efficacy experiments (see **Note 16**).

3. Retrieve from cryostorage cells from established continuous xenografts, as described above **(Subheading 3.1., step 2)**. Inoculate groups of mice with $5 \times 10^6$ cells from primary or secondary engraftments. Starting at wk 2 following inoculation, begin to monitor leukemia engraftment by weekly tail vein bleed (see **Subheading 3.1., steps 3–5**) (see **Note 17**). Drug and the equivalent volume of solvent control treatments should commence when the proportion of human $CD45^+$ cells in the peripheral blood reaches 1%. Before the initial treatment, mice should be randomized to ensure that no bias has been introduced during the initial engraftment period *(19)*. Continue to bleed the mice weekly to monitor leukemia progression in the controls and antileukemic effects in the drug-treated mice. When the proportion of human $CD45^+$ cells in the peripheral blood reaches 50% mice should be sacrificed by cervical dislocation and internal organs examined for leukemia infiltration, as described above.

4. Calculate the mouse event-free survival (EFS) from the initiation of treatment, defined to be when the proportion of human $CD45^+$ cells in the peripheral blood reaches 25%, or when animals exhibit clinical signs of disease (weight loss, lethargy, ruffled fur) associated with high-level leukemic infiltration of bone marrow and spleen at necropsy (see **Note 18**). Mouse EFS can be represented graphically by Kaplan-Meier analysis *(20)*.

5. For statistical comparisons between xenografts and drug treatments, calculate a growth delay factor (GDF) as the difference in median EFS between control and drug-treated mice. GDF values may be >50 d for some xenografts *(18)*.

## 4. Notes

1. If it is not possible to irradiate the mice on the morning of inoculation with leukemia cells, they should be irradiated no more than 24 h prior. We usually autoclave the original container in which the mice arrived and use it to transport the mice to the irradiation suite. If fewer than eight mice are to be irradiated, add sterile 25-g plastic "phantom" mice to a total of eight for the correct dosage to be administered. Dosage should be calculated in consultation with a radiologist.

2. We have been successful in engrafting both bone marrow and peripheral blood biopsies, although for the latter only one sample was attempted *(18)*. Bone marrow biopsies routinely consisted of >85% leukemic blasts, as verified by morphological and immunophenotype analysis. We have also attempted, without success, to engraft leukemia cells from cryopreserved buffy coats from bone marrow biopsies.

3. To obtain the highest viability of cells retrieved from cryostorage, complete medium should be added dropwise for the first 5 mL, to gradually dilute the DMSO in the freezing-down medium.

4. For primary engraftments we aim to inoculate 5 million cells per mouse. However, robust engraftment has been observed at secondary and tertiary passage using as few as 1 million cells.

5. To facilitate the intravenous injection it is important to warm each mouse to dilate the tail vein. The whole box of mice can be placed near the heat lamp at the beginning of the procedure. If the first attempt at inoculation is unsuccessful, we advise that the next attempt be made using the alternate tail vein. This alternative has proven to be very useful, as successive injections in the same tail vein will generally lead to local clotting of the blood, making further attempts difficult. There should be little or no resistance when injecting the cells. Resistance during injection is an indication that the needle may be lodged in the side of the vein. It is possible to observe the cell suspension entering the vein by a pale discoloration of the vein.
6. We have also attempted to use cell lines (e.g., the CEM T-lineage ALL cell line) as in vivo models of disease. However, we observed no dissemination of leukemia cells to the peripheral blood before animals became morbid with disease, and therefore discontinued experiments as engraftment could not be monitored in "real time."
7. We originally bled the animals by creating a nick in the tail using a scalpel blade. However, we subsequently found that use of a 23-gauge needle greatly reduced necrosis of the tail during repeated weekly bleeds. The smaller wound produced by the needle facilitates a more rapid repair of the tail, allowing the mice to be bled weekly for at least 20 wk by experienced personnel. Although it is important to obtain at least 50 µL of blood from each mouse, we do not recommend that piercing of the tail occur more than three times in any one day. Multiple perforations of the veins can cause necrosis, causing great difficulty for future bleeding. These procedures should only be carried out by experienced personnel.
8. Blood samples can be kept at room temperature overnight prior to antibody staining and flow cytometric analysis.
9. At least one sample should be stained with equivalent amounts of IgG isotype control antibodies (APC-conjugated antimouse and FITC-conjugated antimouse, BD Biosciences) to enable accurate setting of the gates during flow cytometry. Despite being antimouse, the APC-conjugated control is recommended for use as an isotype control for direct immunofluorescence staining of human tissue for flow cytometric analysis.
10. At the time of inoculation, a small proportion of the biopsy sample should be stained with antihuman CD45 to verify positive staining. In our experience, one out of 25 biopsy samples stained weakly for CD45. In such a case, use anti-CD19 for B-lineage and anti-CD7 for T-lineage ALL.
11. The 2000 Report of the American Veterinary Medical Association Panel on Euthanasia *(21)* recommends cervical dislocation as a humane technique for the euthanasia of mice. However, the technique should only be performed by properly trained staff, who can consistently apply it humanely and effectively. Alternatively, $CO_2$ asphyxiation may be used, but this may compromise subsequent cardiac puncture.
12. The NOD/SCID strain spontaneously develops thymic lymphomas, and has a reported lifespan of approx 8½ mo *(8)*. The most obvious indication at necropsy

is an enlarged thymus, and should be considered when carrying out prolonged engraftment periods and subsequent passage of cells into secondary and tertiary recipient mice.
13. Bone marrows and spleens of animals that exhibit >50% human CD45$^+$ cells in the peripheral blood are routinely >90% human CD45$^+$ *(18)*. High-level leukemic infiltration of the liver is also routinely observed in this experimental model, with variable infiltration of lungs, kidneys, and meninges.
14. In our experience the recovery of viable cells frozen using containers in isopropanol (e.g., Mr Frosty, Nalgene) placed into the –80°C freezer is comparable to that using a commercially available freezing-down apparatus. We believe this to be due to delays experienced in loading the latter with the large number of vials generated from harvesting engrafted animals (>300 million cells/spleen). The isopropanol containers are designed to control a temperature decrease of 1°C/min for the first hour and, after overnight incubation of the containers at –80°C, vials should be moved into liquid nitrogen storage.
15. We routinely use cells harvested from spleens for engraftment of secondary and tertiary recipient mice, because we have found that these cells engraft as efficiently as cells harvested from the bone marrow. Because of the large numbers of cells harvested from engrafted spleens (300 million–1 billion cells) compared with bone marrow (20–40 million), it is possible to conduct all of our experiments using early-passage cells. In controlled experiments we have not found it necessary to irradiate mice for secondary, tertiary, and subsequent transplantations.
16. In our experience, NOD/SCID mice tend to be more sensitive to established chemotherapeutic drugs compared with SCID mice. For example, the maximum tolerated dose of vincristine in NOD/SCID mice is 0.5 mg/kg once a week for 4 wk, compared with 1 mg/kg for SCID mice *(18,22)*. Dosing schedules that we have established in our laboratory to be suitable for NOD/SCID mice include: vincristine (*Vinca* alkaloid) (0.5 mg/kg ip every 7 d × 4) *(18)*; daunorubicin (anthracycline) (5 mg/kg iv every 7 d × 4) *(23)*; dexamethasone (glucocorticoid) (15 mg/kg ip daily, Mon–Fri, for 4 wk) *(24)*; cytarabine (antimetabolite) (100 mg/kg ip daily, Mon–Fri, repeated every 21 d for 4 courses) *(25)*; and methotrexate (antimetabolite) (5 mg/kg ip daily, Mon–Fri, repeated every 14 d for 4 courses) *(26)*.
17. For large cohorts of mice, and because of the reproducible growth of individual xenografts in this model, we routinely bleed half of each group of mice on alternate weeks until engraftment is evident. Once drug treatments commence, all mice are bled weekly.
18. The dissemination of primary childhood ALL cells into the NOD/SCID peripheral blood is characterized by an initial lag phase, the length of which varies among patient samples, followed by an exponential increase in the proportion of human CD45$^+$ cells in the peripheral blood *(18)*. Because the length of the lag phase varies among different xenografts, we express mouse EFS from the initiation of drug treatment. In some instances it is necessary to inoculate xenografts at different times in order to be able to synchronize the drug treatments. However, for most continuous xenografts, treatments can begin during week 3 or 4 after inoculation.

## Acknowledgments

The Children's Cancer Institute Australia for Medical Research is affiliated with the University of New South Wales and Sydney Children's Hospital.

## References

1. Pui, C.-H., Relling, M. V., Campana, D., and Evans, W. E. (2002) Childhood acute lymphoblastic leukemia. *Rev. Clin. Exp. Hematol.* **6(2),** 161–180.
2. Kersey, J. H. (1997) Fifty years of studies of the biology and therapy of childhood leukemia. *Blood* **90,** 4243–4251.
3. Copelan, E. A. and McGuire, E. A. (1995) The biology and treatment of acute lymphoblastic leukemia in adults. *Blood* **85,** 1151–1168.
4. Chessells, J. M. (1998) Relapsed lymphoblastic leukaemia in children: a continuing challenge. *Br. J. Haematol.* **102,** 423–438.
5. Bhatia, S. (2003) Late effects among survivors of leukemia during childhood and adolescence. *Blood Cells Mol. Dis.* **31,** 84–92.
6. Uckun, F. M., Sather, H. N., Waurzyniak, B. J., et al. (1998) Prognostic significance of B-lineage leukemic cell growth in SCID mice: a Children's Cancer Group study. *Leukemia Lymphoma* **30,** 503–514.
7. Uckun, F. M., Waurzyniak, B. J., Sather, H. N., et al. (1999) Prognostic significance of T-lineage leukemic cell growth in SCID mice: a Children's Cancer Group study. *Leukemia Lymphoma* **32,** 475–487.
8. Shultz, L. D., Schweitzer, P. A., Christianson, S. W., et al. (1995) Multiple defects in innate and adaptive immunologic function in NOD/LtSz-scid mice. *J. Immunol.* **154,** 180–191.
9. Wang, J. C. Y., Lapidot, T., Cashman, J. D., et al. (1998) High level engraftment of NOD/SCID mice by primitive normal and leukemic hematopoietic cells from patients with chronic myeloid leukemia in chronic phase. *Blood* **91,** 2406–2414.
10. Dazzi, F., Capelli, D., Hasserjian, R., et al. (1998) The kinetics and extent of engraftment of chronic myelogenous leukemia cells in non-obese diabetic/severe combined immunodeficiency mice reflect the phase of the donor's disease: an in vivo model of chronic myelogenous leukemia biology. *Blood* **92,** 1390–1396.
11. Rombouts, W. J. C., Martens, A. C. M., and Ploemacher, R. E. (2000) Identification of variables determining the engraftment potential of human acute myeloid leukemia in the immunodeficient NOD/SCID human chimera model. *Leukemia* **14,** 889–897.
12. Hudson, W. A., Li, Q., Le, C., and Kersey, J. H. (1998) Xenotransplantation of human lymphoid malignancies is optimized in mice with multiple immunologic defects. *Leukemia* **12,** 2029–2033.
13. Borgmann, A., Baldy, C., von Stackelberg, A., et al. (2000) Childhood ALL blasts retain phenotypic and genotypic characteristics upon long-term serial passage in NOD/SCID mice. *Pediat. Hematol. Oncol.* **17,** 635–650.

14. Nijmeijer, B. A., Mollevanger, P., van Zelderen-Bhola, S. L., et al. (2001) Monitoring of engraftment and progression of acute lymphoblastic leukemia in individual NOD/SCID mice. *Exp. Hematol.* **29,** 322–329.
15. Dialynas, D. P., Lee, M.-J., Gold, D. P., et al. (2001) Preconditioning with fetal cord blood facilitates engraftment of primary childhood T-cell acute lymphoblastic leukemia in immunodeficient mice. *Blood* **97,** 3218–3225.
16. Steele, J. P. C., Clutterbuck, R. D., Powles, R. L., et al. (1997) Growth of human T-cell lineage acute leukemia in severe combined immunodeficiency (SCID) mice and non-obese diabetic SCID mice. *Blood* **90,** 2015–2019.
17. Baersch, G., Mollers, T., Hotte, A., et al. (1997) Good engraftment of B-cell precursor ALL in NOD-SCID mice. *Klin. Padiat.* **209,** 178–185.
18. Lock, R. B., Liem, N., Farnsworth, M. L., et al. (2002) The nonobese diabetic/severe combined immunodeficient (NOD/SCID) mouse model of childhood acute lymphoblastic leukemia reveals intrinsic differences in biologic characteristics at diagnosis and relapse. *Blood* **99,** 4100–4108.
19. Hanfelt, J. J. (1997) Statistical approaches to experimental design and data analysis of *in vivo* studies. *Breast Cancer Res. Treat.* **46,** 279–302.
20. Kaplan, E. L. and Meier, P. (1958) Nonparametric estimation from incomplete observations. *Am. Statis. Assoc. J.* **53,** 457–481.
21. 2000 Report of the American Veterinary Medical Association Panel on Euthanasia (2000) *JAMA* **218,** 669–696.
22. Millar, J. L., Millar, B. C., Powles, R. L., et al. (1998) Liposomal vincristine for the treatment of human acute lymphoblastic leukaemia in severe combined immunodeficient (SCID) mice. *Br. J. Haematol.* **102,** 718–721.
23. Houba, P. H., Boven, E., van der Meulen-Muileman, I. H., et al. (1999) Distribution and pharmacokinetics of the prodrug daunorubicin-GA3 in nude mice bearing human ovarian cancer xenografts. *Biochem. Pharmacol.* **57,** 673–680.
24. Braunschweiger, P. G., Ting, H. L., and Schiffer, L. M. (1983) Correlation between glucocorticoid receptor content and the antiproliferative effect of dexamethasone in experimental solid tumors. *Cancer Res.* **43,** 4757–4761.
25. Yamagami, K., Fujii, A., Arita, M., et al. (1991) Antitumor activity of 2′-deoxy-2′-methylidenecytidine, a new 2′-deoxycytidine derivative. *Cancer Res.* **51,** 2319–2323.
26. White, L., Haber, M., Brian, M. J., et al. (1989) Therapy-induced drug resistance in a human leukemia line (LALW-2). *Cancer* **63,** 2103–2110.

# 22

## Assessing Growth and Response to Therapy in Murine Tumor Models

### C. Patrick Reynolds, Bee-Chun Sun, Yves A. DeClerck, and Rex A. Moats

#### Summary
Rodent models provide an important means of assessing antitumor activity vs toxicity for new cancer therapies. Tumors are often grown subcutaneously on the flank or back of animals, allowing accurate serial determination of tumor volume with calipers by measuring the tumors in three dimensions. The advantages of assessing tumor volume in subcutaneous tumors must be balanced against the potential artifacts induced by growth of tumor cells in subcutaneous tissue. Various orthotopic models have been developed. However, they are more labor-intensive and generally do not allow accurate assessment of tumor growth and/or response unless investigators have access to small animal cross-sectional imaging. Use of small-animal magnetic resonance imaging (MRI) allows one to assess the growth and response of intracavitary tumors, but the cost and labor-intensive nature of MRI limits its use in drug testing. Another approach to intracavitary solid tumor models is the intravenous injection of tumor cells, which can produce lung, liver, or bone metastases (depending on the cell line used), whereas direct injection of tumor cells into the femur or tibia of mice can cause local growth in bone. Progression of both lung metastases and bone lesions can be assessed by small-animal analog X-ray techniques that are more easily available and less labor-intensive to use, and are proving useful for selected therapeutic and biological studies.

#### Key Words
Mouse xenograft; tumor volume; bone metastases; chemotherapy; radiograph.

### 1. Introduction

Rodent models provide an important means of assessing antitumor activity vs toxicity for new antineoplastic drugs, and they provide a key component of preclinical developmental therapeutics for cancer. Syngeneic rat and mouse tumors played an important role in early cancer drug development *(1–3)*, but these have largely been surpassed by the use of xenografted human solid tumors in athymic (*nu/nu*) mice, in severe combined immunodeficiency (SCID) mice, or in athymic rats *(4–8)*. Human leukemia cells injected intravenously into nod/SCID mice can provide a model of acute lymphoblastic leukemia that is being used for preclinical therapeutic studies *(9–11)*. Although the limitations of rodent models in predicting clinically active agents are well recognized, they still provide an important component of preclinical testing, and significant responses in multiple xenograft models increase the possibility of a new drug having clinical activity *(12)*.

Solid tumors are often grown subcutaneously on the flank or back of animals to allow an accurate serial determination of tumor volume with calipers by measuring the tumors in three dimensions *(13)*. The advantages of assessing tumor volume in subcutaneous tumors must be balanced against the potential artifacts induced by growth of tumor cells in subcutaneous tissue. Various orthotopic models have been developed *(14–19)*, but they are more labor-intensive and generally do not allow the accurate assessment of tumor growth and/or response unless investigators have access to small-animal cross-sectional imaging *(20–22)*. Small-animal magnetic resonance imaging (MRI) allows assessing growth and response of intracavitary tumors *(20–23)*, but the cost and labor-intensive nature of MRI limits its widespread use in preclinical drug testing. However, in brain tumors, where alternatives for assessing tumor response are limited, small animal MRI may see wider application. Micro-computerized tomography (CT) offers another means of assessing intracavitary lesions *(24,25)*, but it is not suitable for intracranial lesions, and the time involved in obtaining and processing images prevents the routine use of micro-CT in drug testing.

Transduction of tumor cells with green fluorescent protein (GFP) is one method for assessing tumor growth and response by use of fluorescence imaging systems that can detect and quantify tumor masses in animals *(26–28)*. However, the potential for GFP transduction to introduce artifacts is considerable, and GFP transduction has been shown to induce oxidative stress and to sensitize tumor cells to a variety of chemotherapeutic drugs *(29)*. An alternative to GFP is to transduce tumor cells with firefly luciferase, which allows the light generated in tumors when the mice are given luciferin to be imaged in special devices *(30–33)*. The potential for luciferase transduction to interfere with tumor growth or sensitize tumor cells to chemotherapy remains unknown. Also, because of the induction of an immune response, either luciferase or GFP marking is limited to use in immunocompromised mice.

Analysis of progression-free survival provides one alternative to intracavitary imaging, but the lack of tumor response data and the inability to exclude tumors that do not engraft from the analysis diminish the usefulness of such models. However, when employing disseminated disease models (tail vein injection) for solid tumors or for leukemias, progression-free survival remains the primary approach for assessing the response of disseminated disease *(9–11,34,35)*.

For tumors in which intravenous injection of tumor cells causes pulmonary or bone metastases, relatively inexpensive analog radiological methods can provide a means of documenting tumor engraftment prior to therapeutic studies, and may also be used to assess response. Intravenous injection or direct injection of some tumor cell lines into the femur or tibia of mice produces bone invasion that can cause lytic lesions evauable with analog radiology *(36)*. Such bone invasion and/or metastasis models have been developed for breast cancer *(37–39)*, prostate cancer *(40)*, and neuroblastoma *(41)*. These models are useful for testing agents that have direct antitumor effects, or agents (such as bisphosphonates) that retard or prevent skeletal events.

We will review here methods for assessing tumor progression and response in subcutaneous murine models with direct measurement. We will also review radiographic techniques currently under development that can be used to assess tumor progression and response to therapy without the use of potentially artifact-inducing transduced cell markers.

## 2. Materials

1. *Mice.* Mice (female, 4–6-wk-old athymic balb/c *(nu/nu)* or homozygous SCID C.B-17/IcrHsd-scid mutant mice can be obtained from a variety of vendors. Mice should be allowed to acclimate to their new environment for 1 wk after arrival.
2. *Animal caging.* Cages require a laminar-flow air delivery system (such as that made by Lab Products, Seaford, DE) or filter cage bonnets on polycarbonate microisolator cages lined with autoclaved bedding to maintain an aseptic environment. Mice should be maintained according to Institutional Animal Care and Use Committee (IACUC) approved experimental protocols. Autoclaved and acidified (pH = 4–6) water and autoclaved standard Purina mouse chow should be provided *ad libitum.*
3. *Medium for suspending tumor cells.* To minimize pH changes during handling of cells outside of a $CO_2$ incubator and to decrease clumping (especially deleterious with intravenous injections), cells are optimally suspended in L-15 (non-bicarbonate-based, non-$CO_2$-requiring medium) that is made without calcium or magnesisum.
4. *Calipers.* Although vernier and dial calipers can be used for measuring subcutaneous tumors, digital calipers (such as those made by Fisher Scientific, Tustin, CA) are the most suitable for the task. Systems for direct entry of caliper data into microcomputers have also been developed *(42)*. However, employing two individuals for the measurements (one to measure, one to transcribe) allows rapid collection of data without the use of computerized calipers.
5. *Injectable anesthetics.* Pentobarbital sodium injection (Abbott Laboratories, North Chicago, IL), given ip at 40 mg/kg is one means of anesthesia. Another is an ip injection of 2.5% Avertin, 0.02 mL 2.5% Avertin/g body weight (ip) for mice,

with a 100% stock solution consisting of 1 g of 2,2,2-tribromoethanol in 1 mL *tert*-amyl alcohol (both made by Sigma-Aldrich, Milwaukee, WI). Mice can also be anesthetized by ip injection of a mixture of ketamine (50 mg/kg) and xylocaine (5 mg/kg).
6. *Inhalational anesthesia.* Isoflurane anesthetic + oxygen is delivered from an inhalational anesthetic apparatus (Abbott Laboratories, North Chicago, IL).
7. *Animal temperature control system.* To prevent hypothermia, one must provide temperature control for the mice during anesthesia. A suitable system for doing this is a water heating pad, the heat therapy system, comprised of a pad (REF TP22GT/PAD) and a pump (T/Pimp TP 500/TP500 C), both made by Gaymar Industries, Orchard Park, NY.
8. *Radiographic system.* Radiographs are generated using a Faxitron MX-20 small-animal X-ray device (Faxitron X-ray Corp., Wheeling, IL). To provide high-resolution radiographs, mammography computed radiography cassettes with high-resolution screens and high-detail single-emulsion mammography film and screens (Fuji EC-MA cassette, Fuji Photo Film Co., Japan) are used *(41)*. Mammography products from other vendors are likely to give similar results.
9. *Software.* Tumor volume measurements, averages and standard deviations, and differences between treated and control animals can be calculated using Microsoft Excel. This program can also be used for creating rudimentary tumor growth-over-time graphs. Macros developed in Excel can also be used to generate Kaplan-Meier (log-rank) assessment of time to progression. Analyzed data can be copied from Excel to SigmaPlot (Jandell Scientific, San Rafael, CA) to create publication-quality graphics.

## 3. Methods

### 3.1. Maintaining Immunocompromised Mice

Mice are allowed to acclimate to their new environment for 1 wk after arrival. Mice are handled under strict aseptic conditions, opening the cage in a laminar-flow hood while wearing a sterile gown and gloves.

### 3.2. Establishing Subcutaneous Xenografts

1. Harvest cells that are 75–80% confluent, highly viable, and in logarithmic growth phase. It is preferred to grow cells in antibiotic-free medium to avoid masking microbial contamination. For neuroblastoma, rhabdomyosarcoma, Ewing's family tumors, retinoblastoma, and certain other tumor types we find that cells can be removed from the substrate using Puck's Solution A plus EDTA (Puck's EDTA), which contains 140 m$M$ NaCl, 5 m$M$ KCl, 5.5 m$M$ glucose, 4 m$M$ NaHCO$_3$, 0.8 m$M$ ethylenediaminetetraacetic acid (EDTA), 13 µ$M$ phenol red, and 9 m$M$ HEPES buffer (pH 7.3) *(43)*, thus avoiding the additional cell damage from trypsin.
2. Viable cell number is determined by hemocytometer counting using trypan blue, and 5–50 million tumor cells (depending on tumorigencity and growth rate) are

injected subcutaneously between the shoulder blades of three to five athyhmic (nu/nu) mice using strict aseptic technique, with a 1-cm$^3$-syringe and a 19-gage needle.
3. For injection, cells are suspended in L-15 medium (Ca$^{2+}$/Mg$^{2+}$-free) culture medium without fetal bovine serum (FBS) such that a total of 200 µL are injected to deliver the desired cell dose.
4. Mice are observed biweekly and tumor growth monitored when tumors become palpable; the lag phase varies from 2 to 12 weeks, depending on the amount of cells injected, the tumor type, and the cell line employed.
5. When tumors reach about 1.5 cm$^3$, two to four mice are sacrificed, the skin over the tumor disinfected with betadine, and the tumors removed under aseptic conditions.
6. The tumor cells are forced through a sterile 80–160-µm stainless-steel mesh strainer, and mixed with cell culture medium to form a slurry, such that injection of 200 µL subcutaneously between the shoulder blades of 20–25 mice delivers a tumor cell dose of approx 5–50 million cells, depending on how aggressive the tumor is (*see* **Note 1**).

## 3.3. Assessing the Volume of Subcutaneous Tumors by Caliper Measurements

1. Tumors should be measured beginning when they are first palpable: the length ($L$ = longest dimension), the width ($W$ = the distance perpendicular to and in the same plane as the length), and the height ($H$ = the distance between the exterior tumor edge and the mouse body). The ellipsoid volume of the tumor, calculated from $0.5 \times L \times W \times H$, provides the most accurate measure of tumor mass *(13)* (**Fig. 1**).
2. For multilobed tumors, or those that grow in irregular shapes, the tumor should be divided visually into two, three, or four lobes of similar dimension that are measured separately (**Fig. 1**). The calculated volume for each lobe can be summed to obtain the volume of the entire mass *(13)*.

## 3.4. Establishing Pulmonary and Bone Metastases by Intravenous Injection

1. Cells are harvested from tissue culture flasks, counted, and suspended in serum-free L-15 (calcium- and magnesium-free) medium at a concentration of $20 \times 10^6$ cells/mL.
2. The mouse should be gently warmed using a heat lamp to increase tail vein circulation, then placed in a suitable restrainer *(10)*, and the tail prepared with betadine and 70% alcohol.
3. The cell suspension is placed into a 1-mL syringe and 100 µL of the cell suspension is injected through a 30-gage needle into the lateral tail vein.

## 3.5. Small Animal Anesthesia (44) (see Note 2)

1. Turn on the oxygen tank. Check the tank meter to ensure that it reads between full and the top of the refill area (red).

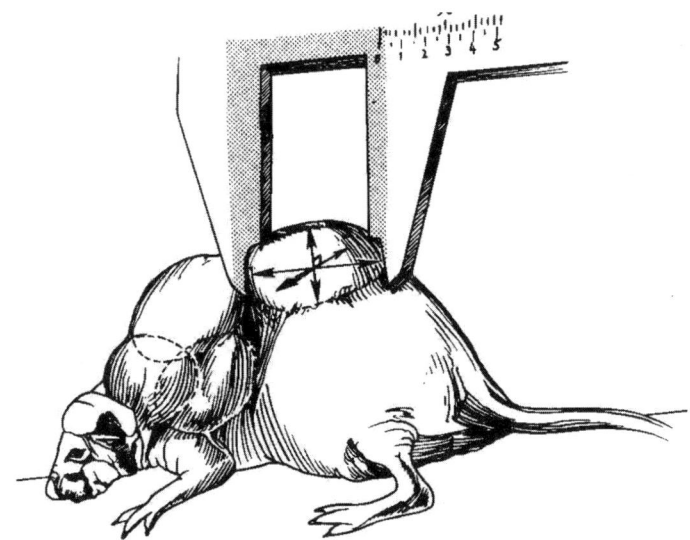

Fig. 1. Illustration of the method for measuring subcutaneous tumors in mice. Tumors are measured in three dimensions, the length (longest dimension), width (shorter dimension, perpendicular to the length), and height (diameter of tumor perpendicular to the length and the width. For multilobed tumors, individual lobes can be measured separately and summed to derive the entire tumor mass.

2. To begin the procedure the oxygen flow meter (green knob on left side of machine) must read 1 L.
3. Turn on (press button) isoflurane vaporizer to achieve 5% for induction. Closely observe the animal and continue until breathing is slow (appropriate anesthesia generally reached within 1 min).
4. After induction, reduce the isoflurane to 2.5% for maintenance of the anesthesia, adjust as necessary, and constantly monitor animals for breathing.
5. To prevent hypothermia, animals must be placed on a body-temperature controller until recovered from the anesthesia.
6. Mice can also be anesthetized by ip injection of a mixture of ketamine (50 mg/kg) and xylocaine (5 mg/kg), or by an ip injection of 2.5% Avertin (300 µL per 25-g mouse body weight). Pentobarbital sodium injection given ip at 40 mg/kg provides a suitable alternative.

### *3.6. Establishing Invasive Bone Tumors by Direct Injection*

1. Injection of certain tumor cell lines into the femur or tibia of immunocompromised mice can result in osteolytic lesions *(40,41)*.
2. To implant cells into the femur, anesthetized mice are placed in a lateral position and the skin overlying the knee and femur cleansed with betadine.

3. A small incision (8–10 mm) is made along the right knee, and the patellar tendon and muscle are split longitudinally to expose the distal femur.
4. A surgical scalpel tip or a 26-gage needle (stabilized with a drill holder) is used to drill a tiny hole in the cortex of the bone.
5. Tumor cells ($1 \times 10^5/\mu L$) are suspended in cell culture medium (without FBS) and 2–5 µL of medium + tumor cells are injected into the bone marrow space slowly via a 30-gage sterile needle attached to a Hamilton 10-µL syringe (Hamilton, Reno, NV).
6. The position of the needle in the marrow cavity can be confirmed by transillumination.
7. After injection, the needle is removed and the hole is sealed with bone wax, the patellar tendon reapproximated, and the skin closed with cyanoacrylate (Nexaband, Veterinary Products Lab, Phoenix, AZ).
8. Mice must be monitored carefully for signs of discomfort, and analgesics can be used immediately after initial surgery and at other times as indicated. Mice are euthanized if they show signs of significant discomfort.
9. A less labor-intensive approach involves injection into the tibia of the mouse, which requires anesthesia but no incision. Mice are maintained under isoflurane anesthesia during the tumor injection procedure.
10. The hair is shaved around the injection site and the skin surface at the injection site is prepped with betadine scrub followed by a 70% alcohol wipe.
11. A 25- or 26-gauge needle is inserted into the proximal joint of the tibia (through the tibial crest) to provide access to the bone marrow and is then removed.
12. Cells (also suspended in serum-free medium at $1 \times 10^5$ µL) are then injected (~2–5 µL) into the marrow cavity of the right hind leg tibial metaphysis, using a 30-gage needle attached to a Hamilton 10-µL syringe.

## *3.7. Determination of Therapeutic Effect in Murine Tumor Models (see Note 3)*

Regardless of whether survival data or tumor measurements are the primary end points, mice should be weighed throughout the course of the experiments, as body weight provides another means of assessing toxicity, usually done in terms of percentage change of body weight from the weight at start of the experiment. Here we will summarize approaches to measuring antitumor effect in both subcutaneous and disseminated disease models, which have been reviewed extensively elsewhere *(2,35,45)*.

### *3.7.1. Intracavitary or Disseminated Disease Models*

These models are attractive in that the tumor cells are often growing in physiologically more relevant tissues than is a subcutaneous xenograft. However, the difficulty (and often impossibility) of measuring the tumor prevents a serial determination of tumor progressive growth in treated vs control animals.

1. Assessing disease burden in leukemia or neuroblastoma can be done using flow cytometry or polymerase chain reaction (PCR) from serial blood samples *(10,34,46)*.
2. Nonetheless, the general end point remains survival from initiation of experiment until the animal is distressed or moribund (*see* **Note 4**).

### 3.7.2. Measures of Antitumor Effect in Disseminated Models

1. Percentage mean or median increase in life span = ratio of the survival time in days of treated animals to the survival time of the untreated control animals. This can be determined as percentage increase in lifespan (% ILS), which is calculated in days from initiation until a moribund state (or death) for treated vs control as % ILS = $[(T - C) / C] \times 100$ *(7)*.
2. An alternative to this is to calculate a $T / C$ ratio for days of survival (or lack of progression).
3. Kaplan-Meier (log-rank) survival analysis can be utilized *(47)*.
4. Net $\log_{10}$ cell kill = $T - C - $ (duration of treatment in days) $/ 3.32 \times T_d$. $T - C$ is the difference in the median day of death (moribund state) between the treated ($T$) and the control ($C$) cohorts *(7)*. The constant 3.32 is the number of doublings required for a population to increase on $\log_{10}$ unit, and $T_d$ is the mean doubling time of the tumor in days, calculated from a log-linear least-squares fit of tumor growth. For disseminated disease models, the latter value is difficult and perhaps impossible to obtain accurately.

### 3.7.3. Subcutaneous Tumor Models

These models have the advantages of (1) providing visual confirmation that 100% of the mice used in an experiment have tumors prior to therapy; and (2) providing a means of assessing tumor response or growth over time, with the latter providing more information than the increase in animal survival that can be measured in intracavitary models.

1. Subcutaneous tumor volumes should be measured as described under **Subheading 3.7.**
2. Data should be presented graphically as shown in **Fig. 2**, in which the growth over time for each mouse in the treated and control groups is shown. Averages of these data can also be displayed or calculated, but it is essential to present each of the mice separately to allow a full assessment of the data *(45)*. Some investigators prefer to do this on a linear scale, while others prefer a semilog scale.
3. For subcutaneous tumors, some experiments involve treating the mice prior to documentation of growing, progressing tumors. These "tumor growth delay" experiments suffer from the same need for high-take rates or large numbers of mice that was discussed under intracavitary models. Again, cross-sectional imaging may prove useful in defining the presence of disease in such models.
4. For models in which treatment begins after tumor growth is documented, often when tumors are at a size of 30–100 mm$^3$, usually two measurements showing

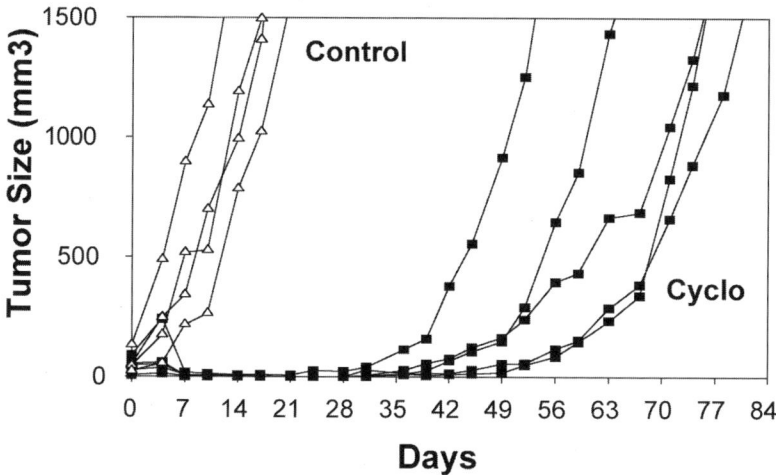

Fig. 2. Example of antitumor activity against a subcutaneous tumor xenograft from the CHLA-136 neuroblastoma cell line *(52)* in a nude mouse as assessed by serial measurements of tumor volume. Each line represents the tumor growth over time for an individual mouse. Shown are control mice (△) and mice treated for 5 d with daily injections (ip) of 156 mg/kg of cyclophosphamide (■).

   increasing tumor size prior to therapy are sufficient to establish tumor engraftment and progression.
5. Tumor volume should be measured twice weekly. The *T/C* ratio can be calculated as a T/C ratio = days to obtain a predefined tumor mass for the treated animals divided by the days to obtain the same size mass in the control animals. For example, with the data shown in **Fig. 2**, the T/C ratio was 3.9.
6. In addition, because the treated animals had a prolonged period without tumor progression, one could also calculate the median time to progression (TTP) at 31 d for the treated animals vs 3 d (first documented progression) for the controls.
7. Data can also be presented as a percent increase in lifespan (% ILS), which is calculated in days from initiation until a moribund state (or death) for treated vs control as % ILS = $[(T - C) / C] \times 100$ *(7)*.
8. Kaplan-Meier (log-rank) analysis of survival or time to progression can also be calculated *(47)*.
9. Analyzing growth of tumors over time has been done using a variety of mathematical approaches *(48–51)*. Although complex models (such as those employing the Gompertz function) are useful for studying growth properties and kinetics of xenografted tumors, they are not generally needed for assessing response to therapy, or in determination of xenograft doubling time, as the latter can usually be done accurately by linear regression *(51)*.

10. For subcutaneously growing tumors, a $\log_{10}$ cell kill can also be calculated as follows:

$$\log_{10} \text{ cell kill} = (T - C \text{ value in days}) / (3.32)(T_d)$$

where $T - C$ (tumor growth delay) = days to reach a defined mass for the treated animals − days to reach the same mass for the control animals; 3.32 is the $\log_{10}$ unit constant; $T_d$ is the doubling time for the tumor in days (derived from the doubling time of the control tumors using a $\log_2$ (linear regression) formula *(51)*.

## 3.8. Radiographic Assessment of Pulmonary Lesions

1. Mice are anesthesized under aseptic conditions and then are placed into Ziplock plastic sandwich bags to provide an aseptic barrier.
2. The Ziplock bags are sealed such that a pocket of the isofluorene/$O_2$ mixture is contained in the bag, providing sufficient gas for the few minutes needed to complete the X-ray.
3. To provide a magnification factor for the radiographs, mice are positioned 10.5 cm below the radiation source, and the film placed at the bottom of the Faxitron, 37.5 cm below the animal. This approach provides a magnification factor of 4 times, with the thoracic cavity of the mouse filling about half the area of the $18 \times 24$-cm mammography film. An example of pulmonary metastases from intravenous injection of a primitive neuroectodermal tumor (PNET) cell line in a SCID mouse is shown in **Fig. 3**.

## 3.9. Radiographic Assessment of Bone Lesions

1. To image bone lesions (direct-injection invasive lesions or metastases), radiographic procedures identical to those described for pulmonary lesions are employed, except that the mouse is positioned to ensure imaging of the lower portion of the mouse, including both legs.
2. We have developed a grading system for bone lesions in mice given direct tumor injection into the femur that provides quantitative scoring of the bone lesions (*see* **Note 5**). The grading system defines four grades: Grade 1 represents a normal bone when compared to the contralateral bone. Grade 2 lesions are asymmetric (relative to contralateral bone) and progressive radiolucent lesions limited to the site of injection. Grade 3 shows asymmetrical and progressive radiolucent areas extending beyond the distal femur. Grade 4 lesions contain a pathological fracture of the bone or a breach in the bone cortex.
3. The time to develop a Grade 4 lesion can be used as a relative end point to determine tumor progression and/or response to therapy *(41)*. An example of a lytic bone lesion from direct injection of a prostate cancer cell line into an athymic mouse is shown in **Fig. 4**.

## 4. Notes

1. Transfer of tumors in this fashion can be repeated many times, but to avoid genetic drift from the original cell line one should limit such transfers to six or less.

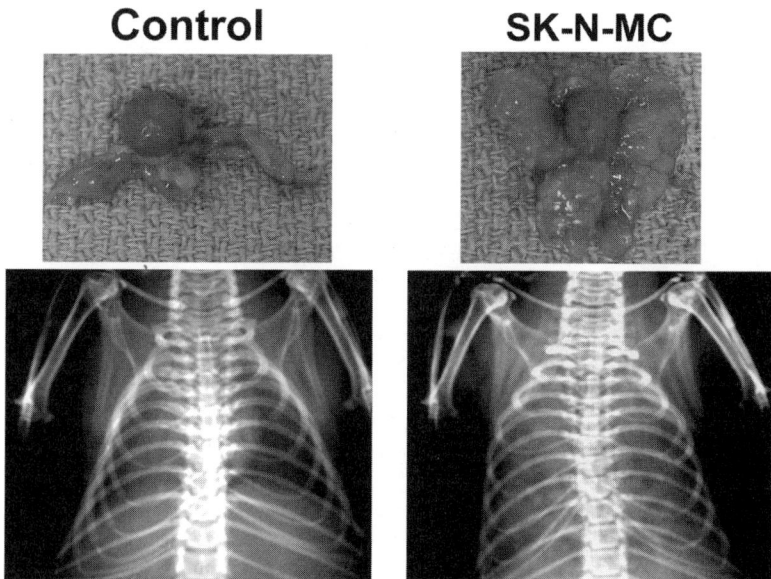

Fig. 3. Radiographic demonstration of experimental pulmonary metastases in a SCID mouse. Mice were injected in the lateral tail vein with $2 \times 10^6$ cells from the SK-N-MC primitive neuroectodermal tumor cell line *(53)*. After 8 wk, multiple pulmonary metastases can be visualized by Faxitron X-ray, which were not seen in the control mice. Postmortem examination confirmed that the lesions seen by X-ray were indeed multiple tumor nodules, visible on gross examination (right panel) and by histopathology (not shown).

2. Ensure that all instruments, animals, and caging are fully prepared before initiating the procedure. Check valves of all tubes and assure open air flow.
3. One approach in the past to measuring a therapeutic effect of a drug was to establish a tumor and then compare survival of treated to untreated mice. However, using actual survival as an end point is no longer acceptable, and mice that become distressed, or in particular those that are moribund, must be euthanized. Similarly, in the case of animals bearing subcutaneous tumors, when a predetermined tumor size (usually for mice this is a tumor $> 1500$ mm$^3$) is reached, the animal must be sacrificed. Thus, all survival data for subcutaneous tumors will reflect a combination of death for toxicity (or other events) and attaining a certain tumor size. By contrast, intracavitary or disseminated disease models will measure survival until death from toxicity, other events, or observation of obvious distress or a moribund state. Death of a treated animal should be presumed to be treatment-related if the animal dies within 15 d of the last therapy, unless death appears to be from tumor progression.
4. A secondary problem with these models is the need for a very high (ideally 100%) success rate for engrafting tumor. The high "take rate" is needed because even a

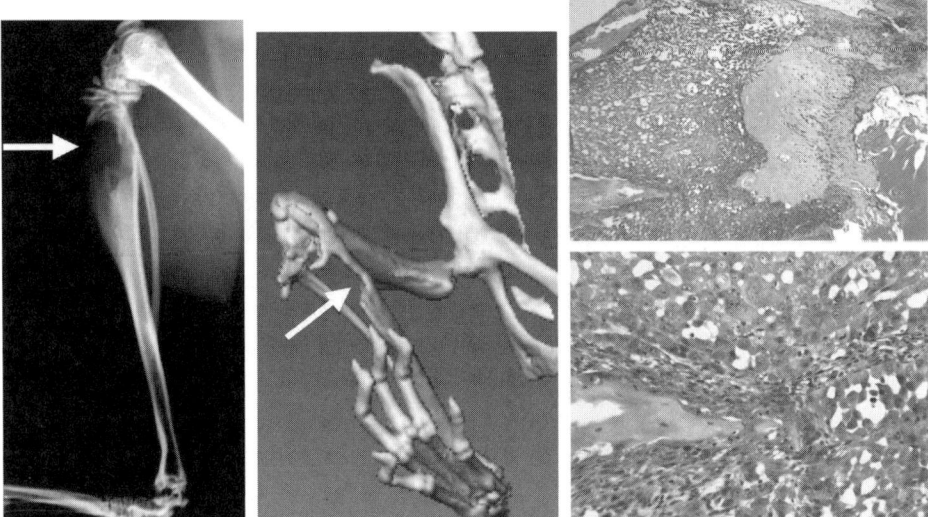

Fig. 4. Lytic lesion in bone of a SCID mouse given an intra-tibial injection of the PC-3 human prostate cancer cell line. Image in left panel from the Faxitron small-animal imager with high-resolution mammography film, middle panel is a 3-D reconstruction of the same lesion from the Micro-Cat CT system. Arrows point to the lytic lesion. Histology (low and high magnification) from the same lesion is shown in the right panel. (Histology photomicrographs courtesy of Hiro Shimada, MD.)

  95% "take rate" can result in the need for very large numbers of mice in any given therapeutic experiment to achieve statistical validity. One approach to overcome this problem would be the use of cross-sectional imaging to confirm disease (in a single observation) prior to starting therapy.
5. The scale is not independent of mouse strain especially at low values, i.e., values of 1 and 2. Thus, care should be taken to customize the scale for your particular strain.

## Acknowledgments

This work was supported in part by the Neil Bogart Memorial Laboratories of the T. J. Martell Foundation for Leukemia, Cancer, and AIDS Research, and by National Cancer Institute Grants CA82830, CA81403, and CA102990.

## References

1. Corbet, T. H., Polin, L., Roberts, B. J., et al. (2002) Transplantable syngeneic rodent tumors: solid tumors in mice, in *Tumor Models in Cancer Research* (Teicher, B. A., ed.), Humana Press, Totowa, NJ, pp 41–71.
2. Harrison, S. (2002) Perspective on the history of tumor models, in *Anticancer Drug Development Guide* (Teicher, B. A., ed.), Humana Press, Totowa, NJ, pp. 3–19.

3. Waud, W. R. (1997) Murine L1210 and P388 leukemias, in *Anticancer Drug Development Guide: Preclinical Screening, Clinical Trials, and Approval* (Teicher, B. A., ed.), Humana Press, Totowa, NJ, pp. 59–74.
4. Fiebig, H. H. and Burger, A. M. (2002) Human tumor xenografts and explants, in *Tumor Models in Cancer Research* (Teicher, B. A., ed.), Humana Press, Totowa, NJ, pp. 113–137.
5. Mattern, J., Bak, M., Hahn, E. W., and Volm, M. (1988) Human tumor xenografts as model for drug testing. *Cancer Metastasis Rev.* **7,** 263–284.
6. Houghton, P. J., Adamson, P. C., Blaney, S., et al. (2002) Testing of new agents in childhood cancer preclinical models: meeting summary. *Clin. Cancer Res.* **8,** 3646–3657.
7. Plowman, J., Dykes, D. J., Hollingshead, M., Simpson-Herren, L., and Alley, M. C. (1997) Human tumor xenograft models in NCI drug development, in *Anticancer Drug Development Guide: Preclinical Screening, Clinical Trials, and Approval* (Teicher, B. A., ed.), Humana Press, Totowa, NJ, pp. 101–125.
8. Shimosato, Y., Kameya, T., and Hirohashi, S. (1979) Growth, morphology, and function of xenotransplanted human tumors. *Pathol. Annu.* **14(pt 2),** 215–257.
9. Lock, R. B., Liem, N., Farnsworth, M. L., et al. (2002) The nonobese diabetic/ severe combined immunodeficient (NOD/SCID) mouse model of childhood acute lymphoblastic leukemia reveals intrinsic differences in biologic characteristics at diagnosis and relapse. *Blood* **99,** 4100–4108.
10. Lock, R. B., Liem, N. L., and Papa, R. A. (2005) Preclinical testing of antileukemic drugs using an in vivo model of systemic disease. *Chemosensitivity; Volume 2. In Vivo Models, Imaging, and Molecular Regulators* (Blumenthal, R. D., ed.), Humana, Totowa, NJ (in press, this volume).
11. Lehne, G., Sorensen, D. R., Tjonnfjord, G. E., et al. (2002) The cyclosporin PSC 833 increases survival and delays engraftment of human multidrug-resistant leukemia cells in xenotransplanted NOD-SCID mice. *Leukemia* **16,** 2388–2394.
12. Johnson, J. I., Decker, S., Zaharevitz, D., et al. (2001) Relationships between drug activity in NCI preclinical in vitro and in vivo models and early clinical trials. [see comment]. *Br. J. Cancer* **84,** 1424–1431.
13. Tomayko, M. M. and Reynolds, C. P. (1989) Determination of subcutaneous tumor size in athymic (nude) mice. *Cancer Chemother. Pharmacol.* **24,** 148–154.
14. Manzotti, C., Audisio, R. A., and Pratesi, G. (1993) Importance of orthotopic implantation for human tumors as model systems: relevance to metastasis and invasion. *Clin. Exp. Metastasis* **11,** 5–14.
15. Kubota,T. (1994) Metastatic models of human cancer xenografted in the nude mouse: the importance of orthotopic transplantation. *J. Cell. Biochem.* **56,** 4–8.
16. Khanna, C., Jaboin, J. J., Drakos, E., Tsokos, M., and Thiele, C. J. (2002) Biologically relevant orthotopic neuroblastoma xenograft models: primary adrenal tumor growth and spontaneous distant metastasis. *In Vivo* **16,** 77–85.
17. Khanna, C., Prehn, J., Yeung, C., Caylor, J., Tsokos, M., and Helman, L. (2000) An orthotopic model of murine osteosarcoma with clonally related variants differing in pulmonary metastatic potential. *Clin. Exp. Metastasis* **18,** 261–271.

18. Shoji, T., Konno, H., Tanaka, T., et al. (2003) Orthotopic implantation of a colon cancer xenograft induces high expression of cyclooxygenase-2. *Cancer Lett.* **195,** 235–241.
19. El Galley, R., Keane, T. E., and Sun, C. (2003) Camptothecin analogues and vinblastine in the treatment of renal cell carcinoma: an in vivo study using a human orthotopic renal cancer xenograft. *Urol. Oncol.* **21,** 49–57.
20. Kikuchi, E., Xu, S., Ohori, M., et al. (2003) Detection and quantitative analysis of early stage orthotopic murine bladder tumor using in vivo magnetic resonance imaging. *J. Urol.* **170,** 1375–1378.
21. Moats, R., Ma, L. Q., Wajed, R., et al. (2000) Magnetic resonance imaging for the evaluation of a novel metastatic orthotopic model of human neuroblastoma in immunodeficient mice. *Clin. Exp. Metastasis* **18,** 455–461.
22. Grimm, J., Potthast, A., Wunder, A., and Moore, A. (2003) Magnetic resonance imaging of the pancreas and pancreatic tumors in a mouse orthotopic model of human cancer. *Int. J. Cancer* **106,** 806–811.
23. Nelson, A. L., Algon, S. A., Munasinghe, J., et al. (2003) Magnetic resonance imaging of patched heterozygous and xenografted mouse brain tumors. *J. Neuro-Oncol.* **62,** 259–267.
24. Paulus, M. J., Gleason, S. S., Easterly, M. E., and Foltz, C. J. (2001) A review of high-resolution X-ray computed tomography and other imaging modalities for small animal research. [Erratum appears in *Lab Anim* (NY) 2001 May;30(5):13]. *Lab Anim* **30,** 36–45.
25. Paulus, M. J., Gleason, S. S., Kennel, S. J., Hunsicker, P. R., and Johnson, D. K. (2000) High resolution X-ray computed tomography: an emerging tool for small animal cancer research. *Neoplasia* (NY) **2,** 62–70.
26. Ito, S., Nakanishi, H., Ikehara, Y., et al. (2001) Real-time observation of micrometastasis formation in the living mouse liver using a green fluorescent protein gene-tagged rat tongue carcinoma cell line. [Erratum appears in *Int. J. Cancer* 2002 Feb 20;97(6):878]. *Int. J. Cancer* **93,** 212–217.
27. Hoffman, R. M. (1024) Visualization of GFP-expressing tumors and metastasis in vivo. *Biotechniques* **30,** 1016–1022.
28. Yang, M., Baranov, E., Jiang, P., et al. (2000) Whole-body optical imaging of green fluorescent protein-expressing tumors and metastases. *Proc. Natl. Acad. Sci. USA* **97,** 1206–1211.
29. Goto, H., Yang, B., Petersen, D., et al. (2003) Transduction of green fluorescent protein increased oxidative stress and enhanced sensitivity to cytotoxic drugs in neuroblastoma cell lines. *Mol. Cancer Ther.* **2,** 911–917.
30. Zhang, L., Hellstrom, K. E., and Chen, L. (1994) Luciferase activity as a marker of tumor burden and as an indicator of tumor response to antineoplastic therapy in vivo. *Clin. Exp. Metastasis* **12,** 87–92.
31. Rice, B. W., Cable, M. D., and Nelson, M. B. (2001) In vivo imaging of light-emitting probes. *J. Biomed. Optics* **6,** 432–440.

32. Edinger, M., Sweeney, T. J., Tucker, A. A., Olomu, A. B., Negrin, R. S., and Contag, C. H. (1999) Noninvasive assessment of tumor cell proliferation in animal models. *Neoplasia* (NY) **1,** 303–310.
33. El Hilali, N., Rubio, N., Martinez-Villacampa, M., and Blanco, J. (2002) Combined noninvasive imaging and luminometric quantification of luciferase-labeled human prostate tumors and metastases. *Lab. Invest.* **82,** 1563–1571.
34. Thompson, J., Guichard, S. M., Cheshire, P. J., et al. (2001) Development, characterization and therapy of a disseminated model of childhood neuroblastoma in SCID mice. *Cancer Chemother. Pharmacol.* **47,** 211–221.
35. Teicher, B. A. (2002) In vivo tumor response end points, in *Tumor Models in Cancer Research* (Teicher, B. A., ed.), Humana Press, Totowa, NJ, pp. 593–616.
36. Menon, K. and Teicher, B. A. (2002) Metastasis models Lungs, spleen/liver, bone, brain, in *Tumor Models in Cancer Research* (Teicher, B. A., ed.), Humana Press, Totowa, NJ, pp. 277–291.
37. Iwasaki, T., Mukai, M., Tsujimura, T., et al. (2002) Ipriflavone inhibits osteolytic bone metastasis of human breast cancer cells in a nude mouse model. *Int. J. Cancer* **100,** 381–387.
38. Yi, B., Williams, P. J., Niewolna, M., Wang, Y., and Yoneda, T. (2002) Tumor-derived platelet-derived growth factor-BB plays a critical role in osteosclerotic bone metastasis in an animal model of human breast cancer. *Cancer Res.* **62,** 917–923.
39. Peyruchaud, O., Winding, B., Pecheur, I., Serre, C. M., Delmas, P., and Clezardin, P. (2001) Early detection of bone metastases in a murine model using fluorescent human breast cancer cells: application to the use of the bisphosphonate zoledronic acid in the treatment of osteolytic lesions. *J. Bone Miner. Res.* **16,** 2027–2034.
40. Corey, E., Quinn, J. E., Bladou, F., et al. (2002) Establishment and characterization of osseous prostate cancer models: intra-tibial injection of human prostate cancer cells. *Prostate* **52,** 20–33.
41. Sohara, Y., Shimada, H, Scadeng, M, et al. (2003) Lytic bone lesions in a human neuroblastoma xenogaft show osteo-clast recruitment and are inhibited by ibandronate. *Cancer Res.* **63,** 3026–3031.
42. Worzalla, J. F., Bewley, J. R., and Grindey, G. B. (1990) Automated measurement of transplantable solid tumors using digital electronic calipers interfaced to a microcomputer. *Invest. New Drugs* **8,** 241–251.
43. Reynolds, C. P., Biedler, J. L., Spengler, B. A., et al. (1986) Characterization of human neuroblastoma cell lines established before and after therapy. *J. Natl. Cancer Inst.* **76,** 375–387.
44. Meyer, R. E., Braun, R. D., and Dewhirst, M. W. (2002) Anesthetic considerations for the study of murine tumor models, in *Tumor Models in Cancer Research* (Teicher, B. A., ed.), Humana Press, Totowa, NJ, pp. 407–431.
45. Begg, A. C. (1980) Analysis of growth delay data: potential pitfalls. *Br. J. Cancer Suppl.* **41,** 93–97.

46. Dialynas, D. P., Shao, L., Billman, G. F., and Yu, J. (2001) Engraftment of human T-cell acute lymphoblastic leukemia in immunodeficient NOD/SCID mice which have been preconditioned by injection of human cord blood. *Stem Cells* **19,** 443–452.
47. Fleming, T. R. and Lin, D. Y. (2000) Survival analysis in clinical trials: past developments and future directions. *Biometrics* **56,** 971–983.
48. G. Gordon Steel. (1977) *Growth Kinetics of Tumoours Cell Population Kinetics in Relations to the Growth and Treatment of Cancer.* Clarendon Press, Oxford.
49. Demicheli, R., Pratesi, G., and Foroni, R. (1991) The exponential-Gompertzian tumor growth model: data from six tumor cell lines in vitro and in vivo. Estimate of the transition point from exponential to Gompertzian growth and potential clinical implications. *Tumori* **77,** 189–195.
50. Rygaard, K. and Spang-Thomsen, M. (1997) Quantitation and gompertzian analysis of tumor growth. *Breast Cancer Res. Treatment* **46,** 303–312.
51. Zwicker, J. I., Proffitt, R. T., and Reynolds, C. P. (1996) A microcomputer program for calculating cell population doubling time in vitro and in vivo. *Cancer Chemother. Pharmacol.* **37,** 203–210.
52. Keshelava, N., Zuo, J. J., Chen, P., et al. (2001) Loss of p53 function confers high-level multi-drug resistance in neuroblastoma cell lines. *Cancer Res.* **61,** 5103–5105.
53. Wang, Y., Einhorn, P., Triche, T. J., Seeger, R. C., and Reynolds, C. P. (2000) Expression of protein gene product 9.5 and tyrosine hydroxylase in childhood small round cell tumors. *Clin. Cancer Res.* **6,** 551–558.

# 23

## Evaluation of Chemosensitivity of Micrometastases with Green Fluorescent Protein Gene-Tagged Tumor Models in Mice

### Hayao Nakanishi, Seiji Ito, Yoshinari Mochizuki, and Masae Tatematsu

#### Summary

The chemosensitivity of micrometastasis is an important factor in therapeutic approaches to micrometastasis. The protocol in this chapter presents procedures capable of examining the drug sensitivity of micrometastases to anticancer agents, especially those in the peritoneal cavity, lymph nodes, and the lung in mice. The protocol consists of green fluorescent protein (GFP) gene-tagged metastasis models in mice and unique detection devices for GFP. The latter include a small, convenient stereo fluorescent microscope for internal visualization of micrometastases at the cellular level with magnification and a handy GFP detection device for external, noninvasive monitoring of therapeutic effect of a drug without magnification. Mice are injected with GFP-tagged tumor cells and divided into an early and a late administration group according to the timing of drug administration. Early administration starts from 1–2 d postinjection for peritoneal and lung metastases and 2–3 wk after subcutaneous injection for lymph node metastasis, when the micrometastasis macroscopically remains invisible—less than 0.5 mm in maximum diameter—as confirmed by the detection device. The results thus obtained indicate that micrometastases are more sensitive to anticancer agents than advanced metastases. This system using GFP-tagged tumor models is an indispensable tool for micrometastasis research.

#### Key Words

Micrometastasis; chemosensitivity; anticancer drug; GFP; peritoneal metastasis; lymph node metastasis; hematogenous metastasis; gastric cancer; colorectal cancer.

### 1. Introduction

Micrometastasis has been defined as a minute metastasis smaller than 2 mm in diameter by UICC. More recently, this term has been divided into two categories: "isolated tumor cells," located in the lumen measuring less than 0.2 mm in diameter; and "micrometastases," which have already invaded the organ (*1*). Prognostic significance of micrometastasis varies in terms of size, tissue localization such as peritoneal cavity, lymph nodes, or blood, and therapeutic status. However, it is generally accepted that metastatic recurrence after curative resection in cancer patients results from free tumor cells in the body fluid and micrometastases in the regional and distant organs that were already present at the time of removal of the primary neoplasm. To decrease the recurrence of cancer patients, the development of diagnostic and therapeutic approaches to identifying such free tumor cells and micrometastases is therefore essential. Recently, much progress has been made in the genetic diagnosis of micrometastases in the peritoneal cavity, lymph nodes and for circulating tumor cells, by using real-time quantitative reverse-transcription polymerase chain reaction (RT-PCR) (*2–4*). For elimination of the micrometastases, postsurgical adjuvant chemotherapy is the treatment of choice. However, the validation of its effectiveness remains controversial, depending on the tumor type. Preclinical studies using an appropriate animal model on the chemosensitivity of free tumor cells and micrometastases to anticancer agents is therefore a leading approach to resolving this discrepancy problem. However, these investigations have been limited by the lack of well-characterized micrometastasis models enabling very small numbers of tumor cells to be specifically detected in the majority of the host tissue background. The chemosensitivity of micrometastases to anticancer agents has remained largely unclear.

The use of tumor cell lines transfected with marker genes such as the *LacZ* gene, encoding a bacterial galactosidase, greatly facilitates specific detection of small numbers of tumor cells (*5–7*). However, it requires fixation and subsequent staining of tissue and cannot visualize metastasis development in living animals. In contrast, green fluorescent protein (GFP), cloned from the genome of the jellyfish *Aequorea victoria* (**8**), is known to yield a bright, stable green fluorescence with no necessity for other substrates or cofactors in live cells. Hoffman et al. have first demonstrated the great advantages of GFP-tagged tumor cells for simple, specific, and sensitive detection of micrometastasis and for monitoring therapeutic effects of anticancer agents on metastasis in living mice (*9–14*). To date, using such marker gene-tagged models, the chemosensitivity of micrometastasis in the gastrointestinal tract, lung, and breast cancers has been evaluated (*7,15–17*). The results indicate that micrometastases at an early stage are more sensitive to anticancer agents than advanced metastases, so that therapeutic approaches targeted to the micrometastasis provide a potentially powerful strategy for protection of patients from metastatic recurrence. The protocol in this chapter describes the procedures based on the authors' in vivo experiments to examine the chemosensitivity of micrometastasis, focusing on those in the peritoneal cavity, lymph nodes, and the lung. Application to examining the chemosensitivity of "isolated tumor cells," a new micrometastasis category, is also covered in this protocol.

## 2. Materials
### 2.1. Animals and Drugs

1. 6–8-wk-old male *nu/nu* nude mice of KSN strain (purchased from Shizuoka Laboratory Animal Center, Hamamatsu, Japan).
2. S-1 (purchased from Taiho Pharmaceutical, Tokyo, Japan).
3. 0.5% carboxymethyl cellulose (CMC).
4. 1-mL syringe, 26-gage needles (Terumo, Tokyo, Japan).
5. Gastric tube.
6. 3-0 surgical suture (Ethicon, USA).
7. 2,2,2-Tribromoethanol anesthesia (Tokyo Kasei, Tokyo, Japan).

### 2.2. Cell Lines

1. GCIY (human gastric adenocarcinoma cell line, from RIKEN cell bank, Tsukuba, Japan); MKN-28 (human gastric adenocarcinoma cell, from RIKEN cell bank); COLM-2, COLM-5 (human colonic adenocarcinoma cell lines, established in our laboratory); RSC3-LM (rat tongue squamous carcinoma cell line, established in our laboratory) *(18)*.
2. GFP-expressing metastatic tumor cell lines; GFP-tagged human gastric cancer cell lines (GCIY-EGFP and MKN28-EGFP) *(17)*; GFP-tagged human colon cancer cell lines (COLM5-EGFP, COLM2-EGFP); GFP-tagged rat tongue cancer cell lines (RSC3LM-EGFP) *(13)*.
3. 0.125% Trypsin/2 m$M$ EDTA solution.
4. Hank's balanced salt solution (HBSS).
5. Dulbecco's Modified Eagle's Medium (DMEM).
6. Culture medium (DMEM supplemented with 10% fetal bovine serum, 100 U/mL penicillin and streptomycin).

### 2.3. Detection and Monitoring Apparatus

1. A small, convenient stereo fluorescent microscope system for GFP observation, model SZ40-GFP (Olympus, Tokyo, Japan), consisting of a stereomicroscope (SZ4045) and a 150-W-high brightness halogen lamp (LG-PS), is used to observe micrometastases internally with incision at magnification ranging from 6.7 to 40×. Under illumination of blue light produced through a bandpass filter (for excitation: 420–480 nm) (Omega Optical Inc., VT, USA) from the halogen source with a flexible guide, emitted GFP fluorescence from metastatic foci is collected through a long-pass cut filter (for emission: 520 nm) on a digital camera (D1H, Nikon, Tokyo, Japan). Oblique white-light illumination is also provided by a fiber-optic light source to enhance brightness **(Fig. 1A)**.
2. Digital images of 2000 × 1312 pixels are captured on a Windows PC with Nikon Capture 3 software.

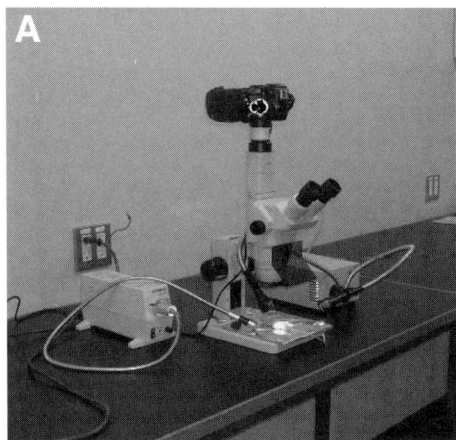 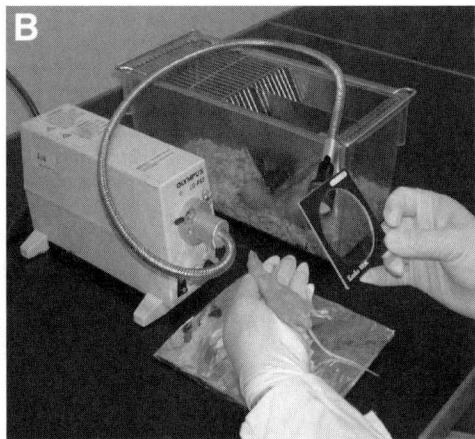

Fig. 1. Illustration of the detection and monitoring systems for GFP used in this study. **(A)** A convenient stereomicroscope system for detecting micrometastases, consisting of a stereomicroscope with 6.7–40-fold magnification and a high-brightness halogen lamp with bandpass filter (right side of the stereomicroscope). Mice are anesthesized and the abdominal wall or the skin is incised. After proper exposure of the omentum or lymph node, micrometastases or isolated tumor cells can be visualized at the cellular level. For enhancement of brightness, oblique white-light illumination by another halogen lamp without filter may also be used (left side of the stereomicroscope). **(B)** A handy GFP-detection device for monitoring the antimetastatic effect of the drug in tumor-bearing mice, consisting of a halogen lamp with a flexible guide and bandpass filter and a gelatin cut filter. Mice are held in the operator's hand, and the metastatic foci in the peritoneum or the inguinal lymph nodes are visualized by external illumination of the blue light in living mice, noninvasively and nonanesthetically.

3. A handy GFP-detection device, consisting of a 100-W halogen lamp (LG-PS2) with bandpass filter and a long-pass gelatin cut filter (Kodak, Rochester, NY), is used for monitoring the antimetastatic effect of the drug in tumor-bearing mice in the animal facility. Mice are held in the operator's hand, and the metastatic foci can be visualized by external illumination of blue light without excision in living mice, noninvasively and nonanesthetically **(Fig. 1B)**.

## 3. Methods
### 3.1. Micrometastasis Models (see Note 1)

1. GFP-tagged tumor cells are isolated by the transfection of tumor cells with the pEGFP-C1 plasmid (Clontech Laboratories, Palo Alto, CA) using the FuGENE6 transfection reagent (Roche Diagnostics, Basel, Switzerland) as described previously *(13)*.

2. Transfectants are first isolated in selection medium supplemented with 1.0-mg/mL geneticin (G418, Wako, Osaka, Japan).
3. G418-resistant colonies are further screened based on the intensity of their GFP fluorescence on the inverted fluorescence microscope (CKX41, Olympus) followed by ring cloning.
4. Resultant cell lines with bright GFP fluorescence are used in the study.

### 3.2. Micrometastasis Formation

1. Exponentially growing GFP-tagged tumor cells are harvested by treatment with 0.125% trypsin/2 m$M$ EDTA solution for 5 min at 37°C.
2. The cells are washed with HBSS twice.
3. The cells are resuspended in 0.2 mL HBSS for subcutaneous (sc) or intravenous (iv) injection and in 0.3 mL HBSS for intraperitoneal injection (ip).
4. Immediately after preparation, $5 \times 10^6$ tumor cell suspension is injected sc in the inguinal region, $1 \times 10^6$ cells iv through the lateral tail vein and $2 \times 10^6$ cells ip through the abdominal wall into the mouse using a 27-gauge syringe.
5. Possible micrometastasis formation is detected and subsequent metastasis development is monitored using GFP detection systems with or without magnification by a stereomicroscope as described above.

### 3.3. Assessment of Chemosensitivity of Micrometastasis vs Advanced Metastasis

#### 3.3.1. Chemosensitivity of Peritoneal Micrometastasis (see **Note 2**)

1. Mice are injected intraperitoneally with $2–3 \times 10^6$ GFP-tagged gastric cancer cells with peritoneal metastatic potential (GCIY-EGFP or MKN28-EGFP) and divided into an early and a late administration group according to the timing of drug administration **(Fig. 2)**.
2. All mice are examined externally, noninvasively and nonanesthetically, with a handy GFP-detection device to confirm metastasis formation at the omentum and mesentery in the peritoneal cavity at 1 d postinjection **(Fig. 3A,C)**.
3. In the early treatment groups, mice ($n = 10$) are administered the drug, for example S-1, an oral 5-fluorouracil [5-FU] derivative, with a gastric tube at a dose of 15–20 mg/kg/d five times per week from d 1 for at least 4 wk.
4. In the late-treatment groups, mice ($n = 10$) are administered the drug orally at the same dose and schedule from d 7 for at least 4 wk.
5. In the control groups, mice are administered vehicle (0.5% CMC) orally in the same manner.
6. Mice are monitored externally at least once a week for qualitative evaluation of inhibitory effects of the drug on peritoneal metastases in terms of nodular size and accumulation of ascites fluid by a handy GFP detection device **(Fig. 3B,D)**.
7. Survival and ascites accumulation of mice are compared between early and late adiministration groups. In our experience using the GCIY-EGFP model, nontreatment control mice died from massive ascites accumulation and subsequent

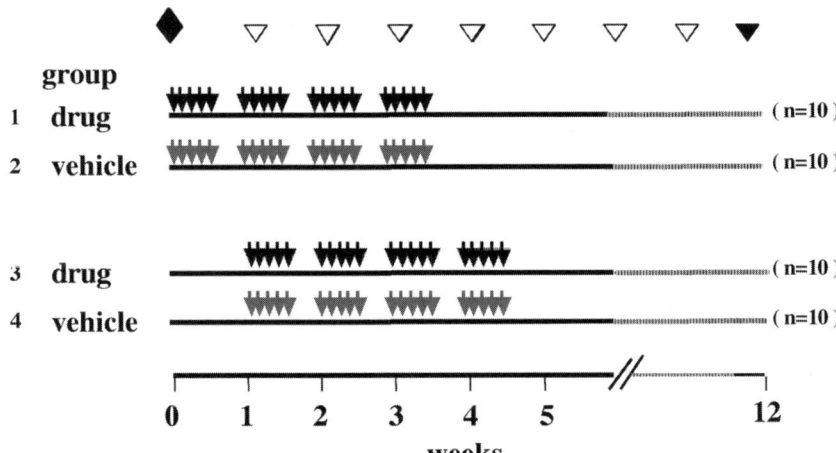

Fig. 2. Schematic representation of experimental protocol for assessment of chemosensitivity of micrometastasis—a peritoneal metastasis case as an example. Mice given an intraperitoneal injection of $2 \times 10^6$ tumor cells are administered the drug at the appropriate doses (group 1) or the vehicle (group 2) starting from d 1 postinoculation for at least 4 wk (early administration group). Mice given $2 \times 10^6$ cells are administered S-1 at the same dose and schedule (group 3 and 4) starting from d 7 postinoculation (late-administration group). (◆) injection of tumor cells. (▼) sacrifice. (▽) fluorescence monitoring by a handy GFP detection device.

intraabdominal hemorrhage within 10 wk postinjection. Late-administered mice survived longer, but all died within 12 wk. In contrast, early-administered mice showed at least in part a complete response without residual tumors or tumor dormancy with a prolonged NC (no change in tumor size) *(17)*.
8. In a separate experiment, mice are sacrificed at 8–10 wk after injection, metastatic nodules with GFP fluorescence and ascites in the peritoneal cavity are removed, and their weights and volumes are compared between groups for assessment of the tumor-diminishing effect of the drug.

### 3.3.2. Chemosensitivity of Lymph Node Micrometastasis (see **Note 3**)

1. Mice are injected subcutaneously into both right and left lower abdominal flanks with $5 \times 10^6$ GFP-tagged colonic and gastric cancer cells with lymph node metastatic potential (COLM5-EGFP or GCIY-EGFP) and divided into an early administration group and a late administration group according to the timing of drug administration.
2. In the early-treatment groups, primary subcutaneous tumors average 7–8 mm in diameter are resected at 2–3 wk postinjection under anesthesia. Before the resection, the inguinal lymph node, a regional lymph node of the subcutaneous tumor, is examined externally or internally through skin incision for micrometastases at

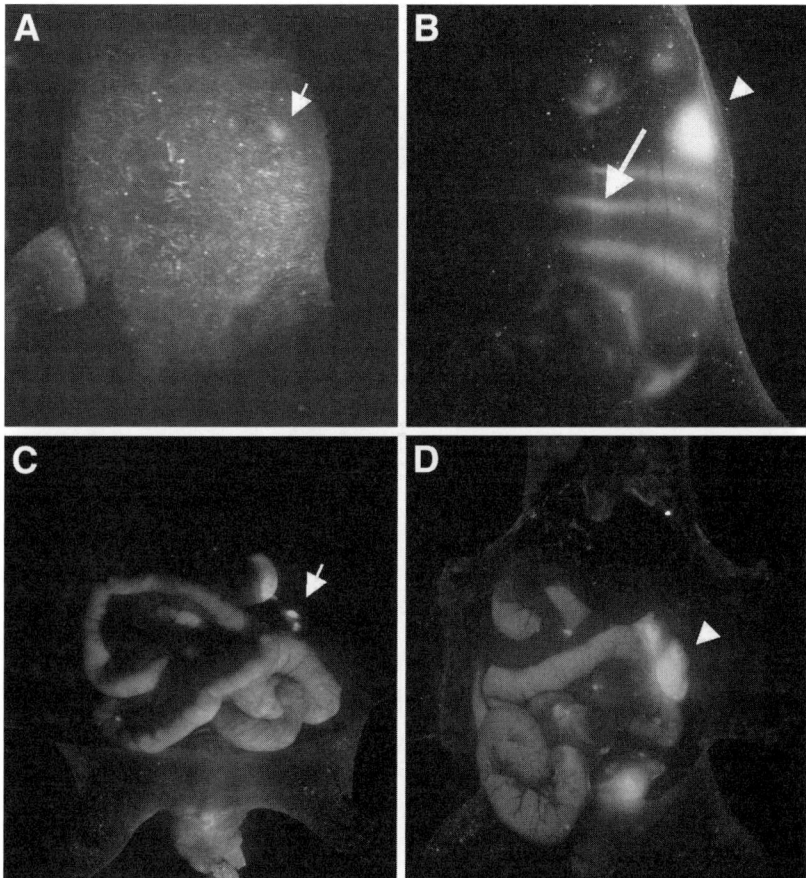

Fig. 3. Visualization of peritoneal micrometastasis after intraperitoneal injection of gastric cancer cells (GCIY-EGFP). External (**A,B**) and internal (**C,D**) visualization of peritoneal metastasis 1 d (**A,C**) and 3 wk (**B,D**) after injection. A small metastatic nodule with GFP fluorescence (small arrows) is observed on the omentum 1 d postinjection. Production of malignant ascites in a stripe-shaped pattern (large arrow) and enlarged metastatic nodules in the omentum (arrowheads) are revealed at 3 wk postinjection. (**C,D**) Photographs show peritoneal cavity after washing with saline.

    the cellular level with a model SZ40-GFP stereo microscope with 20–40X magnification (**Fig. 4A**). If micrometastases are absent, the mice are eliminated from the experimental group. Two days later, mice thus selected for positive micrometastasis ($n = 10$) are administered the drug, for example S-1, orally at a dose of 15–20 mg/kg/d five times per week until 12–13 wk postinjection.
3. In the late-treatment groups, primary tumors are resected at 5 wk postinjection. Before the resection, the presence of metastasis in the inguinal lymph nodes is

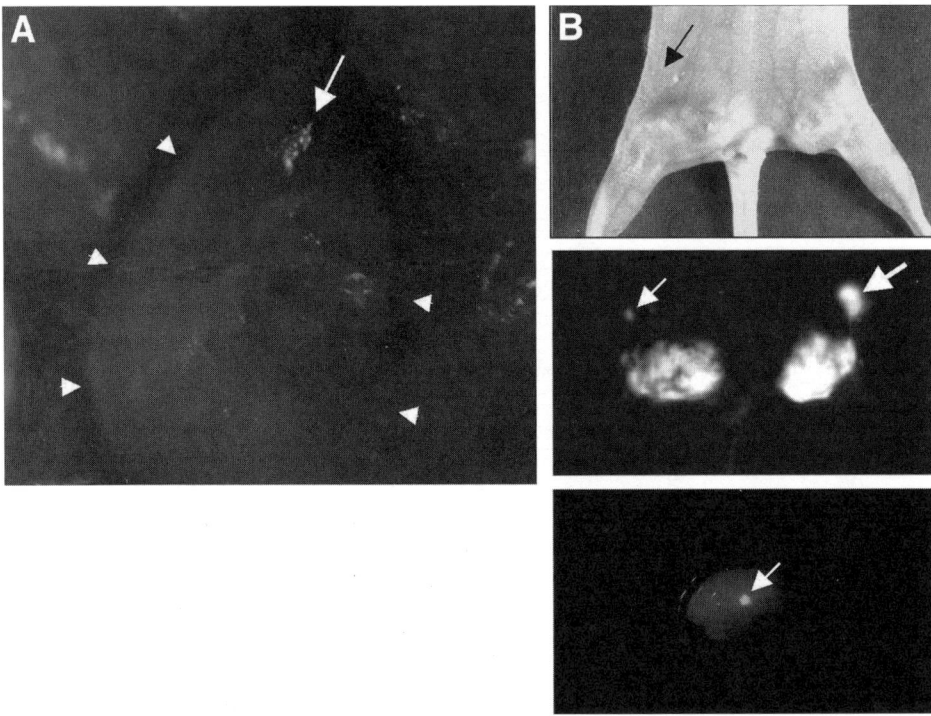

Fig. 4. Visualization of lymph node micrometastasis after subcutaneous injection of colon cancer cells (COLM5-EGFP). **(A)** Internal visualization of micrometastasis or isolated tumor cells in the inguinal lymph node through skin incision 2–3 wk after injection of tumor cells using a SZ40-GFP stereomicroscope with 20× magnification. Single cells and small cell clusters with GFP fluorescence (arrow) are seen in the upper region of a lymph node (arrowheads). **(B)** External visualization of micrometastasis in the inguinal lymph node at 5 wk after injection (upper and middle figure). A pinpoint focus (small arrow) and a macroscopically visible nodule with GFP fluorescence (large arrow) are observed in the right and left inguinal lymph nodes, respectively. Micrometastasis with GFP fluorescence (arrow) in the isolated right inguinal lymph node as shown in the above two figures is seen (lower figure).

confirmed externally with the SZ40-GFP stereomicroscope **(Fig. 4B)**. Two days later, mice ($n = 10$) are administered the drug orally at the same dose and schedule until 12–13 wk postinjection.

4. In the control groups, primary tumors are resected, and mice are administered vehicle (0.5% CMC) orally in the same manner.
5. Mice are monitored externally for inguinal lymph nodes metastasis once a week with a handy GFP detection device for qualitative estimation of the inhibitory effects of the drug on lymph node metastases.

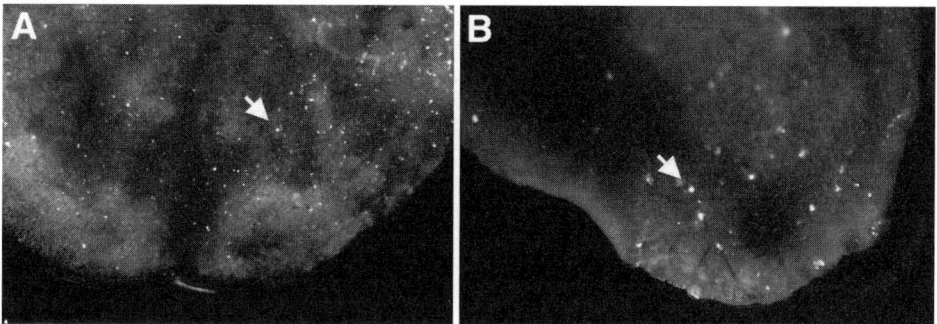

Fig. 5. Visualization of lung micrometastasis after intravenous injection of tongue carcinoma cells (RSC3LM-EGFP). Visualization of metastasis (arrows) in the lung at 1 d (**A**) and 7 d (**B**) after injection using a SZ40-GFP stereomicroscope with 10–20× magnification. Micrometastases increased in size from a single-cell level to small nodules with visible size.

6. At 12–13 wk after injection, mice are sacrificed and the inguinal lymph nodes are removed. Positivity rate for metastasis based on GFP fluorescence and their weight are measured and are compared between the early and late administration groups. Each node is then fixed in buffered formalin and the therapeutic effect is also evaluated histologically. In the COLM5-EGFP model, lymph node weights were significantly reduced by the drug in early-administered mice. Furthermore, positivity rate for lymph node metastasis was decreased by the early drug administration, indicating a complete response to the drug without residual metastasis in the lymph nodes of some mice. In contrast, no such remarkable inhibition was evident in late-administered mice (unpublished results).

### 3.3.3. Chemosensitivity of Lung Micrometastasis (see **Note 4**)

1. Mice are injected intravenously into the lateral tail vein with $1 \times 10^6$ GFP-tagged rat tongue carcinoma cells (RSC3LM-EGFP) and divided into an early administration group and a late administration group according to the timing of drug administration. In this model, many macroscopically invisible but GFP fluorescence-positive metastatic foci are observed on the lung surface at 1 d postinjection by SZ40-GFP stereomicroscope (**Fig. 5A**). This micrometastases model develops visible nodules at 7 d postinjection (**Fig. 5B**).
2. In the early-treatment groups, mice ($n = 10$) are administered the drug, for example S-1, orally at a dose of 15–20 mg/kg/d five times per week from d 1 for 4 wk.
3. In the late-treatment groups, mice ($n = 10$) are administered the drug orally at the same dose and schedule from d 7 for at least 4 wk.
4. In the control groups, mice are administered vehicle (0.5% CMC) orally in the same manner.
5. Survival of mice is compared between the early and late administration groups.

6. In a separate experiment, mice are sacrificed at 4–5 wk after injection, the lungs are removed, and the number of metastatic nodules with GFP fluorescence and lung weights are compared between the two groups.

## 4. Notes

1. For in vivo study using a GFP-tagged metastasis model, it is essential to isolate stable transfectants with bright GFP fluorescence strong enough to allow external monitoring without affecting biological properties of tumor cells. Stable GFP expression is required at least for more than 2 mo in vivo, and the required positivity level of the cells with bright GFP fluorescence is over 80–90%. All steps including transfection with pEGFP plasmid, G418 selection, and further enrichment of GFP-positive cells affect the efficiency of successful isolation of the useful transfectants. Among these, second selection of clones expressing strong GFP fluorescence after G418 selection seems critical. Most laboratories do not have their own cell sorter. Thus, a convenient isolation method is recommended, for example, in which GFP negative or weakly positive cells are removed by mechanical scraping under inverted fluorescence microscopy on a clean bench, followed by the cloning of bright GFP-positive colonies using a stainless ring with silicon grease.
2. In the GCIY-EGFP model, peritoneal metastases can be externally, noninvasively demonstrated selectively in the omentum and mesentery from 1 d postinjection of $2 \times 10^6$ tumor cells by a handy GFP detection device. This omental micrometastasis is less than 0.5 mm in diameter and cannot be easily recognized even after abdominal wall incision without the aid of blue-light illumination. Furthermore, this system can also detect "isolated tumor cells" at a single-cell level using a SZ40-GFP stereomicroscope. However, "isolated tumor cells" are relatively rarely observed in the omentum and thus there is no actual need for routine use of a stereo fluorescence microscope with high magnification for detecting peritoneal micrometastasis. It takes at least 7 d after injection for the omental metastasis to grow into visible nodular masses more than 2 mm in diameter. These findings indicate that the GFP-tagged tumor model in combination with a GFP-detection device is an indispensable tool for peritoneal micrometastasis research.
3. In the COLM5-EGFP model, inguinal lymph node metastases are first observed from 2–3 wk after subcutaneous injection of tumor cells. Such micrometastases vary in size from small cell clusters to nodular masses. Micrometastasis over 0.2 mm in diameter at the skin side of the node can be demonstrated, externally and noninvasively, by a handy GFP detection device. However, "isolated tumor cells" less than 0.2 mm in diameter or micrometastasis located at the opposite (abdominal) side of the inguinal lymph node can possibly be missed by the noninvasive method. Internal blue-light illumination of the inguinal lymph node through a skin incision, along with finger manipulation of the node by pulling or rotation, allows visualization of isolated tumor cells or dislocated micrometastasis in the lymph node with the aid of a SZ40-GFP stereo microscope.

4. In the RSC3LM-EGFP model, lung metastasis formed 1 d after intravenous injection of $1 \times 10^6$ tumor cells consists of a single cell and small cell clusters as visualized by blue-light illumination with a SZ40-GFP stereo microscope. The lung metastases grow and develop into visible nodules 1–2 mm in diameter at 7 d postinjection. However, unlike the two models described above, external detection of lung metastasis *in situ* is difficult with this model because of the disturbance of blue light by the thoracic wall.

## References

1. UICC (1997) *TNM Classification of Malignant Tumors*, 5th ed. (Sobin, L. H. and Wittekind, Ch., eds.), Wiley, New York.
2. Nakanishi, H., Kodera, Y., Yamamura, Y., et al. (2000) Rapid quantitative detection of carcinoembryonic antigen-expressing free tumor cells in the peritoneal cavity of gastric-cancer patients with real-time RT-PCR on the LightCycler. *Int. J. Cancer* **89,** 411–417.
3. Yoshioka, S., Fujiwara, Y., Sugita, Y., et al. (2002) Real-time rapid reverse transcriptase-polymerase chain reaction for intraoperative diagnosis of lymph node micrometastasis: clinical application for cervical lymph node dissection in esophageal cancers. *Surgery* **132(1),** 34–40.
4. Ito, S., Nakanishi, H., Hirai, T., et al. (2002) Quantitative detection of CEA expressing free tumor cells in the peripheral blood of colorectal cancer patients during surgery with real-time RT-PCR on a Light Cycler. *Cancer Lett.* **183(2),** 195–203.
5. Lin, W. C., Pretlow, T. P., Pretlow, T. G. D., and Culp, L. A. (1990) Development of micrometastases: earliest events detected with bacterial *LacZ* gene-tagged tumor cells. *J. Natl. Cancer Inst.* **82,** 1497–1503.
6. Kobayashi, K., Nakanishi, H., Masuda, A., Tezuka, N., Mutai., M., and Tatematsu, M. (1997) Sequential observation of micrometastasis formation by bacterial *lacZ* gene-tagged Lewis lung carcinoma cells. *Cancer Lett.* **112,** 191–198.
7. Nakanishi, H., Kobayashi, K., Nishimura, T., Inada, K., Tsukamoto, T., and Tatematsu, M. (1999) Chemosensitivity of micrometastases and circulating tumor cells to uracil and tegafur as evaluated using *LacZ* gene-tagged Lewis lung carcinoma cell. *Cancer Lett.* **142,** 31–41.
8. Misteli, T. and Spector, D. L. (1997) Applications of the green fluorescent protein in cell biology and biotechnology. *Nat. Biotechnol.* **15,** 961–964.
9. Chishima, T., Miyagi, Y., Wang, X., et al. (1997) Cancer invasion and micrometastasis visualized in live tissue by green fluorescent protein expression. *Cancer Res.* **7(10),** 2042–2047.
10. Yang, M., Baranov, E., Jiang, P., et al. (2000) Whole-body optical imaging of green fluorescent protein-expressing tumors and metastases. *Proc. Natl. Acad. Sci. USA* **97(3),** 1206–1211.
11. Hoffman, R. M. (1999) Orthotopic transplant mouse models with green fluorescent protein-expressing cancer cells to visualize metastasis and angiogenesis. *Cancer Metastasis Rev.* **17,** 271–277.

12. Hoffman, R. M. (2002) Green fluorescent protein imaging of tumour growth, metastasis, and angiogenesis in mouse models. *Lancet Oncol.* **3(9),** 546–556.
13. Ito, S., Nakanishi, H., Ikehara, Y., et al. (2001) Real-time observation of micrometastasis formation in the living mouse liver using a green fluorescent protein gene-tagged rat tongue carcinoma cell line. *Int. J. Cancer* **91,** 212–217.
14. Mochizuki, Y., Nakanishi, H., Kodera, Y., et al. (2004) TNF-α promotes progression of peritoneal metastasis as demonstrated using a green fluorescence protein (GFP)-tagged human gastric cancer cell line. *Clin. Exp. Metastasis* **21,** 39–47.
15. Kurebayashi, J., Nukatsuka, M., Fujioka, A., et al. (1997) Postsurgical oral administration of uracil and tegafur inhibits progression of micrometastasis of human breast cancer cells in nude mice. *Clin. Cancer Res.* **3,** 653–659.
16. Nakanishi, H., Abe, A., Inada, K., Tsukamoto, T., Yasui, K., and Tatematsu, M. (1999) Induction of apoptosis in metastatic foci from human gastric cancer xenografts in nude mice and reduction of circulating tumor cells in blood by 5-FU and 1-hexylcarbamoyl-5-fluorouracil. *J. Cancer Res. Clin. Oncol.* **125,** 660–668.
17. Nakanishi, H., Mochizuki, Y., Kodera, Y., et al. (2003) Chemosensitivity of peritoneal micrometastases as evaluated using a green fluorescence protein (GFP)-tagged human gastric cancer cell line. *Cancer Sci.* **94(1),** 112–118.
18. Takeuchi, S., Nakanishi, H., Yoshida, K., et al. (2000) Isolation of differentiated squamous and undifferentiated spindle carcinoma cell lines with differing metastatic potential from a 4-nitroquinoline N-oxide-induced tongue carcinoma in a F344 rat. *Jpn. J. Cancer Res.* **91,** 1211–1221.

# 24

## $^{99m}$Tc-Annexin A5 Uptake and Imaging to Monitor Chemosensitivity

### Tarik Z. Belhocine and Francis G. Blankenberg

#### Summary

Most anticancer agents act by inducing apoptosis in sensitive tumor cells. Hence, in many types of cancers, significant increase of tumor apoptosis after chemotherapy correlates with tumor chemosensitivity. Theoretically, a reliable evaluation of apoptotic changes, postchemotherapy to baseline, may provide valuable insights into the apoptotic competence of cancers. Until now, assessment of chemosensitivity has usually relied upon histological evidence of tumor response (i.e., partial or complete disappearance of tumor cells) or demonstration of tumor shrinkage by means of morphological imaging (i.e., computed tomography or magnetic resonance imaging). In clinical practice, however, these conventional methods are proving ineffective for monitoring tumor chemosensitivity on a daily basis. Recent developments in molecular imaging have allowed the synthesis of a new radiolabeled agent, $^{99m}$Tc-recombinant human Annexin A5, designed to the assessment of apoptotic response of cancers after a single course of chemotherapy. Such in vivo technique opens promising perspectives for evaluating, noninvasively and early, tumor response to anticancer therapies. Alternative methods for Annexin A5 labeling and imaging may improve the detection of drug-induced apoptosis to monitor chemosensitivity.

#### Key Words

Chemosensitivity; apoptosis; cancer; tumor response; $^{99m}$Tc-Annexin A5.

## 1. Introduction

Tumors are genetically diverse and can be resistant to the cytotoxic effect of any single or combination of anticancer drugs *(1–3)*. As ineffective therapy negatively impacts the patient's survival and may cause severe and irreversible side effects, early and definitive assessment of the efficacy of a specific anticancer therapy would greatly improve the quality of life as well as overall disease management *(4–7)*.

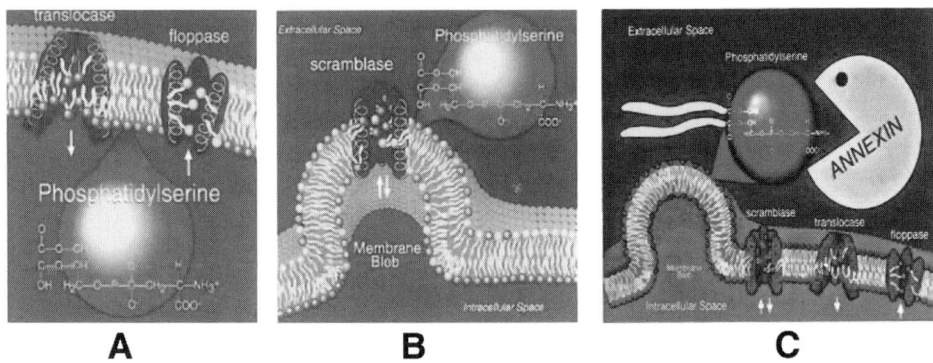

Fig. 1. Molecular basis for Annexin A5 imaging. (**A**) Homeostasis: phosphatidylserine (PS) is normally maintained at the inner leaflet of the cell membrane by translocase and floppase enzymes; (**B**) Apoptosis: externalization of phosphatidylserine to the outer leaflet of cell membrane surface following scramblase activation; event occurring early during the apoptotic cascade (90–120 min); (**C**) Phagocytosis: Calcium-dependent binding of Annexin V to PS with a high affinity ($K_d \approx 5 \times 10^{-10}$ $M$); exposure of PS is also a specific signal for recognition and removal of apoptotic cells by macrophages. (See color insert following p. 238.)

Current response criteria used by most oncology centers, however, rely on gross evaluation of changes in tumor size after weeks of treatments, an interval of time during which a nonresponding tumor may continue to grow while the patient suffers unnecessarily from the side effects of chemotherapy *(8)*. New molecular insights into carcinogenesis and chemosensitivity center on the key role of programmed cell death, also called apoptosis, as the main pathway involved in tumor response to treatment *(9–12)*. Specific molecular events leading to apoptotic cell death following anticancer therapies are attractive checkpoints for the assessment of chemosensitivity. As such, the enzymatically controlled redistribution of phosphatidylserine (PS) from the inner to outer leaflet of the plasma membrane phospholipid bilayer appears to be an ideal target for measuring apoptotic changes early in the course of chemotherapy *(13,14)* (*see* **Fig. 1**).

Recombinant human Annexin A5 (rh-Annexin A5), an endogenous human protein, binds specifically to PS (*see* **Note 1**), which is externalized on the cell surface *(15,16)* (*see* **Fig. 2**). Owing to its nanomolar affinity for PS, fluorescein labeled rh-Annexin A5 has been widely used in flow cytometry for the detection of apoptotic and necrotic cells in vitro *(17)*. More recently, $^{99m}$Tc[technetium]-radiolabeled rh-Annexin A5 was successfully used in several animal and human models to provide noninvasive imaging of programmed cell death in vivo *(18–30)*.

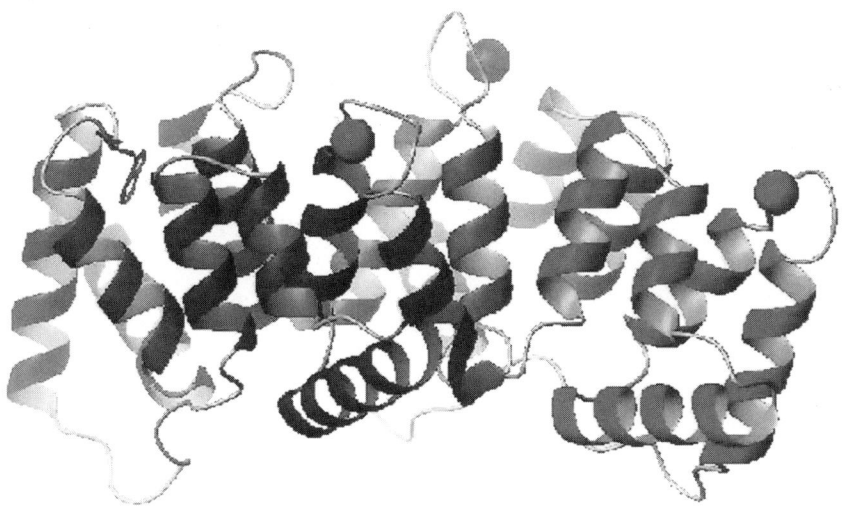

Fig. 2. Molecular structure of human Annexin A5. Crystallographic analysis of human Annexin A5 showed that the protein includes 320 amino acid residues with polypeptide chain folded into a planar cyclic arrangement of four repeats with similar structures of five α-helical segments wound into a right-handed compact superhelix. Three calcium sites (red spheres) have been identified in repeats I (red), II (violin), and IV (blue), while repeat III (green) has a different conformation at this site without any calcium-binding sites. (See color insert following p. 238.)

In this chapter we describe the methodology used in the first pilot study including oncology patients, explored by $^{99m}$Tc-rh-Annexin A5 after a single course of chemotherapy *(31)*. Results of this and other studies using various forms of radiolabeled Annexin A5 are summarized in **Tables 1–3**. We also discuss recent developments in methods and techniques that may help improve Annexin A5 imaging in clinical practice.

## 2. Materials
### 2.1. Radiolabeling of BTAP-rh-Annexin A5

The first clinical oncology imaging study to use $^{99m}$Tc-Annexin A5 was performed in a population of 15 patients with lymphoma and metastatic breast carcinoma of the chest as well as primary lung carcinoma who were undergoing primary chemotherapy *(31)*. The technique relies on the use of the preformed phentioate ligand to obtain the $^{99m}$Tc-rh-AnnexinA5-4.5-bis-thioacetamido-pentanoyl ($^{99m}$Tc-BTAP-rh-Annexin A5) as apoptosis tracer (*see* **Fig. 3A**), a procedure of labeling described by Kasina and Fritzberg as the $N_2S_2$ method *(32)*.

## Table 1
Biodistribution of $^{99m}$Tc-Annexin A5 in Animals (% injected dose per organ)

| % ID/organ | Annexin A5 BTAP-1H | Annexin A5 HYNIC-1H | Annexin A5 EC-30min | Annexin A5 Mutant-117-1H |
|---|---|---|---|---|
| Kidney | 19.11 | 39.16 | 6.97 | 6.17 |
| Liver | 4.67 | 16.59 | 3.95 | 5.97 |
| Bone | 0.42 | 0.18 | ND | 0.14 |
| Spleen | 4.17 | 0.88 | 1.31 | 0.28 |
| Small intestine | 5.08 | 3.31 | 0.20 | 4.18 |
| Large intestine | 5.08 | 0.88 | 0.20 | 1.15 |
| Stomach | 0.44 | 0.88 | 0.25 | 1.69 |
| Lung | 1.04 | 0.61 | 0.54 | 0.40 |
| Heart | 0.51 | 0.14 | ND | 0.07 |
| Thymus | 0.11 | 0.05 | ND | 0.04 |
| Skeletal muscle | 0.12 | 0.03 | 0.09 | 0.03 |
| Brain | ND | 0.01 | ND | 0.02 |
| Carcass | ND | 32.64 | ND | 23.05 |
| Blood | 0.97 | 0.39 | 0.91 | 0.36 |

## Table 2
Biodistribution and Dosimetry of $^{99m}$Tc-Annexin A5 in Humans

| % Injection dose per organ (% ID/organ) | BTAP-Annexin A5[a] (+70 min post-iv) | IM-Annexin A5[b] (+ 4h post-iv) | HYNIC-Annexin A5[c] (+ 3h post-iv) |
|---|---|---|---|
| Kidney | 27.7 ± 8.0 | 21.0 ± 5.6 | 49.7 ± 8.1 |
| Liver | 20.2 ± 4.4 | 12.8 ± 2.2 | 13.1 ± 1.0 |
| Bone marrow | 4.6 ± 2.2 | 4.2 ± 1.6 | 9.2 ± 1.8 |
| Spleen | 2.8 ± 0.8 | 2.5 ± 1.3 | 4.6 ± 1.6 |
| Testes | 0.24 ± 0.08 | 0.51 ± 0.1 | 0.16 ± 0.04 |
| Thyroid | 0.28 ± 0.12 | 0.21 ± 0.11 | 0.14 ± 0.08 |
| Percent blood clearance (half-life) | 87 % (26 ± 5 min) | 52 % (14 ± 6 min) | 92 % (24 ± 3 min) |
| Fraction excreted in urine (% ID) | 57% ± 12 at 20 h | 21.3% ± 6.3 at 20 h | 22.5% ± 3.5 at 24 h |
| Fraction excreted in feces (% ID) | 7 ± 8% at 20 h | 6.6 ± 2% at 20 h | 0.11% ± 0.18 at 24 h |
| Effective dose (µSv/MBq) | 7.6 ± 0.5 | 9.7 ± 1.0 | 11.0 ± 0.8 |
| Biological half-life (h) | 16 ± 7 | 62 ± 13 | 69 ± 7 |
| Radiochemical purity | 96% ± 4% | 82% ± 12% | 94% ± 1.7% |

[a]Annexin A5-4.5-bis-thioacetamido-pentanoyl-Tc$^{99m}$ (Apomate™, Theseus Imaging Corporation, USA).
[b]Annexin A5-(n-1-imino-4-mercaptobutyl)-Tc$^{99m}$ (Mallinckrodt™, Petten, The Netherlands).
[c]Annexin A5-hydrazinonicotinamide-Tc$^{99m}$ (Hynexin™, Theseus Imaging Corporation, USA).

## Table 3
## Radiolabeling Methods Available for Annexin A5 Imaging

| Isotopes | Half-life | Emission types | Nuclear imaging | Linkers | Radiolabeled Annexin A5 for imaging apoptosis |
|---|---|---|---|---|---|
| $^{99m}$Tc | 6.0 h | Gamma | SPECT | BTAP | $^{99m}$Tc-BTAP-Annexin A5 |
| $^{99m}$Tc | 6.0 h | Gamma | SPECT | HYNIC | $^{99m}$Tc-HYNIC-Annexin A5 |
| $^{99m}$Tc | 6.0 h | Gamma | SPECT | IM | $^{99m}$Tc-IM-Annexin A5 |
| $^{99m}$Tc | 6.0 h | Gamma | SPECT | EC | $^{99m}$Tc-EC-Annexin A5 |
| $^{99m}$Tc | 6.0 h | Gamma | SPECT | Directly* | $^{99m}$Tc-Annexin A5-mutant 117 |
| $^{111}$In | 2.80 d | Gamma | SPECT | DTPA-PEG | $^{111}$In-DTPA-PEG-Annexin A5 |
| $^{11}$C | 20 min | Beta + | PET | Directly* | $^{11}$C-Annexin A5 |
| $^{123}$I | 13.2 h | Gamma | SPECT | Directly* | $^{123}$I-Annexin A5 |
| $^{124}$I | 4.18 d | Beta + | PET | –Indirectly**<br>–Directly *** | $^{124}$I-IBA-Annexin A5†<br>$^{124}$I-Annexin A5 |
| $^{68}$Ga | 67.6 min | Beta + | PET | DOTA | $^{68}$Ga-DOTA-Annexin A5 |
| $^{18}$F | 109.7 min | Beta + | PET | –Indirectly¶<br>–Directly* | $^{18}$F-FBA-Annexin A5‡<br>$^{18}$F-(mini)-Annexin A5¶¶ |

Abbreviations and symbols: Gamma, gamma-rays (photons); Beta +, positive beta-particles (positrons); SPECT, single-photon emission tomography; PET, positron emission tomography; BTAP, 4,5-bis (thioacetamido) pentanoyl; HYNIC, hydrazinonicotinamide; IM, n-1-imino-4-mercaptobutyl; EC, L,L-ethylenedicysteine; DTPA-PEG, diethylenetriaminepentaacetic acid-polyethyleneglycol; Directly*, direct labeling with no linker; Indirectly**, indirect method for iodination of Annexin A5 using the N-succinimidyl 3-(4-hydroxy-3-[$^{124}$I]iodophenyl)propionate, also called water-soluble Bolton-Hunter reagent; Directly***, direct method for iodination of Annexin A5 using IodoGen (1,3,4,6-tetrachloro-3,6-diphenylglycouril) or IodoBeads (N-chlorobenzenesulfonamide); †IBA, [$^{124}$I]m-iodobenzoate-Annexin A5; DOTA, 1,4,7,10-tetraazacyclododecane-N,N′,N″,N‴-tetraacetic acid; ¶Indirectly, indirect method for labeling the Annexin A5 protein with [18F] using the Nsuccinimidyl-4-[18F]fluorobenzoate; ‡ FBA: 4-[$^{18}$F]fluorobenzoyl-Annexin A5; ¶¶$^{18}$F-(mini)-Annexin A5, an 8-kDa miniprotein derived from the specific binding domain of annexin A5 for phosphatidylserine was designed for labeling with $^{18}$F using a novel fluorine-labeled maleimide reagent (*see* **ref. 50**).

1. 0.28 mg phenthioate ligand.
2. 45 mg stannous gluconate complex containing sodium gluconate; 0.79 mg stannous chloride dihydrate.
3. 0.16 mL glacial acetic acid–0.2 N hydrochloric acid 1:7 (v/v).
4. Rh-Annexin A5 containing 1.2 mg in 1.2 mL phosphate-buffered saline (PBS).
5. Sephadex G-25 gel filtration columns.
6. 15–30 mCi (555–1110 MBq) sodium pertechnetate Tc99m.

The kit used in this clinical study for the preparation of $^{99m}$Tc-BTAP-rh-Annexin A5 (Apomate™) provided all the nonradioactive reagents needed for reaction with sterile (*see* **Note 2**), nonpyrogenic technetium to obtain $^{99m}$Tc-rh-Annexin A5 tracer suitable for intravenous injection (*see* **Note 3**).

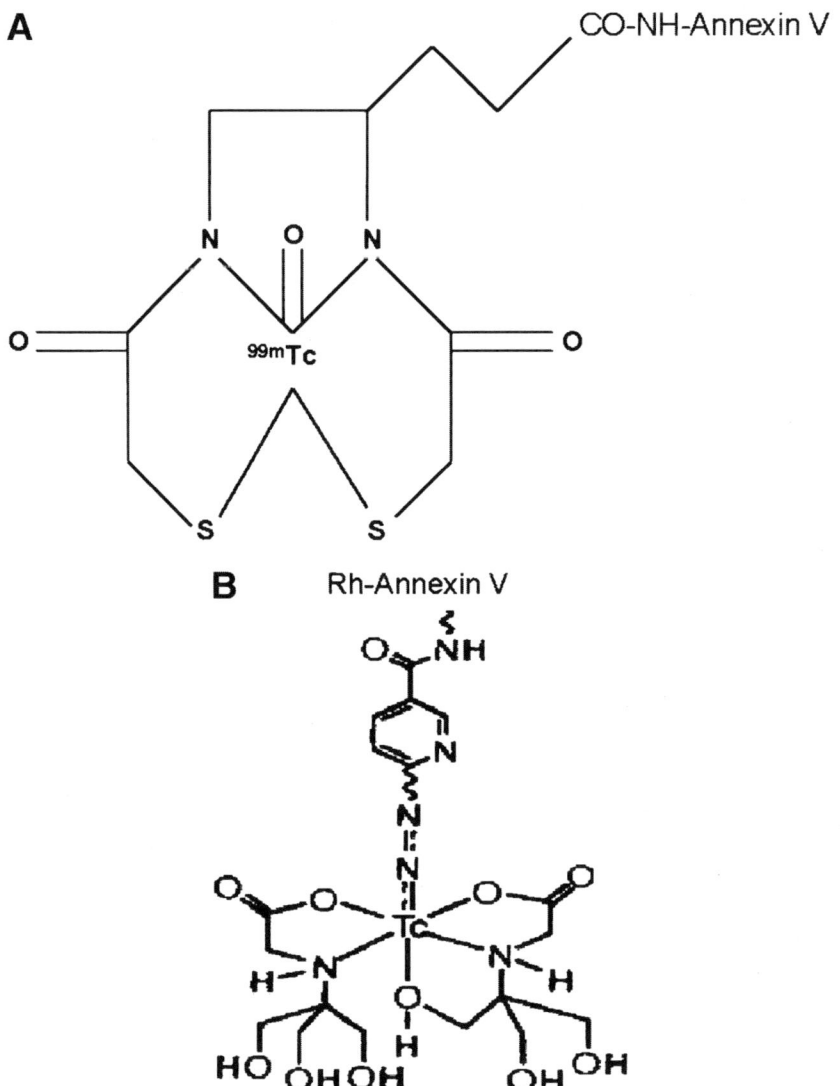

Fig. 3. Chemical structure of $^{99m}$Tc-radiolabeled Annexin A5. (**A**) Structure of $^{99m}$Tc-BTAP-rh-Annexin A5. (**B**) Structure of $^{99m}$Tc-HYNIC-rh-Annexin A5.

## 2.2. Radiolabeling of HYNIC-rh-Annexin A5

The technical limitations inherent to the labeling procedure of $^{99m}$Tc-BTAP-rh-Annexin A5 and its suboptimal biodistribution for imaging have led to the introduction of the HYNIC (hydrazinonicotinamide)-rh-Annexin A5 molecule labeled with $^{99m}$Tc (NAS 2020) (*see* **Note 4** and **Fig. 3B**) for current and future

# Annexin A5 Imaging

clinical trials in the United States and Europe (*see* **Notes 5** and **6**). The details for use of NAS 2020, a clinical kit limited to investigational use are

1. 0.25 mg HYNIC-rh-Annexin A5 conjugate (vial 1).
2. 200 µg stannous chloride dihydrate.
3. 17 mg tricine (N[Tris(hydroxymethyl)methyl]-glycine) (vial 2).
4. 27 mg sodium chloride.
5. 15–25 mCi (555–925 MBq) sodium pertechnetate Tc99m.

## 2.3. Procedural Precautions

1. The user must adhere to strict aseptic procedure during the preparation, withdrawal, and administration of the $^{99m}$Tc rh-Annexin A5 tracer.
2. Accurate measurement of small volumes is required for successful kit preparation, necessitating the use of insulin syringes.
3. The $^{99m}$Tc rh-Annexin A5 labeling depends on maintaining the stannous ion in reduced state. The technetium generator must be eluted at a time that ensures that 120–150 mCi is obtained in a volume of 1.0 mL. Otherwise, an aliquot of high-specific-concentration $^{99m}$Tc material on days an Annexin A5 labeling is scheduled.

## 2.4. Storage Conditions

1. Store all materials in sterile and nonpyrogenic conditions.
2. Store the vials of HYNIC-Annexin A5 solution and the stannous tricine complex (lyophilized) vials in a freezer at –20°C until time for preparation of the radiopharmaceutical for administration to a study subject.

# 3. Methods

The development of a new radiopharmaceutical dedicated to the imaging of drug-induced apoptosis as marker of chemosensitivity requires (1) a correct preparation of the tracer, (2) an appropriate imaging procedure, and (3) optimal timing for imaging cell death following anticancer therapies. These are described under **Subheadings 3.1.–3.3.**

## 3.1. Preparation of the Apoptosis Tracer

### 3.1.1. Procedure for $^{99m}$Tc-BTAP-rh-Annexin A5

The preparation of $^{99m}$Tc-rh-Annexin A5 tracer consists of six major steps:

1. Preliminary preparation of two G-25 Sephadex columns for purification of the $^{99m}$Tc rh-Annexin A5 protein or "column wash."
2. Formulation of ligand by aseptically injecting 0.90 mL of isopropyl alcohol into the phentioate ligand vial.

3. Formation of $^{99m}$Tc ligand ester using 120–150 mCi sodium pertechnetate $^{99m}$Tc solution in a volume of 1.0 mL. The shielded reaction vial is then placed into a shielded water bath at 70°C ± 5°C for 15 min.
4. Reaction of $^{99m}$Tc ligand ester with the protein to form the covalent conjugate. The radioactive reaction mixture is incubated in a shielded container at room temperature for 20 min.
5. Purification of the conjugate on a Sephadex G-25 gel filtration column.
6. Final dilution for patient administration (*see* **Notes 2** and **3**).

### 3.1.2. Procedure for $^{99m}$Tc-HYNIC-rh-Annexin A5

The preparation of $^{99m}$Tc-HYNIC-rh-Annexin A5 tracer consists of two major steps:

1. Aseptic addition of 30–40 mCi $^{99m}$Tc-pertechnetate (1110–1480 MBq) into the HYNIC-Annexin A5 conjugate vial 1; radiolabeling procedure conducted at room temperature (*see* **Note 4**).
2. Reconstitution of the lyophilized stannous tricine (vial 2) with sterile saline; 0.3 mL of the stannous tricine solution is then aseptically added to the HYNIC-Annexin A5 vial.

### 3.1.3. Procedure for Quality Control

1. Radiochemical purity of radiolabeled protein, determined by means of ITLC chromatography, should be ≥ 85%.
2. Range pH of the $^{99m}$Tc-HYNIC-rh-Annexin A5 product should be neutral (6–8).
3. Tracer solution ready for administration should be clear, limpid, and colorless. Any presence of color, particulate matter, or other extraneous material contraindicates its use.
4. The final dosage should be used as soon as possible after preparation but no longer than 6 h.
5. The dose required for injection is 15–25 mCi of $^{99m}$Tc-HYNIC-rh-Annexin A5.
6. The vial or syringe containing the final dosage must be stored shielded at 2–8°C.
7. The tracer is administered intravenously, preferentially through an iv line, in 3–5 min.

## 3.2. Procedure for Imaging Apoptosis with $^{99m}$Tc-rh-Annexin A5

The labeling of recombinant human Annexin A5 with $^{99m}$Tc allows the detection of an apoptotic signal in target tumors with conventional nuclear medicine procedures *(31,33)*. The scintigraphic acquisition may include either dynamic sequences (immediately postinjection) or early static views (+15–30 min). Late static views (+4–6 h) focused on tumor areas initially identified with morphologic imaging (magnetic resonance or computed tomography) as well as whole-body scans may be performed. However, tomographic views in SPECT (single photon emission computed tomography) are strongly recommended (*see*

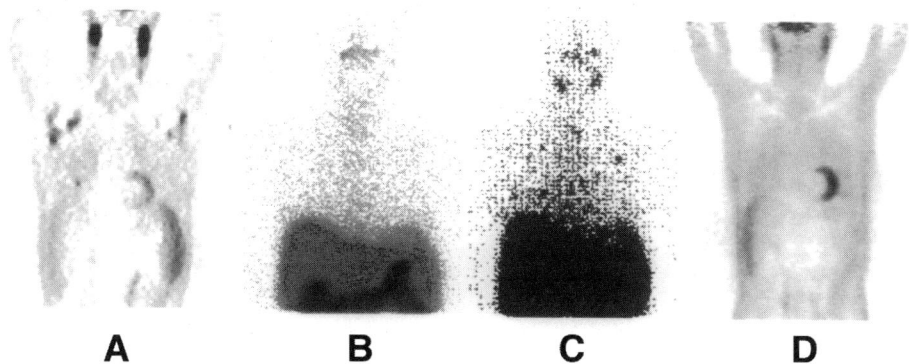

Fig. 4. Increased Annexin A5 uptake in a case of non-Hodgkin's lymphoma with complete response post-CHOP treatment. A pretreatment $^{18}$FDG PET scan detected cervical and axillary lymph nodes (**A**). In comparison to baseline (**B**), $^{99m}$Tc-BTAP-Annexin A5 showed increased uptake of apoptosis tracer at the level of cervical and left axillary nodes 48 h after the first course of chemotherapy (**C**). A follow-up $^{18}$FDG PET scan 6 mo later confirmed complete response to treatment (**D**).

**Notes 5** and **6**). A pretreatment imaging session may serve as in vivo control for comparison to posttreatment imaging sessions (**Fig. 4**), thereby allowing qualitative and quantitative assessment of Annexin A5 uptake (*see* **Notes 7** and **8**). Recently, other chemical forms of radiolabeled Annexin A5 based on different linkers and radionuclides have been designed either for SPECT imaging (*see* **Note 9**) or for positron emission tomography (PET) (*see* **Note 10**). Alternative methods for Annexin A5 labeling and imaging are detailed in **Table 3**.

### 3.3. Optimal Timing for Imaging Apoptosis with $^{99m}$Tc-rh-Annexin A5

Our experience with $^{99m}$Tc-HYNIC-Annexin A5 and $^{99m}$Tc-BTAP-Annexin A5 in animal and human cancer models showed that the optimal timing for imaging drug-induced apoptosis ranged from the 24th to the 72nd hour following the first course of chemotherapy *(13,26,32,35,36)* (*see* **Note 11**). Recent data assessed the dynamics of tracer uptake using the Annexin A5 mutant form 117 at different times after a single injection of Doxorubicin to Balb/c mice (lymphoma-bearing with transgenic tumor cells expressing the luciferase gene for bioluminescent imaging [BLI]) or in untreated mice and naïve mice. A biphasic increase of Annexin A5 uptake at biodistribution confirmed by radionuclide imaging was defined by an initial sharp increase followed by a decrease of Annexin A5 uptake occurring between 1 and 5 h, followed by a lag phase and a second longer sustained rise in Annexin A5 uptake in treated tumors 9–24 h after Doxorubicin injection (*see* **Fig. 5**). A decrease in tumor cell signal as seen by BLI, however, was not detected until 10–16 h posttreatment in vivo, followed by a massive tumor cell loss within 24 h (20% and 10% initial tumor burden at 24 h and 32 h posttreatment, respectively) and complete loss of tumor signal within 4 d (*see* **Fig. 6**). Therefore, Annexin A5 uptake into the tumor is not a gradually increasing process and is undetectable at 48 h, although tumor eradication is not complete at this time. This might reflect the rapid clearance of cells with an inversion of PS by macrophages, a phenomenon that stresses the importance of early Annexin A5 imaging, before tumor cell death and clearance of PS-expressing cells by macrophages (*see* **Note 12**).

## 4. Notes

1. Annexin A5 is a 36-kDa human protein encoded by a gene located on human chromosome 4q26→q28 that spans a region of DNA 28 kb in length containing 13 exons and 12 introns. The active Annexin A5 provided in the kit for investigational purposes is produced by recombinant techniques in *Escherichia coli*. Annexin A5 has selective affinity for PS. The $K_d$ for the binding of Annexin A5 to PS is estimated to be $5 \times 10^{-10}$ $M$. The number of Annexin A5-binding sites on apoptotic tumor cells has been estimated at $6–24 \times 10^6$, while normal red blood cells have as few as 275 Annexin A5-binding sites per cells. The stoichiometry of Annexin A5-binding PS ranges between four and eight Annexin A5 molecules per one PS molecule *(13–16)*. Apomate™ is the trade name of $^{99m}$Tc-BTAP-rh-Annexin A5 (North American Scientific, Theseus Imaging Division, 101 Arch Street, Suite 1762, Boston, MA 02110, USA).

2. The $N_2S_2$ method described in this chapter (**Subheadings 2.1.** and **3.1.1.**) leads to a high labeling rate and a high radiochemical purity yield. This technique, however, remains time-consuming, with six major steps necessitating at least 2 h of preparation and including a boiling step *(31–33)*.

3. One of the major disadvantages of the $N_2S_2$ method, in addition to the complexity and length of the radiolabeling procedure, is the hepatic uptake and excretion of BTAP-Annexin A5 into the digestive system, which precludes imaging within the abdomen *(31,32,34)*.

4. Both animal and human studies showed more favorable biodistribution of HYNIC-Annexin A5 compared to BTAP-Annexin A5, allowing the imaging of apoptosis throughout the entire body (*see* **Tables 1** and **2**). The preparation of $^{99m}$Tc-HYNIC-Annexin A5 takes approximately 30 min and includes only two steps, without the need for boiling *(34–36)*. Multicentric clinical trials are going on to assess its feasibility in oncology patients (NAS 2020 study).

5. SPECT imaging may be particularly useful to localize increased uptake of $^{99m}$Tc-radiolabeled Annexin A5 in three-dimensional space, especially when the apoptotic site is relatively small. Moreover, in some tumor types with high spontaneous apoptosis such as lymphomas, a pretreatment SPECT will be required to determine the uptake of tracer at baseline prior to postchemotherapy imaging *(31,33)*.

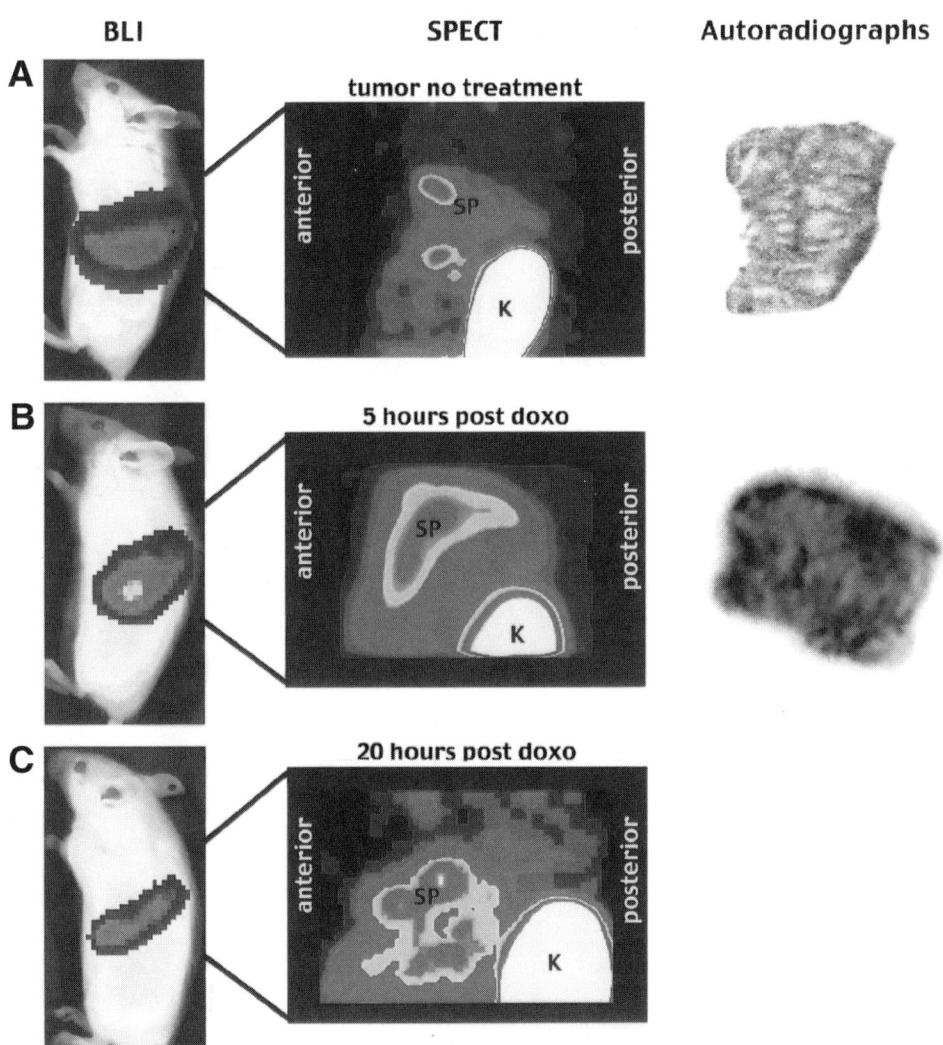

Fig. 5. $^{99m}$Tc-Annexin A5 uptake as seen by SPECT and autoradiography: *(left panel)* BLI left lateral image of a tumor-bearing mouse; *(middle panel)* sagittal small-animal SPECT image from the corresponding mouse; *(right panel)* autoradiographs of a representative frozen section of diseased spleen from the corresponding mouse. Autoradiographs of mouse: (**A**) control, tumor-bearing animal that was left untreated; (**B**) tumor-bearing animal 5 h post-Doxorubicin treatment; (**C**) tumor-bearing animal 20 h post-Doxorubicin treatment. (See color insert following p. 238.)

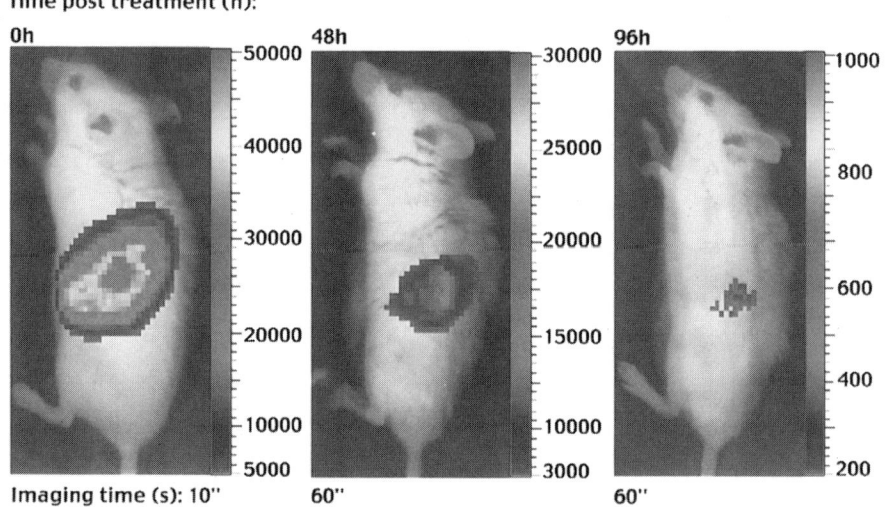

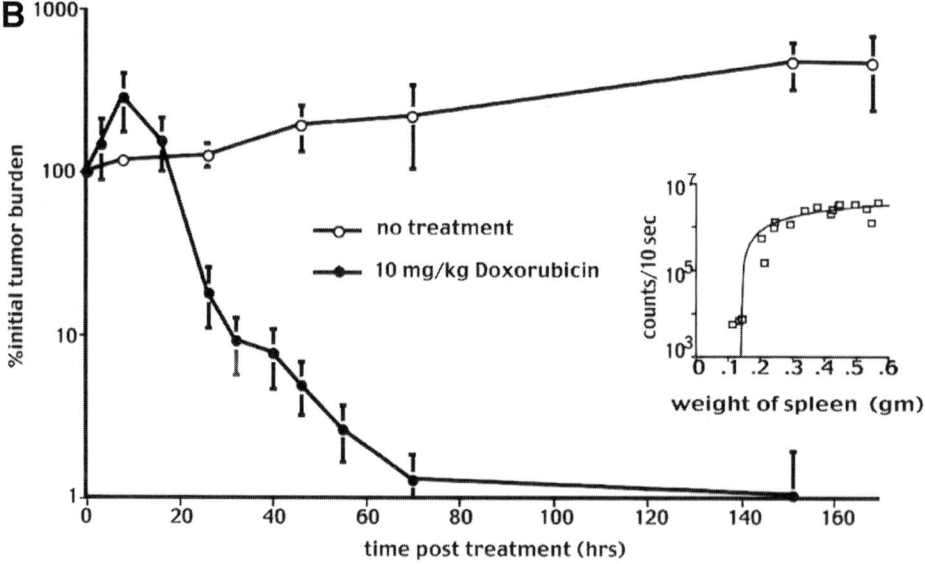

Fig. 6. Evaluation of tumor regression post-doxorubicin treatment by serial BLI. (**A**) Representative example of tumor regression in a single mouse over 4 d. (**B**) Quantification of tumor regression as measured by BLI: $n = 4$ animals in each group. Small insert: correlation between tumor burden measured by BLI and spleen weight in grams ($r^2 = 0.76$; $p = 9.11 \times 10^{-9}$); BLI, bioluminescence imaging. (See color insert following p. 238.)

*Annexin A5 Imaging* 375

6. Apoptotic changes achievable in human solid tumors following chemotherapy most often occur in a limited range (two- to sixfold over prechemotherapy) *(2)*. Even though the minimal mass required for in vivo imaging of cell death is not known, it is likely that SPECT imaging will require significant apoptosis (in at least 10% of cells) to detect the process in a small mass of tissue (~2–3 g) *(21)*. Accordingly, a few apoptotic cells within a large tumor mass may be missed by conventional SPECT imaging because of a poor signal-to-background ratio *(37)*.
7. The contrast level defined by the signal (apoptosis)-to-background (no apoptosis) ratio is the key criterion for any nuclear medicine imaging procedure. $^{99m}$Tc-BTAPrh-Annexin A5 shows high nonspecific renal, liver, spleen, and colon retention, on dynamic radionuclide imaging sequences and whole-body scans producing poor imaging contrast in the abdomen *(31,33,34)*. Recent developments with HYNIC chelator may improve the imaging contrast by reducing bowel uptake, but the high nonspecific renal and liver retention remains problematic *(20,35)*.
8. For oncological applications of the labeled Annexin A5, the accurate determination of apoptotic changes, posttreatment to baseline, is the key element to assess chemosensitivity. Accurate quantification of Annexin A5 uptake requires scrupulous respect of imaging conditions before and after treatment. For instance, the injection dose, the timing of imaging, the type of gamma camera, the acquisition protocol, the software used for digitalized analysis, and also the interpretation criteria, should not significantly differ from a prechemotherapy study to a postchemotherapy study *(31,33)*.
9. Among radiolabeled Annexin A5 forms designed for SPECT imaging, L,L-ethylenedicysteine (EC), the most stable of $N_2S_2$ chelators, has been proposed for labeling the Annexin A5 protein *(38)*. Experimental data showed that EC-Annexin A5 conjugate could be labeled with $^{99m}$Tc easily and efficiently with high radiochemical purity and stability. In addition, a murine model of mammary tumors demonstrated that $^{99m}$Tc-EC-Annexin A5 radionuclide imaging of apoptosis is feasible following irradiation and paclitaxel treatment. Another attractive method uses radiolabeled Annexin A5-117, a self-chelating mutant of Annexin A5 that does not employ specific linkers for $^{99m}$Tc chelation. Annexin A5 117 has been genetically engineered to incorporate an endogenous chelation site for $^{99m}$Tc using glucoheptonate as an exchange reagent. Labeling of Annexin A5 117 is therefore very simple and rapid and can routinely achieve high specific activities. Moreover, $^{99m}$Tc-Annexin A5-117 showed a much lower uptake in the kidney and the liver as compared to HYNIC-Annexin A5 *(39)*. This reduces radiation dose to these target organs and may allow the imaging of renal apoptosis (*see* **Table 1**). In addition, bone marrow uptake is also lower in normal control animals without compromising relative increased uptake of Annexin A5 in response to cyclophosphamide-induced apoptosis. Importantly, there is also less nonspecific uptake in the carcasses of animals injected with Annexin A5-117 mutant as compared to HYNIC-Annexin A5, which may improve target-to-background ratio for most imaging studies. Other authors have proposed the use of polyethyleneglycol (PEG)-Annexin A5 labeled with $^{111}$In (indium-111) to enhance the intratumoral penetration

of Annexin A5. Experimental data showed increased circulating time of $^{111}$In-PEG-Annexin A5 with significant enhancement of its blood extraction toward apoptotic tumor areas *(40)*. Still using conventional nuclear medicine procedures, Annexin A5 was successfully radiolabeled with iodine-123 ($^{123}$I) by means of electrophylic substitution, which gave radiochemical yields up to 70% and specific activities in the range of 7.4–92.5 MBq/µg. Furthermore, $^{123}$I-labeled-rh-Annexin A5 maintained its biological activity, thereby, allowing the imaging of apoptosis *(41)*.

10. An exciting new field of investigation is the radiolabeling of Annexin A5 with β-emitting radionuclides for PET imaging. Recent data report the feasibility of $^{11}$C (carbon-11), $^{124}$I (iodine-124), $^{68}$Ga (gallium-68), and also $^{18}$F (fluorine-18), for labeling the Annexin A5 with a high and stable radiochemical yield *(42–51)*. Experimental data showed that $^{11}$C-Annexin A5, $^{124}$I-Annexin A5, and $^{18}$F-Annexin V were all able to localize at tumor sites treated by proapoptotic drugs *(42–46, 48–51)*. These imaging findings were confirmed by TUNEL and caspase-3 staining of excised target tissues. Since PET is known to be superior to SPECT in terms of spatial resolution and lesion detectability, substantial improvements are expected for qualitative and quantitative imaging of apoptosis (*see* **Table 3**). In addition, hybrid cameras combining PET plus CT in a single device may help apoptotic changes occurring in untreated (spontaneous apoptosis) and treated (induced apoptosis) tumors to be precisely localized at the microscopic and macroscopic levels *(52–54)*.

11. The kinetics of tumor cells death may vary when considering different cancers and therapies. This may be due to factors such as tumor accessibility and the mechanism of tumor cell death, and therefore optimal imaging times may vary for each therapeutic regimen and possibly for different tumor types *(1–3,6,25,31,33,55,56)*. Individual assessment of tumor susceptibility to various proapoptotic drugs may help define the best timing for imaging apoptosis on a patient-by-patient basis. It remains to be determined if multiple posttreatment Annexin A5 scans will improve our assessment of therapeutic efficacy.

12. While no clear explanation is provided yet, the early peak of Annexin A5 uptake prior to tumor cell death is reproducibly observed at several time points (between 1 and 5 h) in repeated animal experiments. The Annexin A5 uptake at 9–24 h postchemotherapy correlates with acute phase of cell death observed by BLI in a murine lymphoma model *(57–60)*. In line with this, recent data with human lymphoma cell cultures treated with Taxol at clinically relevant drug concentrations showed that the apoptosis tracer should be injected in the first 6–12 h after start of treatment, with radionuclide imaging following 4–6 h later *(56,61)*.

## Acknowledgments

The authors thank Drs. Allan Green and Neil Steinmetz (North American Scientific, Theseus Imaging Division) for providing the clinical kits with the recombinant human Annexin A5 to investigational use. The authors also thank Dr. Pierre Rigo (Department of Nuclear Medicine, University Hospital of

Liège, Belgium) for his helpful assistance during the first oncology imaging study with the Annexin A5-BTAP-Tc99m.

## References

1. Staunton, M. J. and Gaffney, E. F. (1995) Tumor type is a determinant of susceptibility to apoptosis. *Am. J. Clin. Pathol.* **103**, 300–307.
2. Symmans, W. F., Volm, M. D., Shapiro, R. L., et al. (2000) Paclitaxel-induced apoptosis and mitotic arrest assessed by serial fine-needle aspiration: implications for early prediction of breast cancer response to neoadjuvant treatments. *Clin. Cancer Res.* **6**, 4610–4617.
3. Ghosh, M., Crocker, J., and Morris, A. (2001) Apoptosis in squamous cell carcinoma of the lung: correlation with survival and clinicopathological features. *J. Clin. Pathol.* **54**, 111–115.
4. Fox, E., Curt, G. A., and Balis, F. M. (2002) Clinical trial design for target-based therapy. *Oncologist* **7**, 401–407.
5. Dive, C., Evans, C. A., and Whetton, A. D. (1992) Induction of apoptosis—new targets for cancer chemotherapy. *Semin. Cancer Biol.* **3**, 417–427.
6. Workman, P. (2002) Challenges of PK/PD measurements in modern drug development. *Eur. J. Cancer* **38**, 2189–2193.
7. Workman, P. and Kaye, S. B. (2002) Translating basic cancer research into new cancer therapeutics. *Trends Mol. Med.* **4 (Suppl.)**, S1–S9.
8. Therasse, P., Arbuck, S. G., Eisenhauer, E. A., et al. (2000) New guidelines to evaluate response to treatment in solid tumors. *J. Natl. Cancer Inst.* **92**, 205–216.
9. Kerr, J. F. R., Winterford, C. M., and Harmon, B. V. (1994) Apoptosis—its significance in cancer and cancer therapy. *Cancer* **73**, 2013–2026.
10. Hickman, J. A. (1992) Apoptosis induced by anticancer drugs. *Cancer Metastasis Rev.* **11**, 121–139.
11. Kaufmann S. H. and Earnshaw W. C. (2000) Induction of apoptosis by cancer chemotherapy. *Exp. Cell Res.* **256**, 42–49.
12. Mow, B. M. F., Blajeski, A. L., Chandra, J., and Kaufman, S. H. (2001) Apoptosis and the response to anticancer therapy. *Curr. Opin. Oncol.* **13**, 453–462.
13. Martin, S. J., Reutelingsperger, C. P., McGahon, A. J., et al. (1995) Early redistribution of plasma membrane phosphatidylserine is a general feature of apoptosis regardless of the initiating stimulus: inhibition by over expression of Bcl-2 and Abl. *J. Exp. Med.* **182**, 1545–1556.
14. Fadok, V. A., Voelker, D. R., Campbell, P. A., Cohen, J. J., Bratton, D. L., and Henson, P. M. (1992) Exposure of phosphatidylserine on the surface of apoptotic lymphocytes triggers specific recognition and removal by macrophages. *J. Immunol.* **148**, 2207–2216.
15. Huber, R., Berendes, R., Burger, A., et al. (1992) Crystal and molecular structure of human annexin V after refinement. Implications for structure, membrane binding and ion channel formation of the annexin family of proteins. *J. Mol. Biol.* **223**, 683–704.

16. Reutelingsperger, C. P. M. (2001) Annexins: key regulators of haemostasis, thrombosis, and apoptosis. *Thromb. Haemost.* **86**, 413–419.
17. Mesner, P. W. and Kaufmann, S. H. (1997) Methods utilized in the study of apoptosis. *Adv. Pharmacol.* **41**, 57–87.
18. Blankenberg, F. G., Katsikis, P. D., Tait, J. F., et al. (1998) In vivo detection and imaging of phosphatidylserine expression during programmed cell death. *Proc. Natl. Acad. Sci. USA* **95**, 6349–6354.
19. Blankenberg, F. G., Katsikis, P. D., Tait, J. F., et al. (1999) Imaging of apoptosis (programmed cell death) with 99mTc Annexin V. *J. Nucl. Med.* **40**, 184–191.
20. Ohtsuki, K., Akashi, K., Aoka, Y., et al. (1999) Technetium-99m HYNIC-annexin V: a potential radiopharmaceutical for the in-vivo detection of apoptosis. *Eur. J. Nuclear Med.* **26**, 1251–1258.
21. Vriens, P. W., Blankenberg, F. G., Stoot, J. H., et al. (1998) The use of technetium Tc 99m annexin V for in vivo imaging of apoptosis during cardiac allograft rejection. *J. Thorac. Cardiovasc. Surg.* **116**, 844–853.
22. Ogura, Y., Krams, S. M., Martinez, O. M., et al. (2000) Radiolabeled Annexin V imaging: diagnosis of allograft rejection in an experimental rodent model of liver transplantation. *Radiology* **214**, 795–800.
23. Blankenberg, F. G., Robbins, R. C., Stoot, J. H., et al. (2000) Radionucleide imaging of acute lung transplant rejection with annexin V. *Chest* **117**, 834–840.
24. D'Arceuil, H., Rhine, W., de Crespigny, A., et al. (2000) $^{99m}$Tc annexin V imaging of neonatal hypoxic brain injury. *Stroke* **31**, 2692–2700.
25. Blankenberg, F. G., Naumovski, L., Tait, J. F., Post, A. M., and Strauss, H. W. (2001) Imaging cyclophosphamide-induced intramedullary apoptosis in rats using $^{99m}$Tc-radiolabeled annexin V. *J. Nucl. Med.* **42**, 309–316.
26. Hofstra, L., Liem, I. H., Dumont, E. A., et al. (2000) Visualisation of cell death in vivo in patients with acute myocardial infarction. *Lancet* **356**, 209–212.
27. Narula, J., Acio, E. R., Narula, N., et al. (2001) Annexin-V imaging for noninvasive detection of cardiac allograft rejection. *Nat. Med.* **7**, 1347–1352.
28. Kown, M. H., Strauss, H. W., Blankenberg, F. G., et al. (2001) In vivo imaging of acute cardiac rejection in human patients using $^{99m}$technetium labeled Annexin V. *Am. J. Transpl.* **1**, 270–277.
29. Hofstra, L., Thimister, P. W. L., DeBruine, A. P., et al. (2001) In vivo detection of apoptosis in an intracardiac tumor. *JAMA* **14**, 1841.
30. Mochizuki, T., Kuge, Y., Zhao, S., et al. (2003) Detection of apoptotic tumor response in vivo after a single dose of chemotherapy with $^{99m}$Tc-Annexin V. *J. Nuclear Med.* **44**, 92–97.
31. Belhocine, T. Z., Steinmetz, N., Hustinx, R., et al. (2002) Increased uptake of the apoptosis-imaging agent (99m)Tc recombinant human Annexin V in human tumors after one course of chemotherapy as a predictor of tumor response and patient prognosis. *Clin. Cancer Res.* **8**, 2766–2774.
32. Kasina, S., Rao, T. N., Srinivasan, A., et al. (1991) Development and biologic evaluation of a kit for preformed chelate technetium-99m radiolabeling of an antibody

Fab fragment using a diamide dimercaptide chelating agent. *J. Nuclear Med.* **32**, 1445–1450.
33. Green, A. M. and Steinmetz, M. D. (2002) Monitoring apoptosis in real time. *Cancer J.* **8**, 82–92.
34. Kemerink, G. J., Boersma, H. H., Thimister, P. W. L., et al. (2001) Biodistribution and dosimetry of $^{99m}$Tc-BTAP-annexin-V in humans. *Eur. J. Nuclear Med.* **28**, 1373–1378.
35. Kemerink, G. J., Liu, X., Kieffer, D., et al. (2003) Safety, biodistribution, and dosimetry of 99mTc-HYNIC-Annexin V, a novel human recombinant Annexin V for human application. *J. Nuclear Med.* **44**, 947–952.
36. Subbarayan, M., Häfeli, U. O., Feyes, D. K., Unnithan, J., Emancipator, S. N., and Mukhtar, H. (2003) A simplified method for preparation of $^{99m}$Tc-Annexin V and its biologic evaluation for in vivo imaging of apoptosis after photodynamic therapy. *J. Nuclear Med.* **44**, 650–656.
37. Blankenberg, F. G., Tait, J., and Strauss, H. W. (2000) Apoptotic cell death: its implications for imaging in the next millennium. *Eur. J. Nuclear Med.* **27**, 359–367.
38. Yang, D. J., Azhdarinia, A., Wu, P., et al. (2001) In vivo and in vitro measurement of apoptosis in breast cancer cells using $^{99m}$Tc-EC-Annexin V. *Cancer Biother. Radiopharm.* **16**, 73–83.
39. Tait, J. F., Brown, D. S., Gibson, D. F., Blankenberg, F. G., and Strauss, H. W. (2000) Development and characterization of Annexin V mutants with endogenous chelation sites for $^{99m}$Tc. *Bioconjugate Chem.* **11**, 918–925.
40. Ke, S., Wen, X., Wu, Q.-P., et al. (2004) Imaging taxane-induced tumor apoptotic using PEGylated, 111in-labeled Annexin V. *J. Nuclear Med.* **45**, 108–115.
41. Lahorte, C., Slegers, G., Philippe, J., Van de Wiele, C., and Dierckx, R. A. (2001) Synthesis and in vitro evaluation of 123I-labelled human recombinant Annexin V. *Bio. Eng.* **17**, 51–53.
42. Ito, M., Tomiyoshi, K., Takahashi, N., et al. (2002) Development of a new ligand, $^{11}$C-labeled Annexin V, for PET imaging of apoptosis. *Proc. SNM 49th Annual Meeting*, No. 1457.
43. Russell, J., O'Donoghue, J. A., Finn, R., Finn, R., et al. (2002) Iodination of Annexin V for imaging apoptosis. *J. Nuclear Med.* **43**, 671–677.
44. Glaser, M., Collingridge, D. R., Aboagye, E., et al. (2003) Iodine-124 labelled Annexin-V as a potential radiotracer to study apoptosis using positron emission tomography. *Appl. Radiat. Isot.* **58**, 55–62.
45. Dekker, B., Keen, H., Zweit, J., et al. (2002) Detection of cell death using $^{124}$I-Annexin V. *Proc. SNM 49th Annual Meeting*, No. 256.
46. Keen, H., Dekker, B., Disley, L., et al. (2003) Iodine-124 labelled Annexin V for PET imaging of in vivo cell death. *Proc. SNM 50th Annual Meeting*, No. 586.
47. Smith-Jones, P. M., Afroze, A., Zanzonico, P., Tait, J., Larson, S. M., and Strauss, H. W. (2003) $^{68}$Ga labelling of Annexin-V: comparison to $^{99m}$Tc-Annexin-V and $^{67}$Ga-Annexin. *Proc. SNM 50th Annual Meeting*, No. 159.

48. Zijlstra, S., Gunawan, J., and Burchert, W. (2003) Synthesis and evaluation of a $^{18}$F-labelled recombinant annexin-V derivative, for identification and quantification of apoptotic cells with PET. *Appl. Radiat. Isot.* **58,** 201–207.
49. Vaidayanathan, G. and Zalutsky, M. R. (1992) Labeling proteins with fluorine-18 using N-succinimidyl 4-[18F] fluorobenzoate. *Int. J. Rad. Appl. Instrum. B* **19,** 275–281.
50. Boisgard, R., Blondel, A., Dolle, F., et al. (2003) A new 18F tracer for apoptosis imaging in tumor bearing mice. *Proc. SNM 50th Annual Meeting*, No. 157.
51. Mease, R. C., Weinberg, I. N., Toretsky, J. A., and Tait, J. F. (2003) Preparation of F-18 labeled Annexin V: a potential PET radiopharmaceutical for imaging cell death. *Proc. SNM 50th Annual Meeting*, No. 1058.
52. Beyer, T., Townsend, D. W., Brun, T., et al. (2000) A combined PET/CT scanner for clinical oncology. *J. Nuclear Med.* **41,** 1369–1379.
53. Townsend, D. W. and Beyer, T. (2002) A Combined PET/CT scanner: the path to true image fusion. *Br. J. Radiol.* **75 (Suppl.),** S24–30.
54. Steinert, H. C. and von Schulthess, G. K. (2002) Initial clinical experience using a new integrated in-line PET/CT system. *Br. J. Radiol.* **75 (Suppl.),** S36–S38.
55. Takei, T., Kuge, Y., Zhao, S., et al. (2003) The time course of apoptotic tumor response following a single dose of chemotherapy: evaluation with $^{99m}$Tc-Annexin V, caspase-3, expression and TUNEL staining in an experimental tumor model. *Proc. SNM 50th Annual Meeting*, No. 583.
56. Blankenberg, F. (2002) To scan or not scan, it is a question of timing: technetium-99m-annexin V radionuclide imaging assessment of treatment efficacy after one course of chemotherapy. *Clin. Cancer Res.* **8,** 2757–2758.
57. Geske, F. J., Monks, J., Lehman, L., and Fadok, V. A. (2002) The role of the macrophages in apoptosis: hunter, gatherer, and regulator. *Int. J. Hematol.* **76,** 16–26.
58. Geske, F. J., Monks, J., Lehman, L., and Fadok, V. A. (2001) Early stages of p53 induced apoptosis are reversible. *Cell Death Differ.* **8,** 182–191.
59. Hammill, A. K., Urh, J. W., and Scheuermann, R. H. (1999) Annexin V staining due to loss of membrane asymmetry can be reversible and precede commitment to apoptotic death. *Exp. Cell Res.* **251,** 16–21.
60. Martin, S., Pombo, I., Poncet, P., David, B., Arock, M., and Blank, U. (2000) Immunologic stimulation of mast cells leads to reversible exposure of phosphatidylserine in the absence of apoptosis. *Int. Arch. Allergy Immunol.* **123,** 249–258.
61. Allman, R., Errington, R. J., and Smith, P. J. (2003) Delayed expression of apoptosis in human lymphoma cells undergoing low-dose Taxol-induced mitotic stress. *Br. J. Cancer* **88,** 1649–1658.

# 25

## Magnetic Resonance Imaging of Tumor Response to Chemotherapy

### Richard Mazurchuk and Joseph A. Spernyak

#### Summary

The breadth and substance of anatomic (structural) and novel physiological (functional) imaging methods to noninvasively monitor and assess anticancer therapies continues to grow. Current techniques span several imaging disciplines including magnetic resonance (MR) imaging, positron emission tomography (PET), computed tomography (CT), ultrasound (US), and optical-based methods using fluorescence and bioluminescence techniques. These methodologies applied in the clinic and/or in animal models offer unique insights into disease processes. Applications affected by imaging include therapeutic response assessment, improved diagnostic evaluations, enhanced delineation of tumor boundaries, elucidation of the underlying mechanisms of therapeutic response and drug resistance, identification of high-risk subpopulations of transgenic animals with specific alterations in their genome leading to abnormal phenotypes, and prediction of therapeutic outcome. This chapter provides a brief introduction to this emerging field, focusing specifically on novel MR applications related to chemotherapeutic response assessment, step-by-step procedures to perform the outlined techniques, and algorithms to analyze resultant data.

#### Key Words

MRI; microvasculature; tumor; BOLD; permeability; perfusion; imaging.

### 1. Introduction

Recent advances in magnetic resonance (MR) imaging and other noninvasive imaging techniques have added dramatically to the arsenal of research tools available to scientists and clinicians for individualized assessment of chemotherapeutic agents. Application of noninvasive functional imaging methods—particularly functional magnetic resonance (fMR) imaging techniques—have yielded: (1) the ability to perform in vivo drug profiling and screening assessments in individual animals, (2) elucidation of underlying mechanism(s) of

From: *Methods in Molecular Medicine, vol. 111: Chemosensitivity:*
*Vol. 2: In Vivo Models, Imaging, and Molecular Regulators*
Edited by: R. D. Blumenthal © Humana Press Inc., Totowa, NJ

therapeutic response and resistance in individual tumors, (3) optimization of both single and combinational therapies, and (4) rapid advances in new drug development and discovery. **Figure 1** depicts a limited overview of existing modalities in relation to their general use, informational content, and chemotherapeutic assessment criteria; techniques including MR data acquisitions are highlighted. Although a detailed description of the MR methods outlined in **Fig. 1** is beyond the scope of this chapter, a representative and integrated fMR imaging module for data acquisition and image processing is represented in **Fig. 2**. Data obtained from each of the outlined fMR methods can then be compared with one another and correlated to standard techniques of chemotherapeutic assessment to provide an early predictive measure of efficacy. MR methods will be discussed in more detail in subsequent sections. MR image data acquired with the module outlined in **Fig. 2A** is typically used for tumor/organ volume measurements, whereas fMR image data acquired using the integrated module as outlined in **Fig. 2B** yields physiological information related to a tumor's microenvironmental status at specific time points following treatment.

In general, MR imaging methods can currently be divided into two categories based on the information each provides **(Fig. 2)**. MR techniques that provide information about tumor anatomy, morphology, or structural characteristics such as the delineation of tumor boundaries (routinely used to assess tumor volume changes) are termed anatomic MR imaging techniques. Acquisition protocols include standard in vivo and ex vivo T1, T2, and proton density-weighted spin echo (SE) and gradient echo (GRE) MR acquisitions yielding either subsecond temporal resolutions or in-plane spatial resolutions of 100–300 µm in 5–15 min or isotropic three-dimensional (3-D) data sets with <110-µm spatial resolution in <14–16 h. Anatomic MR techniques are generally the simplest to perform and interpet because of the existance of well-defined clinical protocols commonly used in standard diagnostic procedures. Conceptually, anatomic-based imaging techniques applied to small animal models of disease are an extension of routine caliper measurements performed using subcutaneously (sc) implanted tumors. Like caliper measurements, MR imaging can be performed longitudinally in time using the same animal studied serially in a noninvasive manner, but with the added advantage of greater accuracy and precision. Unlike caliper measurements, morphometric information from internally

---

Fig. 1. *(see facing page)* Overview of noninvasive, image-based methods currently available for *in vivo* and *ex vivo* assessment of chemotherapeutic efficacy. MR imaging-based methods are currently the only modality that yields both anatomic and physiological information regarding tumor microenvironmental status in a single exam.

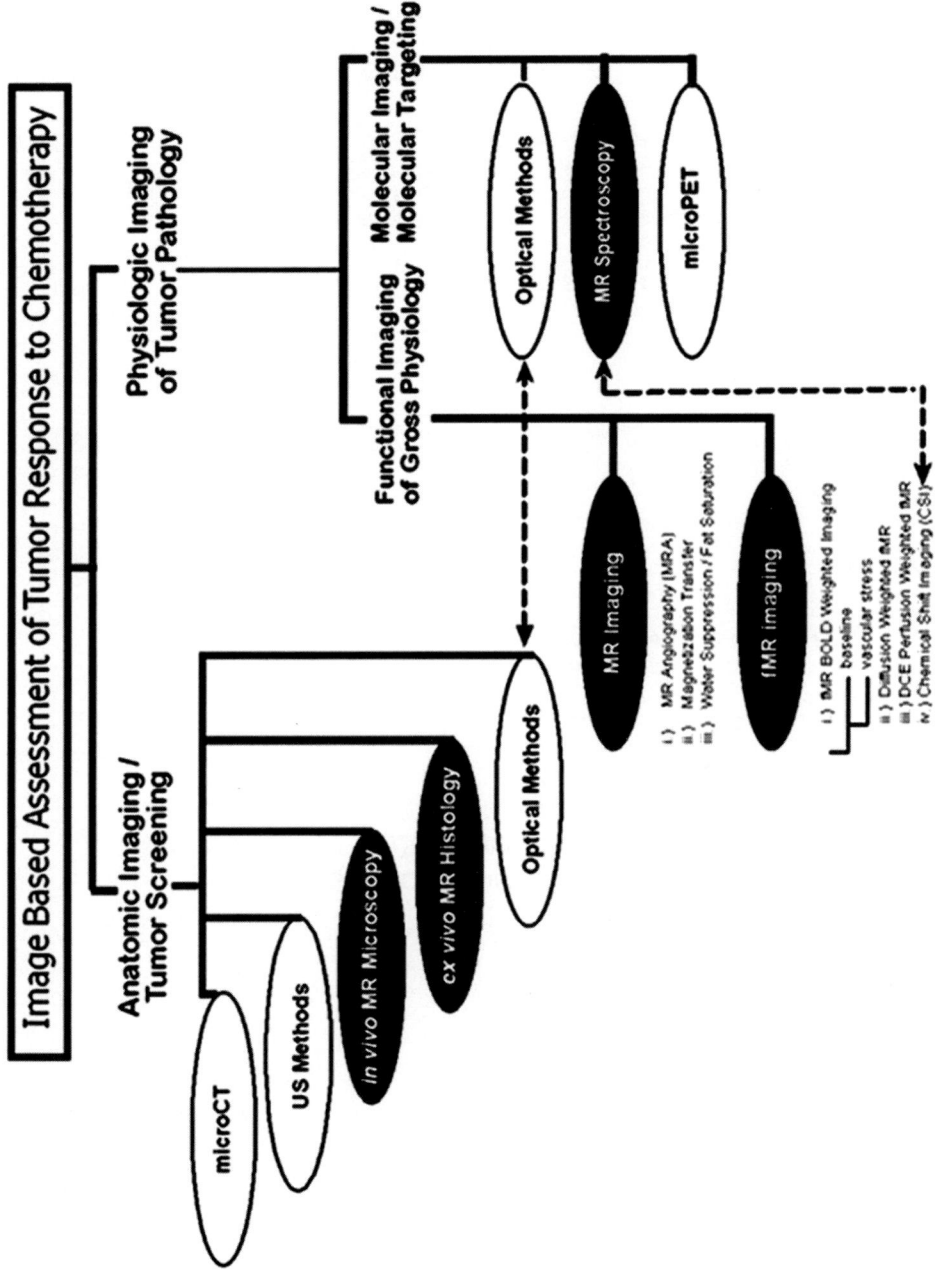

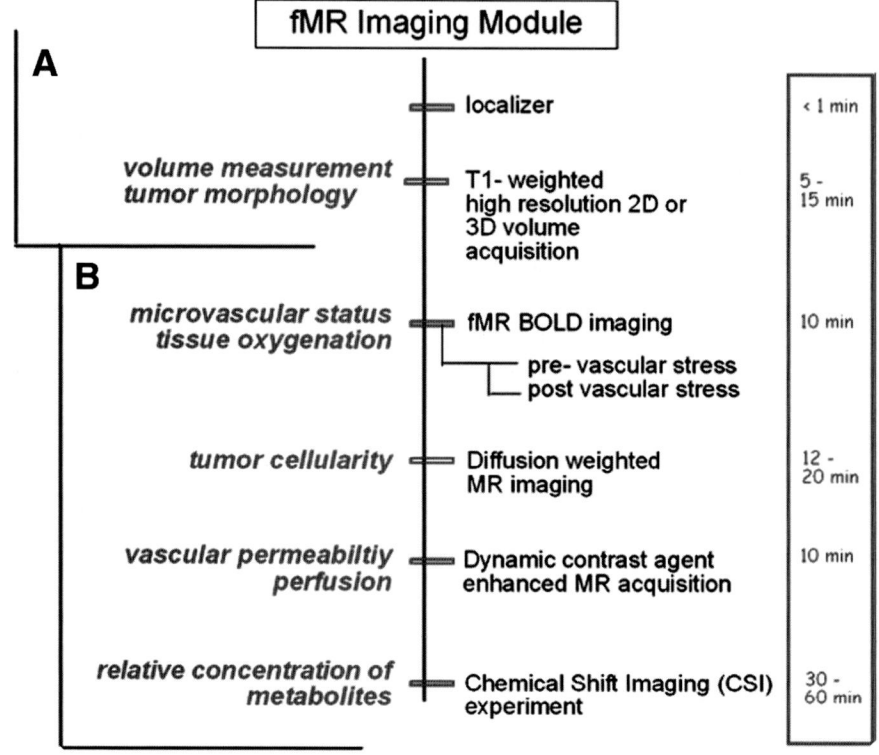

**Integrated MR characterization of vascular permeability, tumor cellularity, microvascular status and metabolite concentrations.**

Fig. 2. Representative fMR tumor imaging module for the assessment of chemotherapeutic efficacy. Methods outlined in (**A**) are used for localization and tumor/organ volume measurements. Methods diagrammed in (**B**) are used for assessing tumor physiology and pathology in animal tumor model systems.

developing tumors is also possible and can be used to assess hemorrhagic areas, major vessels, tumor remodeling processes, etc. Representative ex vivo MR images acquired at 4.7 T are shown in **Fig. 3** as examples of the excellent soft tissue differentiation that can be achieved.

MR imaging techniques that are specifically designed to provide information about tumor pathology and underlying changes in tumor physiology are termed functional MR imaging techniques. These include: (1) techniques that focus on molecular changes and molecular targets termed "molecular sensing" and

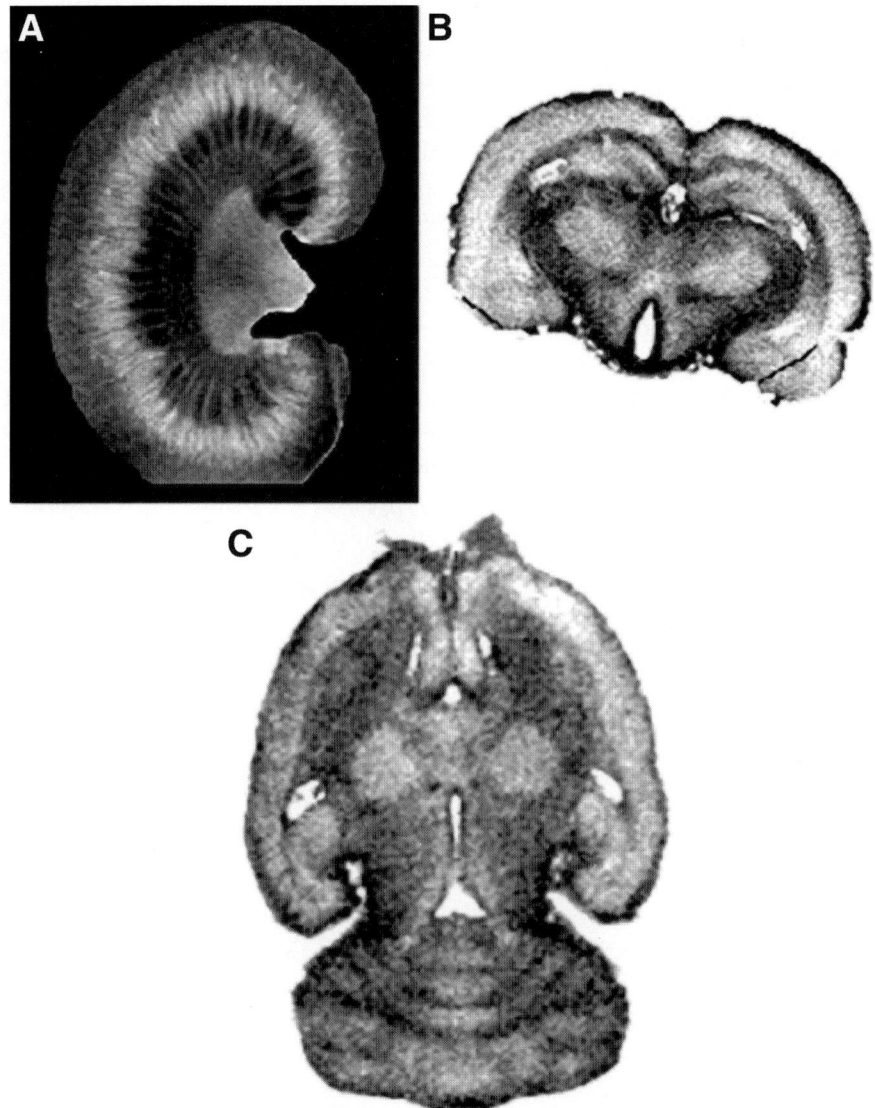

Fig. 3. Ex vivo MR microscopy examples demonstrating excellent soft-tissue contrast from biological samples acquired in less than 30 min at 4.7 T: **(A)** mouse kidney; **(B)** axial section of normal rat brain; **(C)** coronal section of normal rat brain.

(2) techniques that yield information on more general changes (possibly potentiated by a number of molecular changes) occurring in tumor resulting in extracellular vs intracellular pH variations *(1–3)*, increases/decreases in extracellular water content and cellularity *(4)*, relative changes in tumor oxygenation or

hypoxia *(5,6)*, relative metabolite concentrations of a limited number of molecular species (m*M* quantities) *(7,8)*, vascular permeability changes *(9,10)*, vasculogenesis, angiogenesis, etc. *(11)*. To date, fMR generally has not demonstrated the specificity or sensitivity typically associated with positron emission tomography (PET) or optical-based techniques used for molecular targeting experiments or studying alterations in specific metabolic pathways. However, as the field matures, fMR's potential in this area is also expected to develop, e.g., several published reports have demonstrated fMR's feasibility in this realm *(12)*.

The following sections focus on each of the major fMR methods as they currently apply to chemotherapeutic assessment. Results from each of the fMR methods are generally unique and complement results obtained using other techniques. It should be noted that although fMR offers much potential for noninvasive, longitudinal assessment of individual tumors treated using different chemotherapeutic protocols, all fMR methods are still currently in their infancy and their ultimate utility and application for evaluating chemotherapeutic efficacy has not been fully realized.

### 1.1. Blood Oxygenation Level-Dependent (BOLD) Sensitive fMR Imaging of Tumors

The BOLD method provides information related to changes in microvascular status due to changes in tissue oxygenation, blood flow, and metabolic activation after an applied vascular stress. BOLD fMR tehcniques are sensitive to changes in oxyhemoglobin, $HbO_2$ (diamagnetic, higher signal-to-noise ratio, S/N, per unit volume on T2, T2* weighted acquisitions), to deoxyhemoglobin, $dHbO_2$ (less diamagnetic than $HbO_2$ owing to the presence of the paramagnetic deoxy-heme center, lower S/N per unit volume on T2, T2* weighted acquisitions), in metabolically active tumor/tissue regions. However, it should be noted that the dynamic range and sensitivity of observed fMR signal intensity change is proportional to the magnetic field strength at which it is observed and varies with the specific tumor model (including host strain used and the tumor's site of development), vascular perturbation applied, and the MR pulse sequence used for data acquisition. Moreover, the specific data analysis and rendering scheme(s) used for data visualization can also lead to invalid interpretation of results. Therefore, care must be taken to ensure valid input, modeling/characterization, and output of data, taking into account all parameters influencing data acquisition. In general, the higher the magnetic field strength, $B_0$, the greater the degree of MR signal intensity change (dynamic range) observed from a BOLD sensitive acquisition and the greater the sensitivity of the technique to tumor microvascular status. To characterize microvascular tumor changes, at least two data sets of BOLD fMR sensitive images are required. First, a baseline data set is collected. Then, a second set of images using identical fMR parameters is acquired while a systemically applied microvascular "stress" is administered in the form of an injectable agent (e.g., acetazolamide) or gaseous mixture (e.g., carbogen at 5–7% $CO_2$, 95–93% $O_2$). The raw data collected are then analyzed with respect to the observed signal intensity change from baseline values. This procedure can be repeated as time permits (i.e., alternating applied microvascular stress/nonstress data acquisitions) to improve S/N and reproducibility. Interpretation of BOLD fMR results include the following assumptions: (1) Metabolically active tumor regions require increased oxygenation, blood flow, and/or blood volume for continued development. (2) To sustain tumor growth, the vascular system in mammals generally supplies an overabundance of oxyhemoglobin and nutrients to these areas (Fick's law) *(13–15)*. (3) Excess oxyhemoglobin spills over into venous blood pools, raising the oxyhemoglobin/deoxyhemoglobin ratio resulting in a localized elevation of MR signal intensity from these regions on BOLD sensitive fMR data acquisitions. To a first approximation, these physiological processes are believed to be the primary cause of signal intensity change in a fMR experiment. However, tumor regions with increased blood flow velocities as compared to baseline values that exceed the ability of a given pulse sequence to label flowing spins during the course of the MR acquisition, or metabolic requirements that exceed available blood supply, will yield decreased fMR signal intensities compared to baseline values, making data interpretation more difficult. Still, the advantage of applying these techniques to small-animal tumor models is that experimental tumors generally develop very rapidly (days–weeks), compared to human tumors observed in the clinic (weeks–years). Consequently, vasculature in animal tumor models does not have time to develop normally (i.e., tumor vessels are generally characterized as being tortuous, leaky, and typically lack autoregulatory control mechanisms [Steal effect] associated with normal-functioning mature vessels) *(16,17)*. The working fMR hypothesis is that rapidly developing tumor regions (rich in vasculogeneic or angiogeneic vessels) are unable to shunt blood to other areas when perturbed by systemically induced increases in blood flow and blood volume. Subsequently, abnormal tumor vessels demonstrate a unique MR signature that is discernable during a fMR BOLD sensitive experiment. In this manner, fMR BOLD sensitive imaging is able to differentiate well-perfused tumor regions with immature vasculature and rich in oxygenation from more mature, normal-functioning vessels (bulk tumor) and tumor regions containing principally apoptotic/necrotic areas **(Figs. 4–6)**. In these examples, vessel physiology is used to assess microvascular tumor status and optimize the observed dynamic range of their BOLD fMR signal intensity change calculated from baseline values (i.e., MR signal intensity changes for angiogeneic vessels > bulk tumor vessels > apoptotic/necrotic tumor regions). To date, BOLD sensitive fMR imaging applications have demonstrated apparent correlations with microvessel density (MVD) and vessel diameter measurements *(18,19)*, tumor oxygenation measurements, and tumor regions characterized as metabolically active from immunohistochemical staining techniques *(20)*. Moreover, BOLD fMR methods have been used to noninvasively assess microvascular functioning, determine angiogeneic regions within tumor, and to assess antiangiogeneic, antimetastatic, and chemotherapeutic strategies directed against cancer *(21–25)*.

### 1.2. Diffusion-Weighted fMR Imaging of Tumors

The diffusion-weighted fMR method typically provides information associated with changes in tumor cellularity and cellular boundary conditions as related to changes in bulk water content. Specifically, the diffusion of water in tissues is a complex process that is mediated by water mobility in intra- and extracellular spaces, the relative volume of these spaces, and cellular/vascular membrane integrity and permeability. Increases in tissue water mobility as measured by diffusion-weighted fMR imaging can be quantitatively expressed in three dimensions as an "apparent diffusion coefficient" (ADC), which reflects these processes as a relative measure of bulk water *vs* bound water compartments. Results suggest that increases in tumor ADCs observed at early time points following chemotherapy are associated with subsequent decreased tumor cellularity per unit volume, often observed in dead and dying tissues. To measure these changes, ADCs are obtained by applying varying gradient pulse strengths and radiofrequency (RF) pulses that are designed to diminish MR signals from "mobile proton spins" while preserving MR signals from "stationary proton spins." Diffusion fMR imaging has been used successfully to stage tumor growth and aggressiveness noninvasively in several animal models of disease (**Fig. 7**) and is currently undergoing clinical evaluation for its ability to assess tumor progression and response to therapy *(26–30)*.

---

Fig. 4. *(see facing page)* (**A**) T1-weighted axial MR image of a nude mouse implanted sc bilaterally with human squamous cell carcinoma of the head and neck growing 7–10 d (~200 mg) treated with a combination of irinotecan (100 mg/kg/wk × 3) followed 24 h later by 5-FU (50 mg/kg/wk × 3). On d 5 post-initial treatment, BOLD-sensitive fMR images were obtained (**B**). The mouse was then sacrificed, tumor harvested and fixed in zinc fixative. Immunohistological staining was done on sequential sections. (**C**) H&E (morphology). (**D**) Hypoxia (pimonidazole staining detecting pO2 < 10 mm Hg). (**E**) CAIX (innate hypoxia marker detected by MAb M75). (**F**) CD31 (blood vessel staining). T2-weighted SE BOLD fMR imaging depicts a generally well-perfused tumor with heterogeneous vascular regions demonstrating a high correlation to histology results (*see* **Fig. 5**).

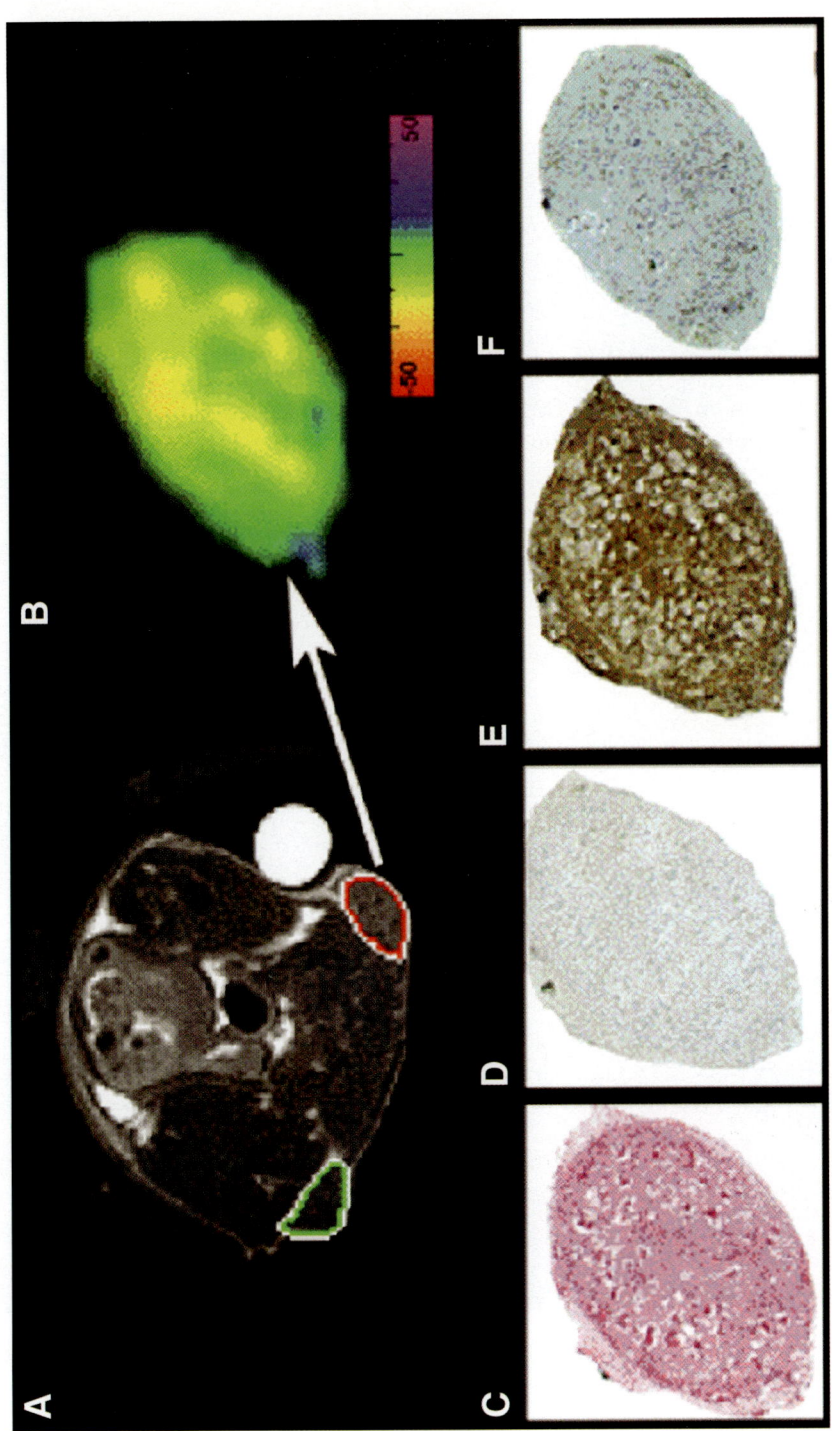

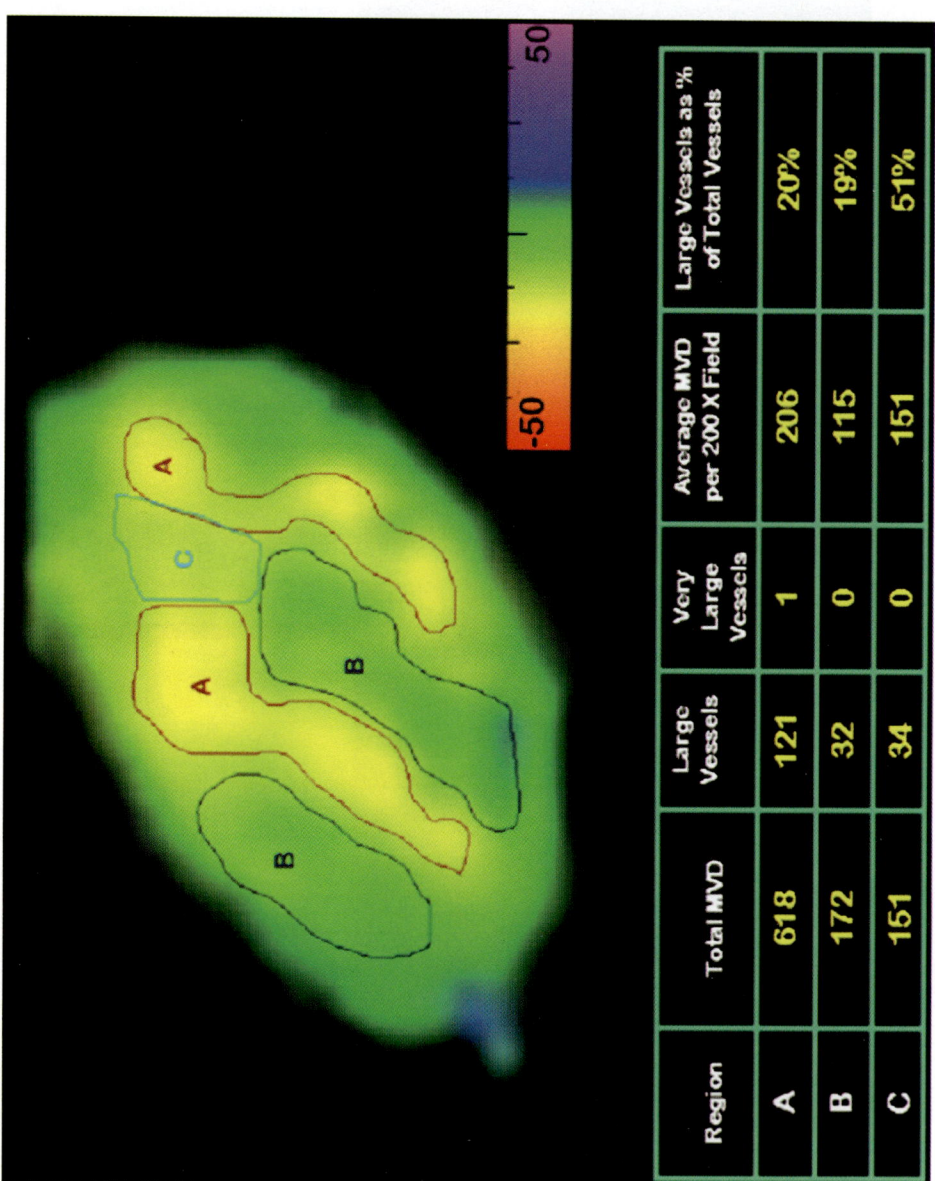

## 1.3. Dynamic Contrast-Enhanced (DCE) Perfusion-Weighted fMR Imaging

The DCE method typically provides information pertaining to changes in vascular permeability within tumors and has been routinely used to assess relative changes in tumor perfusion as a function of time and treatment. However, with the advent of novel MR agents custom designed for specific cellular phenotypes and/or genotypes, the method has expanded in importance and potential application. The number of available agents undergoing in vitro/in vivo characterization has grown to the point where high-throughput screening of promising compounds is now underway using MR as well as in combination with other modalities. In general terms, a MR contrast-enhancing agent is administered and rapid MR data acquisitions obtained to monitor the dynamic change in MR signal intensity as a function of time and injected dose (**Fig. 8**). To date, many variations of this technique exist for small animal imaging and include an array of MR pulse sequences, magnetic field strengths, and contrast-enhancing agents designed for single or multiple molecular targets in order to quantitatively answer detailed questions related to normal vs abnormal physiology *(31–42)*. In general, results, data analysis, and subsequent interpretation of results appear to be dependent on the specific physiochemical properties of the MR contrast-enhancing agent used, including its charge and molecular weight (MW), attached functional groups, number of receptor sites, etc., as well as the mode (oral, ip, iv), concentration, rate, volume, and duration of administered dose.

## 1.4. Localized In Vivo MR Spectroscopy and Chemical Shift Imaging (CSI)

These spectroscopic methods typically provide information concerning the relative concentration of specific metabolites within tumors compared to normal tissue. Subsequent changes in tumor metabolite concentration as a function of time and treatment may be indicative of therapeutic response and overall tumor status. For example, the concentration of lactate, a by-product of glycolysis, is a reliable biochemical indicator of anaerobic metabolism. Lactate is formed from

---

Fig. 5. *(see opposite page)* BOLD-sensitive fMR image (from **Fig. 4**) with regions of interest (ROIs) outlining areas where microvessel density (MVD) measurements were performed on histological samples. Regions visualized as bright yellow (**A**) demonstrated the highest MVD and number of vessels characterized as large and very large vessel diameters. Regions visualized as pale green with several blue areas (**B**) yielded lower MVDs and percentage of large vessels expressed as a percentage of total number of vessels. Regions visualized as pale yellow (intermediate fMR signal intensity measurements) (**C**) yielded intermediate average MVDs.

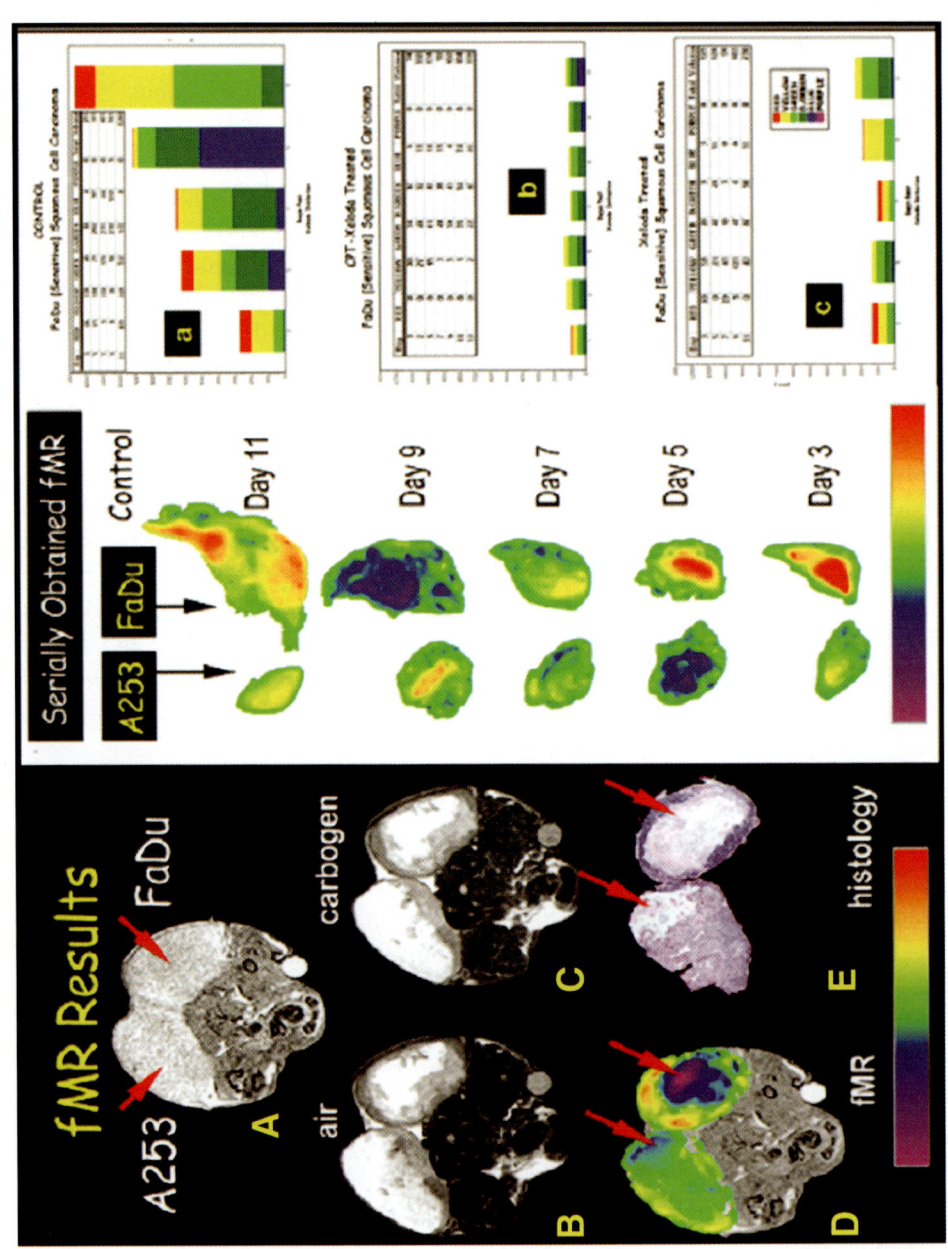

pyruvate in the cytosol in a reversible reaction catalyzed by the enzyme lactate dehydrogenase. If the amount of oxygen is limited, as typically occurs in tumors, much of the pyruvate is reduced to lactate that can be visualized using localized in vivo MR spectroscopy or CSI techniques. Observed changes in lactate concentration, either alone or in combination with other altered metabolite concentrations, has been used as a marker to assess therapeutic response *(43–53)*. Although various magnetically sensitive nuclei can be used for data acquisition (including $^{19}$F, $^{13}$C, $^{23}$Na, $^{7}$Li, $^{39}$K, $^{17}$O, and $^{14,15}$N), $^1$H and $^{31}$P techniques are almost exclusively employed because of their MR sensitivities, ease of study, and because they provide information related to tissue energetics and metabolic status. $^1$H metabolites commonly studied include: N-acetylaspartate (NAA), γ-aminobutyric acid (GABA), lactate (lac), γ-glutamate, (Glu), asparatate (Asp), phosphocholine (PCho), phosphocreatine (PCr), creatinine (Cr), and

---

Fig. 6. *(see opposite page)* Representative fMR imaging data of serially acquired data set as a function of time. Mouse tumored sc with both resistant (A253) and sensitive (FaDu) human squamous cell carcinoma of the head and neck. (*Left panel*): (a) Axial T1-weighted SE MR image of an untreated animal (slice thickness = 1 mm) approx midline through both tumors. (b, c) T2-weighted SE images with the mouse breathing room air for 5 min (b) followed by carbogen breathing (c) for 5 min applied as a "vascular stress." fMR imaging results calculated as a normalized percent change from baseline values obtained from (b,c) are shown in (d) and compared to standard H&E histology results (e). Clearly demonstrated are heterogeneous areas depicting regions of well-perfused aggressively growning tumors as well as poorly perfused regions with diminished oxygenation and blood flow containing dead and dying cells. FMR signal intensity changes (red/yellow) are shown to contain an increased density of young, immature blood vessels indicative of angiogenesis, while signal intensity changes (blue/purple) are indicative of decreased blood flow, decreased cellularity, and increased extracellular water content. Green regions represent little change from baseline values and are associated with bulk tumor. Arrows illustrate the correlation between fMR (d) and histology (e). (*Right panel*): fMR data obtained in this manner can be serially acquired noninvasively from the same animal and visualized as images. Graphs depict total tumor volume change (total bar height) with the volume contribution of each segmented color shown as a function of time and treatment. Uncontrolled tumor growth (increased red/yellow components) shown for untreated tumor. (f) Results for irinotecan/5-FU-treated tumor (g) demonstrate significant reductions in all color components, representing maximal decreases in oxygenation, blood flow, perfusion, and metabolic rate as compared to baseline control values. More important, although total tumor volume measurements for irinotecan/5-FU (g) and 5-FU alone- (h) treated FaDu tumors are similar, their physiological composition appears to be quite different (i.e., significantly less red/yellow components are observed for irinotecan/5-FU- vs 5-FU-treated tumors on d 7–11 post-initial treatment).

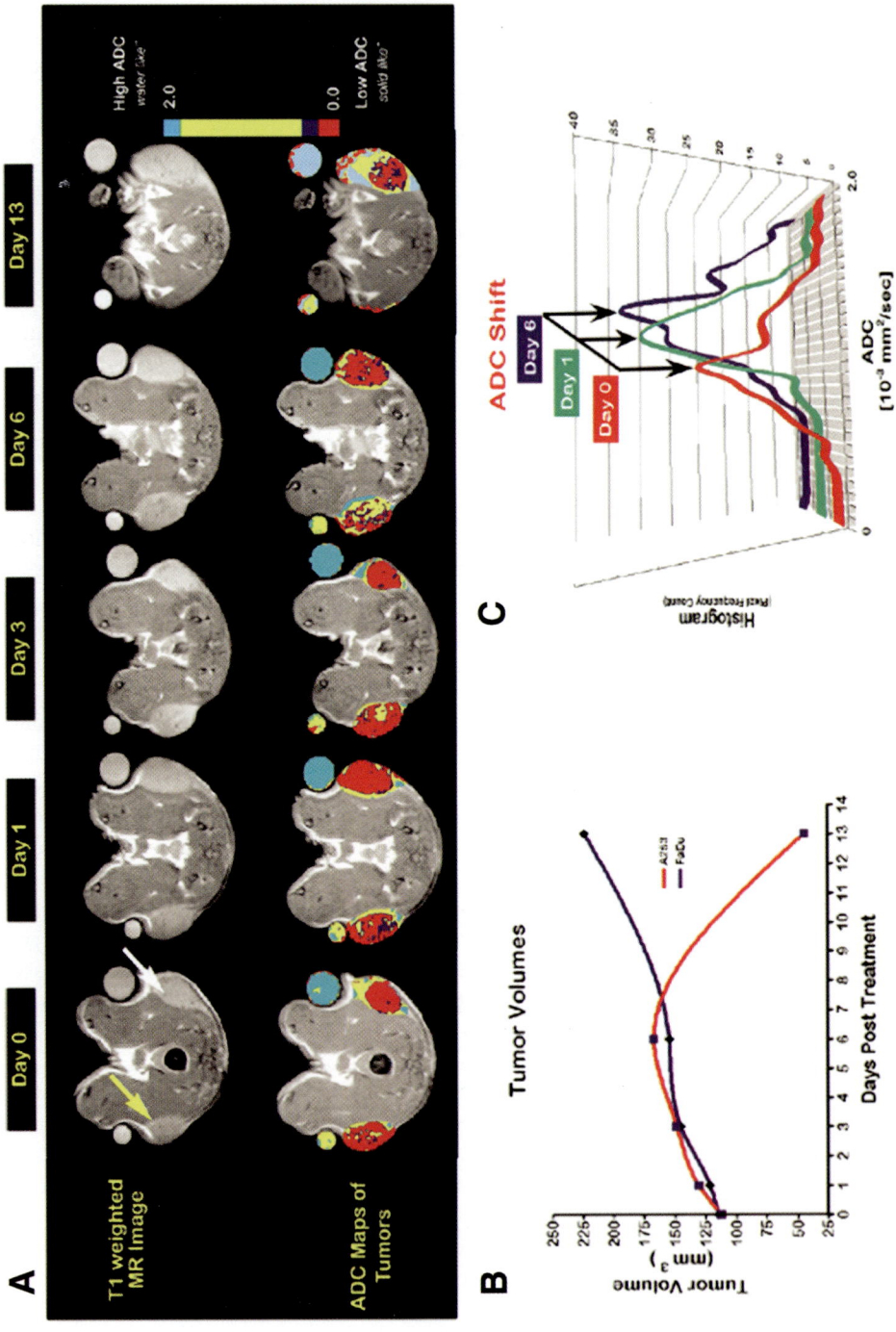

lipids **(Fig. 9)**. Moreover, the ability to determine rate constants for specific metabolic processes occurring during and after treatment is possible, e.g., monitoring formation of α-fluoro-β-alanine (FBAL) from the degradation of 5-fluorouracil (5-FU) after its administration *(54–60)*. However, the relatively long acquisition times required for adequate signal-to-noise ratio (S/N) using CSI, and to a lesser extent, localized in vivo spectroscopy techniques limit the utility of the method for routine screening assessments at this time. In general, most spectroscopic protocols are incorporated into general scanning procedures with total acquisition times less than 40 min to 1 h in an attempt to maintain clinical relevance. Active areas of research in this area include schemes for decreasing acquisition times (e.g., automatic shimming procedures and water suppression techniques) and/or improving the quality (e.g., S/N) and specificity of the information in a data set. It should also be noted that an emerging field demonstrating much excitement and potential impact for tumor assessment is the study of small molecules from body fluids such as urine, blood, etc. The method has been termed "metabonomics" or "metabolic profiling" and uses MR spectroscopic and multivariate analysis techniques to elucidate the principle components of a sample contributing to abnormal vs normal parameter characteristics *(61)*.

## 2. Materials
### 2.1. General Considerations

Small-animal fMR imaging techniques generally require the same materials as those required for "good" clinical MR studies—with a few added require-

---

Fig. 7. *(see opposite page)* **(A)** T1-weighted axial MR image of a nude mouse implanted sc bilaterally with two histologically different human squamous cell carcinomas 7–10 d postimplantation (~200 mg) and subsequently treated with combination irinotecan (100 mg/kg/wk × 1) followed 24 h later by 5-FU (100 mg/kg/wk × 1). ADC maps were generated (regions containing both tumors, calibration standards containing water, and a water-based lubricant) and results overlaid on T1 MR images for localization. **(B)** Tumor volume measurements for both tumors as a function of time posttreatment corresponding to time points of serial MR diffusion-weighted acquisitions. **(C)** Histogram results of pixel frequency counts vs ADC values in range from 0.0 to $2.0 \times 10^{-3}$ mm$^2$/s demonstrating shift in ADC values for A253 tumor regions from lower values (more "solidlike") toward higher values (more "waterlike") as a function of time and treatment, suggesting a decrease in cellularity as a function of time post treatment. This example demonstrates the potential use of this method as a "prognostic marker" for assessing successful chemotherapeutic response. It should be noted that in this particular instance, A253 (tumor on the left, which is generally characterized as being more chemoresistant) responded better than FaDu (tumor on the right, which is generally characterized as being more chemosensitive to this combinational chemotherapy).

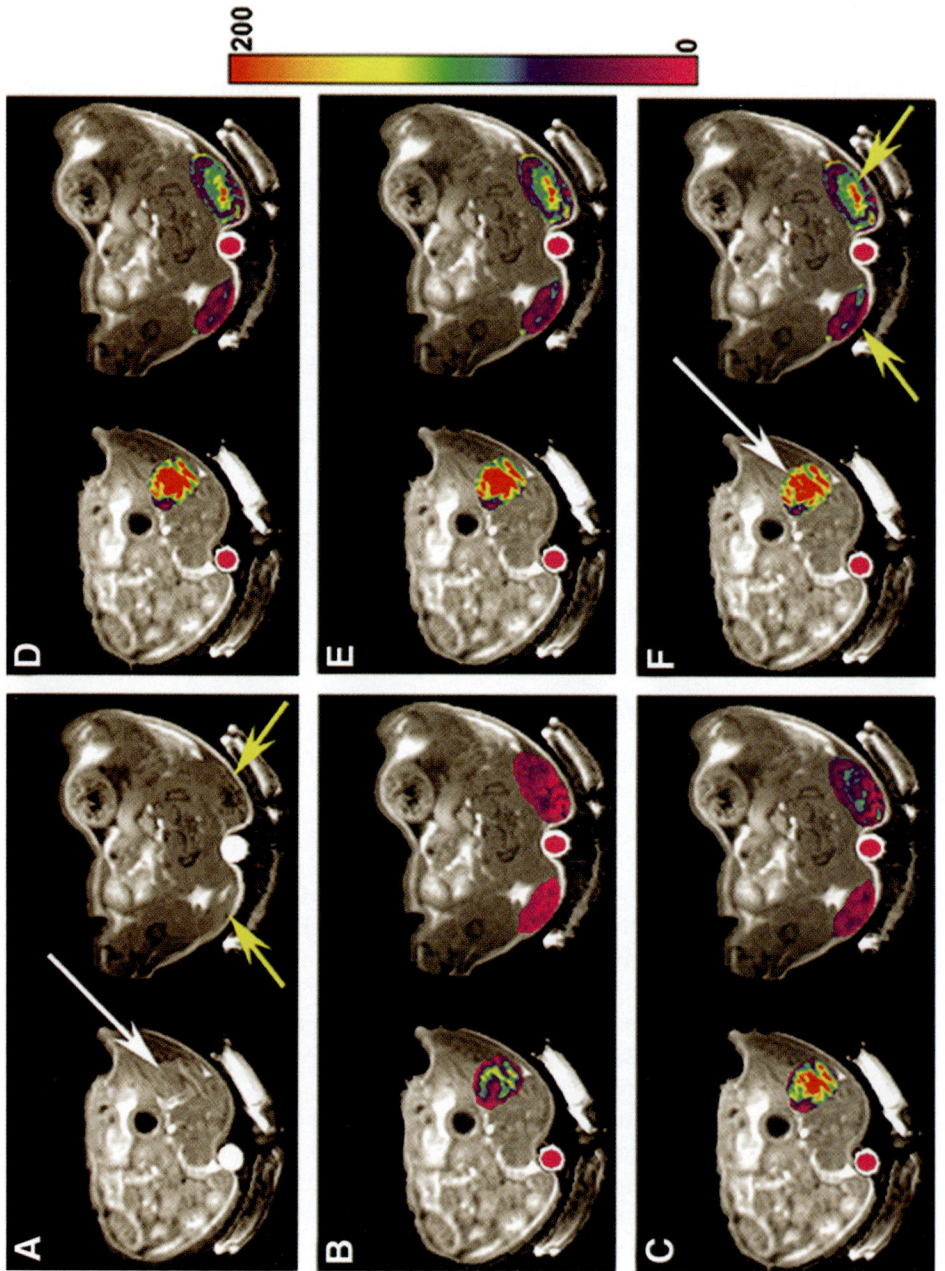

ments. It is suggested that the MR system, whenever possible, include a homogeneous, high-field-strength magnet (superconducting magnet), fast and reliable gradients with minimal eddy currents, and digital electronics for data acquisition. Customized small-animal RF transceiver or receive-only coils are routinely used by most research sites for optimal S/N, depending on specific application needs and study goals. Minimizing animal motion during data acquisition is paramount for all MR studies—especially fMR studies because of the potential for inducing image artifact that could alter analysis and interpretation of data. In this regard, the suitable use of an animal restraining device(s) and/or applied anesthetic(s) (either injectable or gaseous anesthetics) cannot be overemphasized. Maintaining the core body temperature of an animal throughout the duration of an MR acquisition is also critically important. Because many gradient coil systems are water-cooled to dissipate excess gradient heat, the use of an isothermal blanket or circulating heated water bath is highly recommended. The lowering of core body temperature in a small animal rapidly results in constriction of surface blood vessels and a shunting of blood to internal organs. Additionally, instrumentation for triggering MR acquisitions to various portions of the cardiac or respiratory cycle to reduce motion artifacts can greatly improve the quality of MR and fMR data sets. Most of these items are now available commercially and can be custom-configured for specific MR systems and application needs by third-party venders. The use of physiological monitoring devices for assessing body temperature, respiration, cardiac cycle, etc., is suggested whenever possible. Suitable reference standards must be included for quantification of fMR

Fig. 8. *(see opposite page)* (**A**) T1-weighted axial MR images depicting kidney (white arrow) and tumor regions (yellow arrows) of a nude mouse implanted sc bilaterally with two histologically different human squamous cell carcinomas of the head and neck (A253 shown on left side of the mouse, and FaDu shown on right side of the mouse). Images were acquired approx 7–10 d post-tumor implantation with tumor weights ~approx 200 mg. A MR calibration standard and water bath to maintain body temperature is present below the abdominal sections. Subsequent dynamic contrast-enhanced (DCE) perfusion-weighted fMR acquisitions were obtained following administration of Gd-DTPA administered iv via a tail vein catheter and MR-compatible MR injector at a dose of 0.3 mmol/kg. Regions of interest containing tumors and standard were then processed and fused to the T1-weighted MR data set. ROIs are visualized as a percent change from baseline values obtained in (**A**) and shown as a function of time post-contrast-enhancing agent administration (**B–F**). Clearly depicted (**F**) is lower MR signal intensity change from A253 (left side of mouse), a less vascularized tumor (from MR and histology results) demonstrating a higher degree of chemotherapeutic resistance as compared to the FaDu tumor (right side of mouse), which has increased vascularization and typically demonstrates a better chemotherapeutic response.

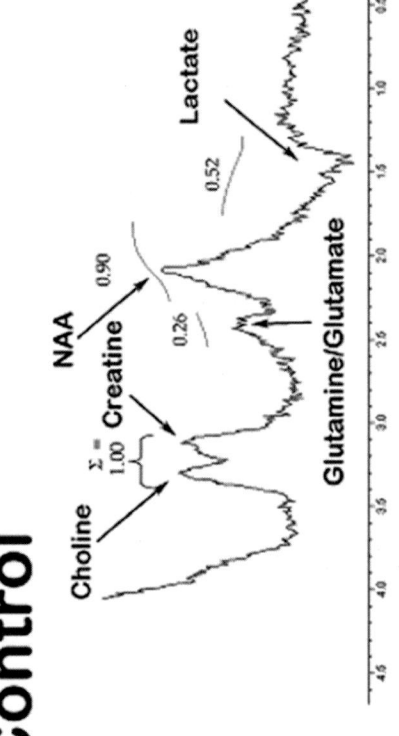
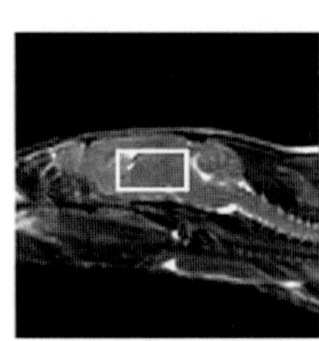
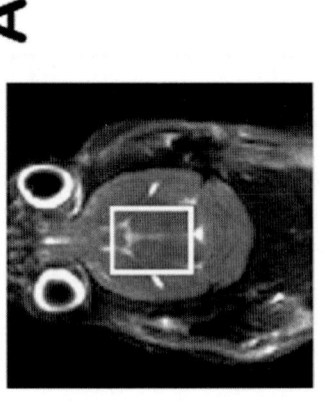

# MR Imaging of Tumor Response to Chemotherapy

results and system calibration of S/N, chemical shift information, origin of image artifact, and/or magnetic field "drift" over time.

## 2.2. Anatomic Imaging Protocols

1. T1, T2, T2*, proton-density-weighted spin-echo or gradient-echo pulse sequences.
2. Gadolinium-based contrast agent (optional) for delineating tissue borders. Contrast agents are discussed in detail under **Subheading 3.4.**
3. Software for post acquisition processing of raw data.

## 2.3. Blood Oxygenation Level-Dependent (BOLD) Sensitive fMR Imaging of Tumors

1. Carbogen (7–5% $CO_2$, 93–95% $O_2$) medical gas mixture or injectable (e.g., acetazolamide, an inhibitor of carbonic anhydrase) for inducing microvascular stress during data acquisition.
2. BOLD-sensitive fMR pulse sequence (generally a T2 or T2* weighted MR pulse sequence).
3. Software for post acquisition processing of raw data.

## 2.4. Diffusion-Weighted fMR Imaging of Tumors

1. Diffusion-weighted MR pulse sequences sensitive to water diffusion in $x$, $y$, and/or $z$ directions.
2. Diffusion-weighted MR reference standard (external) containing tubes of water and olive oil embedded in 0.5–1.0% agarose.
3. Software for post acquisition processing of raw data.

## 2.5. Dynamic Contrast-Enhanced (DCE) Perfusion-Weighted fMR Imaging

1. A rapid-acquisition MR pulse sequence such as a fast low–angle shot (FLASH), echo planar imaging (EPI) sequence, fast spin echo (FSE) techniques, keyhole imaging, or various standard SE and GRE sequences with suitable echo times (TEs) and repetition times (TRs).
2. A MR contrast-enhancing agent containing a paramagnetic metal chelate (*see* **Note 1**).
3. An iv catheter designed specifically for mouse tail vein injections (Strategic Applications, IL). Alternatively, a catheter can be constructed from a 27–30-gage needle inserted into a flared end of PE 10 tubing (polyethylene tubing, 0.28 mm

---

Fig. 9. *(see opposite page)* Examples of high-resolution MR imaging (**A**) saggital section and (**B**) coronal section of mouse brain with regions indicating location of magnetic resonance spectroscopic (MRS) acquisitions. Localized in vivo MR spectra acquired at 4.7 T from the brains of an experimental $Pdha1^{\Delta ex8}/Pdha^{WT}$, $Cre^{br+}$ female mouse (**C**) and control $Pdha1^{flox8}/Pdha^{WT}$, $Cre^{br-}$ age-matched female (**D**).

(0.011 in) ID, 0.61 mm (0.024-in) OD Intramedic Clay Adams Brand, Becton Dickinson) prefilled with isotonic sterile saline.
4. MR-compatible injector designed for use within a strong magnetic field interfaced to a computer for precise and accurate administration of a small volume of contrast media.
5. MR reference standard (external standard preferred when available—if not, use internal tissue minimally perturbed by administration of the contrast-enhancing agent, e.g., muscle) for signal intensity calibration.
6. Software for post-image acquisition data processing of raw data. A variety of commercial software packages are available (e.g., Mathematica, Wolfram Research, Champaign, IL; Matlab, MathWorks, Natick, MA; AnalyzePC, Biomedical Imaging Resource, Mayo Clinic, Rochester, MN; IDL Software, Research Systems, Boulder, CO; etc.).

### 2.6. Localized In Vivo MR Spectroscopy and Chemical Shift Imaging (CSI)

1. MR spectroscopic pulse sequence(s) sensitive to localized chemical shift information while providing adequate water suppression and magnetic field homogeneity (*see* **Note 2**).
2. A reference standard for qualitative/quantitative comparisons containing a known concentration of a metabolite under defined conditions (pH, temperature, etc.) (*see* **Note 3**).
3. Software for post-acquisition processing of raw spectral data (e.g., XWinNMR, Bruker, Billerica, MA; WinNuts, Acorn NMR, Livermore, CA).

## 3. Methods
### 3.1. Anatomic Imaging Protocols
#### 3.1.1. Localizer

1. Set up SE or GRE acquisition with flip angle $30° < X < 60°$ and short TE, TR, and short total acquisition time, large FOVs, image acquisition in a plane perpendicular/parallel to major axis of tumor, and single/multislice acquisitions to define subsequent region(s) of interest for tumor analysis (*see* **Notes 4** and **5**).
2. Anesthetize mice by either ip injection of 100 mg/kg ketamine HCl + 10 mg/kg xylazine or the administration of gaseous isoflurane.
3. Imaging preparations are usually performed in a sterile, vented hood and include placement of an iv catheter if subsequent blood sampling or DCE MR is to be performed.
4. The mice are then placed in an acrylic animal positioning/restraining device machined to fit into the center of a RF transceiver coil concentric with the main magnetic field and gradient coils.
5. Several hoses are attached to the acrylic mouse holder. One hose is placed near the nose for administration of room air or gaseous anesthesia during data acquisition.

Another hose is connected to a vacuum outlet (low pressure) at the opposite side for gas exhaust. Other hoses are available for input of additional medical gas mixtures (such as carbogen) typically used for functional MR imaging purposes. This design ensures adequate ventilation during data acquisition and facilitates the administration of isoflurane, as needed, throughout the procedure.
6. Physiological monitoring (cardiac/respiratory) and the triggering of data acquisitions (to reduce motion artifacts) of individual animals are performed as per available equipment and requirements. If isoflurane is used, the exhaust gases are passed through a scrubber before being exhausted.
7. Determine optimal MR acquisition parameters using semiautomated algorithms or manual adjustment.
   a. Optimize magnetic field homogeneity across volume of interest.
   b. Set resonant frequency for nuclei under study and determine chemical shift of molecular species to be characterized. For $^1$H-MR imaging, this will be the water or fat resonance.
   c. Set transmit gain for 90° flip (maximal signal) or 180° flip (minimal signal) and set receiver gain to maximize dynamic range of data without signal clipping.
   d. Typical MR parameters used at 4.7 T (sagittal or coronal plane): TE/TR = 10/200 ms, 128 × 128 matrix, 50-kHz bandwidth, 2000-ms excitation and refocusing pulse length, 64 × 32-mm FOV, 2-mm slice thickness with interlaced data acquisition, 5–15 slices, 1 echo, 1 NEX with a total data acquisition time of approx 26 s. Using a whole-body 35-mm-diameter RF transceiver coil and shielded gradient coils, the resulting data set yields in-plane spatial resolutions of 500 × 250 mm$^2$ with adequate S/N and soft-tissue differentiation (T1-weighted contrast).

### 3.1.2. High-Resolution T1-Weighted SE or GRE Acquisition

1. Typical MR parameters for SE at 4.7 T (axial plane): TE/TR = 8/400 ms, 256 × 192 matrix, 40-kHz bandwidth, 3000-ms excitation and 1860-ms refocusing pulse length, 32 × 32-mm FOV, 1-mm slice thickness with interlaced data acquisition, 5–21 contiguous slices, 4 NEX with a total data acquisition time of < 5 min 10 s. Using a 35-mm-diameter RF transceiver coil designed for whole-body murine imaging, the resulting data set yields an in-plane spatial resolution of 125 × 167 mm$^2$ with adequate S/N and soft-tissue differentiation.
2. Additional inversion recovery, fat suppression, magnetization transfer, and/or other pulses and motion-suppression techniques are commonly used as necessary for enhanced tumor boundary discrimination.

### 3.1.3. High-Resolution Moderately T2-Weighted SE, Fast SE, or GRE Acquisition

1. MR imaging parameters are generally adjusted and optimized for each MR acquisition in order to maximize tumor/tissue conspicuity.

2. Tumor volume changes are monitored longitudinally in individual mice as a function of time and treatment by iterative repetitions of the above protocol. It is expected that MR exams not exceed one scan every 1–2 wk for determining tumor onset and one time point not more than every 1–2 d (fast-growing tumors) to 1 wk (slower-growing tumors) for assessment of tumor growth.
3. Tumor volume measurements are performed using T1-, T2-, or proton density-weighted SE or GRE MR pulse sequences with or without the administration of a contrast-enhancing agent for high-contrast anatomical differentiation of tumor boundaries.
4. Typical MR parameters for fast SE at 4.7 T (axial plane): TE/TR = 10/2424 ms, 192 × 128 matrix, 50-kHz bandwidth, 2000-ms excitation and refocusing pulse length, 32 × 32-mm FOV, RARE factor = 8 echoes yielding a $TE_{eff}$ = 41.05 ms, 1-mm slice thickness with interlaced data acquisition, 5–21 contiguous slices, 8 NEX with a total data acquisition time of < 5 min 20 s. The resulting data set yields an in-plane spatial resolution of 167 × 250 mm$^2$ with adequate S/N and soft-tissue differentiation (*see* **Note 6**).
5. Postacquisition image processing of raw data: Using techniques published previously *(62)*, MR images are generally segmented by visual inspection of the image using thresholding and "seed-growing" algorithms, whereby a user selects a pixel of interest and the software connects adjacent pixels in two or three dimensions having a defined signal intensity range. The accuracy of tumor boundary definition is then generally assessed and adjusted on a slice-by-slice basis (*see* **Note 7**).
6. Finally, pixels visually determined to contain tumor are summed in three dimensions (voxels) using automated analysis programs yielding a measurement of total tumor volume.
7. Tumors of a minimum size of < 10–20 mm$^3$ can be detected using high-resolution MR scanners and artifact-free data sets. Auto segmentation algorithms are becoming increasingly available, user-friendly, and robust.

## 3.2. Blood Oxygenation Level-Dependent (BOLD) Sensitive fMR Imaging of Tumors

1. Typical MR parameters for T2-weighted MR imaging data acquisitions (*see* **Note 8**): TE/TR = 35/4500 ms, 128 × 128 matrix, 50-kHz bandwidth, 2000-ms excitation and refocusing pulse length, 32 × 32-mm FOV, RARE factor = 4 echoes yielding a $TE_{eff}$ = 79.66 ms, 1-mm slice thickness with interlaced data acquisition, 5–21 contiguous slices, 2 NEX with a total data acquisition time of < 4 min 55 s. Using a whole-body 35-mm-diameter RF transceiver coil, the resulting data set yields an in-plane spatial resolution of 250 mm$^2$ with adequate S/N and BOLD sensitivity.
2. Baseline MR data is first acquired (animal breathing room air) and then repeated after an applied vascular stress (such as carbogen or acetazolamide) (*see* **Note 9**).
3. Postacquisition image processing of raw data (*see* **Notes 10** and **11**). The workflow paradigm utilizes at least two sequentially acquired fMR data sets, one set used for baseline vascular status and another set acquired while administering a

vascular stimulus to the animal. A map of the pixel-by-pixel change in signal intensity of baseline values compared to the applied vascular stress is calculated from the BOLD-sensitive fMR acquisition for either the whole MR data set, or more commonly, for specific regions of interest that have been segmented into "objects" (tumors, organs, phantoms, etc.).
4. The resultant functional MR map of signal intensity change can then be saved as a floating-point volume and individual ROIs examined statistically.
5. To enhance visualization of specific regions of change, a color lookup table (lut) is applied to the functional map, and an anisotropic diffusion filter (iterations = 4–6, time interval = 0.25) and/or low-pass filter (kernel 3 × 3 × 1) applied in order to reduce systemic noise while preserving internal tumor boundary regions.
6. The resultant colorized functional map can then be overlaid upon a T1-weighted scan for high-resolution localization of anatomic and physiological information.
7. The resultant data set containing anatomic and physiological information can also be rendered for 2-D/3-D display and saved as a series of single-slice 2-D TIFF (tagged image file format) images or rendered as a surface or 3-D projection through the data set for hardcopy or publication.
8. The following parameters should be adjusted as needed:
   a. Color lookup table applied to functional map.
   b. Dynamic range of lookup table.
   c. Opacity of regions containing physiological information overlaid on image containing morphological/anatomic information.
   d. Spatial filter parameters (including but not limited to kernel size, iterations, kappa).

## *3.3. Diffusion-Weighted fMR Imaging of Tumor*

### *3.3.1. Isotropic Diffusion-Weighted Acquisitions for ADC Calculations*

1. The following MR parameters are typical values for multislice, multidiffusion-weighted SE at 4.7 T (axial plane): TE/TR = 30/1200 ms, 128 × 128 matrix, 50-kHz bandwidth, 2000-ms excitation and refocusing pulse length, 32 × 32-mm FOV, diffusion gradient pulse = 14 ms, diffusion gradient strength (4) = 8.00, 128.00, 256.00, 384.0 mT/m, diffusion $B$ value (4) = 3.236, 569.065, 2263.023, 5082.565 s/mm$^2$, diffusion gradient duration = 6 ms, diffusion gradients applied in $x$, $y$, and $z$ directions, 1.5-mm slice thickness with 0.5-mm slice gap, pulse shape for imaging = sinc3, 2 NEX with a total data acquisition time of < 20 min 25 s. Using a whole-body 35-mm-diameter RF transceiver coil, the resulting data set yields an in-plane spatial resolution of 250 × 250 mm$^2$ with adequate S/N (*see* **Note 12**).

### *3.3.2. Postacquisition Image Processing of Raw Data*

1. The degree of diffusion weighting is frequently related to the strength of the diffusion gradient in mT/m. A quantitative representation of diffusion weighting (without gradient cross-terms) is expressed in the $B(i)$ value term ($B$) using the equation $S(B) = S_0 \, e^{[-(ADC)*B)]} + C$, where $S(B)$ is the signal intensity dependent on

$B$, $S_0$ is the signal obtained without diffusion gradient ($B = 0$), ADC = apparent diffusion coefficient, $B = \gamma^2 * \mathrm{dgs}^2 * \mathrm{dd}^2 * (\mathrm{db} - \mathrm{dd}/3)$ and is expressed in s/mm² and dgs = amplitude of the diffusion gradient pulse; dd = duration of each diffusion gradient pulse; db = duration between the start of the first diffusion gradient pulse and the start of the second diffusion gradient pulse, and $C$ is the offset from zero as $B \rightarrow \infty$. From this equation it follows that signal attenuation due to diffusion is influenced by three parameters: (a) diffusion gradient duration, (b) diffusion gradient strength, and (c) db.

2. After acquiring a series of diffusion-weighted images, a map of the diffusion coefficients, or ADC map, can be generated from the raw data by solving algebraic expressions relating resultant data to the parameters used for acquisition. Although it is an oversimplification of the biophysics involved, in general, ADC values are inversely related to the cellularity of tumors. ADC maps can be calculated from the raw data by solving the above diffusion equation for $D$ on a pixel-by-pixel basis using nonlinear regression analysis of MR signal intensity vs $B$ value. Algorithms for data calculations are currently available on most MR acquisition software packages, or ADC calculations can be performed offline using commercially available software (e.g., Mathematica, Wolfram Research, Champaign, IL; Matlab, MathWorks, Natick, MA; IDL Software, Research Systems, Boulder, CO; etc.) (*see* **Note 13**).

## 3.4. Dynamic Contrast-Enhanced (DCE) Perfusion-Weighted fMR Imaging

### 3.4.1. Acquisition

1. Place iv catheter in tail vein.
2. Acquire MR localizer image for selection anatomic reference.
3. Set up and begin acquiring MR data using preselected dynamic acquisition or fast acquisition protocol. Typical SE parameters at 4.7 T for fast-acquisition perfusion-weighted imaging: TE/TR = 8.1/234 ms, 192 × 128 matrix, 42-kHz bandwidth, 3000-µs excitation and 1860-µs refocusing pulse length, 32 × 32-mm FOV, 1.0-mm slice thickness, 1 NEX with a total data acquisition time of < 30 min for 20–60 evolutions (or approx 10–30 s per image or faster, depending on the desired acquisition speed, infusion parameters, S/N required, etc). Using a whole-body 35-mm-diameter RF transceiver coil, the resulting data set yields an in-plane spatial resolution of 167 × 250 µm² with adequate S/N (*see* **Note 14**). Acquire several baseline scans before initiating contrast-enhancing agent infusion.
4. Initiate infusion of contrast-enhancing agent. Whenever possible, use low volume with a high concentration of the selected agent (so as to model biodistribution and pharmacokinetics using well characterized tracer kinetic algorithms commonly used for PET) (*see* **Note 15**).

### 3.4.2. Postacquisition Image Processing of Raw Data

1. After acquiring a series of DCE perfusion-weighted images, the resultant images can be visualized as a movie of individual image slices played back in a time-

ordered fashion related to their MR acquisition. The capability is routinely available on most MR scanners.
2. More elaborate and detailed analysis can be performed offline on the raw data by calculating on a pixel-by-pixel basis the percentage change from baseline values, the percentage change from the average of a range of images immediately preceding the slice of interest, the absolute signal intensity change from baseline, the T1 and/or the T2 contribution of the contrast enhancing agent (if relaxivity measurements were also performed), etc. (*see* **Notes 16** and **17**).

## 3.5. Localized In Vivo MR Spectroscopy and Chemical Shift Imaging (CSI)

### 3.5.1. Acquisition

1. Ensure that the animal is positioned so that the tumor or volume under study is as close to magnetic field isocenter as possible and concentric with the sensitive volume of the RF coil used.
2. Set transceiver gains: With water suppression pulses off, determine transmitter and receiver gains for 90° and/or 180° flip angles.
3. Shimming: Adjust first-order $X$, $Y$, and $Z$ magnetic field gradient power supply shims for optimal magnetic field homogeneity across volume of interest (*see* **Note 18**).
4. If available, repeat the above procedure for higher-order magnetic field gradient power supply values. The FWHH (full width at half-height) linewidth for water in an in vivo sample at 4.7 T should be < 7–12 Hz across the volume of interest.
5. Water suppression: Ensure that the offset frequency for water is set correctly.
6. Acquiring MR spectroscopic data: Typical MR acquisition parameters for PRESS at 4.7 T; TE/TR = 80/2000 ms, 50-kHz bandwidth, 1000-ms excitation pulse length, excitation pulse shape = hermite, 2048 NEX with a total data acquisition time of < 1 h 8 min 16 s. Voxel size is determined primarily by the tissue, organ, or tumor being investigated. Using a whole-body 35-mm diameter RF transceiver coil, the resulting data set yields a localized voxel for data sampling with adequate S/N (*see* **Notes 19** and **20**).

### 3.5.2. Postacquisition Image Processing of Raw Data

1. Processing of spectroscopic data sets is input specific and varied (*see* **Note 21**).
2. Some typical parameters used for enhancing digitally acquired spectroscopic data sets:
   a. Exponential multiplication (EM) with line broadening (LB) = 1–3 Hz improves S/N.
   b. Zero filling (ZF) of the raw data (e.g., 2K data points) improves digital resolution.
   c. Fourier transformation (FT) converts amplitude-vs-time acquired data to amplitude-vs-frequency data, thereby resolving individual frequency components in raw data.

d. Phasing raw data (ph0, ph1) minimizes phase errors in resultant data set due to acquisition imperfections, system errors, etc.

e. Baseline correction (BC) fits resultant data set to a polynomial or other function to improve integration accuracy of resultant frequency components.

3. Chemical shift offset (usually in hertz) to a known reference standard such as water peak for comparison and calibration of results as a function of magnetic field strength (generally in parts per million, ppm). This allows results obtained at different magnetic field strengths to be readily compared and analyzed.

## 4. Notes

1. The most commonly used contrast-enhancing agents contain gadolinium [Gd(III)] because of its seven unpaired electrons and large paramagnetic moment. At present, three similar Gd(III)-derived MR contrast-enhancing agents have been approved for clinical use in the United States, the bis-*N*-methylglucamine salt of Gd(III)diethylenetriaminepentaacetic acid (DTPA) (Magnavist®), the bis *N*-methylamide of Gd(III) DTPA (Omniscan®), and the Gd(III) chelate of 20 (2-hydroxypropyl) derivative of 1,4,7,10-tetraazacyclododecane-*N,N2',N",N"'*-1,4,7-tetraacetic acid (Prohance®). All three of these agents are low-molecular-weight, carboxylate-containing, water-soluble complexes. After intravenous injection of a Gd(III)-containing agent, a transient MR signal increase is observed on T1-weighted scans as these agents first reside in the vascular space and then penetrate the "leaky" capillary beds common in many tumors (nonspecific uptake/retention). However, the effects of these agents are relatively short-lived, as they are rapidly excreted through the kidneys by glomerular filtration (plasma half-life < 15 min). Although a growing number of MR contrast-enhancing agents have been designed and are currently undergoing evaluation to improve agent specificity by targeting defined metabolic pathways, cellular receptors or physiological environmental conditions, no specific tumor-avid MR contrast-enhancing agent is clinically available to date. Still, it is important to note that preliminary results from several agents look extremely promising and might yield a clinical impact in the not so distant future. It should also be noted that several experimental macromolecular contrast-enhancing agents are commercially available for studies using animal models of disease. These agents, while not fully characterized or intended for ultimate clinical use, have and will continue to demonstrate unique insights into chemotherapeutic questions assessing drug delivery, drug resistance, vascular effects vs direct cell kill, etc. Historically, several pharmaceutical or chemical companies have listed partial summaries of available MR agents including their predominant effects, indications for usage, and their stage of development, e.g., follow the links at www.amershamhealth.com. As indicated, both "positive-contrast" (e.g., $Gd^{3+}$-based) and "negative-contrast" (e.g., $Fe^{2+,3+}$, Dy-based) MR imaging enhancers are available from various sources in limited supplies for specific indications. For example, MacroGd™ and other agents are commercially available exclusively for small animal research (PharmaIn, Buffalo Grove, IL).

MacroGd™ is a macromolecular long-circulating gadolinium-containing contrast agent (MethoxyPEG succinyl-poly-L-lysine-DTPA, Gd salt) with a molecular weight (MW) of approx 500 kDa for fMR quantitation of tumor angiogenesis, vascular structures and abnormal vascular permeability in cancer, inflammation, arthritis, etc. Another agent is human serum albumin (HSA) linked to Gd-DTPA or one of its derivatives with a MW of approx 40 kDa *(63)*. In general, higher-MW macromolecular agents tend to demonstrate prolonged plasma half-lives, thereby increasing S/N per unit time and decreasing many of the problems associated with rapid-acquisition MR techniques such as artifacts due to phase-encoding errors. A growing number of agents developed specifically for multi-modality-based "molecular targeting" and in rapid development include monocrystalline iron oxide nanoparticles (MION), polycrystalline iron oxide nanoparticles (PION), and "magnetic nanosensing crosslinked iron oxide (CLIO) particles. CLIO particles consist of a small (5-nm) monocrystalline superparamagnetic iron oxide cores stabilized by a cross-linked (CL), aminated dextran coating, resulting in an overall particle size of 45 nm, to which specific peptides can be attached for cellular/molecular targeting *(64)*. These experimental MR contrast-enhancing media and other related MR agents will, when fully realized, yield improved visualization of vascular structures, specific cell types and cellular markers, etc. A subset of these agents will no doubt be important for future assessment, design, and optimization of chemotherapeutic protocols as well as for determining their ultimate efficacy in both clinical and preclinical environments.
2. In general, four distinct methods have emerged for 3-D in vivo localization of spectral data. These include (a) point-resolved spectroscopy (PRESS), (b) stimulated echo acquisition mode (STEAM), (c) image-selected in vivo spectroscopy (ISIS), and (d) magnetic resonance spectroscopic imaging (MRSI), sometimes called chemical-shift imaging (CSI) methods. Each of these methods has its own advantages and disadvantages. For example, unlike STEAM, PRESS acquisitions retain the entire possible signal available from an acquisition. A disadvantage of PRESS is that a series of RF pulses must be applied in the presence of an orthogonal gradient field, thereby prohibiting TE times as short as those possible using STEAM, so that proton metabolites with rapidly decaying signals cannot be observed.
3. A reference standard should be used whenever possible for comparing chemical shift, concentration, and local environmental factors that influence MR spectral signatures (preferably an internal reference standard should be used, but even an external standard can document reproducibility criteria and magnetic field homogeneity across the region of interest).
4. Representative images of each patient/sample/animal should be outputted to high-quality, extremely durable media, either onto film or dye-sublimation paper. Several medical photography companies offer suitable equipment (Codonics, Middleburg Heights, OH; Sony Business Solutions & Systems, New York, NY). Media must be resistant to fading or damage. Critical to each hardcopy is unique

identification of each scan and the date acquired. Additionally, important acquisition parameters such as TE/TR, resolution, and a distance scale are recommended as print area allows.

5. All data acquired must be archived for long-term storage on optical media, either CD-recordable (CDRs) or DVD-recordable (DVD±R). Rewritable optical media or magnetic media such as tape is not recommended for long-term archival because of their lower reliability. Alternatively, data may be transferred over a network to a large-capacity, RAID array for online storage, granted that the array is routinely backed up. A database of all archived data should be included in any archival strategy and should be searchable for numerous fields (patient ID or name, date of acquisition, keywords, etc.) to facilitate fast retrieval from archive media.

6. Additional preparatory pulses and/or motion-suppression techniques can be used as necessary for enhanced tumor boundary discrimination.

7. A large amount of postprocessing entails defining regions of interest and delineating anatomic boundaries. As such, postprocessing software should contain a reasonable toolbox for defining regions, including rectangular and circular functions, spline tools, seeded-growth algorithms, and manual trace and edit functions. Although there will continue to be advances in the field of automated image processing, it has been our experience that accurate measurements still require manual editing and fine-tuning of region-defining algorithms.

8. In studies in which the applied vascular stress is global, such as the administration of acetazolamide or carbogen, changes in the microvasculature may not be immediate and would require a delay be present between administration and data acquisition. It is also expected that the microvascular state may not return immediately to baseline status, and thus prevent repeating the experiment and consistent results. With this in mind, it is recommended that multiple baseline images be acquired prior to administration of the vascular stress agent and examined to determine if acquisition-to-acquisition artifacts exist.

9. Care must be taken to minimize any possible animal movement and to maintain identical MR acquisition parameters before, during, and immediately after applied vascular stress.

10. For processing BOLD-sensitive fMR data acquisitions, several commercially available software packages exist for developing customized analysis routines. Our laboratory has developed interactive fMR analysis algorithms interfaced to commercial image analysis and display software (AnalyzePC 5.0, Mayo Clinic, Rochester, MN). The module is dynamic, allowing researchers to process and explore functional MR data sets interactively.

11. Another possible pitfall in BOLD studies is the reconstruction of the raw data to an image, often saved in 8-, 16-, or 32-bit gray-scale color depth. Despite identical acquisition parameters in serially acquired scans, the intensity levels in the resultant images may vary as a result of inconsistent image reconstruction, often performed automatically by scanner software to maximize image contrast and to avoid "clipping" of the raw data. To this end, it is recommended that investigators

have an intimate knowledge of the image reconstruction methods used, and fully characterize scan-to-scan variability of signal intensity using suitable phantoms. It is also recommended a sealed phantom be in place during all live animal scans to act as an external standard for consistency.
12. Because the apparent diffusion coefficient (ADC) of water is highly dependent on the temperature of the sample under study, care must be taken to minimize any possible change in tumor temperature or animal movement during acquisition of diffusion data.
13. ADC calculations are often obtainable with commercially available packages obtained from MR imager vendors. However, individual researchers may find these packages too constricting or proprietary and may wish to calculate ADC values in an external program as discussed under **Subheading 3.3.2.** We offer some concerns over issues that should be addressed and some tips to aid in determining ADC values.

As shown under **Subheading 4.1.3.**, the signal intensity in a diffusion-weighted image is determined by the equation $S(B) = S_0 e^{[-(ADC)*B]} + C$. A paramount practical concern is the inclusion of the concept of a plateau, represented by the variable $C$, which accounts for system noise. At high diffusion gradient strengths (high $B$ values), systemic noise can account for a relatively significant portion of signal intensity, and failure to account for system noise may result in inaccurate calculations of ADC values. We recommend including within a diffusion experiment an acquisition that contains very high $B$ values (diffusion gradient strengths), which will result in a "noise image" that can then be subtracted from the other images acquired in the experiment, such that $S(B) - C = S_0 e^{[-(ADC)*B]}$.

Calculating the ADC values can be achieved in a number of ways. As mentioned under **Subheading 3.3.2.**, one can fit the acquired data using nonlinear regression analysis, which requires at least three different $B$ values and resulting images. It also requires appropriate initial estimation of $S_0$, $C$, and ADC values for the calculating function to converge. An alternative method involves applying the natural log (ln) to the equation, resulting in a linear equation $\ln[S(B) - C] = -(ADC) * B$. ADC can then be calculated with only two differing $B$ values, reducing experiment time and still providing accurate ADC calculations. Accounting for system noise, however, remains essential.
14. Care must be taken to minimize any possible animal movement and to maintain identical MR acquisition parameters before, during, and immediately after contrast-enhancing agent administration.
15. Be careful to minimize unwanted effects, toxicities, and confounding results caused by variations in pH, temperature, injection volume, viscosity, osmolarity, aggregation, solubility, etc.
16. For comparing longitudinal scans and/or postacquisition signal intensity quantification, time = 0 should correspond to the first image demonstrating signal intensity change in referenced anatomy (e.g., change in major vessel such as the aorta or vena cava, or signal intensity change in an organ such as the kidney or initial change in tumor). This will minimize systematic errors due at least in part to variations in

catheter length, injection volume, minor variations in the rate of infusion, etc.
17. It is often advantageous to visualize the change in signal intensity from DCE imaging as a percent change from baseline values, i.e., precontrast administration, and apply a color lookup table to facilitate visualization of the degree of change in intensity. Often subtle distinctions in intensity changes that can be missed by the human eye with a gray-scale image are seen readily when they are colorized. Also, as DCE imaging requires increased temporal resolution and shorter imaging times, phase artifacts are magnified and tend to obscure global changes in the anatomy with volatility of image intensities between scans. To reduce volatility and improve visual esthetics, we suggest applying either a low-pass or median filter with a $1 \times 1 \times 3$ or $1 \times 1 \times 5$ kernel to "smooth" out volatility between sequential scans (it is assumed that the Z direction is time, not space). Again, a number of commercially available software packages are available for performing these calculations and for visualizing the results as individual images or movie files.
18. Remember that this procedure must be performed in an iterative manner, because changes in one parameter are intimately coupled to results obtained in three dimensions.
19. It should be noted that a primary concern with in vivo spectroscopy of tumors is the near-identical chemical shifts of lactate, commonly used as a measure of anaerobic metabolism, and lipids present within or at the periphery of the tumor. To account for this, MR spectroscopy experiments are generally carried out with variable echo times. Because of the considerably shorter TE time of lipids, signal arising from the lipids is minimized at higher TEs, and a more accurate assessment of lactate concentration can then be determined.
20. Care must be taken to minimize any possible animal movement and to minimize unwanted signal contributions from bone and/or fat compartments.
21. The breadth and complexity of spectroscopic processing techniques prohibit detailed discussion in this chapter, and researchers can obtain thorough treatments elsewhere *(65,66)*.

## References

1. Gillies, R. J., Raghunand, N., Karczmar, G. S., and Bhujwalla, Z. M. (2002) MRI of the tumor microenvironment. *J. Magn. Reson. Imaging* **16,** 430–450.
2. Bhujwalla, Z. M., Artemov, D., Aboagye, E., et al. (2001) The physiological environment in cancer vascularization, invasion and metastasis. *Novartis. Found. Symp.* **240,** 23–38.
3. Bhujwalla, Z. M., Artemov, D., Ballesteros, P., Cerdan, S., Gillies, R. J., and Solaiyappan, M. (2002) Combined vascular and extracellular pH imaging of solid tumors. *NMR Biomed.* **15,** 114–119.
4. Ross, B. D., Zhao, Y. J., Neal, E. R., et al. (1998) Contributions of cell kill and posttreatment tumor growth rates to the repopulation of intracerebral 9L tumors after chemotherapy: an MRI study. *Proc. Natl. Acad. Sci. USA* **95,** 7012–7017.

5. Howe, F. A., Robinson, S. P., Rodrigues, L. M., and Griffiths, J. R. (1999) Flow and oxygenation dependent (FLOOD) contrast MR imaging to monitor the response of rat tumors to carbogen breathing. *Magn. Reson. Imaging* **17,** 1307–1318.
6. Robinson, S. P., Collingridge, D. R., Howe, F. A., Rodrigues, L. M., Chaplin, D. J., and Griffiths, J. R. (1999) Tumour response to hypercapnia and hyperoxia monitored by FLOOD magnetic resonance imaging. *NMR Biomed.* **12,** 98–106.
7. Griffiths, J. R. and Glickson, J. D. (2000) Monitoring pharmacokinetics of anticancer drugs: non-invasive investigation using magnetic resonance spectroscopy. *Adv. Drug Deliv. Rev.* **41,** 75–89.
8. Ackerstaff, E., Glunde, K., and Bhujwalla, Z. M. (2003) Choline phospholipid metabolism: a target in cancer cells? *J. Cell Biochem.* **90,** 525–533.
9. Bhujwalla, Z. M., Artemov, D., Natarajan, K., Ackerstaff, E., and Solaiyappan, M. (2001) Vascular differences detected by MRI for metastatic versus nonmetastatic breast and prostate cancer xenografts. *Neoplasia* **3,** 143–153.
10. Bhujwalla, Z. M., Artemov, D., Natarajan, K., Solaiyappan, M., Kollars, P., and Kristjansen, P. E. (2003) Reduction of vascular and permeable regions in solid tumors detected by macromolecular contrast magnetic resonance imaging after treatment with antiangiogenic agent TNP-470. *Clin. Cancer Res.* **9,** 355–362.
11. Lewin, M., Bredow, S., Sergeyev, N., Marecos, E., Bogdanov, A. Jr., and Weissleder, R. (1999) In vivo assessment of vascular endothelial growth factor-induced angiogenesis. *Int. J. Cancer* **83,** 798–802.
12. Weissleder, R. and Mahmood, U. (2001) Molecular imaging. *Radiology* **219,** 316–333.
13. Boxerman, J. L., Bandettini, P. A., Kwong, K. K., et al. (1995) The intravascular contribution to fMRI signal change: Monte Carlo modeling and diffusion-weighted studies in vivo. *Magn. Reson. Med.* **34,** 4–10.
14. Bandettini, P. A., Kwong, K. K., Davis, T. L., Tootell, R. B., Wong, E. C., and Fox, P. T. (1997) Characterization of cerebral blood oxygenation and flow changes during prolonged brain activation. *Hum. Brain* Mapp. *5, 93–109.*
15. Davis, T. L., Kwong, K. K., Weisskoff, R. M., and Rosen, B. R. (1998) Calibrated functional MRI: mapping the dynamics of oxidative metabolism. *Proc. Natl. Acad. Sci. USA* **95,** 1834–1839.
16. Howe, F. A., Robinson, S. P., McIntyre, D. J., Stubbs, M., and Griffiths, J. R. (2001) Issues in flow and oxygenation dependent contrast (FLOOD) imaging of tumours. *NMR Biomed.* **14,** 497–506.
17. Bott, G. (1985) Vasodilators and regional blood flow. *Indian J. Pharmacol.* 1985.
18. Mazurchuk, R., Zhou, R., Straubinger, R. M., Chau, R. I., and Grossman, Z. (1999) Functional magnetic resonance (fMR) imaging of a rat brain tumor model: implications for evaluation of tumor microvasculature and therapeutic response. *Magn. Reson. Imaging* **17,** 537–548.
19. Zhou, R., Mazurchuk, R., and Straubinger, R. M. (2002) Antivasculature effects of doxorubicin-containing liposomes in an intracranial rat brain tumor model. *Cancer Res.* **62,** 2561–2566.

20. Bhattacharya, A., Toth, K., Mazurchuk, R., et al. (2004) Lack of microvessels in well-differentiated regions of human head and neck squamous cell carcinoma A253 is associated with fMR imaging detectable hypoxia, limited drug delivery and resistance to irinotecan therapy. *Clin. Cancer Res.* **10,** 8005–8017.
21. Neeman, M. and Dafni, H. (2003) Structural functional, and molecular MR imaging of the microvasculature. *Annu. Rev. Biomed. Eng.* **5,** 29–56.
22. Neeman, M., Dafni, H., Bukhari, O., Braun, R. D., and Dewhirst, M. W. (2001) In vivo BOLD contrast MRI mapping of subcutaneous vascular function and maturation: validation by intravital microscopy. *Magn. Reson. Med.* **45,** 887–898.
23. Shaharabany, M., Abramovitch, R., Kushnir, T., et al. (2001) In vivo molecular imaging of met tyrosine kinase growth factor receptor activity in normal organs and breast tumors. *Cancer Res.* **61,** 4873–4878.
24. Artemov, D., Solaiyappan, M., and Bhujwalla, Z. M. (2001) Magnetic resonance pharmacoangiography to detect and predict chemotherapy delivery to solid tumors. *Cancer Res.* **61,** 3039–3044.
25. Fenton, B. M., Lord, E. M., and Paoni, S. F. (2000) Enhancement of tumor perfusion and oxygenation by carbogen and nicotinamide during single- and multifraction irradiation. *Radiat. Res.* **153,** 75–83.
26. Chenevert, T. L., Meyer, C. R., Moffat, B. A., et al. (2002) Diffusion MRI: a new strategy for assessment of cancer therapeutic efficacy. *Mol. Imaging* **1,** 336–343.
27. Ross, B. D., Moffat, B. A., Lawrence, T. S., et al. (2003) Evaluation of cancer therapy using diffusion magnetic resonance imaging. *Mol. Cancer Ther.* **2,** 581–587.
28. Chenevert, T. L., Stegman, L. D., Taylor, J. M., et al. (2000) Diffusion magnetic resonance imaging: an early surrogate marker of therapeutic efficacy in brain tumors. *J. Natl. Cancer Inst.* **92,** 2029–2036.
29. Stegman, L. D., Rehemtulla, A., Hamstra, D. A., et al. (2000) Diffusion MRI detects early events in the response of a glioma model to the yeast cytosine deaminase gene therapy strategy. *Gene Ther.* **7,** 1005–1010.
30. Chenevert, T. L., McKeever, P. E., and Ross, B. D. (1997) Monitoring early response of experimental brain tumors to therapy using diffusion magnetic resonance imaging. *Clin. Cancer Res.* **3,** 1457–1466.
31. Daldrup-Link, H. E. and Brasch, R. C. (2003) Macromolecular contrast agents for MR mammography: current status. *Eur. Radiol.* **13,** 354–365.
32. Choyke, P. L., Dwyer, A. J., and Knopp, M. V. (2003) Functional tumor imaging with dynamic contrast-enhanced magnetic resonance imaging. *J. Magn. Reson. Imaging* **17,** 509–520.
33. Padhani, A. R. (2002) Dynamic contrast-enhanced MRI in clinical oncology: current status and future directions. *J. Magn. Reson. Imaging* **16,** 407–422.
34. Roberts, T. P., Turetschek, K., Preda, A., et al. (2002) Tumor microvascular changes to anti-angiogenic treatment assessed by MR contrast media of different molecular weights. *Acad. Radiol.* **9 (Suppl. 2),** S511–S513.
35. Roberts, T. P., Helbich, T. H., Ley, S., et al. (2002) Utility (or not) of Gd-DTPA-based dynamic MRI for breast cancer diagnosis and grading. *Acad. Radiol.* **9 (Suppl. 1),** S261–S265.

36. Roberts, H. C., Roberts, T. P., Brasch, R. C., and Dillon, W. P. (2000) Quantitative measurement of microvascular permeability in human brain tumors achieved using dynamic contrast-enhanced MR imaging: correlation with histologic grade. *Am. J. Neuroradiol.* **21,** 891–899.
37. Gossmann, A., Helbich, T. H., Kuriyama, N., et al. (2002) Dynamic contrast-enhanced magnetic resonance imaging as a surrogate marker of tumor response to anti-angiogenic therapy in a xenograft model of glioblastoma multiforme. *J. Magn. Reson. Imaging* **15,** 233–240.
38. Stiskal, M., Demsar, F., Muhler, A., et al. (1999) Contrast-enhanced MR imaging of two superparamagnetic RES-contrast agents: functional assessment of experimental radiation-induced liver injury. *J. Magn. Reson. Imaging* **10,** 52–56.
39. Pham, C. D., Roberts, T. P., van Bruggen, N., et al. (1998) Magnetic resonance imaging detects suppression of tumor vascular permeability after administration of antibody to vascular endothelial growth factor. *Cancer Invest.* **16,** 225–230.
40. Brasch, R., Pham, C., Shames, D., et al. (1997) Assessing tumor angiogenesis using macromolecular MR imaging contrast media. *J. Magn. Reson. Imaging* **7,** 68–74.
41. Aksoy, F. G. and Lev, M. H. (2000) Dynamic contrast-enhanced brain perfusion imaging: technique and clinical applications. *Semin. Ultrasound CT MR* **21,** 462–477.
42. Padhani, A. R., Gapinski, C. J., Macvicar, D. A., et al. (2000) Dynamic contrast enhanced MRI of prostate cancer: correlation with morphology and tumour stage, histological grade and PSA. *Clin. Radiol.* **55,** 99–109.
43. Kurhanewicz, J., Swanson, M. G., Nelson, S. J., and Vigneron, D. B. (2002) Combined magnetic resonance imaging and spectroscopic imaging approach to molecular imaging of prostate cancer. *J. Magn. Reson. Imaging* **16,** 451–463.
44. Mueller-Lisse, U. G., Vigneron, D. B., Hricak, H., et al. (2001) Localized prostate cancer: effect of hormone deprivation therapy measured by using combined three-dimensional 1H MR spectroscopy and MR imaging: clinicopathologic case-controlled study. *Radiology* **221,** 380–390.
45. Males, R. G., Vigneron, D. B., Star-Lack, J., et al. (2000) Clinical application of BASING and spectral/spatial water and lipid suppression pulses for prostate cancer staging and localization by in vivo 3D 1H magnetic resonance spectroscopic imaging. *Magn. Reson. Med.* **43,** 17–22.
46. Yu, K. K., Scheidler, J., Hricak, H., et al. (1999) Prostate cancer: prediction of extracapsular extension with endorectal MR imaging and three-dimensional proton MR spectroscopic imaging. *Radiology* **213,** 481–488.
47. Scheidler, J., Hricak, H., Vigneron, D. B., et al. (1999) Prostate cancer: localization with three-dimensional proton MR spectroscopic imaging—clinicopathologic study. *Radiology* **213,** 473–480.
48. Artemov, D., Pilatus, U., Chu, S., Mori, N., Nelson, J. B., and Bhujwalla, Z. M. (1999) Dynamics of prostate cancer cell invasion studied in vitro by NMR microscopy. *Magn. Reson. Med.* **42,** 277–282.
49. Kaji, Y., Kurhanewicz, J., Hricak, H., et al. (1998) Localizing prostate cancer in the presence of postbiopsy changes on MR images: role of proton MR spectroscopic imaging. *Radiology* **206,** 785–790.

50. Parivar, F., Hricak, H., Shinohara, K., et al. (1996) Detection of locally recurrent prostate cancer after cryosurgery: evaluation by transrectal ultrasound, magnetic resonance imaging, and three-dimensional proton magnetic resonance spectroscopy. *Urology* **48,** 594–599.
51. Kurhanewicz, J., Vigneron, D. B., Hricak, H., et al. (1996) Prostate cancer: metabolic response to cryosurgery as detected with 3D H-1 MR spectroscopic imaging. *Radiology* **200,** 489–496.
52. Kurhanewicz, J., Vigneron, D. B., Hricak, H., Narayan, P., Carroll, P., and Nelson, S. J. (1996) Three-dimensional H-1 MR spectroscopic imaging of the in situ human prostate with high (0.24–0.7-cm$^3$) spatial resolution. *Radiology* **198,** 795–805.
53. Kurhanewicz, J., Vigneron, D. B., Nelson, S. J., et al. (1995) Citrate as an in vivo marker to discriminate prostate cancer from benign prostatic hyperplasia and normal prostate peripheral zone: detection via localized proton spectroscopy. *Urology* **45,** 459–466.
54. Blackstock, A. W., Lightfoot, H., Case, L. D., et al. (2001) Tumor uptake and elimination of 2′,2′-difluoro-2′-deoxycytidine (gemcitabine) after deoxycytidine kinase gene transfer: correlation with in vivo tumor response. *Clin. Cancer Res.* **7,** 3263–3268.
55. Brix, G., Bellemann, M. E., Gerlach, L., and Haberkorn, U. (1998) Intra- and extracellular fluorouracil uptake: assessment with contrast-enhanced metabolic F-19 MR imaging. *Radiology* **209,** 259–267.
56. Vion-Dury, J., Machy, P., Confort-Gouny, S., Leserman, L., and Cozzone, P. J. (1993) Specific in vitro labeling of cells with a fluorine-19 probe encapsulated in antibody-targeted liposomes: a F-19 NMR spectroscopy study. *Magn. Reson. Med.* **29,** 252–255.
57. Wolf, W., Albright, M. J., Silver, M. S., Weber, H., Reichardt, U., and Sauer, R. (1987) Fluorine-19 NMR spectroscopic studies of the metabolism of 5-fluorouracil in the liver of patients undergoing chemotherapy. *Magn. Reson. Imaging* **5,** 165–169.
58. Yamada, K., Matsuzawa, T., Sato, T., et al. (1986) In vivo F-19 NMR imaging and the influence of oxygenation on relaxation time. *Sci. Rep. Res. Inst. Tohoku Univ. [Med.]* **33,** 44–48.
59. Kanazawa, Y., Momozono, Y., Ishikawa, M., et al. (1986) Metabolic pathway of 2-deoxy-2-fluoro-D-glucose studied by F-19 NMR. *Life Sci.* **39,** 737–742.
60. Raleigh, J. A., Franko, A. J., Treiber, E. O., Lunt, J. A., and Allen, P. S. (1986) Covalent binding of a fluorinated 2-nitroimidazole to EMT-6 tumors in Balb/C mice: detection by F-19 nuclear magnetic resonance at 2.35 T. *Int. J. Radiat. Oncol. Biol. Phys.* **12,** 1243–1245.
61. Nicholson, J. K., Connelly, J., Lindon, J. C., and Holmes, E. (2002) Metabonomics: a platform for studying drug toxicity and gene function. *Nat. Rev. Drug Discov.* **1,** 153–161.

62. Mazurchuk, R., Glaves, D., and Raghavan, D. (1997) Magnetic resonance imaging of response to chemotherapy in orthotopic xenografts of human bladder cancer. *Clin. Cancer Res.* **3,** 1635–1641.
63. Ostrowitzki, S., Fick, J., Roberts, T. P., et al. (1998) Comparison of gadopentetate dimeglumine and albumin-(Gd-DTPA)30 for microvessel characterization in an intracranial glioma model. *J. Magn. Reson. Imaging* **8,** 799–806.
64. Schellenberger, E. A., Bogdanov, A. Jr., Hogemann, D., Tait, J., Weissleder, R., and Josephson, L. (2002) Annexin V-CLIO: a nanoparticle for detecting apoptosis by MRI. *Mol. Imaging* **1,** 102–107.
65. Peter Bigler. *NMR Spectroscopy: Processing Strategies*, 2nd ed., Wiley-VCH, New York, 2000.
66. de Graaf, RA. *In Vivo NMR Spectroscopy*, Wiley, New York, 1988.

# 26

# Metabolic Monitoring of Chemosensitivity with $^{18}$FDG PET

## Guy Jerusalem and Tarik Z. Belhocine

### Summary

Accurate and early evaluation of tumor response to chemotherapy is a growing clinical need for optimal management of oncology patients. This is even more warranted by the lack of appropriate response evaluation criteria to new molecularly targeted anticancer therapies. In the two last decades, new developments in the field of nuclear oncology have allowed the introduction of various radiopharmaceuticals to be used on dedicated imaging devices. In the present chapter, we report the added value that positron emission tomography (PET) with $^{18}$F-fluorodeoxyglucose ($^{18}$FDG) may offer to assess tumor response to treatment. PET is a high-end imaging technology using 18FDG as metabolic tracer that mimics the biochemical behavior of the natural glucose molecule. Because most tumor types exhibit increased glucose metabolism, the imaging of $^{18}$FDG uptake within cancer tissues prior to any treatment enables the metabolic technique to follow tumor responsiveness sequentially after one or several courses of chemotherapy. Moreover, metabolic tumor response evaluated by $^{18}$FDG PET often precedes morphological tumor changes measured by computed tomography or magnetic resonance imaging. So far, the suboptimal properties of $^{18}$FDG tracer and the lack of standardized methodology in PET imaging remain objective limitations for qualitative and quantitative assessment of chemosensitivity using the metabolic method.

### Key Words

Metabolic imaging; $^{18}$FDG; PET; cancer; chemosensitivity.

## 1. Introduction

Most tumor types exhibit increased glucose metabolism (*see* **Note 1**) *(1,2)*. Such a pathological feature is mediated by an increase of glucose transporters (GLUT), especially GLUT-1, GLUT-3, and GLUT-5 *(3)*. The malignant process is also characterized by quantitative and qualitative enzymatic changes affect-

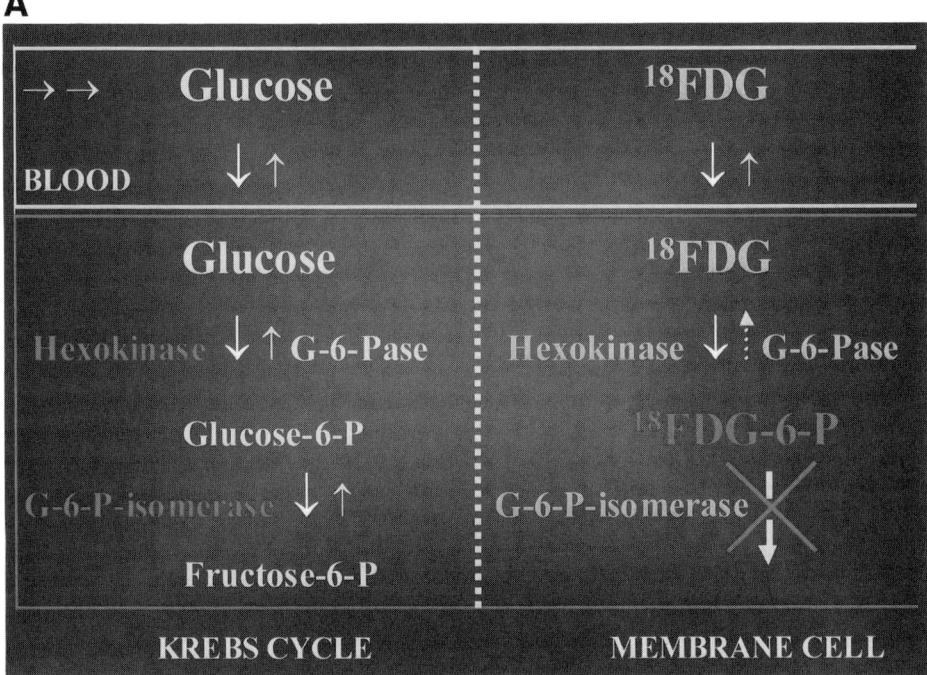

Fig. 1A. Glucose uptake into tumor cells. The glucose molecule is avidly taken up into tumor cells via facilitative (energy-independent) glucose transporters (GLUTs) and phosphorylated by hexokinase. The glucose-6-phosphate is then substrate for glucose-6-phosphate-isomerase, thereby, leading to fructose-6-phosphate. In anaerobic conditions, fructose-6-phosphate is engaged into the pyruvate and lactate pathways, while in aerobic conditions, the compound enters into the Krebs cycle. (See color insert following p. 238.)

ing key enzymes of the glycolytic pathway, such as hexokinase, phosphofructokinase, and pyruvate kinase *(4,5)* (*see* **Fig. 1A**).

The glucose tropism of tumor cells has been exploited for the imaging of cancers by using a radiolabeled glucose analog (**Fig. 1B**), 18F-fluoro-2-deoxy-D-glucose ($^{18}$FDG) (*see* **Note 2**), with positron emission tomography (PET) *(6,7)*. In many malignancies, the value of $^{18}$FDG PET is nowadays well recognized, either for staging the extent of disease prior to any treatment or for detecting recurrences in follow-up *(8,9)*.

Another field of interest provided by $^{18}$FDG PET is the possibility to monitor chemosensitivity by the assessment of the metabolic response of cancers *(10)*. Indeed, in various animal and human cancer models, $^{18}$FDG uptake has been shown to correlate with tumor cell proliferation and/or viability (*see* **Note 3**)

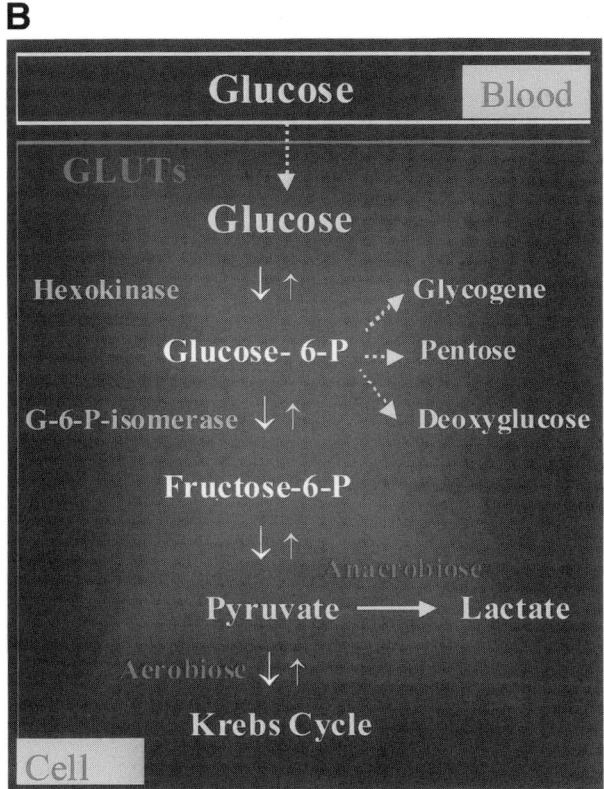

Fig. 1B. $^{18}$FDG uptake into tumor cells. The FDG molecule follows the metabolic pathways involving the same GLUT transporters and glycolytic enzymes. Unlike natural glucose, however, FDG-6-phosphate cannot be targeted by glucose-6-phosphate isomerase, an enzyme that requires the presence of an atom of oxygen on carbon 2 ($-C_2$) to be active. As the activity of the reverse enzyme (glucose-6-phosphatase) is negligible, FDG-6-phosphate bearing a negative charge accumulates in tumor cells without further significant degradation. Therefore, the tissue concentration of $^{18}$FDG tracer, a radiolabeled glucose analog, reflects quite faithfully that of FDG, which is ultimately an indicator of the glycolytic activity related to the endogenous glucose. (See color insert following p. 238.)

*(11–14)*. As treatment dose is linearly correlated with the log of the surviving fraction of sensitive tumor cells, the metabolic tracer may help assess chemosensitivity through the rate of cells surviving *(15)*. In addition, metabolic response of cancers assessed by $^{18}$FDG PET often precedes tumor shrinkage as determined by conventional morphological imaging *(16,17)*.

Several preclinical and clinical studies have assessed various protocols based on the use of $^{18}$FDG PET for monitoring chemosensitivity *(18)*. The qualitative

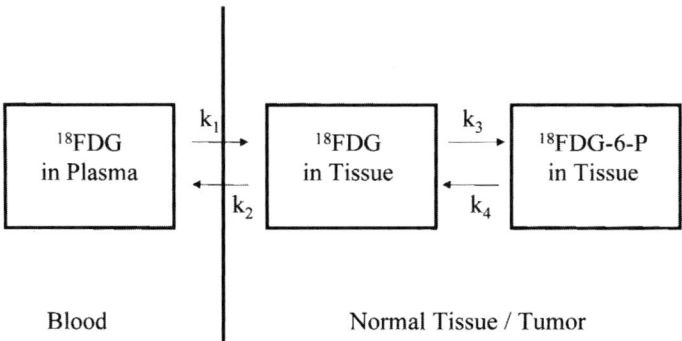

Fig. 2. Quantitative assessment of $^{18}$FDG uptake using a compartmental model. Nonlinear regression is considered the method of reference for the quantitative assessment of $^{18}$FDG uptake. This kinetic approach is derived from Sokoloff's brain model and allows the determination of four kinetic constants related to $^{18}$FDG uptake and metabolism into tumor and nontumor tissues ($k_1$ = input function; $k_2$ = output function; $k_3$ = phosphorylation (hexokinase); $k_4$ = dephosphophrylation (glucose-6-phosphatase); $k_4$ constant is assumed to be negligible in irreversible models ($k_4 = 0$).

assessment of tumor responsiveness is done roughly by imaging the tumor burden on the whole body *(19,20)*. So far, visual interpretation has been subjective and often operator-dependent (*see* **Note 4**). The quantification of $^{18}$FDG uptake into tumor tissues has been proposed to achieve more accurate and reproducible assessment of chemosensitivity *(18,20,21)*. Reference quantitative approaches were originally based on kinetic methods requiring arterial blood sampling either for complex compartmental models or for simplified graphical analyses (*see* **Note 5**) *(22–25)*. **Figure 2** shows the compartmental analysis derived from Sokoloff's brain model to measure the kinetic constants related to $^{18}$FDG uptake and metabolism into tumor and nontumor tissues. Other authors suggested more practical methods based on the standardized uptake value body weight (SUV-BW) as the measurement of the $^{18}$FDG concentration normalized to the injected activity and to the body weight *(26,27)*. Further technical refinements have been derived from SUV-BW to quantify $^{18}$FDG uptake into tumor tissues using more independent and reproducible metabolic indexes *(28–35)*. However, the varying protocols of available clinical data prevent the definition of a well-standardized metabolic method for monitoring oncology patients *(17,18,20,22)*. **Tables 1** and **2** summarize the spectrum of methods for monitoring chemosensitivity with $^{18}$FDG PET.

In the present chapter, we report a practical method that may be easily implementable in clinical practice. Based on our experience in monitoring var-

## Metabolic Imaging

ious kinds of tumors such as lymphomas, breast cancers, lung cancers, and uterine cancers, we describe the methodological steps for qualitative and quantitative assessment of tumor responsiveness using $^{18}$FDG PET *(36–43)*. Nonetheless, various factors may alter the accuracy of metabolic assessment of chemosensitivity (*see* **Table 3**). In particular, the suboptimal properties of the $^{18}$FDG tracer stress the need for more specific and accurate methods to monitor chemosensitivity (*see* **Notes 6–9**).

## 2. Materials

1. $^{18}$F-fluorodeoxyglucose ($^{18}$FDG), 150–370 MBq (*see* **Note 10**).
2. Positron emission scanner (PET scanner) tomography, preferably a dedicated device (*see* **Note 11**).
3. Intravenous (iv) catheter for continuous infusion.
4. 0.9% NaCl, 500-mL solution.
5. Diazepam (Valium™), 5–10-mg tablets.
6. Mebeverine (Duspatalin™), 5–10-mg tablets.
7. Furosemide (Lasix™), 20-mg (2 mL) ampoules.
8. Glucometer, strips for rapid determination of patient's glycemia.
9. Insulin with rapid action (Actrapid™), to be used when necessary.

## 3. Methods

The assessment of chemosensitivity by means of $^{18}$FDG PET implies correct patient preparation, adequate imaging technique, and a reliable quantitative approach. Last but not least, the timing for appropriate assessment of metabolic tumor response to anticancer therapies according to the clinical needs should be taken into account. This latter condition, however, remains a matter to controversy. As stated above, we chose to describe a practical method based on a static, whole-body imaging, and a simple semiquantitative evaluation of $^{18}$FDG tumor uptake. Each step for a good procedure is detailed under **Subheadings 3.1., 3.2.,** and **3.3.**

### 3.1. Patient Preparation

1. Patients should fast for at least 6 h to diminish physiological glucose utilization and reduce insulin levels to near basal levels. (Fasting reduces $^{18}$FDG uptake by the heart and muscles, which optimizes the imaging quality in PET oncology.)
2. Access to medications and sugar-free solutions (coffee, water, etc.) is allowed.
3. Patients should ideally be installed in a quiet environment.
4. Place an iv line (in patients with breast cancers, perfusion should preferably be put in on the opposite side of the primary tumor).
5. Measure blood glucose level rapidly using instantaneous glucometer.
    a. Nonfasted diabetic patients should be appropriately medicated, and properly equilibrated.

## Table 1
## Qualitative and Quantitative Assessment of Chemosensitivity Using $^{18}$FDG PET

| Methods | Advantages | Limitations | Dependencies |
|---|---|---|---|
| Visual | 1. Static acquisition<br>2. Whole-body imaging<br>3. No blood sampling<br>4. Shorter scan times<br>5. ± Transmission scan | 1. Nonquantitative<br>2. Operator-dependent<br>3. Tumor-to-background ratio varies with activity<br>4. "Oversimplification" of dynamic tumor process<br>5. Lower counting statistics | 1. Uptake time<br>2. Glucose levels<br>3. Partial volume effects |
| Kinetic methods<br>Nonlinear regression (compartmental model)<br>Patlak graphical analysis | 1. Reference methods<br>2. Kinetic analysis<br>3. Dynamic acquisition<br>4. Quantitative<br>5. Less dependence on uptake time | 1. Arterial blood sampling required<br>2. Longer scan times (approx 1 h)<br>3. Localized views<br>4. Transmission scan required<br>5. Complex measurements<br>6. Difficult to implement in clinical practice | 1. Partial volume effects<br>2. Quality of arterial blood sampling |
| Simplified kinetic method (SKM) or Hunter method | 1. Static acquisition<br>2. Venous blood sampling<br>3. Quantitative<br>4. Simple relation between $K_i$ and SUV | 1. Blood sampling required<br>2. Longer scan times (approx 1 h)<br>3. Localized views<br>4. Transmission scan required<br>5. Difficult to implement in clinical practice | 1. Partial volume effects<br>2. Pool of nondiabetic patients required for reference values |
| SUV (standardized uptake value) or DUR (differential uptake ratio) or DAR (differential absorption ratio) | 1. Static acquisition<br>2. Whole-body imaging<br>3. No blood sampling<br>4. Semiquantitative<br>5. Easy computation<br>6. Implementable in clinical practice | 1. Various SUV-based methods<br>2. "Oversimplification" of dynamic tumor process<br>3. Lower counting statistics<br>4. Transmission scan required<br>5. Less accurate for small changes<br>6. No consensus for interpretation of SUV changes | 1. Uptake time<br>2. Glucose levels<br>3. Body weight<br>4. Partial volume effects |
| Tumor-to-nontumor ratio (T/N) | 1. Static acquisition<br>2. Whole-body imaging<br>3. No blood sampling<br>4. Semiquantitative<br>5. Easy computation | 1. "Oversimplification" of dynamic tumor process<br>2. Lower counting statistics<br>3. Less accurate for small lesions | 1. Reference values for nontumor area<br>2. Uptake time<br>3. Glucose levels<br>4. Body weight |

*(continued)*

## Table 1 (continued)

| Methods | Advantages | Limitations | Dependencies |
|---|---|---|---|
| | 6. Transmission not required<br>7. Implementable in clinical practice | 4. Less accurate for lesions located in boundary areas | 5. Partial volume effects |
| Total lesion evaluation (TLE) or 2ROIs—6P FDG model or Wu method | 1. Volumetric method<br>2. Dynamic method<br>3. Calculation of metabolic index ($K_i$)<br>4. Calculation of volumetric index<br>5. More accurate therapeutic follow-up | 1. Blood sampling required<br>2. Transmission scan required<br>3. Complex measurements<br>4. Method used for research purposes<br>5. Difficult to implement in clinical practice | 1. References values required<br>2. Volumetric volume dependent on number of voxels<br>3. Partial volume effects |
| Total lesion glycolysis (TLG) or Larson-Ginsberg index | 1. Volumetric method<br>2. Calculation of SUV<br>3. Calculation of volumetric index<br>4. Calculation of delta TLG | 1. Various SUV definitions<br>2. "Oversimplification" of dynamic tumor process<br>3. Method used for research purposes | 1. References values required<br>2. Partial volume effects<br>3. Respiratory motion effects |

    b. Fasted diabetics should be studied as first patients of the day, with medications delayed.
    c. Glucose level should be < 140 mg/dL.
    d. $^{18}$FDG PET scan should be postponed if glucose level > 200 mg/dL.
    e. For intermediate levels (140–200 mg/dL), scan is possible after medical adjustment using subcutaneous (sc) or intravenous (iv) insulin.
    f. Insulin-based adjustment schemes for normalization of glycemia are defined on a patient-by-patient basis, knowing that high serum insulin levels increase $^{18}$FDG uptake in muscles. Also, the radiolabeled tracer should not be injected earlier than 1 h for iv or 2 h for sc after the last insulin injection.
6. Measure weight and height.
7. Record all clinical data, current medications, and/or previous treatments (radiotherapy, chemotherapy, surgery).
8. Patients should be well hydrated before and after $^{18}$FDG injection.
9. Prescription of medications is left to the discretion of the physician.
10. 5–10 mg diazepam may be given orally, especially in patients with lymphomas or head and neck cancers, to minimize muscular tension.
11. 10–20 mg furosemide may be injected through the iv line within 15 min of $^{18}$FDG injection to force diuresis, a medication aimed to reduce both urinary stasis and bladder radiation exposure.

## Table 2
## Standardized Uptake Values: Definitions and Characteristics

| Standardized uptake value (SUV) | Definitions | Characteristics |
|---|---|---|
| SUV-body weight (BW) | SUV – BW = $Q \times W/Q_{inj}$<br>$Q$ = radioactive concentration (MBq/L)<br>$W$ = body weight (kg)<br>$Q_{inj}$ = activity injected (MBq) | 1. Simple<br>2. Easy computation<br>3. Dependent on weight and height |
| SUV-body surface area (BSA) | SUV – BSA = $Q \times BSA/Q_{inj}$<br>$Q$ = radioactive concentration (MBq/L)<br>BSA = body surface area (m$^2$)<br>BSA = $W^{0.425} \times H^{0.725} \times 0.00718$<br>$W$ = body weight (kg)<br>$H$ = height (cm)<br>$Q_{inj}$ = activity injected (MBq) | 1. SUV of choice<br>2. Most independent SUV with regard to weight and height<br>3. Best correlation with kinetic methods (reference methods) |
| SUV-ideal body weight (IBW) | SUV – IBW = $Q \times IBW/Q_{inj}$<br>$Q$ = radioactive concentration (MBq/L)<br>IBW = 45.5 + 0.91 ($H$ – 152)<br>$Q_{inj}$ = activity injected (MBq) | 1. IBW calculated from the formulas of Zasadny and Wahl<br>2. Dependent on weight and height |
| SUV-lean body mass (LBM) | SUV – LBM = $Q \times LBM/Q_{inj}$<br>$Q$ = radioactive concentration (MBq/L)<br>LBM = lean body mass (kg)<br>LBM = $(1.07 \times W) - 148 (W/H)^2$<br>$W$ = body weight (kg)<br>$H$ = height (cm)<br>$Q_{inj}$ = activity injected (MBq) | 1. Calculation of LBM required<br>2. SUV – LBM < SUV – BW<br>3. Less dependent on weight and height than SUV-BW |
| Glycemia-corrected SUV (SUV corr) | SUV – Corr = SUV × Gly<br>Gly = glycemia (g/L) | 1. No consensus for SUV-corr<br>2. Correction suggested in patients with increased glycemia or with hyperinsulinemia<br>3. Correction in patients with diabetes or pancreatic cancer |

12. 5–10 mg mebeverine may be administrated orally to reduce bowel retention of tracer.
13. Inject 150–370 MBq $^{18}$FDG via the iv line (*see* **Note 12**).
14. Wash the line with 0.9% NaCl perfusion.

**Table 3**
**Factors Influencing the Uptake of 18FDG into Tissues**

1. Tracer activity administrated
2. Biodistribution of tracer (uptake in target and nontarget tissues)
3. Density of glucose transporters (GLUTs)
4. Rate of glycolytic kinases (hexokinases I-II, phosphofructokinase, pyruvate kinase PK-M2) and glucose-6-phosphatase
5. Blood perfusion of tissues
6. Tracer supply into tumors
7. Clearance of tracer
8. Patient's body weight
9. Body fat component
10. Endogenous competition (blood glucose levels)
11. Tumor cell viability and/or proliferation
12. Tumor microenvironment (hypoxia, inflammation tissues)
13. Time of uptake determination (interval time after tracer administration)
14. Times of PET scanning (pretreatment vs posttreatment, or after one or several courses of chemotherapy)

15. Patients should drink at least 500 mL water, especially after tracer injection.
16. Patients should be isolated about 1 h in a single room, an interval that optimizes the $^{18}$FDG uptake for static whole-body imaging.

## *3.2. PET Procedure*

### *3.2.1. Data Acquisition*

1. Static whole-body acquisition should be performed as usual in routine practice.
2. Pretreatment and posttreatment PET scans should be performed under similar technical conditions (injection dose, latency time, acquisition time).
3. Emission scans should be performed 45 ± 15 min post-tracer injection.
4. The performance of transmission scans for attenuation correction is recommended for optimal visual interpretation and more accurate semiquantification (*see* **Note 13**).
5. Segmentation of transmission images is recommended, especially at the thoracic level, for better localization of tumor sites.
6. Hybrid imaging systems (combined PET and computerized tomography [CT] scans) may improve the reliability of qualitative interpretation; care should be taken, however, for quantitative interpretation (*see* **Note 14**).

### *3.2.2. Data Reconstruction*

1. Iterative reconstruction methods are recommended for a better quality of attenuation-corrected images (*see* **Note 15**).

2. Reconstruction parameters should be defined and kept constant for treatment monitoring (i.e., two iterations, eight subsets for ordered subset expectation maximization).
3. Similar reconstruction algorithms should be applied pretreatment and posttreatment.

### 3.2.3. Quality Assurance

1. Qualitative and quantitative assessment using $^{18}$FDG PET should be performed under optimal technical conditions, which requires randoms, scatter, and attenuation corrections as well as measuremnts of imaging quality (*see* **Note 16**).
2. Adequate PET scanner calibration should be performed for reliable metabolic monitoring of chemosensitivity, especially in terms of reproducibility of quantitative measurements (*see* **Note 17**).

### *3.2.4. Qualitative Assessment of Chemosensitivity*

The visual reading of whole-body $^{18}$FDG PET images is most often sufficient for the assessment of chemosensitivity. Although quite simple, this process requires methodological steps as described below.

1. Compare metabolic status of tumors postchemotherapy to baseline (*see* **Fig. 3A**).
2. Assess visually metabolic response of tumors to chemotherapy on whole-body images (*see* **Note 4**).
3. Analyze carefully all PET images, including attenuation and non-attenuation-corrected images, as well as transmission images (*see* **Note 18**).
4. Review CT or magnetic resonance imaging (MRI) data when necessary to identify anatomical details precisely.
5. Final interpretation of PET data should be preferentially based on attenuation-corrected images.

### *3.2.5. Semiquantitative Assessment of Chemosensitivity*

As tumor response to chemosensitivity is intrinsically complex, any method aiming at the quantification of $^{18}$FDG tumor uptake remains approximate *(8,10,12,18,20)*. Therefore, the simpler the quantification approach, the easier will be its implementation in clinical practice. Based on this principle, we report a simple semiquantitative method with easy computation based on the standardized uptake value (SUV), a reproducible index that has been shown to correlate well with the net rate of influx of $^{18}$FDG ($K_i$) as gold standard defined from kinetic methods *(17,18,21)*.

1. Use attenuation-corrected PET images.
2. Display transaxial slices, in a form of $128^2$ matrix, from the "SUV function" available in PET softwares.
3. Select consecutive transaxial slice levels showing high $^{18}$FDG tumor uptakes.

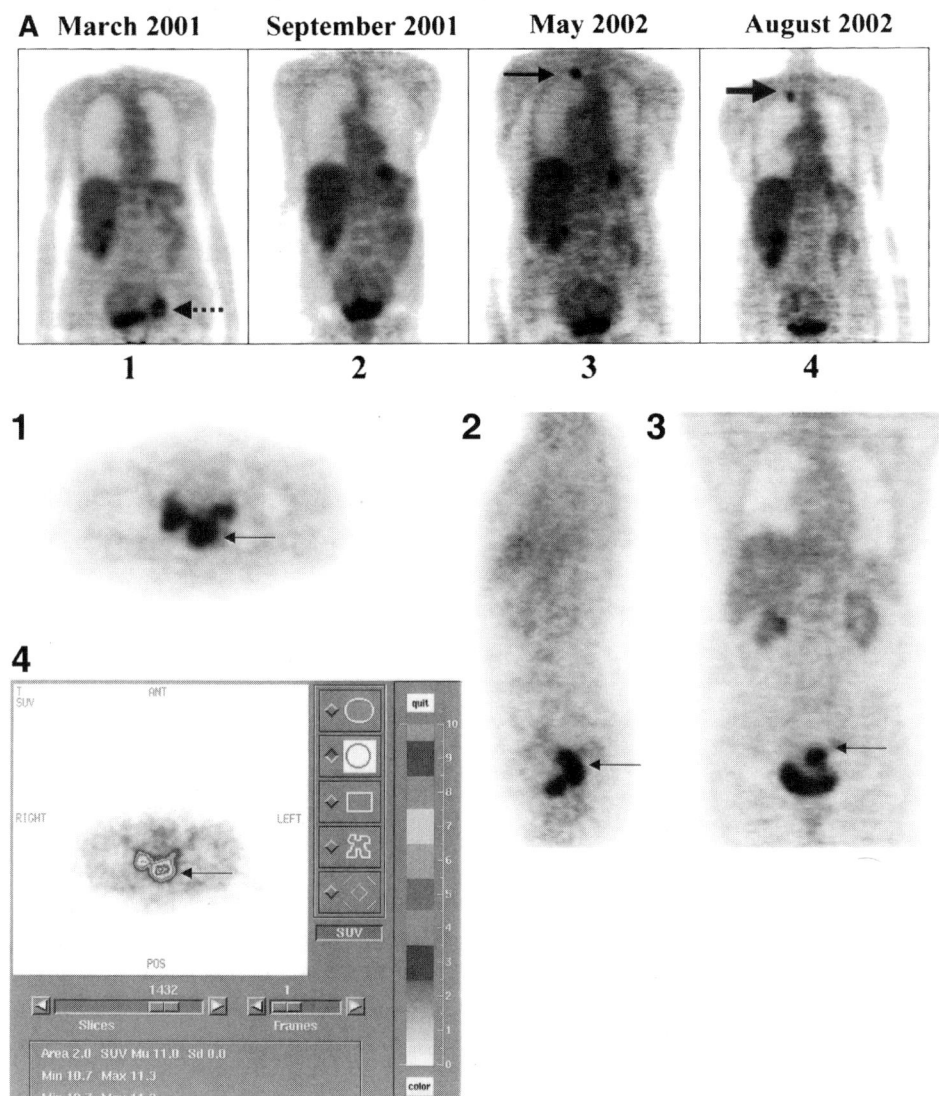

Fig. 3. Monitoring of cervical cancer treated by concomitant chemotherapy and radiation with $^{18}$FDG PET. **(A)** Qualitative assessment of treatment efficacy over time: 1, detection of a pelvic recurrence (dashed arrow); 2, normal PET study after surgical resection; 3, detection of a lung recurrence (thin arrow); 4, persistence of a lung recurrence after chemo-radiation (thick arrow). **(B)** Semiquantitative assessment of $^{18}$FDG uptake within the primary cervical tumor: 1, transaxial slice; 2, sagittal slice; 3, coronal slice; 4, standardized uptake values (SUV max = 11.3; SUV mean = 11.0; SUV min = 10.7). (See color insert following p. 238.)

**Table 4**
**Response Evaluation Criteria in $^{18}$FDG PET Oncology (EORTC Recommendations)**

| Response evaluation criteria | 1999 EORTC recommendations |
| --- | --- |
| Complete metabolic response | 1. Tumor no longer identifiable |
| Partial metabolic response | 1. Decrease in SUV > 15–25% after one cycle of chemotherapy and > 25% decrease after more than one cycle |
| | 2. No reduction in extent of $^{18}$FDG uptake required |
| Stable metabolic response | 1. Increase in SUV < 25% |
| | 2. Decrease in SUV < 15% |
| | 3. No visible increase in extent of $^{18}$FDG tumor uptake (< 20% in longest diameter) |
| Progressive metabolic response | 1. SUV > 25%. |
| | 2. Visible increase in the extent of $^{18}$FDG tumor uptake (> 20% in the longest dimension) or the appearance of new $^{18}$FDG uptake in metastatic lesions |

4. A color "SUV scale" may help to visualize the map of $^{18}$FDG uptakes after adequate calibration.
5. Draw one or several regions of interest (ROIs) over tumor sites by using preferably automatized circular ROIs.
6. Peak of $^{18}$FDG uptake should be sampled by ROIs defined over tumor areas.
7. Size of ROIs in terms of pixels (in 2-D ROIs) or voxels (in 3-D ROIs) should be kept constant before treatment and after one or several courses of chemotherapy.
8. The size of ROIs should be defined as a trade-off between accuracy and reproducibility.
9. The minimal size of ROIs allowing the quantification of radioactivity into a small tumor deposit should correspond to a spherical volume with a diameter equal to twice spatial resolution (i.e., resolution = 6 mm; diameter = 12 mm $\Rightarrow$ ROI = 3 pixels of 4 mm).
10. Record mean and maximal SUV-BW as indexes automatically computed (*see* **Fig. 3B**).
11. Calculate mean and maximal SUV-BSA (MBq/L) as indexes, preferably recommended by the EORTC PET study group (*see* **Table 4**) (*see* **Note 19**).
12. Repeat the same calculation process on different organs with tumor involvement (*see* **Notes 20** and **21**).
13. Keep the same calculation parameters to quantify the $^{18}$FDG uptake sequentially over time (*see* **Fig. 4**).

# Metabolic Imaging

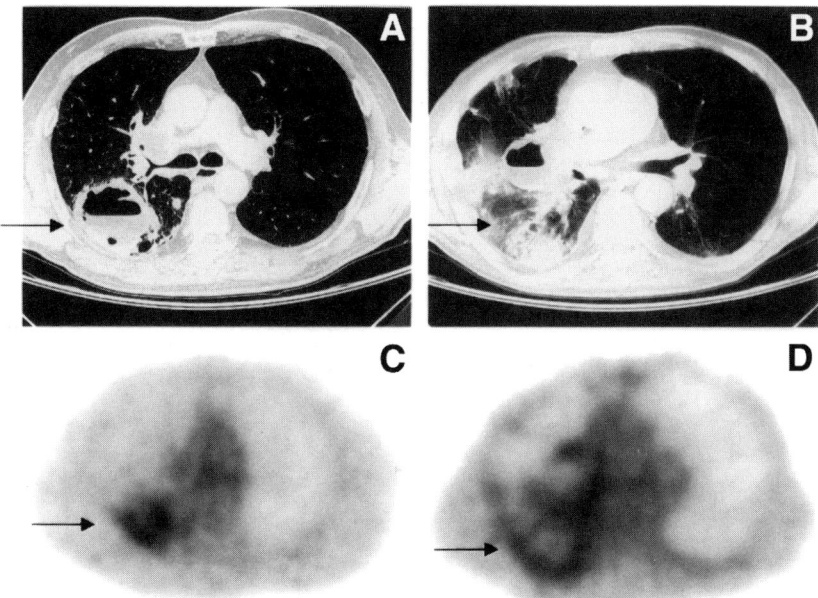

Fig. 4. Monitoring of a Stage IV non-small-cell lung cancer treated by MIP protocol with $^{18}$FDG PET. **(A)** Pretreatment thoracic CT scan showed a right lung cancer with a necrotic component. **(B)** After one cycle of chemotherapy (+ 3 mo), thoracic CT scan showed the progression of disease (MIP, mitomycin-ifosfamide-platinum). **(C)** Pretreatment PET scan showed a right lung cancer with a necrotic component. **(D)** After one course of chemotherapy (+ 1 mo), PET scan showed the progression of disease.

### 3.3. Timing for Metabolic Monitoring of Chemosensitivity

The optimal timing for the assessment of chemosensitivity with metabolic imaging remains to be defined. Indeed, no standardized scheme exists, and recommendations are based on a few preclinical and clinical studies with a limited number of patients and varying study designs *(10,17,18)*.

1. Pretreatment PET scan should be performed within 2 wk prior to starting the first course of chemotherapy (**Fig. 5**).
2. Inflammatory cells within a tumor mass may induce increased $^{18}$FDG uptake by macrophage-rich areas early after chemotherapy (*see* **Note 22**).
3. Transcient stunning of tumor cells may induce decreased $^{18}$FDG uptake early after chemotherapy (*see* **Note 23**).
4. Posttreatment PET scan should be performed at least 2 wk, preferably 4 wk, following primary treatment, to avoid inaccurate changes of $^{18}$FDG uptake into tumor

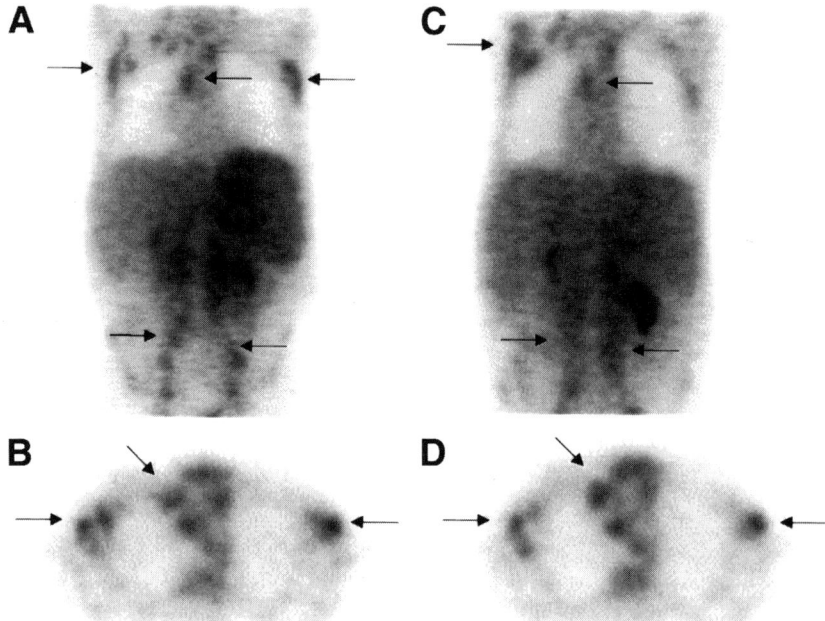

Fig. 5. Monitoring of a Stage IV non-Hodgkin's lymphoma treated by MCE protocol with $^{18}$FDG PET. **(A,B)** Pretreatment PET scan showed a disseminated lymph node involvement (coronal and transaxial slices). **(C,D)** After one cycle of chemotherapy (+ 3 mo), PET scan showed a stable disease with the persistence of nodal involvement (coronal and transaxial slices). MCE, melphalan-cyclolal-endoxan.

tissues, a misinterpretation that may flaw the assessment of chemosensitivity using the metabolic technique (*see* **Note 24**).

## 4. Notes

1. Increase in glucose consumption is a typical feature of malignant cells. Such a characteristic is exhibited by nearly all mammalian cells. The glycolytic phenotype likely reflects the genetically selected tendency of tumor cells for carcinogenesis and tumor invasion *(1,2)*.
2. $^{18}$F-fluoro-2-deoxy-D-glucose ($^{18}$FDG) is a glucose analog (FDG) labeled with a β-emitting positron ($^{18}$F)*. The tracer is synthesized in small hospital-based

---

*$^{18}$F is a positron emitter (β+) with a maximal energy of 635 keV and a half-life of 110 min. In the body, $^{18}$F produces two annihilations photons (γ) of 511 keV per disintegration after β+ (antimatter)/e– (matter) reaction. The two γ are emitted nearly simultaneously in opposite directions. According to the positron emission tomography principle, the two annihilations photons are detected by a ring of detectors placed in coincidence.

cyclotrons. $^{18}$FDG offers clear advantages over other PET tracers because of its longer half-life (110 min for $^{18}$F vs 20 min for $^{11}$C, 10 min for $^{13}$N, 2 min for $^{15}$O), which makes radiochemistry feasible for clinical oncology imaging purposes. In addition, large production and commercial distribution of $^{18}$FDG has become quiet widespread, thereby allowing easy access to this tracer in most major oncology centers in Europe and United States.
3. In neoplastic tissues, $^{18}$FDG has been shown to correlate mainly with the number of viable tumor cells, including both proliferating and nonproliferating cells. Accumulation of $^{18}$FDG has also been demonstrated in nonneoplastic tissues such as inflammatory cells, especially after treatment. (On the other hand, fibrotic tissues or scars do not take up the glucose tracer *(11–14)*.
4. Visual interpretation relies mainly on the experience of the nuclear physician. As a consequence, the qualitative reading of PET scans may be a source of errors, especially during the learning curve. In addition, subtle changes in $^{18}$FDG patterns may be a matter for equivocal interpretation even among experienced nuclear physicians.
5. The method of choice to estimate the net $^{18}$FDG phosphorylation rate constant ($K_i$) (mL/min/g) is based on the original three-compartmental model developed by Sokoloff for the measurement of local cerebral glucose utilization *(22)*. Using a nonlinear regression approach or estimates from Patlak graphical analysis, the glucose metabolic rate (MR$_{glu}$) is defined by: MR$_{glu}$ = [$k_1 \times k_3 / (k_2 + k_3)$] $\times C_P / L_C$ = $K_i \times (C_P / L_C)$, where $K_i = k_1 \times k_3 / (k_2 + k_3)$; $k_1$ and $k_2$ refer to forward and reverse capillary transport of $^{18}$FDG; $k_3$ refers to phosphorylation of $^{18}$FDG; $C_P$ is the plasma glucose concentration; $L_C$ is the lumped constant, a correction factor for differences in transport and phosphorylation kinetics between glucose and $^{18}$FDG. Of note, except for hepatocellular carcinoma and cholangiocarcinoma, the dephosphorylation of $^{18}$FDG-6-phosphate to $^{18}$FDG by phosphatase is assumed to be negligible. Therefore, the dephosphorylation constant ($k_4$) is not taken into account (i.e., $k_4 = 0$) (*see* Fig. 2).
6. $^{18}$FDG PET is a metabolic technique that explores the glycolytic changes occurring in tumor cells. Early after chemotherapy, however, $^{18}$FDG uptake by nontumor cells such as inflammatory cells (macrophages, fibroblasts, leucocytes, neutrophile granulocytes) may broadly overlap the area of $^{18}$FDG uptake due to tumor cells. Therefore, $^{18}$FDG is not the ideal tracer to monitor chemosensitivity.
7. In the arena of PET tracers, $^{18}$F-fluorothymidine ($^{18}$FLT) is increasingly being investigated to monitor chemosensitivity instead of $^{18}$FDG *(44–48)*. Indeed, $^{18}$FLT may be used for imaging tumor proliferation by providing insights into the DNA synthetic pathway. $^{18}$FLT is phosphorylated by cytosolic S-phase-specific thymidine kinase-1 (TK1), a key enzyme of the proliferative pathway, into $^{18}$FLT-6-phosphate. The latter molecule is trapped in tumor cytosol with negligible incorporation into DNA, which, in turn, makes the use of $^{18}$FLT particularly attractive to assess tumor response to antiproliferative therapies. Preclinical and clinical studies found a close correlation between $^{18}$FLT tumor changes and proliferative indexes such as Ki-67 and PCNA (proliferative cell nuclear antigen). Semiquantitative analyses showed

more pronounced and earlier changes of $^{18}$FLT uptake in comparison to $^{18}$FDG uptake.

8. Tumor response to cytotoxic drugs is nowadays acknowledged to be mediated by specific pathways involving the apoptotic cascade. Recent data highlighted alternative tracers that may assess more specifically the genetic ability exhibited by some cancers to respond apoptotically to antitumor therapies. For instance, radiolabeled recombinant human Annexin V has been shown to localize at tumor sites with histologically proven apoptosis; a significant increase of tracer uptake was detected as early as 24 h following the first course of chemotherapy *(49–51)*.

9. In recent years, the detection of tumor hypoxia has become another means to assess the ability of sensitive cancer cells to respond to treatment. That is, hypoxia is usually associated with resistance to antitumor therapies and poor prognosis. Accordingly, newly designed PET tracers such as $^{18}$F-FMISO (fluorine-18 fluoromisonidazole) and $^{60}$Cu-radiolabeled ATSM [diacetyl-bis(N$^4$-methylthiosemicarbazone] have been shown to accumulate significantly in hypoxic tissues *(52)*. $^{60}$Cu-ATSM offers, however, the advantage of being rapidly washed out from non-hypoxic tissues, thereby providing a good signal-to-background ratio for imaging purposes. In a pilot clinical study, $^{60}$Cu-ATSM was found to accurately predict tumor responsiveness in patients with lung cancers treated by chemotherapy and/or radiation. If these preliminary results are confirmed on large series, $^{60}$Cu-ATSM may play a pivotal role in monitoring oncology patients treated by various antihypoxic therapies *(53,54)*.

10. The $^{18}$FDG doses depend first on the type of PET cameras (dedicated or adapted devices). The acquisition mode (2-D or 3-D) also influences the injection doses: in 2-D mode (with lead septa collimating the annihilation photons), higher activities are allowed (typically, 370 MBq in adult patients or 6 MBq/kg in children or obese patients); in 3-D mode (without septa, resulting in higher count rates), lower doses are advised for cost saving or to avoid detector saturation (150–250 MBq for dedicated PET to 100–200 MBq for adapted SPECT devices).

11. Cameras dedicated to the PET imaging offer better performance than SPECT devices adapted to the use of $^{18}$FDG. In particular, the sensitivity, the lesion detectability, and to a lesser extent the spatial resolution achieved by dedicated PET scanners are known to be better than those obtained with transformed conventional cameras *(55)*.

12. The use of $^{18}$FDG should comply to the general radioprotection rules in terms of shipment and transport of radioactive materials, tracer preparation in the "hot" room of the nuclear medicine unit, patient administration, and storage of wastes.

13. In most conventional PET devices, a transmission scan is obtained with an external radioactive source ($^{137}$Cs or $^{68}$Ge), which allows the determination of attenuation correction factors (ACFs). In general, the resulting attenuation-corrected emission images provide more reliable information for visual interpretation. Transmission scans are also required for more accurate semiquantitative assessment of $^{18}$FDG uptake. In hybrid PET-CT scanners, ACFs may be easily obtained from the

CT scan. This allows a more rapid transmission scan with lower statistical noise and finally a highly qualitative CT-based attenuation correction *(56)*.
14. Combined PET-CT systems provide, in the same space/time, both metabolic and anatomical information, which may be particularly valuable to improve the diagnostic accuracy for oncological applications *(56–58)*. However, quantitative radioactive values obtained from CT-based attenuation correction have been shown to be significantly higher than the $^{68}$Ge-based transmission values (conventional PET)—an overestimation by an average 11% in bone lesions and 2.1% in soft tissues. As a result, without the implementation of correction algorithms, care should be taken for comparison of quantitative data obtained with varying PET systems (single vs hybrid cameras) *(59,60)*.
15. The use of iterative reconstruction methods is preferred in PET because it results in better imaging quality. Main iterative algorithms are based on statistical modeling of the true information as well as the degrading effects contained in collected raw images. In comparison to conventional analytic methods such as filtered back projection (FBP), iterative methods such as ordered-subset expectation maximization (OSEW) and derivative-algorithms (attenuation weighted-OSEM) lead to a significant improvement in data measurement and processing. Overall, final images are less noisy and more rapidly reconstructed *(61)*.
16. PET performance should be verified, especially for sensitivity, spatial resolution, counting statistics, and noise equivalent count. Measurements should be done according to national or international standards *(62,63)*.
17. Accurate quantification of $^{18}$FDG uptake requires an adequate calibration of PET scanners, a process that establishes the relationship between the measured count rate per volume and the true activity concentration. Usually, calibration procedures are based on scanner manufacturer guidelines, and rely on the use of standard phantoms containing a certified activity of $^{68}$Ge. Whenever possible, independent calibration procedures are preferable to test the accuracy of PET measurements. This may be implemented in practice by sampling an aliquot of the phantom, thereby checking the well counter by measuring its activity with the on-site dose calibrator *(64)*.
18. Visual interpretation of PET scans for qualitative assessment of chemosensitivity should be done with full knowledge of normal distribution of the $^{18}$FDG tracer and its physiological variants. Of note, the radiolabeled glucose analog is avidly taken up by the brain (gray matter), and inconstantly by the heart (depending on the fasting state). In addition, $^{18}$FDG is moderately taken up into the liver, the spleen, and the digestive system (stomach and bowels), and is excreted through the kidneys and the bladder. $^{18}$FDG uptakes into the thymus, the thyroid, and the muscles may be seen in particular clinical circumstances (i.e., young patients < 30 yr, thyroiditis, diabetics, muscular tension, or respiratory failure, respectively).
19. According to the European Organization for Research and Treatment of Cancer (EORTC) PET study group recommendations, SUV normalized to body surface area (SUV-BSA) is the more reliable SUV index in terms of reproducibility and

independency with regard to weight and height *(65)*. In a recent study, however, a comparison between different analytical methods concluded that, in addition to Patlak graphical analysis and simplified kinetic method (SKM), SUV normalized to lean body mass (SUV-LBM), rather than SUV-BSA, could be possible alternatives to nonlinear regression (NLR) as gold standard *(66)*. Some authors have proposed the use of a threshold method (i.e., 60% SUV max and, better, 75% SUV max) to improve standardized uptake value reproducibility *(67)*. Such a computerized technique yields more stable quantitative parameters that are more independent from region size and shape, which in turn minimizes operator bias. Other authors have suggested the noninvasive measurement of the net influx constant ($K_i$) by means of a simple mathematical formula that correlates $K_i$ to SUV: $K_i$ = SUV × $k_p$ × $V_0$, where $k_p$ is the plasma clearance rate and $V_0$ is the initial distribution volume of $^{18}$FDG. $K_i$ appears feasible for standardization in clinical routine with more reliable assessment of $^{18}$FDG tumor uptake than SUV *(68)*.

20. $^{18}$FDG uptake into tumor tissues may vary considerably from one organ to another, with various quantitative profiles, a pattern related mainly to individual tumor behavior. Regardless of the available practical methods recommended for quantification purposes (Patlak analysis, simplified kinetic method, and SUV), lower agreement with nonlinear regression (reference method) was found for bone metastases *(66)*.

21. The same technical conditions (injection doses, acquisition times, data reconstruction, and processing) and response evaluation criteria should be used over time for accurate metabolic monitoring of chemosensitivity *(17,18,21,65,69)*.

22. Inflammatory cells within tumor tissues may cause an increase of $^{18}$FDG uptake, especially under activation conditions (i.e., after chemotherapy or radiotherapy). Autoradiographic studies localized this phenomenon in macrophage-rich areas, which may avidly take up the glucose tracer *(12,14,70)*. In some cases, this process may overlap the area covered by tumor cells, thereby leading to falsely increased $^{18}$FDG uptake. To overcome this confusing bias in estimating the true tumor glucose metabolism, some authors have proposed a dual-time method aimed to measure changes over time ($\Delta$SUV). Accordingly, inflammatory or benign cells will exhibit decreased or stabilized $^{18}$FDG uptake (i.e., SUV $t_{45\,min}$ vs SUV $t_{+90\,min}$, or SUV $t_0$ vs SUV $t_{+30\,min}$), while $^{18}$FDG uptake into tumor cells will increase over two time points *(37,71)*.

23. Early after initiation of chemotherapy, tumor cells may be stunned by cytotoxic or cytostatic drugs. When mechanisms of glucose membrane transport and enzymatic pathways for its metabolism are temporarily blocked, no or lower $^{18}$FDG uptake into tumor cells, in comparison to baseline, may be falsely interpreted as a response to anticancer therapies *(36,72)*. Therefore, soon after treatment (up to 3 wk following primary chemotherapy), caution should be taken before considering the normalization of $^{18}$FDG uptake as actual response to treatment *(73)*. Of note, tumors presenting with a low rate of proliferation, such as well-differentiated carcinoids or low-grade lymphomas, may have a low (or no) uptake of $^{18}$FDG

regardless of the timing of PET imaging *(43,74)*. Ultimately, microscopic cancer cells or small tumor residues arising from malignancies that have responded macroscopically to chemotherapy may be overlooked because they are below the spatial resolution of currently available PET scanners *(36,39)*.
24. Varying and contradictory $^{18}$FDG patterns have been reported in the 2–3 wk after induction of chemotherapy. Some of them reflect a "flare phenomenon," a process that is likely related to increased uptake of $^{18}$FDG by inflammatory cells, although its clinical significance is not completely elucidated yet *(12,70,75)*. On the other hand, experimental studies showed a dose- (mono vs combination therapy) and time-dependent (1-, 2-, 3-, 4-h delay on d 1, 2, and 3 after chemotherapy) increase of $^{18}$FDG uptake after therapy *(76)*. In a SCID mice model inoculated with Daudi cells (B-cell leukemia cell line of human origin), autoradiographic and histological correlations were performed on tumor tissues at different time points postinjection of cyclophosphamide (d 0, +1, +3, +5, +8, +10, and +15) *(12)*. A decreasing percentage of viable tumor cells was initially observed after chemotherapy from d 0 to d +3 along with reduction of SUVs. $^{18}$FDG uptake into tumor tissues, however, stabilized at d +8 and d +10, while a lower fraction of viable cells was detected. This correlated with an increased reaction of host stromal and necrotic cells. The amount of viable tumor cells increased again at d +15, which was accurately predicted by increase in SUV. At this later time point, tumor weight remained stable although the host response and the necrotic component fell strongly. As a consequence, in oncology practice, the quantification of $^{18}$FDG uptake during at least the first 2 wk following chemotherapy does not reflect glycolytic changes within tumor cells only, but also includes in nonnegligible part some host and necrotic components as well. Therefore, one should recommend assessing metabolic tumor changes by means of $^{18}$FDG PET beyond the first 2–3 wk, preferably 4 wk, after chemotherapy.

## Acknowledgments

Many thanks to Dr. Pierre Rigo for sharing his invaluable experience in the field of $^{18}$FDG PET imaging (University Hospital of Liège, Division of Nuclear Medicine, 1998–2000). The authors also thank Dr. Karoline Spaepen for helpful discussions.

## References

1. Warburg, O. (1956) On the origin of cancer cells. *Science* **123,** 309–314.
2. Gatenby, R. A. and Gawlinski, E. T. (2003) The glycolytic phenotype in carcinogenesis and tumor invasion. *Cancer Res.* **63,** 3847–3854.
3. Hatanaka, M. (1974) Transport of sugars in tumor cell membranes. *Biochem. Biophys. Acta* **355,** 77–104.
4. Weber, G. (1977) Enzymology of cancer cells (first of two parts). *N. Engl. J. Med.* **296,** 486–492.

5. Weber, G. (1977) Enzymology of cancer cells (second of two parts). *N. Engl. J. Med.* **296,** 541–551.
6. Pauwels, E. K. J., Ribeiro, M. J., Stoot, J. H. M. B., McCready, V. R., Bourguignon, M., and Mazière, B. (1998) FDG accumulation and tumor biology. *Nuclear Med. Biol.* **25,** 317–322.
7. Wahl, R. L., Hutchins, G. D., Buchsbaum, D. J., Liebert, M., Grossman, H. B., and Fisher, S. (1991) 18F-2-deoxy-D-glucose uptake into human tumor xenografts—feasibility studies for cancer imaging with positron emission tomography. *Cancer* **67,** 1544–1550.
8. Kubota, K. (2001) From tumor biology to clinical PET: a review of positron emission tomography (PET) in oncology. *Ann. Nuclear Med.* **15,** 471–486.
9. Maisey, M. N. (2002) Overview of clinical PET. *Br. J. Radiol.* **75,** S1–S5.
10. Smith, T. A. D. (1998) FDG uptake, tumour characteristics and response to therapy: a review. *Nuclear Med. Commun.* **19,** 97–105.
11. Waki, A., Fujibayashi, Y., and Yokoyama, A. (1998) Recent advances in the analyses of the characteristics of tumors on FDG uptake. *Nuclear Med. Biol.* **25,** 589–592.
12. Spaepen, K., Stroobants, S., Dupont, P., et al. (2003) [$^{18}$F]FDG PET monitoring of tumour response to chemotherapy: does [$^{18}$F]FDG uptake correlate with the viable tumour cell fraction? *Eur. J. Nuclear Med. Mol. Imaging* **30,** 682–688.
13. Higashi, K., Clavo, A. C., and Wahl, R. L. (1993) Does FDG uptake measure proliferative activity of human cancer cells? In vitro comparison with DNA flow cytometry and tritiated thymidine uptake. *J. Nuclear Med.* **34,** 414–419.
14. Kubota, K., Kubota, R., and Yamada, S. (1993) FDG accumulation in tumor tissue. *J. Nuclear Med.* **34,** 419–421.
15. Skipper, H. E., Schabel, F. M. Jr., and Wilcox, W. S. (1964) Experimental evaluation of potential anticancer agents: XII. On the criteria and kinetics associated with "curability" of experimental leukaemia. *Cancer Chemother. Rep.* **35,** 1–111.
16. Yoshioka, T., Takahashi, H., Oikawa, H., et al. (1997) Influence of chemotherapy on FDG uptake by human cancer xenografts in nude mice. *J. Nuclear Med.* **38,** 714–717.
17. Giannopoulou, C. (2003) The role of SPET and PET in monitoring tumour response to therapy. *Eur. J. Nuclear. Med.*
18. Hoekstra, C. J., Paglianiti, I., Hoekstra, O. S., et al. (2000) Monitoring response to therapy in cancer using [$^{18}$F]-2-fluoro-2-deoxy-D-glucose and positron emission tomography: an overview of different analytical methods. *Eur. J. Nuclear Med.* **27,** 731–743.
19. Coleman, R. E. (2000) FDG imaging. *Nuclear Med. Biol.* **27,** 689–690.
20. Coleman, R. E. and Graham, M. M. (2002) Is quantification necessary for oncological PET studies. *Eur. J. Nuclear Med.* **29,** 133–135.
21. Eckelman, W. C., Tatum, J., L., Kurdziel, K. A., and Croft, B. Y. (2000) Quantitative analysis of tumor biochemistry using PET and SPECT. *Nuclear Med. Biol.* **27,** 633–635.
22. Sokoloff, L., Reivich, M., Kennedy, C., et al. (1977) The [$^{14}$C]deoxyglucose method for the measurement of local cerebral utilization: theory, procedure, and normal values in the conscious and anesthetized albino rat. *J. Neurochem.* **28,** 897–916.

23. Reivich, M., Kuhl, D., Wolf, A., et al. (1979) The [$^{18}$F]fluorodeoxyglucose method for the measurement of local cerebral utilization in man. *Circ. Res.* **44,** 127–137.
24. Phelps, M. E., Huang, S. C., Hoffman, E. J., Selin, C., Sokoloff, L., and Kuhl, D. E. (1979) Tomographic measurement of local cerebral glucose metabolism rate in humans with (F-18)2-fluoro-2-deoxy-D-glucose: validation of method. *Ann. Neurol.* **6,** 371–388.
25. Patlak, C. S., Blasberg, R. G., and Fenstermacher, J. D. (1983) Graphical evaluation of blood-to-brain transfer constants from multiple-time uptake data. *J. Cereb. Blood Flow Metab.* **3,** 1–7.
26. Strauss, L. G. and Conti, P. S. (1991) The application of PET in clinical oncology. *J. Nuclear Med.* **32,** 801–820.
27. Weber, W. A., Ziegler, S. I., Thodtmann, R., Hanauske, A. R., and Schwaiger, M. (1999) Reproducibility of metabolic measurements in malignant tumors using FDG PET. *J. Nuclear Med.* **40,** 1771–1777.
28. Huang, H. S.-C. (2000) Anatomy of SUV. *Nuclear Med. Biol.* **27,** 643–646.
29. Zasadny, K. R. and Wahl, R. L. (1993) Standardized uptake values of normal tissues at PET with 2-[fluorine-18]-fluoro-2-deoxy-D-glucose: variations with body weight and a method for correction. *Radiology* **189,** 847–850.
30. Kim, C. K., Gupta, N. C., Chandramouli, B., and Alavi, A. (1994) Standardized uptake values of FDG: body surface area correction is preferable to body weight correction. *J. Nuclear Med.* **35,** 164–167.
31. Sugawara, Y., Zasadny, K. R., Neuhoff, A. W., and Wahl, R. L. (1999) Reevaluation of the standardized uptake value for FDG: variations with body weight and methods for correction. *Radiology* **213,** 521–525.
32. Hunter, G. J., Hamberg, L. M., Alpert, N. M., Choi, N. C., and Fishman, A. J. (1996) Simplified measurement of deoxyglucose utilization rate. *J. Nuclear Med.* **37,** 950–955.
33. Sadato, N., Tsuchida, T., Nakaumra, S., et al. (1998) Non-invasive estimation of the net influx constant using the standardized uptake value for quantification of FDG uptake of tumours. *Eur. J. Nuclear Med.* **25,** 559–564.
34. Thie, J. A., Hubner, K. F., and Smith, G. T. (1999) Standardized uptake value and influx constant: relationships and variabilities, with model interpretation and clinical implications. *Clin. Pos. Imag.* **2,** 99–104.
35. Larson, S. M., Erdi, Y., Akhurst, T., et al. (1999) Tumor treatment response based on visual and quantitative changes in global tumor glycolysis using PET-FDG imaging: the visual response score and the changes in total lesion glycolysis. *Clin. Pos. Imag.* **2,** 159–171.
36. Rigo, P., Paulus, P., Kaschten, B. J., et al. (1996) Oncological applications of positron emission tomography with fluorine-18 fluorodeoxyglucose. *Eur. J. Nuclear Med.* **23,** 1641–1674.
37. Hustinx, R., Smith, R. J., Benard, F., et al. (1999) Dual time point fluorine-18 fluorodeoxyglucose positron emission tomography: a potential method to differentiate malignancy from inflammation and normal tissue in the head and neck. *Eur. J. Nuclear Med.* **26,** 1345–1348.

38. Belhocine, T., De Barsy, C., Hustinx, R., and Willems-Foidart, J. (2002) Usefulness of 18 F-FDG PET in the post-therapy surveillance of endometrial carcinoma. *Eur. J. Nuclear Med.* **29,** 1132–1139.
39. Belhocine, T., Thille, A., Fridman, V., et al. (2002) Contribution of whole-body $^{18}$FDG PET imaging in the management of cervical cancer. *Gynecol. Oncol.* **87,** 90–97.
40. Jerusalem, G., Belhocine, T., Silvestre, R. M., et al. (2001) Role of positron emission tomography in the early treatment evaluation of patients with breast cancer. *Med. Nucleare Imagerie fonctionnelle et métabolique* **25,** 341–346.
41. Jerusalem, G., Belhocine, T., Beguin, Y., et al. (2001) Positron emission tomography using 18F-fluorodeoxyglucose for monitoring chemotherapy in metastatic breast cancer. *Proc. Am. Soc. Clin. Oncol.* **20,** 47b (abstr. 1935).
42. Jerusalem, G., Beguin, Y., Fassotte, M. F., et al. (2003) Early detection of relapse by whole-body positron emission tomography in the follow-up of patients with Hodgkin's disease. *Ann. Oncol.* **14,** 123–130.
43. Jerusalem, G., Beguin, Y., Fassotte, M. F., et al. (2000) Persistent tumor 18F-FDG uptake after a few cycles of polychemotherapy is predictive of treatment failure in non-Hodgkin's lymphoma. *Haematologica* **85,** 613–618.
44. Grierson, J. R., Muzik, O., Stayanoff, J. C., Lahwhorn-Crews, J. M., Obradovich, J. E., and Mangner, T. J. (2002) Kinetics of 3′-deoxy-3′-[$^{18}$F]fluorothymidine uptake and retention in dogs. *Mol. Imag. Biol.* **4,** 83–89.
45. Dittmann, H., Dohmen, B. M., Kehlbach, R., et al. (2002) Early changes in [$^{18}$F]FLT uptake after chemotherapy: an experimental study. *Eur. J. Nuclear Med. Mol. Imaging* **29,** 1462–1469.
46. Wagner, M., Seitz, U., Buck, A., et al. (2003) 3′-[$^{18}$F]Fluoro-3′-deoxythymidine ([$^{18}$F]-FLT) as positron emission tomography tracer for imaging proliferation in a murine B-cell lymphoma model and in the human disease. *Cancer Res.* **63,** 2681–2687.
47. Vesselle, H., Grierson, J., Muzi, M., et al. (2002) In vivo validation of 3′ deoxy-3′-[(18)F]fluorothymidine ([(18)F]FLT) as a proliferative imaging tracer in humans: correlation of [(18)F]FLT uptake by positron emission tomography with Ki-67 immunohistochemistry and flow cytometry in human lung tumor. *Clin. Cancer Res.* **8,** 3315–3323.
48. Barthel, H., Cleij, M. C., Collingridge, D. R., et al. (2003) 3′-Deoxy-3′-[$^{18}$F]-fluorothymidine as a new marker for monitoring tumor response to antiproliferative therapy in vivo with positron emission tomography. *Cancer Res.* **63,** 3791–3798.
49. Belhocine, T. Z., Steinmetz, N., Hustinx, R., et al. (2002) Increased uptake of the apoptosis-imaging agent (99m)Tc recombinant human Annexin V in human tumors after one course of chemotherapy as a predictor of tumor response and patient prognosis. *Clin. Cancer Res.* **8,** 2766–2774.
50. Green, A. M. and Steinmetz, M. D. (2002) Monitoring apoptosis in real time. *Cancer J.* **8,** 82–92.

51. Mochizuki, T., Kuge, Y., Zhao, S., et al. (2003) Detection of apoptotic tumor response in vivo after a single dose of chemotherapy with $^{99m}$Tc-Annexin V. *J. Nuclear Med.* **44,** 92–97.
52. Koh, W-J., Rasey, J. S., and Evans, M. L. (1992) Imaging of hypoxia in human tumors with [18F]fluoromisonidazole. *Int. J. Radiat. Oncol. Biol. Phys.* **22,** 199–212.
53. Fujibayashi, Y., Taniuchi, H., Yonekura, Y, Ohtani, H., Konishi, J., and Yokoyama, A. (1997) Copper-62-ATSM: a new hypoxia imaging agent with high membrane permeability and low redox potential. *J. Nuclear Med.* **38,** 1155–1160.
54. Dehdashti, F., Mintun, M. A., Lewis, J. S., et al. (2003) In vivo assessment of tumor hypoxia in lung cancer with $^{60}$Cu-ATSM. *Eur. J. Nuclear Med. Mol. Imaging* **30,** 844–850.
55. Delbeke, D., Patton, J. A., Martin, W. H., and Sandler, M. P. (1999) FDG PET and dual-head gamma camera positron coincidence detection imaging of suspected malignancies and brain disorders. *J. Nuclear Med.* **40,** 110–117.
56. Cohade, C. and Wahl, R. L. (2003) Applications of positron emission tomography/computed tomography image fusion in clinical positron emission tomography-clinical use, interpretation methods, diagnostic improvements. *Semin. Nuclear Med.* **23,** 228–237.
57. Townsend, D. W. and Beyer, T. (2002) A combined PET/CT scanner: the path to true image fusion. *Br. J. Radiol.* **75,** S24–S30.
58. Israel, O., Mor, M., Gaitini, D., et al. (2002) Combined functional and structural evaluation of cancer patients with a hybrid camera-based PET/CT system using $^{18}$F-FDG. *J. Nuclear Med.* **43,** 1129–1136.
59. Nakamoto, Y., Osman, M., Cohade, C., et al. (2002) PET/CT: Comparison of quantitative tracer uptake between germanium and CT transmission attenuation-corrected images. *J. Nuclear Med.* **43,** 1137–1143.
60. Kamel, E., Hany, T. F., Burger, C. N., et al. (2002) CT vs (68)Ge attenuation correction in a combined PET/CT system: evaluation of the effect of lowering the CT tube current. *Eur. J. Nuclear Med. Mol. Imaging* **29,** 346–350.
61. Vandenberghe, S., D'Asseler, Y., Van de Walle, R., et al. (2001) Iterative reconstruction algorithms in nuclear medicine. *Comput. Med. Imag. Graph.* **25,** 105–111.
62. Daube-Witherspoon, M. E., Karp, J. S., et al. (2002) PET performances measurements using the NEMA NU 2-2001 Standard. *J. Nuclear Med.* **43,** 1398–1409.
63. International Electrotechnical Commission. (1998) EC Standard 61675-1: Radionuclide Imaging Devices—Characteristics and Test Conditions. Part 1. Positron Emission Tomographs. International Electrotechnical Commission, Geneva, Switzerland.
64. Geworski, L., Knoop, B. O., de Wit, M., Ivanèeviæ, V., Bares, R., and Munz, D. L. (2002) Multicenter comparison of calibration and cross calibration of PET scanners. *J. Nuclear Med.* **43,** 635–639.
65. Young, H., Baum, R., Cremerius, U., et al. (1999) Measurement of clinical and subclinical tumour response using [$^{18}$F]-fluorodeoxyglucose and positron emission tomography: review and 1999 EORTC recommendations. *Eur. J. Cancer* **35,** 1773–1782.

66. Krak, N. C., van der Hoeven, J. M., Hoekstra, O. S., Twisk, J. W. R., van der Wall, E., and Lammertsma, A. A. (2003) Measuring [$^{18}$F]FDG uptake in breast cancer during chemotherapy: comparison of analytical methods. *Eur. J. Nuclear Med. Mol. Imaging* **30,** 674–681.
67. Lee, J. R., Madsen, M. T., Bushnel, D., and Menda, Y. (2001) A threshold method to improve standardized uptake value reproducibility. *Nuclear Med. Commun.* **21,** 685–690.
68. Sadato, N., Tsuchida, T., Nakaumra, S., et al. (1998) Non-invasive estimation of the net influx constant using the standardized uptake value for quantification of FDG uptake of tumours. *Eur. J. Nuclear Med.* **25,** 559–564.
69. Beaulieu, S., Kinahan, P., Tseng, J., et al. (2003) SUV varies with time after injection in $^{18}$F-FDG PET of breast cancer: characterization and method to adjust for time differences. *J. Nuclear Med.* **44,** 1044–1055.
70. Kubota, R., Yamada, S., Kubota, K., Ishiwata, K., Tamahashi, N., and Ido, T. (1992) Intratumoral distribution of fluorine-18-fluorodeoxyglucose in vivo: high accumulation in macrophages and granulation tissues studied by autoradiography. *J. Nuclear Med.* **33,** 1972–1980.
71. Zhuang, H., Pourdehnad, M., Lambright, E. S., et al. (2001) Dual time points 18F-FDG PET imaging for differentiating malignant from inflammatory processes. *J. Nuclear Med.* **42,** 1412–1417.
72. Ichiya Y., Kuwabara, Y. Otsuka, M., et al. (1991) Assessment of response to cancer therapy using fluorine-18-fluorodeoxyglucose and positron emission tomography. *J. Nuclear Med.* **32,** 1655–1660.
73. Cremerius, U., Effert, P. J., Adam, G., et al. (1998) FDG PET for detection and therapy control of metastatic germ cell tumor. *J. Nuclear Med.* **39,** 815–822.
74. Belhocine, T., Foidart, J., Rigo, P., et al. (2002) Fluorodeoxyglucose positron emission tomography and somatostatin receptor scintigraphy for diagnosing and staging carcinoid tumours: correlations with the pathological indexes p53 and Ki-67. *Nuclear Med. Commun.* **23,** 727–734.
75. Findlay, M., Young, H., Cunningham, D., et al. (1996) Noninvasive monitoring of tumor metabolism using fluorodeoxyglucose and positron emission tomography in colorectal cancer liver metastases: correlation with tumor response to fluorouracil. *J. Clin. Oncol.* **14,** 700–708.
76. Haberkorn, U., Reinhardt, M., Strauss, L. G., et al. (1992) Metabolic design of combination therapy: use of enhanced fluorodeoxyglucose uptake caused by chemotherapy. *J. Nuclear Med.* **33,** 1981–1987.

# Index

$^{18}$FDG- PET, 417
2D gel electrophoresis, 273
5-fluorouracil (5-FU), 259, 305
$^{99m}$Tc-annexin-A5, 364

**A**

acute lymphoblastic leukemia, 327
analytical gel, 273
anatomic imaging, 382
angiogenesis inhibitor , 300
animal model, 285
antileukemic drugs, 323
antisense oligonucleotides, 307
apoptosis, 43, 55, 69, 79, 138, 186, 364

**B**

Bak, 85
Bax, 85
Bcl-2, 85
Bcl-X, 85
Bid, 85
Bim, 85
bone metastasis, 339

**C**

camptothecin, 305
caspase activity, 74
cDNA microarray, 201
cell cycle, 35, 137
cell metabolism, 109
cell synchronization, 34
ceramidases, 191
ceramide, 187
chromosome loss, 21

cisplatin, 306
colonic implantation, 311
cytosine analogs, 303

**D**

diphenylamine assay, 80
disseminated model, 342
DNA diffusion assay, 58
DNA fragmentation, 39, 79
DNA repair, 135
drug efflux, 154
drug resistance, 127
drug retention, 156
drug transport, 156
drug transporters, 128

**F**

fission yeast, 241
flow cytometry, 37, 47, 155
fluorescence microscopy, 314
fluorescent labeling, 208
fluorochromes, 151

**G**

gene disruption, 241
gene expression profile, 197, 237
glycosylceramide synthase, 190
green fluorescent protein (GFP), 313, 351
GSH-dependent system, 132

**H**

hybridization, 203

## I

image analysis, 274
imaging, 363
immunodetection, 85
immunofluorescence microscopy, 48
immunoprecipitation, 86
interferon, 306
intracardiac injection, 290
intracarotid injection, 290
intrahepatic, 311
isoelectric focusing, 272

## L

lipid analysis, 184
lung cancer, 312

## M

magnetic resonance imaging (MRI), 399
mammary fat pad, 289
mass spectrometry, 275
metabolic imaging, 417
metalloproteinase inhibitor, 302
Metamouse, 297
metastastic breast cancer, 285
microgels, 59
micrometastases, 351
micronucleus assay, 7
MR spectroscopy, 405
MRK 16 antibody, 169
mRNA, 257
multidrug resistance (MDR), 167
mutagenesis, 244

## N

NOD/SCID mouse, 327

## O

orthotopic implantation, 298
oxygenation, 399

## P

pancreatic cancer, 312
PARP cleavage, 73
P-glycoprotein, 169
preparative gel, 273
prostate, 311
proteomics, 237

## R

radiograph, 344
radiolabeling, 365
real time RT-PCR, 257
red fluorescent protein (RFP), 313
RNA isolation, 204

## S

silicon sensors, 11
silver staining, 273
sphingomyelin, 188
sphingomyelinase, 189
support vector machine, 235

## T

telomerase, 97
tissue culture, 46
transformation, 248
TRAP assay, 101
TRF assay, 104
tumor slices, 119
tumor volume, 339
TUNEL assay, 50

## W

whole body imaging, 314

## X

xenograft, 338